A Guide to Genetic Counseling

A Guide to Genetic Counseling

Third Edition

Edited by

Vivian Y. Pan

Jane L. Schuette

Karen E. Wain

Beverly M. Yashar

WILEY Blackwell

Library of Congress Cataloging-in-Publication Data
Names: Pan, Vivian Y., editor. | Schuette, Jane L., 1956– editor. |
    Wain, Karen E., editor. | Yashar, Beverly M., editor.
Title: A guide to genetic counseling / edited by Vivian Y. Pan,
    Jane L. Schuette, Karen E. Wain, Beverly M. Yashar.
Description: Third edition. | Hoboken, NJ : Wiley-Blackwell, 2025. |
    Includes index.
Identifiers: LCCN 2024031740 (print) | LCCN 2024031741 (ebook) | ISBN
    9781119892083 (paperback) | ISBN 9781119892076 (Adobe PDF) | ISBN
    9781119892106 (epub)
Subjects: MESH: Genetic Counseling–methods
Classification: LCC RB155.7 (print) | LCC RB155.7 (ebook) | NLM QZ 52 |
    DDC 616/.042–dc23/eng/20240909
LC record available at https://lccn.loc.gov/2024031740
LC ebook record available at https://lccn.loc.gov/2024031741

Cover Design: Wiley
Cover Image: © OsakaWayne Studios/Getty Images

Set in 10/12pt Times LT Std by Straive, Pondicherry, India

Contents

**10 Health Disparities and Opportunities for Equity
in Genetic Counseling**   **319**

*Nadine Channaoui, Altovise T. Ewing-Crawford, Barbara W. Harrison,
and Vivian Y. Pan*

**11 Genetic Counselors in the Healthcare Ecosystem:
Navigating Policies, Payment and Professional Advocacy**   **355**

Gillian W. Hooker and Katie Lang

List of Contributors

Patient-Centered Communication and Providing Information in Genetic Counseling

JEHANNINE (J9) AUSTIN, PhD, FCAHS, CGC   Professor, UBC Departments of Psychiatry and Medical Genetics, Vancouver, BC, Canada

Inclusion, Inclusivity, and Inclusiveness in Genetic Counseling: On Being an Authentic and Collaborative Community of Providers

ANNIE K. BAO, MS, LMFT   Educator, Mental Health & Well-Being Consultant, Columbia University, Vagelos College of Physicians and Surgeons, Chicago, IL, USA

Building a Working Alliance Through Culturally Conscious Interviewing

GAYUN CHAN-SMUTKO, MS, CGC   Associate Director, Associate Professor, MGH Institute of Health Professions, Boston, MA, USA

Health Disparities and Opportunities for Equity in Genetic Counseling

NADINE CHANNAOUI, MS, CGC   Genetic Counselor, Mass General Brigham, Boston, MA, USA

Ethical Genetic Counseling Practice

CURTIS R. COUGHLIN II, PhD, MS, MBE, CGC   Associate Professor of Pediatrics, Section of Clinical Genetics and Metabolism, Department of Pediatrics and The Center for Bioethics and Humanities, University of Colorado Anschutz Medical Campus, Aurora, CO, USA

Inclusion, Inclusivity, and Inclusiveness in Genetic Counseling: On Being an Authentic and Collaborative Community of Providers

DEANNA R. DARNES, MS, LCGC   Genetic Counselor/Clinical Trial Specialist, Scripps Research Translational Institute, Kansas City, MO, USA

Examining Our Work through Case Presentations

RICHARD DINEEN, MS, CGC   Genetic Counselor, RUSH University Medical Center, Chicago, IL, USA

Understanding the Counseling in Genetic Counseling Practice

LUBA DJURDJINOVIC, MS   Director of Ferre Genetics, Executive Director of Ferre Institute, Inc., Binghamton, NY, USA

Health Disparities and Opportunities for Equity in Genetic Counseling

ALTOVISE T. EWING-CRAWFORD, PhD, LCGC   Global Health Equity Portfolio Lead, Genentech, San Francisco, CA, USA

Health Disparities and Opportunities for Equity in Genetic Counseling

BARBARA W. HARRISON, MS, CGC   Assistant Professor, Department of Pediatrics, Division of Medical Genetics, Howard University College of Medicine, Washington, DC, USA

Thinking it all Through: Case Preparation and Management

LAUREN E. HIPP, MS, CGC   Genetic Counselor, University of Michigan, Department of Internal Medicine, Ann Arbor, MI, USA

Genetic Counselors in the Healthcare Ecosystem: Navigating Policies, Payment and Professional Advocacy

GILLIAN W. HOOKER, PhD, ScM, CGC   Chief Scientific Officer, Concert; Adjunct Associate Professor, Department of Medicine, Vanderbilt University School of Medicine, Nashville, TN, USA

Inclusion, Inclusivity, and Inclusiveness in Genetic Counseling: On Being an Authentic and Collaborative Community of Providers

LIANN H. JIMMONS, MS, LCGC   Genetic Counselor, Valley Children's Hospital, Fresno, CA, USA; Honolulu, HA, USA (Kingdom of Hawai'i)

Examining Our Work through Case Presentations

LOGAN B. KARNS, MS, CGC   Senior Genetic Counselor and Lecturer, Department of Obstetrics and Gynecology, University of Virginia School of Medicine, Charlottesville, VA, USA

Family History: An Essential Tool

DIANE R. KOELLER, MS, MPH, CGC   Senior Genetic Counselor, Dana-Farber Cancer Institute, Boston, MA, USA

Genetic Counselors in the Healthcare Ecosystem: Navigating Policies, Payment and Professional Advocacy

KATIE LANG, MS, CGC   Senior Associate in Medicine, Department of Medicine, Vanderbilt University Medical Center, Nashville, TN, USA

Clinical Supervision: Strategies for Receiving and Providing Direction, Guidance, and Support

MONICA MARVIN, MS, CGC   Clinical Professor, University of Michigan, Departments of Human Genetics and Internal Medicine, Ann Arbor, MI, USA

Ethical Genetic Counseling Practice

KELLY E. ORMOND, MS, CGC   Research Scientist, Health Ethics & Policy Lab, Department of Health Sciences and Technology, ETH Zurich, Zurich, Switzerland; Adjunct Professor, Department of Genetics and Stanford Center for Biomedical Ethics, Stanford University School of Medicine, Stanford, CA, USA

Health Disparities and Opportunities for Equity in Genetic Counseling

VIVIAN Y. PAN, MS, CGC   Senior Genetic Counselor, University of Illinois Chicago, Chicago, IL, USA

The Medical Genetics Evaluation

SHANE C. QUINONEZ, MD   Clinical Associate Professor, University of Michigan Departments of Internal Medicine and Pediatrics, Ann Arbor, MI, USA

Professional Identities, Evolving Roles, Expanding Opportunities

ERICA RAMOS, MS, CGC   VP, Advisory Services, Genome Medical, Inc., San Diego, CA, USA

The Practice and Profession of Genetic Counseling

ROBERT G. RESTA, MS, LCGC   Independent Scholar, Seattle, WA, USA

Family History: An Essential Tool and Examining Our Work through Case Presentations

JANE L. SCHUETTE, MS, CGC   Clinical Genomics Variant Science Team Lead & Certified Genetic Counselor, Variantyx Inc., Framingham, MA, USA

Genetic Counseling Research: Understanding the Basics

SARAH SCOLLON, MS, CGC Assistant Professor, Baylor College of Medicine and Texas Children's Hospital, Houston, TX, USA

Evaluating and Using Genetic Testing

NATASHA STRANDE, PhD, FACMG Senior Associate Consultant, Mayo Clinic, Rochester, MN, USA

Examining our Work through Case Presentations

MATTHEW J. THOMAS, ScM, CGC Genetic Counselor and Lecturer, University of Virginia School of Medicine, Department of Pediatrics, Charlottesville, VA, USA

Examining our Work through Case Presentations

BARRY S. TONG, MS, MPH, CGC Genetic Counselor Supervisor, University of California San Francisco, Helen Diller Family Comprehensive Cancer Center, San Francisco, CA, USA

Thinking it all Through: Case Preparation and Management

WENDY R. UHLMANN, MS, CGC Clinical Professor, University of Michigan, Departments of Internal Medicine and Human Genetics, Ann Arbor, MI, USA

Evaluating and Using Genetic Testing

KAREN E. WAIN, MS, CGC Genetic Counselor, Consultant, K.E. Wain Consulting, LLC, Otsego, MN, USA

Genetic Counseling Research: Understanding the Basics

BEVERLY M. YASHAR, MS, PhD, CGC Clinical Professor, Emeritus, University of Michigan, Department of Human Genetics, Ann Arbor, MI, USA

Preface

Welcome to the newest edition of *A Guide to Genetic Counseling*. The third edition of this textbook provides learners with a comprehensive overview of genetic counseling and explains the fundamental principles applicable to its practice. We emphasize the patient-care process, highlighting theoretical frameworks, technologies, and contextual realities that impact care. Our goal is to help learners appreciate the diverse perspectives, approaches, and areas of expertise that embody the genetic counseling profession and build knowledge and skills for success as practitioners. Using the American Board of Genetic Counseling core competencies as a scaffold, the book's content covers the genetic counseling process from case initiation to completion, addresses critical professional issues, and considers the profession's historical journey, current advances, and future challenges. This book is designed to serve as a foundational and introductory text for genetic counseling students and as a comprehensive reference for anyone seeking to understand the practice of genetic counseling.

Our goal has remained the same as the first two editions—to codify the knowledge in the field of genetic counseling and facilitate academic instruction. You may ask: "Has the practice of genetic counseling really changed?" The short answer is both yes and no. Many of the chapters in this edition have a similar focus to that of the second edition; however, all the content has been updated and new chapters have been added to reflect current principles and practices in clinical care, the expanded landscape of genetic counseling practice, and to directly address the topics of inclusivity and health disparities. The chapters are organized to help learners focus on the development of counseling skills, envision practical aspects of working as a genetic counselor, and foster contextual self-awareness and professional development as one considers the role of the individual, society, and the profession.

In embarking on this third edition, it became evident that the practice of genetic counseling has grown more complex than it was when the first edition was published in 1998 and the second edition in 2009. Beyond technological advances, the profession is reckoning with how to respond to social injustices, inequities, and health disparities. This is hard work (and heart work); we encourage readers to engage and re-engage with this textbook throughout their education and their career. Creating and editing the third edition was a learning journey for each of us as we worked to understand and learn from the unique perspectives we held about the practice of genetic counseling. Our intentional approach to this textbook extends to decisions on content, approach, and language. We acknowledge that practices evolve and what might be considered acceptable today, may change tomorrow. This necessitates constant reflection and adaptation. We firmly believe that words matter and that understanding the nuances of language is a crucial aspect of effective communication. We encourage readers to reflect on why and in what context specific terminologies are used. We humbly acknowledge that no textbook can include all relevant content, perspectives, or clinical approaches, and as editors, we do not represent all views, knowledge, and experiences. We have therefore sought to engage authors who bring diversity across personal characteristics, perspectives, and expertise. Consequently, we hope that learners and educators will appreciate the importance of curiosity and openness to differing perspectives as important aspects of learning, applying, and mastering the provided content. We urge all users of this text to embrace the value of being a lifelong learner, a key skill in maintaining competence and growing professionally.

Finally, we dedicate this third edition of *A Guide to Genetic Counseling* to genetic counseling students and all who strive to teach, mentor, support, and affirm them. You are the future of genetic counseling. May this text provide you with a framework for developing your skills, your professional self, and your dedication to the provision of high-quality genetic counseling services for all people.

Vivian Y. Pan, MS, CGC
Jane L. Schuette, MS, CGC
Karen E. Wain, MS, CGC
Beverly M. Yashar, MS, PhD, CGC

Acknowledgment

We have many to thank for helping us bring this book to completion. Our profound gratitude extends to the chapter contributors to this third edition of *A Guide to Genetic Counseling*. They generously shared their knowledge, innovation, and persistence, which is invaluable to the success of this book. The laborious task of crafting a chapter or case presentation often goes unnoticed—undertaken behind the scenes, after work hours, and frequently during personal time. We recognize their unspoken dedication, for many during personal difficulties, and commend their courage to share their vulnerabilities. Such efforts are a testament to the contributors' profound commitment to the field of genetic counseling and their belief in the crucial role of genetic counseling education. We express our sincere thanks for their dedication and contributions.

As we sought to make the textbook more inclusive, we extend special appreciation to Annie Bao, Deanna Darnes, and Liann Jimmons. They engaged in critical discussions with us around author compensation and the DEIJ-factors that lead to the exclusion of marginalized individuals in efforts like this textbook, including the altering or erasing of authentic voices, input, and truths. Annie, Deanna, and Liann pushed us to advocate for a more just arrangement. We thank them for raising their voices, maintaining unwavering integrity, and challenging the oppressive norms and inertia that prevent progress. We would also like to convey gratitude and acknowledgement specifically to Ginger Tsai, whose suggestion of using sensitivity reading introduced a novel and important aspect of enhancing the quality of this text. This new editorial process helps to ensure the content is not only accurate but also sensitive and inclusive. Deepti Babu, Nadine Channaoui, Gayun Chan-Smutko, Altovise Ewing, Barbara Harrison, Erica Ramos, Michelle Takemoto, and Vivian Ota Wang offered invaluable guidance and feedback to individual editors early in the process, which shaped our approach to inclusivity related content. We also express appreciation to Wiley for their openness, curiosity, and collaborative approach in navigating these contractual arrangements.

Finally, we deeply appreciate the groundwork laid by contributors to the first and second editions. Without their pioneering efforts, our current work would not have been possible, and we recognize the lasting impact of their scholarship on the field. Sincere thanks to these predecessors, as our endeavors stand firmly on the solid foundation they established.

1

The Practice and Profession of Genetic Counseling

Robert G. Resta[1]

GENETIC COUNSELING—A CLINICAL ACTIVITY AND A PROFESSION

Change, if you will, is in the DNA of genetic counseling. The *clinical activity* of genetic counseling began in the early decades of the twentieth century. It then continued to evolve in response to advances in the understanding of the principles of genetics and the expansion of biomedical technology and bioinformatics. This in turn led to a greater understanding of genetic disease etiology, manifestations, variability, and treatment, along with new genetic testing capabilities such as genomic analysis, prenatal testing, and pre-implantation genetic diagnosis. Equally important advances occurred in the study of human behavior and psychology, public health policy, ethical analysis, and counseling theory. These have occurred in the context of shifting social and ethical norms, reproductive patterns

[1] This chapter is adapted from an earlier edition of this book, authored by Ann Walker.

A Guide to Genetic Counseling, Third Edition. Edited by Vivian Y. Pan, Jane L. Schuette, Karen E. Wain, and Beverly M. Yashar.
© 2025 John Wiley & Sons Ltd. Published 2025 by John Wiley & Sons Ltd.

like the decades long unwavering trend in delayed child-bearing in many Westernized countries, and new philosophies of medical care such as patients assuming greater responsibility for their health care management and owning their medical records.

It is only since the 1970s, however, that the *profession* of genetic counseling has arisen. The education and practice of genetic counseling professionals involves expertise in all the above elements, enabling them to function as members of genetics health care teams and working with diverse specialists. Beyond medical clinics, genetic counselors work in genetic testing laboratories, educational institutions, research, private practice groups, and health insurance companies, to name a few. Today's genetic counselor provides a unique service, distinct from the contributions of other specialists, for patients and families who seek to understand, adapt to, and cope with the genetic, medical, and—most critically—psychological aspects of conditions they confront.

Fifty years after the first master's degrees were awarded in genetic counseling, genetic counselors have achieved a prominent place in genetic health care delivery, education, laboratory services, and public policy development. Around the globe they have formed professional organizations and developed mechanisms for accrediting genetic counselors and creating training programs.

The definition, goals, and scope of genetic counseling are tied to time and place. What constituted genetic counseling a century ago appears quite different than it does in 2023, and contemporary genetic counseling can look and sound different across the globe. There is no one "right way" to practice genetic counseling, some Platonic ideal against which all comers are to be measured. Instead, the practice of genetic counseling is continually shaped and reshaped by its regional, social, economic, scientific, medical, historical, and ethical context. Today's "best practices" and professional codes of ethics are tomorrow's discarded approaches and ethical shortcomings. The measures of success in genetic counseling in the UK or US might be different than the measures in Saudi Arabia or China or India.

In order to understand how genetic counseling arrived where it is we must understand what it is and where it has come from. This chapter provides an overview of defining genetic counseling, the history of genetic counseling as a practice and as a profession, its ethos and philosophy, and the current practice of genetic counseling. Because of the historical focus of this chapter, some terms are used that were common or considered appropriate at the time that they were written but are now considered offensive. I have set these terms in quotation marks to alert the reader that they are being used strictly for historical context.

DEFINING GENETIC COUNSELING

The term "genetic counseling" was coined in 1947 by Sheldon Reed, a PhD geneticist at the Dight Institute for Human Genetics at the University of Minnesota and one of the first clinical geneticists. He defined it quite tersely as "a kind of genetic social work without eugenic connotations." (Resta, 1997b). While this definition is lacking in specifics, it does capture the general essence of the idealized concept of genetic counseling.

The American Society of Human Genetics 1975 Definition

Various authors proposed their own brief definitions of genetic counseling in the 1950s and 1960s, but it was not until the early 1970s that a more formal definition was proposed by a committee of the American Society of Human Genetics (ASHG), and was subsequently adopted by ASHG in 1975:

> Genetic counseling is a communication process which deals with the human problems associated with the occurrence or risk of occurrence of a genetic disorder in a family. This process involves an attempt by one or more appropriately trained persons to help the individual or family to: (1) comprehend the medical facts including the diagnosis, probable course of the disorder, and the available manage-ment, (2) appreciate the way heredity contributes to the disorder and the risk of recurrence in specified relatives, (3) understand the alternatives for dealing with the risk of recurrence, (4) choose a course of action which seems to them appropriate in their view of their risk, their family goals, and their ethical and religious standards and act in accordance with that decision, and (5) to make the best possible adjust-ment to the disorder in an affected family member and/or to the risk of recurrence of that disorder. (ASHG, 1975)

This definition held up quite well for several decades, articulating as it does several central features of genetic counseling. The first is the two-way nature of the interaction—quite different from the "advice-giving" of the eugenic period or the supposedly neutral and objective information-based counseling characteristic of the mid-twentieth century. The second is that genetic counseling is a *process,* ideally taking place over a period of time and across the lifespan so the client can gradually adapt to and assimilate complex or distressing information regarding diagnosis, prognosis, and risk and formulate age-appropriate decisions or clinical and social strategies. The third is the emphasis on the client's autonomy in decision-making related to reproduction, testing, or treatment, and the recognition that such decisions will appropriately be different depending on the personal, family, and cultural contexts in which they are made. The fourth acknowledges that the occurrence or risk for a genetic disorder can have a family-wide impact different from that of other kinds of diseases and indicates that there should be a psychotherapeutic component of genetic counseling to help people explore and manage the implications of often rare disorders. Implicit in the words "appropri-ately trained persons" is the admonition that genetic counseling requires special knowledge and skills distinct from those needed in other medical and counseling interactions.

No master's level genetic counselors were on the committee that crafted this definition. This was primarily the result of the profession being so new; the first class of genetic counselors graduated in 1972, just as the ASHG committee was first convening. But the lack of genetic counselor input may also have been partially due to the fact that genetic counselors, who were often called genetic associates in the 1970s, were initially regarded as having an ancillary role in the genetics clinic (Heimler, 1997).

2006 NSGC Definition of Genetic Counseling

Because genetic counseling has continued to evolve, in 2003 the National Society of Genetic Counselors (NSGC) appointed a task force to re-visit the definition of genetic counseling. Recognizing that many types of professionals provide genetic counseling, the group's charge was to define *genetic counseling*, rather than to describe various *professional roles* of genetic counselors (Resta et al., 2006). In reviewing the literature, the task force found 20 previous definitions of genetic counseling. They also considered the purposes for which a genetic counseling definition might be used. Among these are marketing the profession, not only to potential clients but also to insurance companies, hospital administrators, and health maintenance organizations; increasing public, professional and media awareness of genetic counseling; developing practice guidelines and legislation for licensure; and providing a basis for research in genetic counseling. They settled on a succinct definition that would be readily understandable, broad enough to apply to the variety of settings in which genetic counseling may be practiced, and that acknowledges the increasing importance of genetic counseling for common and complex diseases. As approved by the NSGC Board of Directors, the definition reads:

> Genetic counseling is the process of helping people understand and adapt to the medical, psychological, and familial implications of genetic contributions to disease. This process integrates the following:
>
> * Interpretation of family and medical histories to assess the chance of disease occurrence or recurrence.
> * Education about inheritance, testing, management, prevention, resources, and research.
> * Counseling to promote informed choices and adaptation to the risk or condition.

Note that the definition does not include references to eugenics, the health of the gene pool, or assessing reproductive decisions. Of course, this is the way that just one branch of a profession has chosen to define its core clinical activity. Genetic counselors from other geographic locales or other genetic professionals might define it differently, though none has done so formally and the NSGC definition is still widely cited.

HISTORICAL OVERVIEW OF GENETIC COUNSELING

The commonly told origin story often begins in August of 1947 when Sheldon Reed coined the term genetic counseling. But 1947 is more of a historical pivot point that shifted genetic counseling on its current trajectory rather than a true origin. The groundwork for Reed's vision was laid down nearly a century before.

Eugenic Roots of Medical Genetics and Genetic Counseling

A convenient historical starting point for the story of genetic counseling can be somewhat arbitrarily assigned to 1883 when the British polymath Francis Galton, Charles Darwin's half-first cousin, coined the word *eugenics* and defined it somewhat abstrusely as "a brief word to express the science of improving stock, which is by no means confined to questions of judicious mating, but which, especially in the case of man, takes cognizance of all influences that tend in however remote a degree to give to the more suitable races or strains of blood a better chance of prevailing speedily over the less suitable than they otherwise would have had" (Galton, 1883).

Eugenics did not emerge out of the blue in 1883 from the head of Galton, however. For example, in 1872, John Humphrey Noyes described what he called a science of "rational reproduction" for the religious Oneida Community that he founded in New York State (Noyes and Noyes, 1872). Another source of eugenic thought in the mid-nineteenth century were the asylums for the "insane." Directors of these institutes in North America and Europe were alarmed by the surge in the patient populations of these institutions and began suggesting that people with a family history of insanity should refrain from reproduction because of what they perceived to be the social, economic, and human costs of psychiatric conditions (Porter, 2018). Concerns about the economic and social "threat" of the growing numbers of lower socioeconomic status people during the Industrial Revolution were not limited to just a few intellectuals. Think of Ebenezer Scrooge's attitude toward the poor in Charles Dicken's *A Christmas Carol* from 1843: "If they [the poor] would rather die," said Scrooge, "they had better do it, and decrease the surplus population." Galton provided focus and scientific legitimacy to ideas and beliefs that had been voiced by others in the prior decades.

In the United States, the focal point of eugenics was the Eugenics Record Office (ERO) at Cold Spring Harbor in New York, headed by Charles Davenport, a well-respected PhD geneticist, and Harry Laughlin who served as its Superintendent. The ERO staff collected pedigrees in an effort to demonstrate what they felt was the Mendelian inheritance of physical, psychological, and behavioral traits. The pedigrees were intended to distinguish between "good families" and "dysgenic families," the latter characterized by undesirable traits such as low IQ, poverty, alcoholism, unemployment, and "loose" sexual behavior. The pedigrees used by today's genetic counselors are direct descendants of, and nearly indistinguishable in format from, the ERO pedigrees.

The ERO advocated for anti-miscegenation and mandatory sterilization laws, along with immigration restriction to protect the "true" American racial stock, which largely implied people of Northern and Western European origin. Fear of immigration and replacement of "native" American stock (as distinct from Native Americans) was viewed as a threat to society a century ago, just as it is often viewed by some today. Ultimately, mandatory sterilization laws targeting socially and genetically undesirable individuals were passed in more than 30 states and resulted in more than 60,000 legally mandated sterilizations that continued well into the second half of the twentieth century.

A common misconception about eugenics is that it was identified primarily with ultra-conservative and racist viewpoints. While it is certainly true that eugenics was used as both a justification and tool of racist policies, eugenics was embraced to varying degrees across the sociopolitical spectrum (Paul, 1984). Eugenics was often viewed as a policy that could help people who were socioeconomically deprived. Progressives may have been opposed to some eugenic goals and policies, but they were not necessarily critical of all eugenic policies, particularly those that could help achieve what they thought of as more positive and helpful outcomes; for example, reducing poverty and undesirable social behaviors such as criminality and alcoholism. Eugenics was a global phenomenon, although it manifested differently in different countries depending on local circumstances. Advocacy of eugenics was not confined to upper middle class White Western Europeans and Americans; support for eugenics could be found across Asia, Latin America, African Americans, and Jews (Bashford and Levine, 2010).

The most extreme and reprehensible application of eugenic measures took place in Nazi Germany during the 1930s and 1940s, measures which borrowed directly from, and with the support of, prominent American and English eugenicists (Kühl, 1994). The result was the horrific treatment and deaths of millions across Europe, including Jews, Roma, Sinti, people with disabilities, homosexuals, and criminals, among others. The moral revulsion at these profound abuses and misapplications of genetic principles contributed to the demise of classical eugenics. It also led many geneticists to reject eugenics, though not as completely and clearly as is typically claimed (Paul, 1997).

The seeds of the specialty of medical genetics—and the clinical practice of genetic counseling—were sown in this field of eugenics. The genetic counseling that took place in the early genetics clinics was shaped by a conscious and stated rejection of classical eugenics and its overt racism and abuses. The post-World War II story of genetic counseling pivots to its modern trajectory in 1947 when Sheldon Reed coined the term *genetic counseling*. Reed and nearly all the other medical geneticists were highly educated, financially secure white males whose social and economic status and biases were reflected in how they formulated the developing ethos of genetic counseling. They shifted the focus of genetic counseling from race- and class-based eugenics to the goal of protecting the health of the human gene pool and to nondirective parental education about reproductive risks as one way of protecting the gene pool. Implicit in this approach is an assumption that the lives of some people with genetic conditions were somehow a threat to the future of humanity. At the same time that they were espousing nondirectiveness, geneticists felt that properly counseled parents would make the "right" decisions and refrain from reproduction if they were at increased risk of having a child with a genetic condition (Paul, 1997). The tension between these seemingly conflicting approaches is illustrated in the contrasts between these two quotations from Sheldon Reed from the 1950s (note that some of vocabulary in these quotes that are out of place with current perspectives):

> We try to explain thoroughly what the genetic situation is but the decision must be a personal one between the husband and wife, and theirs alone.
>
> (Sheldon Reed, cited in Resta (1997a))

> If our observation is generally correct, that people of normal mentality will behave in the way that seems correct to society as a whole, then an important corollary follows. It could be stated as a principle that the mentally sound will voluntarily carry out a eugenics program which is acceptable to society if counseling in genetics is available to them.
>
> (Sheldon Reed, cited in Resta (1997a))

This idea of genetic counseling as a sort of informed and voluntary eugenics continued to shape the practice up until the 1970s. Many ASHG presidents during this time gave vocal and strong support to "protecting" the human gene pool through reproductive and other measures (Resta, 2020). James Neel, an ASHG president and a towering early figure in the field of medical genetics, even titled his autobiography *Physician to the Gene Pool* (Neel, 1994). By the 1970s, geneticists started to subtly switch the focus of genetic counseling from protecting the gene pool to "disability prevention" through counseling about reproductive decisions. Nearly every study that assessed the effectiveness of genetic counseling, whether performed by physicians or master's level genetic counselors, from the 1960s to the 1990s, looked at its impact on disability and reproduction (Resta, 2019).

Genetic Testing Technology and Genetic Counseling Grew Hand in Hand

Up until 1956, few diagnostic tests were available. Knowledge of the physical structure of DNA was only three years old; there was no means of prospectively identifying unaffected *carriers* of genetic conditions; and given that it was still thought that there were 48 chromosomes in the human genome, the basis for chromosomal syndromes was unknown. Even with the goal of preventing genetic disorders, there was little for genetic counseling to offer families beyond information, sympathy, and the option to avoid childbearing.

The capabilities of genetics changed dramatically over the next 10 years as the correct human diploid complement of 46 chromosomes was reported by Tjio and

Levan (Tjio and Levan, 1956) and the cytogenetic basis of Down syndrome (Lejeune et al., 1959), Klinefelter syndrome (Jacobs and Strong, 1959), Turner syndrome (Ford et al., 1959) and trisomies 13 (Patau et al., 1960) and 18 (Smith et al., 1960; Edwards et al., 1960) were elucidated. Over this decade it also became possible to identify carriers for alpha or beta thalassemia (Kunkel et al., 1957; Weatherall, 1963); a host of abnormal hemoglobins; and metabolic diseases such as galactosemia (Hsia et al., 1958), Tay-Sachs disease (Volk et al., 1964), and G6PD deficiency (Childs et al., 1958), among others. Amniocentesis was first utilized for prenatal diagnosis—initially for sex determination using Barr body analysis (Serr et al., 1955)—and then for karyotyping (Steele and Breg, 1966). In 1968 Henry Nadler reported the first diagnosis of a fetal chromosome condition— Down syndrome as the result of an inherited D/G chromosomal translocation—as well as galactosemia and mucopolysaccharidoses (Nadler, 1968).

These advances in genetics meant that families had more options to better assess their risks and possibly avoid having a child with a genetic condition if they so desired. But the choices were by no means straightforward. Tests were not always informative. Prenatal diagnosis was novel and its potential pitfalls were incompletely understood. Explaining the technologies and the choices was time-consuming. However, clinical genetics' tenet of nondirective counseling was echoed elsewhere as medicine began to shift from its paternalistic approach toward promoting patient autonomy in decision-making. The emphasis in genetic counseling shifted too, from simply providing information that families would presumably use to make "rational" decisions (thereby preventing genetic disorders), towards a more interactive process in which individuals were not only educated about risks, but also helped with the difficult tasks of exploring issues related to the disorder in question, and of making decisions about reproduction, testing, or management that were consistent with the needs, resources, and values of patients and their families. To achieve this, genetic counselors needed to acquire the skills to understand the psychological meaning of their patients' beliefs, words, and actions (Tips and Lynch, 1963; Kessler, 1997). This environment helped to create the need for a dedicated genetic counseling profession and the development of post-graduate training programs to teach the necessary counseling skills and technical knowledge to work with patients. Equally important, this training needed to instill a clinical self-confidence in the value of a genetic counselor that newly minted counselors would need to advocate for themselves in creating employment opportunities and a professional identity separate from medical geneticists.

THE GENETIC COUNSELING PROFESSION

The professional non-MD trained genetic counselor emerged in the United States in the early 1970s. A profession typically has multiple components, including certified training programs, professional certification of individuals to assure competency, a professional organization to advocate for the profession's interests, a means to obtain licensure or registration, employment opportunities, a scope of practice and a clearly defined core skill set. This section discusses these components.

Genetic Counseling Training Programs in The United States

The first graduate program to educate master's level professionals in human genetics and genetic counseling was established at Sarah Lawrence College in 1969 and graduated its first class in 1972 (Stern, 2012). By the end of that decade, there were 10 such training programs, though some were short-lived (Stern, 2012).

It is somewhat surprising that Sarah Lawrence College would serve as the birthplace of the profession. Located about a half hour north of New York City, Sarah Lawrence is a small liberal arts college that had no formal affiliations with medical centers or a vigorous genetics research program. No medical geneticists were on its faculty. The genetic counseling training program grew out of the vision of two people: Melissa Richter and Joan Marks. Richter was a former riveter and welder at a machine plant, and a sergeant in the Women's Army Corps. She went on to obtain a doctorate in psychology and eventually served as Dean of Graduate Studies at Sarah Lawrence. She claimed to have developed the idea of a genetic counseling training program after reading Sheldon Reed's book *Counseling In Medical Genetics* (Reed, 1955; Stern, 2012). Joan Marks, a psychiatric social worker, assumed directorship of the Sarah Lawrence program in 1974 after Richter's untimely death from breast cancer. Marks was responsible for incorporating a significant psychosocial component into genetic counseling training.

The number of genetic counseling training programs has increased regularly, with a notable rise in the last five years. In 2023 in the United States there are over 50 genetic counseling graduate training programs. Most training programs take about two years to complete, with some variation among programs. The curriculum combines clinical training involving rotations at clinics, laboratories, and other relevant institutions along with coursework in the principles of human genetics/genomics, genetic counseling, and clinical genetics; basic counseling skills; ethical, legal, and social issues; research methodology; principles and basics of some common medical specialties such as oncology, pediatrics, neurology, and obstetrics; laboratory methods; client education, communication and counseling; health care delivery systems and principles of public health; and professional development.

Accreditation for genetic counseling training programs is the responsibility of the Accreditation Council for Genetic Counseling (ACGC) (www.gceducation. org). Collaboration between program directors is coordinated by the Genetic Counselor Educators Association (formerly known as the Association of Genetic Counseling Program Directors), whose mission is "to promote collaborative interactions between individuals involved in genetic counseling graduate education and to support the highest standards of practice" (https://educategc.org).

In 1994, the newly created American Board of Genetic Counseling (ABGC) sponsored a meeting that included directors of all existing genetic counseling programs, the ABGC Board, and consultants from outside the genetic counseling field who had expertise in clinical supervision and accreditation. The goal was to develop consensus about what new graduates should be able to do. By analyzing the counselor's role in various clinical scenarios, participants identified areas of required knowledge and skills (Fine et al., 1996) and from these analyses, 27 "competencies" were described. These were revised in 2015 and 2023. Since helping students to develop these competencies is what this book is all about, the 2023 version of this description is appended to this chapter.

Genetic Counseling Training Around the Globe

Global expansion of the genetic counseling training programs began in the 1980s, starting with Canada (1985), South Africa (1989), the UK and the Netherlands (1992), Australia (1995), and then spread to the rest of the world. In 2023, outside of the US, more than 20 countries on five continents offer more than 60 programs of advanced training in genetic counseling (Abacan et al., 2019). Not all countries offer a master's degree in genetic counseling specifically and instead may offer alternative degrees or certificate programs. In the Netherlands, for example, experienced genetic counselors can earn a master's degree as a Physician Assistant. Programs in India offer a master's degree as well as one-year diploma and certificate programs (Abacan et al., 2019).

Directors of many of these programs met as a group for the first time in Manchester, England in May 2006 to learn about each other's curricula and experiential training, genetics service delivery models, and mechanisms for genetic counselor credentialing. A Transnational Alliance of Genetic Counseling (with the clever acronym TAGC) was born at this meeting, and one outcome is that information about training programs around the world can now be found on the TAGC website (https://sc.edu/study/colleges_schools/medicine/centers_and_institutes_new/transnational_alliance_for_genetic_counseling/index.php).

Professional Organizations

A milestone in the evolution of any profession is the formation of its own society. For genetic counselors, this came in 1979 when the NSGC was incorporated. The goals of the new society were "to further the professional interests of genetic counselors, to promote a network of communication within the genetic counseling profession and to deal with issues related to human genetics" (Heimler, 1997). In 1980, the newly formed NSGC—then numbering only about 200 members—lobbied successfully for genetic counselors to be included among subspecialties that would be certified by the newly created American Board of Medical Genetics (ABMG) (starting in 1993, certification fell to the American Board of Genetic Counseling; refer to below discussion). NSGC has helped achieve representation by genetic counselors on the Boards of Directors and on numerous committees of the ASHG, the American College of Medical Genetics and Genomics (ACMG), and various government advisory boards. The NSGC sponsors an annual education conference to provide continuing education for its members and a forum for discussing research and clinical issues of interest. Since 1992, it has published its own journal, the *Journal of Genetic Counseling*, which has become the primary national and international venue for communicating research about genetic counseling. In 1991, the NSGC developed a professional code of ethics. Most importantly, the Society has become recognized as the voice of the profession and serves as a resource for information about genetic counseling issues for the media, the public, and other health, public policy, and genetics professionals.

Similar organizations have been formed around the world, such as the Canadian Association of Genetic Counsellors, the Professional Society of Genetic Counselors in Asia, the Australasian Society of Genetic Counsellors, the French Association of Genetic Counselors, the Japanese Society of Genetic Counselors (which publishes the *Japanese Journal of Genetic Counseling*), and, in the UK, the Association of Genetic Nurses and Counsellors.

Professional Certification in Genetic Counseling

As noted above, until 1992, genetic counselors in the United States were certified by the ABMG (now known as the American Board of Medical Genetics and Genomics), the organization that also certified medical geneticists. In the early 1990s, the ABMG petitioned the American Board of Medical Specialties (ABMS) for the creation of an American College of Medical Genetics (Epstein, 1992). The ABMS agreed but only on the condition that genetic counselors, who are not physicians and did not typically hold PhDs, be excluded. After much, at times, bitter debate, genetic counselors elected to "secede" from ABMG and in 1993 formed their own certification organization, the American Board of Genetic Counseling (ABGC). The ABGC has certified genetic counselors in the US since then. ABGC requires applicants to have graduated from a genetic counseling training program that was accredited by the Accreditation Council for Genetic Counseling. Candidates must pass a written examination to achieve board certification. Certification must be renewed every five years, either through continuing education or re-examination. Genetic counselors trained outside of the US may be eligible for ABGC certification if they hold a current certification/registration from an international body and have earned a master's degree from a genetic counseling program that has achieved accreditation/recognition from an ABGC-approved accrediting body (www.abgc.net).

Internationally, a number of different organizations provide certification for genetic counselors, such as the Canadian Association of Genetic Counselors, the European Board of Medical Genetics, the Human Genetics Society of Australasia, and the Japanese Society of Genetic Counselors. Requirements for certification vary with each organization. In some countries, the terms certification and registration are used interchangeably.

Licensure and Registration

In 2000, California became the first state to pass legislation creating licensure for genetic counselors, though the bill was not actually signed until 2010 and the first licenses were issued in 2012. In 2002, Utah became the first state to actually issue licenses. In the US, hospitals and other health care organizations generally expect that their providers will be licensed or registered, as do many third-party payers such as health insurance companies and publicly funded medical programs. Usually, a state's legislature decides if a group should be licensed to protect the interests of the citizens it represents. As of August 2023, 33 states have passed licensure laws and the number is expected to increase in the future. Genetic counselors are not recognized Medicare providers, but efforts are underway to pass federal legislation that would provide this status.

Outside of the US, licensure or registration requirements and granting bodies vary with each country. In many countries, genetic counselors are not yet eligible for licensure or registration.

Employment of Genetic Counselors

In seeking employment, the first genetic counselors who graduated from Sarah Lawrence and other programs carved out new positions for themselves in medical centers and universities around the country. Initially most of the jobs were in pediatric genetics clinics where they worked closely with medical geneticists. Sometimes professional tensions arose when some of these bright, well-trained counselors were treated as physician-helpers and relegated to mundane tasks such as obtaining medical records, coordinating patient appointments, and reviewing the medical literature to provide the physician with the latest information on genetic conditions. As these genetic counselors demonstrated their considerable knowledge, skills, and unique role in patient care, they gained more clinical freedom and respect and began advocating for themselves and demanding greater responsibilities commensurate with their training. When prenatal diagnosis started integrating its way into obstetric care in the late 1970s and early 1980s, many counselors migrated to prenatal testing centers, often working with obstetricians who typically gave greater clinical responsibilities to genetic counselors, who had the sophisticated knowledge of genetics and the training to work with patients who were considering or undergoing amniocentesis.

Since the 1970s, genetic counselors have greatly increased their presence across medical specialties and employment settings. According to the 2024 NSGC Professional Status Survey (NSGC, 2024) genetic counselors in the United States were employed in many settings, such as university medical centers, private and public hospitals/medical facilities, commercial and university laboratories, health maintenance organizations, not-for-profit organizations, solo private practice, private genetic counseling companies, and government organizations and agencies. Fifty-six percent of survey respondents worked in direct patient care, 25% worked in nondirect patient care (typically in a commercial diagnostic laboratory), and 19% had a mixed position. In addition to patient care, genetic counselors hold roles as educators, clinical coordinators, student supervision, genetic variant analysts, marketing and sales, management, and research. They work with a wide range of providers, including, but not limited to, clinical geneticists, primary health care providers, oncologists, ophthalmologists, cardiologists, surgeons, obstetricians, nephrologists, immunologists, endocrinologists, dermatologists, psychiatrists, social workers, laboratory scientists, and hospital administrators.

Employment outside of the United States is dictated by local circumstances. In Canada, the UK, Australia, and New Zealand, genetic counselors work in many of the same settings as their US counterparts, with many employed by the public health services in those countries. In some countries, such as Israel, they must work under the supervision of a clinical geneticist. Genetic counselors are not recognized health care providers in some countries, such as Germany, Belgium, and Austria (Abacan et al., 2019).

Scope of Practice and Core Skill Set

A 2007 NSGC task force developed a complementary document to define genetic counselors' scope of practice and to capture the broad range of activities involved in genetic counseling. "Scope of practice" is a term frequently used in the context of licensing nonphysician medical professionals—particularly those with advanced practice degrees such as physician assistants, nurse practitioners, or audiologists. A scope of practice describes activities that an appropriately trained and qualified member of a profession should be able (and allowed) to do. It is usually developed by one or more organizations representing the profession as a means of educating others about their training, skills, their unique place in service delivery, and for encoding in regulatory language the tasks a licensed or registered professional should be entitled to perform. Sometimes the scopes of practice of different professional groups overlap—occasionally causing tension if a newer professional group begins to provide services that historically have been the sole province of another. To some extent this has occurred with the ACMG, the primary professional organization for clinical geneticists but which also includes genetic counselors in its membership.

Defining a scope of practice is often viewed as an important step in a profession's development. While this was part of the reason the NSGC undertook the task, a more urgent one was to provide a document that could be used in efforts to educate legislators about the need for genetic counselor licensure and to assist states in developing licensure regulations that would be as uniform as possible. The NSGC scope of practice (refer to Appendix 2) describes elements of the genetic counselor's role as they relate to clinical genetics, to counseling and communication, and to professional ethics and values.

A profession also needs a clearly articulated core set of skills in order to meet the demands of its scope of practice. To that end, in 2008, the NSGC Core Skills Task Force (CSTF) was charged with identifying a list of core skills for genetic counselors who work in clinical and nonclinical positions that, taken together, differentiate genetic counselors from other health professionals. The Task Force identified six key skills, which are listed in Table 1-1:

TABLE 1-1. Core skills of genetic counselors

Core Skills of Genetic Counselors	Benefits of Skill to Employer/Audience	Examples of these Skills
Deep and broad knowledge of genetics	Improve quality of services/products	Broad range of specialty areas where GCs practice (prenatal risk assessment; pediatric and adult diagnosis; presymptomatic risk assessment for hereditary and common disease)
Ability to tailor, translate, and communicate complex information in a simple, relevant way for a broad range of audiences	Transfer specialized knowledge to others (customer, other professionals, patients, etc.	Patient education; physician education; case summaries; public speaking & education; journal and public press writing; creating education and marketing materials
Strong interpersonal skills, emotional intelligence, and self-awareness	Promote teamwork, collaboration and consensus-building	Cross-functional team-building and collaboration; networking to expand available resources; motivating others; people management and development
Ability to dissect and analyze a complex problem	Find solutions to problems	Risk assessment; results interpretation; family history assessment; analysis of counseling session to provide relevant information and follow-up; utilizing data to make supported conclusions
Research skills (self- education)	Meet deadlines and provide timely answers	Identifying information sources including medical literature and experts and extracting relevant information for audience; self-study
In-depth knowledge of health care delivery	Solutions are clinically feasible, applicable & fiscally responsible	Develop clinical protocols and policies; identify relevant benefits of genetic services for marketing purposes

Source: https://www.nsgc.org/Portals/0/Docs/Secure/Core%20Skills%20of%20Genetic%20Counselors. pdf?ver=t2DhGtVx2tW2O4CE54eAOw%3d%3d.

Because of the many potential future directions of genetic counseling, it is anticipated that the scope of practice and core skill set will be revised periodically to reflect how the practice and profession of genetic counseling are changing. The NSGC website should be accessed for the most up-to-date versions.

OTHER PROVIDERS OF GENETIC COUNSELING

In addition to master's level genetic counselors, other health care providers include genetic counseling as part of their clinical practice.

Clinical Geneticists

Physicians (MD and DO) who have completed accredited residency and/or fellowship programs in North America may become eligible for certification in clinical genetics by the ABMG or the Canadian College of Medical Geneticists (CCMG). In the past, many of these physicians first trained in pediatrics, internal medicine, obstetrics, or another specialty before entering genetics. Recognition of the ABMG by the American Board of Medical Specialties in the early 1990s meant that residencies could have clinical genetics as the *primary* specialty. Some institutions also offer one or more combined residencies with both genetics and another specialty as the focus. There are several such programs in the US and in Canada (where clinical genetics training is under the aegis of the CCMG and the Royal College of Physicians). ABMG currently offers certification in clinical genetics and genomics, clinical biochemical genetics, laboratory genetics and genomics, as well as the subspecialties of medical biochemical genetics and molecular genetic pathology.

Board certification in clinical genetics requires the physician to have knowledge and experience in diagnosing and treating genetic conditions and birth defects, as well as a thorough understanding of the underlying genetics principles. Genetic counseling is assumed to be part of their fellowship training, though there is no certification in genetic counseling *per se*. Clinical geneticists often have specialized areas of interest, such as dysmorphology, neurogenetics, metabolic, or adult disorders, but should also be able to provide expertise on diagnosis and management for a wide range of genetic conditions.

Applicants seek ABMG certification in biochemical genetics and laboratory genetics and genomics if they intend to be involved in those clinical activities—either working with patients or carrying out diagnostic testing—so even laboratory-oriented certification examinations assess knowledge of genetic counseling in addition to expertise in the appropriate subspecialty(ies). Historically, the ABMG has been unusual among medical specialty boards in certifying PhDs as well as MDs.

Genetics Nurses

There are enough nurses working in genetics to have their own professional society, The International Society of Nurses in Genetics, (ISONG), although relatively few are certified in *genetic counseling*. This is because eligibility for both the ABGC and ABMG requires master's level training in genetics, usually from an accredited genetic counseling program. However, advanced practice and other specialty nurses work in pediatric and adult clinics and programs where genetic and congenital conditions are diagnosed and treated. Many have acquired their knowledge of genetics through years of clinical experience, and a few actually hold a graduate degree in genetics nursing from one of the handful of programs that have provided such training. Nurses' additional skills in physical and psychosocial assessment, case management, patient education, clinic administration, and community health are highly valued in specialty and outreach clinics, and in genetics screening programs. Those with specialization in areas such as infant special care, oncology, or midwifery may be astute "case-finders" of patients in need of genetics services and helpful allies in their care.

The Genetics Nursing Credentialing Commission uses a portfolio-based mechanism for appropriately prepared nurses to become credentialed in genetic nursing. Those with a graduate degree from an accredited program and 300 hours of training in a practice, at least half devoted to genetics, can qualify for a credential as an Advanced Practice Nurse in Genetics (APNG) by providing a logbook of 50 genetics cases, an in-depth written description of four cases, and by documenting sufficient recent genetics coursework or continuing education. Nurses with a Bachelor of Nursing degree can qualify as a Genetics Clinical Nurse (GCN) through a similar process. This portfolio-based approach to credentialing is similar to that used for genetic counselors in the UK and some other countries that do not have examination-based certification.

PHILOSOPHY AND ETHOS OF GENETIC COUNSELING

Genetic counseling has continued to try to consciously distance itself from eugenic goals, as reflected in the philosophy and ethos of modern genetic counseling. In addition, the expansion of genetic counseling services to specialties such as oncology and cardiology, where the focus of counseling is on lifelong health issues rather than primarily reproductive issues, has helped genetic counseling branch out from its eugenics roots. Some of the core ethical and philosophical principles of genetic counseling practice are briefly reviewed below.

Voluntary Utilization of Services

Genetic counseling operates on a number of assumptions and principles. Among these are that the decision to utilize genetics services should be entirely voluntary. Society at large and other entities such as insurance companies clearly have economic and potentially eugenic interests in promoting prevention of genetic disease. However, in many countries, the prevailing philosophy is that information should be made available and tests offered when appropriate, but that patients and families should have the right to make their own decisions—particularly about genetic testing and reproduction—unencumbered by pressure or by the implication that they are being fiscally or socially irresponsible if they chose *not* to try to prevent the birth of a child with a hereditary disease, or not to pursue a hereditary cancer test, or to decline risk-reducing surgery.

In reality, of course, patients sometimes are referred to genetics services not at their own request but by virtue of a care provider's fear of litigation, or because they have been identified through a screening program about which they were not adequately educated. Furthermore, decisions about testing or reproduction are often influenced by financial considerations. Genetic disorders usually come with additional health care costs, which may or may not be covered by health insurance or public medical assistance programs. In some cases, insurers consider newer genetic tests to be "experimental" or regard genetic counseling as unnecessary outside of the context of pregnancy. To assume that families can always make voluntary decisions about utilizing genetic services, reproductive choices, or cope with being at increased risk of developing cancer or cardiomyopathy, based solely on their preferences, personal goals, and moral views is, at best, naïve. In order to maximize the ability of families to benefit from advances in genetics, it is incumbent on genetic counselors to educate insurers about the value of genetics services and testing, to advocate for access to these services, and to be involved in developing public policies that promote responsible use of genetics, assure that patients will be able to *make* choices, access appropriate medical and social services for them and their families, adapt to having or being at risk for a genetic condition, and protect them from misuse of genetic information.

Diversity, Justice, Equity, Inclusion

Ideally, genetics services, including counseling, diagnosis, and treatment, should be equally and readily available to all who need and choose to use them. Compared with other medical specialties, however, genetics services are more likely to be accessed by people living in heavily populated areas who have some sort of health insurance coverage, enough education or medical sophistication to know that such services exist, and the ability to advocate for themselves in the health care system. As capabilities continue to expand and genetic testing for more common conditions like cancer and cardiovascular disease integrate their way into routine health care, equitable access to genetic services needs to be improved. Particularly in the last few years, there has been increasing acknowledgment among genetic counselors that their patient populations do not adequately reflect the diversity of the larger population in the US and elsewhere, resulting in underserving of many people, particularly those who are not cis-gendered, have lower incomes, or come from non-Northern and Western European backgrounds (Yip et al., 2019; Hallford et al., 2020; Bellaiche et al., 2021; Rouse et al., 2021; Uebergang et al., 2021; Young et al., 2021).

Notably, genetic counselors themselves in the United States are more likely to be from the middle-to-upper income and White segment of the population and, in 2024, ~92% identify as women, 6% as men, and 2% as gender-nonconforming

(NSGC, 2024). This demographic skewing is found in most countries where genetic counselors are recognized professionals. Genetic counselors, students, and applicants to genetic counseling training programs who identify as a non-White or not cis-gender report significant experiences of racism, bias, microaggressions, and insensitivity, as well as difficulty applying to and getting into genetic counseling training programs (Alvarado-Wing et al., 2021; Carmichael et al., 2021; Dewey et al., 2021; Young et al., 2021; Pollock et al., 2022).

The NSGC, along with efforts of individual and groups of genetic counselors, have made clear and specific formal commitments to increasing the diversity and inclusiveness, ethnic and otherwise, of the patients they serve and of the profession itself (NSGC, 2021a). The Minority Genetics Professional Network (MGPN) is one group that is trying to address these disparities by serving "as an organized way for genetic professionals of racial and ethnic minority backgrounds to connect with one another to address these issues together" (https://www.westernstatesgenetics.org/mgpn-resources/). This has come as part of a larger social reckoning on racial and ethnic bias as well as the intentional and unintentional harms that have resulted from this lack of diversity, justice, equity, and inclusion. This is particularly critical for genetic medicine and counseling, where eugenics has not been the only source of ethical shortcomings. For example, racism has resulted in the undertreatment, mismanagement, and greater suffering of individuals diagnosed with, or carriers of, sickle cell anemia (Wailoo, 2001). While the damage of the past cannot be undone, hopefully a greater understanding of the history of genetics along with efforts to reduce the inequities and injustices that result from racism, ableism, and gender discrimination will reduce the chances of similar harms being repeated.

Client Communication

One of the core features of genetic counseling is a belief in the importance of educating clients about genetic conditions. However, the verb "educate" suggests a one-way process whereby the counselor teaches the client and that creates a power differential of the counselor over the client rather than the counselor and client working together as equals. But a genetic counseling session is more typically a two-way process in which the counselor and the patient are educating each other. Clients educate counselors about their family histories, their understanding of disease etiology, their goals, concerns, and values; and the counselor modifies and adapts the information accordingly. Therefore, consistent with the most recent guidelines from the Accreditation Council of Genetic Counseling (refer to Appendix 1), the term "communication" is used here rather "education." In order to be good educators, counselors need to be good communicators.

Expanding on the NSGC definition, this communication typically includes information about: 1) the features, natural history and range of variability of the condition in question; 2) its genetic (or nongenetic) basis; 3) how it can be diagnosed and managed; 4) the chances it will occur or recur in various family members; 5) the economic, social, and psychological impact—positive as well as negative—that it may have; 6) resources available to help families deal with the challenges it presents; 7) strategies that can ameliorate or prevent it if the family so wishes; and 8) relevant research that may contribute to understanding the disorder or better treatment.

As important as communication is to genetic counseling, most studies have shown that patients have limited recall of the information that was provided, especially over time (Resta, 2019). This does not mean that patients are incapable of understanding technically complex information. Rather, patients will integrate and adapt this information into their unique world views and life experiences to make it psychologically meaningful. For this reason, studies that assess the effectiveness of genetic counseling should not rely primarily on patient recall of information as a good measure.

In providing education about diagnosis and related issues, most geneticists and genetic counselors subscribe to the belief that all relevant information should be disclosed. Being selective in what one tells a client is viewed as paternalistic—and disrespectful of the person's autonomy and competence. There is wide disagreement, however, both in philosophy and in practice, on what geneticists or counselors view as "relevant". Most would probably concur that a competent patient should be given the facts about their own diagnosis—even in a challenging scenario such as informing a patient with androgen insensitivity syndrome and who was assigned female at birth about their XY karyotype.

But there is less consensus about what should be done with other dilemmas, like disclosing misassigned paternity revealed through DNA testing when it does not affect risk assessment. Nor is it clear if a counselor should be obligated to address issues of potential genetic significance that are not related to the reason for referral (e.g., a familial cancer history uncovered in the context of prenatal diagnosis counseling). This is particularly true for genomic testing of infants and children, which might reveal information about adult-onset conditions unrelated to the reason for referral—what are sometimes called incidental or secondary findings—or for autosomal dominant conditions, information about cancer, or other health risks faced by the parents. Currently the ACMG recommends more than 90 such secondary conditions be reported out when clinical exome and genome testing is performed, and the list continues to grow (www.ncbi.nlm.nih.gov/clinvar/docs/acmg/). This is an area for which there is not universal agreement and policies will continue to evolve.

As testing capabilities and understanding of genetic mechanisms have become more extensive and complex, clients have become more diverse in their cultural backgrounds, education, and health literacy. Concomitantly, the time available for counseling has often decreased. In the 1980s and early 1990s, when a typical session might last an hour and a half and most clients were college educated, middle class, and English speaking, a "genetics lesson" was a prominent feature of genetic counseling. We believed that clients needed a basic understanding of genes, chromosomes, and how the test would be done in order to make informed decisions. Now, however, with burgeoning genetic knowledge and technology, the pressure to increase the patient load, to speed up the counseling session, to schedule clients more as soon as possible, and a more frequent need to work through interpreters, achieving this level of client education is often impractical. Moreover, full disclosure of all "relevant information" could paralyze even the most sophisticated patient. Despite these pressures, however, it will always be critical for the counselor to disclose any information relevant to decision-making and the medical and social management of genetic conditions in ways that the client can interpret and act on.

Nondirective Counseling

Adherence to a nonprescriptive (often less appropriately referred to as "nondirective") approach is perhaps the most defining feature of genetic counseling. The philosophy stems from the belief that genetic counseling should, insofar as is possible, be based in patient autonomy and devoid of eugenic motivation. That being said, autonomy itself can be constrained by social and economic factors; the choices available to people who are non-Western and/or low-income may not be the same as those available to upper income people from the ethnic majority. In addition, not all cultures value individual autonomy and put greater emphasis on familial or group autonomy (Resta, 2021).

Although nondirectiveness is a time-honored tradition, it can be counterproductive for the counselor and counselees to try to avoid expressing *any* opinions. It can also show a lack of counseling skills on the part of the genetic counselor. This is especially true when a genetics evaluation reveals *personal* health risks, such as an increased liability to specific diseases that could be reduced by particular interventions (e.g., aggressive screening, chemoprevention, or prophylactic surgery to reduce breast or ovarian cancer risk due to a pathogenic *BRCA1/2* variant; monitoring serum iron, dietary modifications, or therapeutic phlebotomy in a person with hemochromatosis) (Kessler, 1992; Jamal et al., 2020).

A measure of directiveness can even be appropriate in certain situations involving reproductive decision-making—an area where genetic counselors have historically shied away from expressing opinions or offering advice. If a risk could be reduced by various actions (e.g., avoiding exposure to a teratogenic drug, taking folate supplements, or achieving good diabetic control prior to pregnancy), few counselors would hesitate to advise the client accordingly. A client should expect a genetics professional to be able to provide guidance when the genetic and medical issues are complex, if there is limited data or medical opinions conflict, and even when choices raise problematic moral or psychosocial issues. Failing to share our knowledge and experience out of fear that we will be perceived as directive is simply poor genetic counseling.

One challenge to the notion that genetic counseling is nondirective—particularly in the context of prenatal testing—stems from criticisms by some (but not all) people with disabilities, their advocates, and disability rights scholars and activists

(Wilson, 2021). In these critics' views, the very availability of prenatal testing and abortion is a form of directiveness in as much as it suggests that there is a socially condoned "right" decision. Why else would testing be available, particularly for conditions in which prenatal testing does not improve medical or developmental outcomes? These critics further argue that prenatal testing and selective termination for Down syndrome and other conditions devalues and dehumanizes people with disabilities and is largely a manifestation of eugenics lurking beneath an ethical justification of patient choice.

Genetic counselors may counter-argue that they do not try to influence decisions about whether to undergo prenatal testing and abortion, and that patient decisions one way or another are voluntary and always supported by the genetic counselor. Nonetheless, many genetic counseling jobs in clinics and laboratories depend on the existence of prenatal testing; if prenatal testing disappeared overnight, so too would many genetic counseling positions. This conflict of interest can make it difficult to assert or maintain a position of neutrality.

These critiques raise a number of important issues that genetic counselors have not fully and adequately addressed. Genetic counselors are in the seemingly contradictory positions of acting as strong advocates for people with disabilities, while also working in prenatal testing programs and laboratories that, intentionally or not, result in a reduction in the number of births of people with Down syndrome and other conditions (de Graaf et al., 2017). This will continue to be an important issue for genetic counselors to address as the number of people who undergo prenatal testing, and the number and variability of conditions that are screened for, continues to expand at a rapid pace around the globe (Ravitsky et al., 2021).

Confidentiality and Protection of Privacy

Respecting confidentiality and protecting personal health information has always been an essential part of any medical interaction, but it has become even more critical since the passage of The Health Insurance Privacy and Accountability Act (HIPAA) in 1996. However, genetic counseling raises additional issues with regard to confidentiality and privacy protection. Information about an individual's family history, carrier status, diagnosis, or risk of genetic disease in themselves or their offspring is potentially stigmatizing. With the advent of law enforcement and immigration databases, direct to consumer genetic testing, and samples containing DNA being stored for many reasons, concerns have been raised about the *privacy* of genetic information. Genetic material obtained for one purpose (ancestry studies, newborn screening, or military identification) can also reveal information about unrelated features of the genotype (e.g., risk for late-onset disease, misattributed paternity) that may be both unwanted and damaging, and may even unknowingly be used to help solve criminal investigations (Kling et al., 2021). The privacy of genetic information increasingly will become a cause for both litigation and legislation.

Concerns have also been raised that information about genetic risk could lead to discrimination in employment or difficulties in obtaining or retaining insurance.

For these reasons it is especially critical that genetic information be kept confidential. In the United States, the Genetic Information Nondiscrimination Act (GINA) of 2008 provides protection against using genetic information of healthy people in obtaining health insurance and employment. Notably, GINA is not applicable to members of the military, federal employees enrolled in the Federal Employees Health Benefits program, military veterans obtaining health care through the Veterans Administration, and individuals covered under the Indian Health Service, although many of these individuals have similar protections under other laws and policies. In addition, employers with fewer than 15 employees are exempt. GINA also does not provide protection from discrimination in long-term care, disability, life, mortgage, and other types of insurance.

On the other hand, knowing a person's diagnosis or genotype sometimes provides information not only about their *own* risk, but also that of family members who may be only remotely related. This can create a conflict between the client's right to privacy and the benefit to relatives of knowing about their potential risk. If the risk is substantial or serious, and when options are available to prevent harm, some have argued that the client—and sometimes the counselor—may have an ethical duty to warn relatives. There are only a few other situations in medicine (e.g., a serious infectious disease or threat to another's safety disclosed in the course of psychotherapy) where breaching confidentiality is warranted if the client refuses to share information with those at risk. (Refer to Chapter 12 for additional discussion.)

Psychological and Affective Dimensions of Genetic Counseling

Just providing information does not necessarily promote client autonomy. To succeed in empowering individuals to cope with and adapt to a genetic condition or risk, and to make difficult decisions, the counselor needs to encourage clients to regard themselves as competent and help them project how various events or courses of action could affect them and their family. This cannot be done without knowing something of their social, cultural, educational, economic, emotional, and experiential circumstances. The client's ability to attend to, understand, interpret, and utilize information will be influenced by all of these factors. An effective counselor will be attuned and responsive to affective responses and able to explore not only the client's understanding of information, but also what it means to them, and what impact they feel it will have within their social and psychological framework.

THE PRACTICE OF GENETIC COUNSELING

Genetic counseling has traditionally been conducted via in-person meetings with patients and their families within the physical space of clinic offices, examination rooms, and hospital wards and supplemented by telephone interactions.

This approach is now being enhanced by internet-based genetic counseling sessions (discussed below). But wherever genetic counseling is carried out, the patient interaction shares some common and essential components.

Who Comes for Genetic Counseling?

People come to genetic counseling for many reasons. Some are looking for a diagnosis or testing for their own condition or disease or for the condition of a family member, such as cancer, cardiovascular disease, or a neurological disorder. For some, it may come as an unanticipated surprise, such as when a routine screening colonoscopy of a healthy person reveals a large number of colon polyps. Some are looking for more information after already having had testing performed by another health professional or a commercial laboratory. Some come before they are pregnant to get a better understanding of the conditions any future children may be at risk for and to learn about their reproductive, testing, and risk-reducing options. Others come during pregnancy to decide if they should undergo prenatal screening or have already had a positive prenatal test result. Some are parents seeking a diagnosis, prognosis, and treatment options for their newborn infant or child. Some are in emotional and/or medical crisis and are desperately seeking psychological help or medical direction, such as a young *BRCA1* variant carrier who has been diagnosed with breast cancer and is trying to decide about prophylactic bilateral mastectomy and explore options for preserving fertility. Increasingly, more patients with no apparent risk factors have elected to undergo genetic testing to help identify otherwise unanticipated health risks, such as cancer and cardiovascular disease (Kelly et al., 2021, Majumder et al., 2021).

Components of the Genetic Counseling Interaction

Because of this great variety of reasons for referral for genetic counseling, there is no one set of uniform components for all genetic counseling sessions. What follows is a discussion of some of the most common components, recognizing that any given component may play minimal or no role in any one particular genetic counseling session.

Contracting   Of critical importance to counseling success is learning about the client's or family's understanding about the reason for referral and their expectations about what will be gained through the consultation. Each genetic counseling session should begin with what is sometimes called contracting—asking the patient why they have sought genetic counseling and what they expect out of it and the counselor explaining what they can or cannot offer along those lines. Determining the family's beliefs about causation and assessing emotional, experiential, social, educational, and cultural issues that may affect their perception of information is a process that should be ongoing throughout the course of the evaluation.

Information-Gathering   An integral part of genetic evaluation is the family history. This usually is recorded in the form of a pedigree to clarify relationships and note phenotypic features that may be relevant to the diagnosis or condition that the patient may be at risk for. Additional family history of potential genetic significance (e.g., consanguinity, infertility, birth defects, late-onset diseases, psychiatric disorders) may also be obtained depending on the reason for referral, though there are no strict guidelines about what medical information should or should not be included. Adherence to conventions for symbols notating gender, sex, biologic relationships, pregnancy outcomes, and genotypic information, when known, will assure that any pedigree can be readily and accurately interpreted (Bennett et al., 2022). Taking a pedigree also can provide insight into a patient's understanding of disease etiology as well as the dynamic of the family relationships.

Many genetic counseling clinics are collecting family histories prior to the counseling appointment using electronic pedigree tools and virtual conversation agents (i.e., chatbots) when patients have access to, and familiarity using, internet-based technology (Welch et al., 2018; Ponathil et al., 2020; Wang et al., 2021). This allows patients to gather their family histories at a more leisurely pace and to verify information from relatives, birth and death certificates, and medical records. This also gives the counselor the opportunity to review the pedigree prior to the appointment, research information about specific conditions in the family, and focus clinic time on counseling patients instead of collecting information.

Pertinent medical information routinely obtained may include obstetric history, disease history, and testing history. Often, clinical features or medical history important to a diagnosis must be confirmed—even before the visit—by obtaining medical records not only on the patient, but also on relevant family members previously evaluated or treated. In the context of cancer genetic counseling, it may be important to obtain not only records (such as pathology reports or test results) but actual tissue samples or slides from affected individuals to verify a diagnosis, particularly for uncommon tumors or conditions that may require the expertise of a specialist.

Establishing or Verifying Diagnosis   Although a genetic diagnosis can sometimes be established or ruled out solely by reviewing medical records, evaluation usually involves at least one clinic visit. This might be for a diagnostic procedure, as in the case of prenatal testing, or for a physical examination by the clinical geneticist or other specialist experienced with the condition. Confirming or excluding a clinically suspected diagnosis can require additional assessments, such as imaging studies, evaluations by other specialists, or examinations of particular family members. Increasingly, however, genetic and genomic testing alone may be sufficient not only to diagnose an affected individual or carrier, but also to provide important information about prognosis or severity. With many genetic tests commercially available, genetic diagnoses can now often be made or confirmed by the primary care physician or a specialist in a field other than genetics. Some commercial genetics laboratories have aggressively marketed genetic tests to nongeneticists and even directly to consumers, so testing increasingly is occurring outside of the context of genetics evaluation. This sometimes creates difficult situations in which genetic counseling must be provided *post hoc* to a client who was inadequately educated about testing or its implications, or who may have undergone inappropriate testing.

The NSGC's Scope of Practice even indicates that genetic counselors may "order tests and perform clinical assessments in accordance with local, state and federal regulations." This is more likely to be appropriate in the context of prenatal diagnosis counseling or cancer risk assessment than in a general genetics clinic.

Risk Assessment   In many cases, the client's concerns center not around diagnosis of an affected individual but on assessing future reproductive or personal health risk or risks to children and other relatives. The counselor can sometimes make such an assessment by analyzing the pedigree—taking into account the pattern of inheritance and the client's relationship to individuals with the condition. Statistical calculations may be needed to incorporate additional information (e.g., carrier frequencies, test sensitivity and specificity, numbers of affected and unaffected individuals, the client's age) to modify the risk. Questions about carrier or genetic condition status may be resolved with appropriate laboratory tests. When a condition has a multifactorial basis or is genetically heterogeneous, the best risk estimates may come from epidemiologic data on other families with affected individuals. Answering concerns about potentially mutagenic or teratogenic exposures also usually relies on empirical data about the agent in question, and on evaluating the timing, duration, and dose of the exposure. In some areas of genetic counseling, such as cancer risk assessment, factors such as reproductive history, hormone use, and lifestyle issues such as smoking, obesity, or alcohol use are also important variables in risk assessment. Polygenic risk scores, which entail simultaneous analysis of many single nucleotide polymorphisms at multiple loci, are sometimes employed in clinical practice to assess the risk of common conditions such as cancer and cardiovascular disease (Wray et al., 2021).

Information-Giving   Once a diagnosis or risk is determined, the client and/or family needs to understand how it was arrived at and what the implications are for the affected person and other family members. This includes describing the condition, its variability, its natural history, and its uncertainties—making sure that the family's prior perception of the genetics and treatment of the disorder (if any) is still appropriate. It is appropriate to make sure that, depending on the situation, the client, parents, or family is told about medical, surgical, social, and educational interventions that can correct, prevent, or alleviate symptoms. Discussions should also include available financial and social resources (e.g., support groups) to help treat and cope with the condition. When appropriate, it may be important to describe reproductive options (e.g., prenatal or pre-implantation diagnosis) that could reduce risk or provide information during pregnancy. Clearly this depth of discussion would neither be warranted nor feasible in the time available for a routine prenatal session, but once a specific fetal diagnosis is made or suspected, the prospective parents should have access to as much information as they need to make an informed decision about their course of action. Follow-up review letters sent to the patient can be helpful in giving the patient the time and additional opportunity to process complex information.

Psychological Counseling and Support   Being given a diagnosis or learning about a personal health or reproductive risk often generates powerful emotional responses that must be acknowledged and dealt with if the information is to be assimilated. Part of counseling is preparing clients for these responses and helping them adapt to them, often over a period of months or years. Sometimes, as in a fetal or neonatal diagnosis, critical decisions must be made rapidly on the basis of new and distressing data. In other situations, carrier or presymptomatic testing may reveal that a person is *not* at increased risk to develop a disease or have affected children. If this new knowledge overturns long-held beliefs, it can be quite disorienting. Clients often need help in trying possible scenarios "on for size" to help them imagine how various courses of action—including just the decision to *undergo* diagnostic testing—may affect them and their family. Counselors must be knowledgeable about resources that can help families adjust to the reality of a condition or risk, be alert to reactions that are beyond their skills to treat, and be able to make an effective referral when necessary.

Attention to the psychological and affective dimensions of patients, along with a notable lack of a goal of eugenics or protecting the gene pool, is captured in the Reciprocal Engagement Model (REM) of genetic counseling. As the models' developers state: "*Model of practice* refers to why and how the service is delivered to patients, as described by tenets, goals, strategies, and behaviors" (Veach et al., 2007). Another paper nicely summarizes the basis of the REM: "The REM is built on the tenets of patient-centered communication and counseling, understanding and appreciation of the patient's unique situation, support and guidance to patients to build rapport and trust, and facilitative decision-making. The REM incorporates the patient's values, prior knowledge, beliefs, and experiences, and allows for the development of a mutual relationship, which is at the core of the genetic counseling process" (Schmidlen et al., 2018). This model makes clear that the emotional and medical wellbeing of patients and families are the primary focus of genetic counseling.

Alternative Service Delivery Models

In part spurred on by the Covid pandemic, a growing number of genetic counselors provide counseling using internet-based video and audio platforms (Amendola et al., 2021). This approach allows greater access to genetic counseling in urban and particularly rural settings where geographic distances to medical centers can be a deterrent to utilizing genetic counseling services. It also permits greater flexibility to genetic counselors in where they perform their work and where their employer is based, as the position may not require a regular need to work from an employer's office or to be in the same state (provided they meet local licensure requirements) or time zone as their patients.

As genetic testing has become more widely available beyond a limited number of laboratories, nongenetics providers, general practitioners, as well as specialists, have become increasingly involved in providing some or all aspects of genetic counseling. This has led to alternative service delivery models in which the genetic counselor may play a supporting, consulting, or educational role for the ordering provider (Trepanier and Allain, 2020; Brown-Johnson et al., 2021; Lemke et al., 2021).

THE MANY ROLES OF GENETIC COUNSELORS

Genetic counseling historically had a significant focus on reproduction and pediatric evaluation. This has changed considerably over the years, and genetic counselors are now engaged in a wide range of roles, some of which are discussed here (Figure 1-1).

Genetic Counseling for Reproductive Issues

According to the 2022 Professional Status Survey, nearly half of all genetic counselors practice in the prenatal and preconception/reproductive arenas.

Patients may seek counseling *before* they conceive because of concerns about the reproductive implications of their family history, or may seek screening or help with result interpretation for carrier status for an ever-growing list of conditions. Others may come as part of an evaluation for infertility or fetal loss, or for donor screening if they are considering using assisted reproductive techniques. With the growing use of pre-implantation genetic diagnosis—not only for known genetic disorders, but also to enhance the likelihood of a successful pregnancy after *in vitro* fertilization—some "prenatal" counseling may occur before conception.

Genetic counseling also commonly takes place during pregnancy among patients who are considering various prenatal screening and diagnostic testing or after they have undergone such testing. These testing options can include amniocentesis, chorionic villus sampling (CVS), ultrasonography, maternal serum screening of analytes, and analysis of cell-free DNA (cfDNA) and can be used to test for common chromosomal aneuploidies as well as a rapidly expanding range of genetic and congenital conditions utilizing karyotyping, microarrays, genomic analysis, and other testing modalities.

The American College of Obstetrics and Gynecology (ACOG) recommends that noninvasive prenatal testing (NIPT) and other forms of prenatal screening be

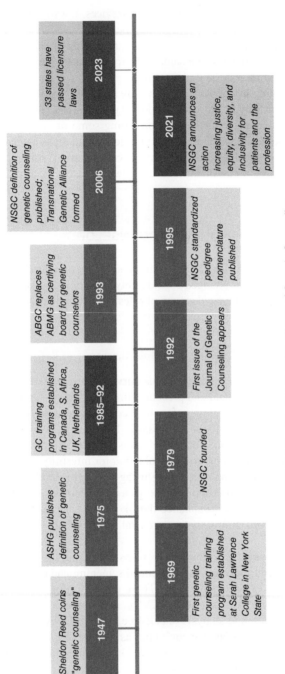

FIGURE 1-1. Key Events in The History of Genetic Counseling

1947 — Sheldon Reed coins "genetic counseling"

1975 — ASHG publishes definition of genetic counseling

1985–92 — GC training programs established in Canada, S. Africa, UK, Netherlands

1993 — ABGC replaces ABMG as certifying board for genetic counselors

2006 — NSGC definition of genetic counseling published; Transnational Genetic Alliance formed

2023 — 33 states have passed licensure laws

1969 — First genetic counseling training program established at Sarah Lawrence College in New York State

1979 — NSGC founded

1992 — First issue of the Journal of Genetic Counseling appears

1995 — NSGC standardized pedigree nomenclature published

2021 — NSGC announces an action increasing justice, equity, diversity, and inclusivity for patients and the profession

made available to all pregnant people, regardless of age or other risk factors (www.acog.org/advocacy/policy-priorities/non-invasive-prenatal-testing/current-acog-guidance). Discussing the host of prenatal screening options has become so complicated that it is daunting for both the care provider and the pregnant person. In spite of this complexity, blood for first trimester screening is often drawn in the primary care setting in the context of "routine prenatal blood work," sometimes without the patient fully understanding the implications of screening. Consequently, a patient who embarked on a pregnancy with no known risk factors may unexpectedly find themselves in the genetic counselor's office discussing multiple testing options after fetal ultrasound or other screens suggest an increased chance of Down syndrome or other conditions.

Genetic Counseling in Neonatology and Pediatrics

Most genetic conditions and birth defects appear after an uncomplicated pregnancy and in the absence of a family history of the condition or other identifiable risk factors. Genetic counselors have an important role to play after the birth or stillbirth of a baby born with multiple or serious anomalies, or when an infant with a genetic condition dies. According to the 2024 Professional Status Survey, about 23% of genetic counselors work with pediatric patients (NSGC, 2024). Increasingly, when these conditions are diagnosed prenatally, genomic testing is initiated prenatally with the intention of guiding neonatal management (Mellis et al., 2022). Genomic testing can also play a critical role in diagnosing and managing young children who have genetic conditions (Elliott, 2020). The counselor can help the family understand the cause of the problem (when known), aid parents in understanding how prenatal or postnatal genomic testing might help guide their baby's medical care, and help them grieve for the baby's death or the "loss" of the normal child they had anticipated. At a time when families may feel abandoned by previously trusted professionals and friends who are uncomfortable dealing with a baby's death or a birth defect, the counselor can provide not only information, but also ongoing emotional support that can sometimes continue through subsequent pregnancies.

Many genetic conditions are not suspected until later in childhood or adolescence. In some situations, as with delayed physical or cognitive development, clinical manifestations may only become evident over time. In others, a newly recognized health problem or feature of a disorder may prompt concerns about a particular diagnosis. Genetic counseling in these circumstances includes gathering information relevant to establishing the diagnosis, anticipating its impact on the patient or family, addressing their fears and distress, educating them about the condition and its implications, and ensuring that they access necessary medical and social services. Because genetic counselors understand the unique, genetic, psychological, and medical issues that attend many chronic conditions, they are often part of teams of professionals who provide ongoing management for diseases such as cystic fibrosis, craniofacial or bleeding disorders, muscular dystrophies, inherited metabolic conditions, and hemoglobinopathies.

Genetic Counseling for Adult-Onset Diseases

Another arena for genetic counseling is in genetic testing for conditions that develop later in life. As per the 2024 NSGC Professional Status Survey, nearly 60% of genetic counselors work primarily with adult patients, with the majority of this group working with patients who are at risk for or have developed a hereditary cancer (NSGC, 2024). As molecular tests have become available for disorders such as Huntington disease, familial amyotrophic lateral sclerosis, and numerous hereditary cancer predispositions, healthy individuals who are at risk may consider learning about their genotype to diminish anxiety, remove uncertainty, or make personal and medical decisions. Numerous complex genetic and psychosocial issues arise in helping families consider testing and coping with results. Many physicians who traditionally have cared for affected individuals in these families feel ill equipped to provide the necessary communication and counseling that should surround testing. Consequently, genetic counselors now find themselves working in settings such as cancer centers, dialysis units, and specialties such as ophthalmology, neurology, cardiology, psychiatry, pharmacogenetics, endocrinology, immunology, and dermatology that historically may not have had established relationships with genetics. Many counselors now work more closely with oncologists, neurologists, surgeons, or cardiologists than they do with clinical geneticists.

In these work settings genetic counselors are removed from the traditional "genetics team" and may be looked to for diagnostic expertise that formerly was provided by clinical geneticists. Until recently, diagnosing most genetic conditions required the skill in physical diagnosis and acumen in synthesizing complex historical and laboratory information that physicians have. For some genetic conditions, this undoubtedly will always be the case. However, with the increasing use of genomic testing, genetic counselors have the skills and training to play a critical role in interpreting the diagnostic, prognostic, and treatment implications of genomic results. The NSGC has indicated that ordering diagnostic tests and other clinical assessments, "in accordance with local, state and federal regulations" is within the genetic counselor's scope of practice.

Genetic Counselors Working Outside of Hospitals and Other Medical Facilities

The most rapidly expanding role for genetic counselors has been with established commercial and university-based genetic testing laboratories and start-up companies (Field et al., 2016; Rabideau et al., 2016; Cho and Guy, 2020). The 2024 NSGC Professional Status Survey reports that about 65% of counselors are employed by a medical facility, 17% of genetic counselors are employed by a commercial or noncommercial laboratory, and the rest are employed in a variety of settings such as insurance companies, private practice groups, research institutions, and pharmaceutical companies (NSGC, 2024). Genetic counselors provide technical expertise in genetic test development and interpretation, case management, reporting test results, education of other laboratory staff and students as well as outreach to the clinical community, filling sales and marketing roles, business development and managerial positions. Some lab-based genetic counselors provide pre- and (more commonly) post-test genetic counseling to patients who have had or are considering genetic testing through the laboratory. Some laboratories allow patients to bypass physicians when ordering a genetic test and so the lab genetic counselor can be an important resource for such patients.

Genetic Counselors in Research

While genetic counselors have always been involved in research activities, over the last 10 years they have taken on increasingly important roles in research about genetic counseling and genetic counseling outcomes (Senter et al., 2020). The 2024 NSGC Professional Status Survey reports that about 20% of genetic counselors engage in some type of research (NSGC, 2024). In addition, most graduate training programs require students to complete a masters' thesis or capstone project that entails some research component.

Genetic counselors are often involved with helping people decide if they wish to participate in research projects and explaining test results if the research involves clinical testing. But beyond this important role, genetic counselors also design, conduct, and obtain funding for research projects, as well as analyzing data. They often collaborate with specialists in areas such as cardiology, oncology, obstetrics, neurology, pathology, laboratory medicine, public health, epidemiology, statistics, research design, and the social sciences in conducting research studies that have wider implications for the delivery of medical care and our understanding of basic human psychology and behavior.

PROFESSIONAL GROWTH AND SKILL ACQUISITION

While genetic counselors enter the field with an impressive armamentarium of skills and knowledge, two years of training cannot prepare them for all counseling situations or for future developments in genetics that cannot even be imagined today. Ongoing self-education is critical, and counselors must stay abreast of the literature, routinely attend professional meetings (virtually or in person), and communicate with genetics colleagues in order to provide quality service. Current examples of advances in technology and in genetic testing that might require additional technical education and training in counseling approaches, especially for genetic counselors who graduated more than a few years ago, include polygenic scores (using multiple single nucleotide variants to predict the likelihood of a trait or condition), whole genome testing, and the development of sophisticated chatbots that utilize a generative language model to mimic human conversation and generate well-written texts on many technical subjects.

Furthermore, professional recertification and, in some states, licensure, require genetic counselors to obtain continuing education credits throughout their careers.

Special Interest Groups

The NSGC has special interest groups (SIGs) for many subspecialty areas. In 2023, there are 22 SIGS, many of which have active e-mail listservs that provide invaluable information and a forum to learn, ask questions, and discuss issues of common interest. Many SIGs sponsor workshops at the NSGC Annual Conference and regular webinars throughout the year to update their members and other counselors on recent advances and changes in counseling practice.

Maintaining membership in professional societies and being active on their committees afford opportunities to work with colleagues from around the country and to develop leadership skills. Involvement in education, advocacy, and political activism can also bring personal rewards and lead to recognition in the community and beyond.

Applying Genetic Counseling Skills Outside of The Medical Clinic

The 2024 NSGC Professional status survey reported that genetic counselors are finding new and exciting ways to apply their counseling skills and knowledge base, such as "working in administration, basic and behavioral research, public and professional education, educational content development and editing, public health, private industry, laboratory support, public policy, public relations and consulting" (NSGC, 2024). They have also helped establish genetic counseling start-ups and form new commercial testing laboratories. This has created opportunities for career advancement, professional development, personal satisfaction, and higher salaries beyond those found in direct clinical settings. Some counselors have obtained additional graduate degrees, such as an MBA or PhD, or additional training in psychotherapy and social work, to help further their careers and open up new opportunities.

CONCLUDING REMARKS

Genetic counseling and genetic counselors have come a long way since 1947. Both the practice and the profession have evolved from a vaguely defined clinical activity carried out by handful of practitioners scattered in a few specialized clinics, to thousands of genetic counselors around the globe with clearly defined and ever-expanding roles at the cutting edge of medicine and who have become integrated into nearly all aspects of health care. The journey has not been without its challenges, but confronting and moving past those challenges has spurred genetic counselors to achieve greater personal and professional growth. More importantly, our patients have benefited both psychologically and medically from this progress. We have made their lives better, sometimes in small and sometimes in profound ways. We have been there with them on their journeys, sharing their joy, grief, hope, despair, laughter, anger, certainty, and confusion. Whatever the work setting, genetic counselors are nominally there to help patients; but patients have always guided us more than we have guided them, something we should never lose sight of. They have taught us much, and have so much more to teach us, as long as we are willing to listen. And that is what genetic counseling is all about.

APPENDIX 1

Practice-Based Competencies for Genetic Counselors, from the website of the Accreditation Council for Genetic Counseling, downloaded 9/28/2023 (https://www.gceducation.org/forms-resources/). Refer to the website for examples and further explication of these competencies.

Practice-Based Competencies for Genetic Counselors

Embedded within the seven competencies are 27 sub-competencies that support the attainment of the practice-based competencies. These competencies, along with the Accreditation Council for Genetic Counselors' Standards of Accreditation, provide guidance for the training of genetic counselors and for evaluating train-ees' knowledge and skills. The didactic and experiential components of a genetic counseling training curriculum must support the development of proficiency in the following competencies: 1) Genetics and Genomics Expertise, 2) Risk Assessment, 3) Counseling, 4) Communication, 5) Research, 6) Healthcare Systems, and 7) Professional Identity. These competencies and skills, as defined by the sub-competencies, describe the minimal skill set of a genetic counselor which should be applicable across practice settings.

Genetics and Genomics Expertise

1. Apply knowledge of genetics and genomics principles, genetic conditions, and testing technologies to the practice of genetic counseling.
   1a. Demonstrate knowledge of genetics and genomics principles and concepts.
   1b. Apply knowledge of genetic conditions to the delivery of genetics services.
   1c. Demonstrate knowledge of genetic testing methodologies and variant interpretation.

Risk Assessment

2. Evaluate personalized genetic risk.
   2a. Analyze family history to estimate genetic risk.

2b. Calculate risk using probability methods and risk models.

2c. Integrate clinical and laboratory data into risk assessment.

2d. Order genetic tests guided by client-centered risk assessment.

Counseling

3. Promote integration of psychosocial needs and client-centered decision-making into genetic counseling interactions.

3a. Use applicable counseling skills and theories.

3b. Establish a working alliance with client.

3c. Promote psychosocial adaptation.

3d. Facilitate client's decision-making process.

Communication

4. Communicate genetics and genomics information to clients, colleagues, and other community partners.

4a. Tailor communication to specific individuals and audiences.

4b. Use a variety of approaches to communicate genetics and genomic information.

4c. Convey probabilities based on client's risk perception and numeracy.

Research

5. Synthesize the evidence base relevant to genetic counseling.

5a. Critically interpret data and literature.

5b. Apply data and literature considering its strengths, weaknesses, and limitations.

5c. Demonstrate knowledge of how genetic counselors engage and contribute to the research process.

Healthcare Systems

6. Demonstrate how genetic counselors fit within the larger healthcare system.

6a. Demonstrate how disparities, inequities, and systemic bias affect access to healthcare for diverse populations.

6b. Describe the financial considerations in the delivery of genetic services.

6c. Advocate for continuity of care.

6d. Collaborate with members of the Care Team, clients, and other Community Partners.

Professional Identity

7. Embody the values of the genetic counseling profession.

   7a. Adhere to the genetic counselor scope of practice.

   7b. Follow applicable professional ethical codes.

   7c. Exhibit behaviors that promote an inclusive, just, equitable, and safe environment for all individuals and communities.

   7d. Engage in self-reflective practice to promote ongoing growth and development.

APPENDIX 2

Genetic Counselors' Scope of Practice (NSGC 2007)

"This "Genetic Counselors' Scope of Practice" statement outlines the responsibilities of individuals engaged in the practice of genetic counseling. Genetic counselors are health professionals with specialized education, training and experience in medical genetics and counseling who help people understand and adapt to the implications of genetic contributions to disease. Genetic counselors interact with clients and other healthcare professionals in a variety of clinical and non-clinical settings, including, but not limited to, university-based medical centers, private hospitals, private practice, and industry settings. The instruction in clinical genetics, counseling, and communication skills required to carry out the professional responsibilities described in this statement is provided in graduate training programs accredited by the Accreditation Council of Genetic Counseling (ACGC), as well as through professional experience and continuing education courses.

The responsibilities of a genetic counselor are threefold: (i) to provide expertise in clinical genetics; (ii) to counsel and communicate with patients on matters of clinical genetics; and (iii) to provide genetic counseling services in accordance with professional ethics and values. Specifically:

Section I: Clinical Genetics

1. Explain the nature of genetics evaluation to clients. Obtain and review medical and family histories, based on the referral indication, and document the family history using standard pedigree nomenclature.

2. Identify additional client and family medical information relevant to risk assessment and consideration of differential diagnoses, and assist in obtaining such information.

3. Research and summarize pertinent data from the published literature, databases, and other professional resources, as necessary for each client.

4. Synthesize client and family medical information and data obtained from additional research as the basis for risk assessment, differential diagnosis,

genetic testing options, reproductive options, follow-up recommendations, and case management.

5. Assess the risk of occurrence or recurrence of a genetic condition or birth defect, using a variety of techniques, including knowledge of inheritance patterns, epidemiologic data, quantitative genetics principles, statistical models, and evaluation of clinical information, as applicable.

6. Explain to clients, verbally and/or in writing, medical information regarding the diagnosis or potential occurrence of a genetic condition or birth defect, including etiology, natural history, inheritance, disease management and potential treatment options.

7. Discuss available options and delineate the risks, benefits and limitations of appropriate tests and clinical assessments. Order tests and perform clinical assessments in accordance with local, state and federal regulations.

8. Document case information clearly and concisely in the medical record and in correspondence to referring physicians, and discuss case information with other members of the healthcare team, as necessary.

9. Assist clients in evaluating the risks, benefits and limitations of participation in research, and facilitate the informed consent process.

10. Identify and access local, regional, and national resources such as support groups and ancillary services; discuss the availability of such resources with clients; and provide referrals, as necessary.

11. Plan, organize and conduct public and professional education programs on medical genetics, patient care and genetic counseling issues.

Section II: Counseling and Communication

1. Develop a genetic counseling agenda with the client or clients that includes identification and negotiation of client/counselor priorities and expectations.

2. Identify individual client and family experiences, behaviors, emotions, perceptions, values, and cultural and religious beliefs in order to facilitate individualized decision making and coping.

3. Assess client understanding and response to medical information and its implications, and educate client appropriately.

4. Utilize appropriate interviewing techniques and empathic listening to establish rapport, identify major concerns and engage clients in an exploration of their responses to the implications of the findings, genetic risks, and available options/interventions.

5. Identify the client's psychological needs, stressors and sources of emotional and psychological support in order to determine appropriate interventions and/or referrals.

6. Promote client-specific decision making in an unbiased non-coercive manner that respects the client's culture, language, traditions, lifestyle, religious beliefs and values.
7. Use knowledge of psychological structure to apply client-centered techniques and family systems theory to facilitate adjustment to the occurrence or risk of occurrence of a congenital or genetic disorder.

Section III: Professional Ethics and Values

1. Recognize and respond to ethical and moral dilemmas arising in practice, identify factors that promote or hinder client autonomy, and understand issues surrounding privacy, informed consent, confidentiality, real or potential discrimination and potential conflicts of interest.
2. Advocate for clients, which includes understanding client needs and perceptions, representing their interests in accessing services, and eliciting responses from the medical and social service systems as well as the community at large.
3. Recognize personal limitations in knowledge and/or capabilities and seek consultation or appropriately refer clients to other providers.
4. Maintain professional growth, which includes acquiring relevant information required for a given situation, keeping abreast of current standards of practice as well as societal developments, and seeking out or establishing mechanisms for peer support.
5. Respect a client's right to confidentiality, being mindful of local, state and federal regulations governing release of personal health information.

This Scope of Practice statement was approved in June 2007 by the National Society of Genetic Counselors (NSGC) - the leading voice, advocate and authority for the genetic counseling profession. It is not intended to replace the judgment of an individual genetic counselor with respect to particular clients or special clinical situations and cannot be considered inclusive of all practices or exclusive of other practices reasonably directed at obtaining the same results. In addition, the practice of genetic counseling is subject to regulation by federal, state and local governments. In a subject jurisdiction, any such regulations will take precedence over this statement. NSGC expressly disclaims any warranties or guarantees, express or implied, and shall not be liable for damages of any kind, in connection with the information set forth in this Scope of Practice statement or for reliance on its contents.

Genetic counseling is a dynamic profession, which undergoes rapid change with the discovery of new genetic information and the development of new genetic tests and treatment options. Thus, NSGC will periodically review and, where appropriate, revise this statement as necessary for consistency with current practice information."

REFERENCES

Abacan M, Alsubaie L, Barlow-Stewart K, et al. (2019) The global state of the genetic counseling profession. *Eur J Hum Genet* 27:183–197.

Alvarado-Wing TE, Marshall J, Best A, et al. (2021) Exploring racial and ethnic minority individuals' journey to becoming genetic counselors: mapping paths to diversifying the genetic counseling profession. *J Genet Couns* 30:1522–1534.

Amendola LM, Golden-Grant K & Scollon S. (2021) Scaling genetic counseling in the genomics era. *Annu Rev Genomics Hum Genet* 22:339–355.

ASHG (1975) Genetic counseling. *Am J Hum Genet* 27:240–242.

Bashford A & Levine P. (2010) Introduction: Eugenics and The Modern World. *The Oxford Handbook of The History of Eugenics*, Oxford: Oxford University Press.

Bellaiche MMJ, Fan W, Walbert HJ, et al. (2021) Disparity in access to oncology precision care: a geospatial analysis of driving distances to genetic counselors in the U.S. *Front Oncol* 11:689927.

Bennett RL, French KS, Resta RG, & Austin J. (2022) Practice resource-focused revision: Standardized pedigree nomenclature update centered on sex and gender inclusivity: A practice resource of the National Society of Genetic Counselors. *J Genet Couns* 10.1002/jgc4.1621, 10.1002/jgc4.1621.

Brown-Johnson CG, Safaeinili N, Baratta J, et al. (2021) Implementation outcomes of humanwide: integrated precision health in team-based family practice primary care. *BMC Fam Pract* 22:28.

Carmichael N, Redlinger-Grosse K, & Birnbaum S. (2021) Examining clinical training through a bicultural lens: experiences of genetic counseling students who identify with a racial or ethnic minority group. *J Genet Couns* 31(2):411–423.

Childs B, Zinkham W, Browne EA, et al. (1958) A genetic study of a defect in glutathione metabolism of the erythrocyte. *Bull Johns Hopkins Hosp* 102:21–37.

Cho MT & Guy C. (2020) Evolving roles of genetic counselors in the clinical laboratory. *Cold Spring Harb Perspect Med* 10(10):a036574.

De Graaf G, Buckley F, Dever J, & Skotko BG. (2017) Estimation of live birth and population prevalence of Down syndrome in nine U.S. states. *Am J Med Genet A* 173:2710–2719.

Dewey C, McCarthy Veach P, Leroy B, & Redlinger-Grosse K. (2021). Experiences of United States genetic counseling supervisors regarding race/ethnicity in supervision: a qualitative investigation. *J Genet Couns* 31(2):510–522.

Edwards JH, Harnden DF, Cameron AH, et al. (1960) A new trisomic syndrome. *Lancet* 1:787–790.

Elliott AM. (2020) Genetic counseling and genome sequencing in pediatric rare disease. *Cold Spring Harb Perspect Med* 10(3):a036632.

Epstein CJ. (1992) Organized medical genetics at a crossroad. *Am J Hum Genet* 51: 231–234.

Field T, Brewster SJ, Towne M, & Campion MW. (2016) Emerging genetic counselor roles within the biotechnology and pharmaceutical industries: as industry interest grows in rare genetic disorders, how are genetic counselors joining the discussion? *J Genet Couns* 25:708–719.

Fine BA, Baker DL, Fiddler MB, & Consortium ACD. (1996) Practice-based competencies for accreditation of and training in graduate programs in genetic counseling. *J Genet Couns* 5:113–121, 10.1007/BF01408656.

Ford CE, Jones KW, Polani PE, et al. (1959) A sex-chromosome anomaly in a case of gonadal dysgenesis. *Lancet* 1:711–713,

Galton F. (1883) *Inquiries into Human Faculty and its Development*, London: Macmillan.

Hallford HG, Coffman MA, Obregon-Tito AJ, et al (2020) Access barriers to genetic services for Spanish-speaking families in states with rapidly growing migrant populations. *J Genet Couns* 29:365–380.

Heimler A. (1997) An oral history of the National Society of Genetic Counselors. *J Genet Couns* 6:315–336.

Hsia DY, Huang I. & Driscoll SG. (1958) The heterozygous carrier in galactosemia. *Nature* 182:1389–1390.

Jacobs PA & Strong J. (1959) A case of human intersexuality having a possible XXY sex-determining mechanism. *Nature* 183:302–303.

Jamal L, Schupmann W, & Berkman BE. (2020) An ethical framework for genetic counseling in the genomic era. *J Genet Couns* 29:718–727.

Kelly MA, Leader JB, Wain KE, et al. (2021) Leveraging population-based exome screening to impact clinical care: the evolution of variant assessment in the Geisinger MyCode research project. *Am J Med Genet C Semin Med Genet* 187:83–94.

Kessler S. (1992) Psychological aspects of genetic counseling: VII. Thoughts on directiveness. *J Genet Couns* 1:9–17.

Kessler S. (1997) Psychological aspects of genetic counselling: IX. Teaching and Counseling. *J Genet Couns* 6:287–295.

Kling D, Phillips C, Kennett D, & Tillmar A. (2021) Investigative genetic genealogy: current methods, knowledge and practice. *Forensic Sci Int Genet* 52:102474.

Kühl S. (1994) *The Nazi Connection: Eugenics, American Racism, and German National Socialism*, New York: Oxford University Press.

Kunkel HG, Cappellini R, Müller-Eberhard U, & Wolf J. (1957) Observations on the minor basic hemoglobin component in the blood of normal individuals and patients with thalassemia. *J Clin Invest* 36(11):1615–1625

Lejeune J, Gautier M, & Turpin R. (1959) Etude des chromosomes somatiques de neuf enfants mongolien. *Compt Rend* 248:1721–1722.

Lemke AA, Amendola LM, Thompson J, et al (2021). Patient-reported outcomes and experiences with population genetic testing offered through a primary care network. *Genet Test Mol Biomarkers* 25:152–160.

Majumder M, Guerrini C, & McGuire A. (2021) Direct-to-consumer genetic testing: value and risk. *Annu Rev Med* 72:151–166.

Mellis R, Oprych K, Scotchman E, et al (2022) Diagnostic yield of exome sequencing for prenatal diagnosis of fetal structural anomalies: a systematic review and meta-analysis. *Prenat Diagn* https://doi.org/10.1002/pd.6115

Nadler HL. (1968) Antenatal detection of hereditary disorders. *Pediatrics* 42:912–918.

Neel JV. (1994) *Physician to the Gene Pool: Genetic Lessons and Other Stories*, New York, NY: Wiley.

Noyes JH & Noyes TR. (1872) *Essay on Scientific Propagation, with an Appendix Containing the Health Report of the Oneida Community*, Oneida, NY: The Oneida Community.

NSGC. (2024) *2024 Professional Status Survey* [Online]. Available: https://www.nsgc. org/Policy-Research-and-Publications/Professional-Status-Survey Accessed June 14, 2024.

Paul D. (1984) Eugenics and the left. *J Hist Ideas* 45: 567–590, 10.2307/2709374.

Paul D. (1997) From eugenics to medical genetics. *J Policy Hist* 9: 96–116.

Patau K, Smith DW, Therman E, et al. (1960) Multiple congenital anomaly caused by an extra autosome. *Lancet* 1:790–793.

Pollock B, Wetherill L, Delk P, et al. (2022) Diversity training experiences and factors associated with implicit racial bias among recent genetic counselor graduates of accredited programs in the United States and Canada. *J Genet Couns* 31(3):792–802.

Ponathil A, Ozkan F, Welch B, et al. (2020) Family health history collected by virtual conversational agents: an empirical study to investigate the efficacy of this approach. *J Genet Couns* 29:1081–1092.

Porter TM. (2018) *Genetics in the Madhouse - The Unknown History of Human Heredity*, Princeton, NJ: Princeton University Press.

Rabideau MM, Wong K, Gordon ES, & Ryan L. (2016) Genetic counselors in startup companies: redefining the genetic counselor role. *J Genet Couns* 25: 649–57.

Ravitsky V, Roy MC, Haidar H, et al. (2021) The emergence and global spread of noninvasive prenatal testing. *Annu Rev Genomics Hum Genet* 22:309–338.

Reed SC. (1955) *Counseling in Medical Genetics*, Philadelphia, PA: W.B. Saunders.

Resta RG. (1997a) Eugenics and nondirectiveness in genetic counseling. *J Genet Couns* 6:255–258.

Resta RG. (1997b) The historical perspective: Sheldon Reed and 50 years of genetic counseling. *J Genet Couns* 6:375–377.

Resta RG. (2019) What have we been trying to do and have we been any good at it? A history of measuring the success of genetic counseling. *Eur J Med Genet* 62:300–307.

Resta RG. (2020) Selective amnesia, Part 2: Guardians of the gene pool. The DNA Exchange. Available from: https://thednaexchange.com/2020/06/28/selective-amnesia-part-2-guardians-of-the-gene-pool/ Accessed January 18, 2022.

Resta R. (2021) Complicated shadows: the limits of autonomy in genetic counseling practice. In: Bonnie S LeRoy, Patricia M Veach, & Nancy P Callanan (Eds) *Genetic Counseling Practice: Advanced Concepts and Skills* Second edition, Hoboken, NJ: Wiley Blackwell.

Resta R, Biesecker BB, Bennett RL, et al. (2006) A new definition of genetic counseling: National Society of Genetic Counselors' Task Force report. *J Genet Couns* 15(2):77–83.

Rouse SL, Florentine MM, Taketa E, & Chan DK. (2021) Racial and ethnic disparities in genetic testing for hearing loss: a systematic review and synthesis. *Hum Genet* 141(3–4):485–494

Schmidlen T, Sturm AC, Hovick S, et al. (2018). operationalizing the reciprocal engagement model of genetic counseling practice: a framework for the scalable delivery of genomic counseling and testing. *J Genet Couns* 27:1111–1129.

Senter L, Austin JC, Carey M, et al. (2020) Advancing the genetic counseling profession through research: identification of priorities by the National Society of Genetic Counselors research task force. *J Genet Couns* 29:884–887.

Serr DM, Sachs L, & Danon M. (1955) Diagnosis of sex before birth using cells from the amniotic fluid. *Bull Res Counc Isr* 5B(2):137–8.

Smith DW, Patau K, Therman E, & Inhorn SL. (1960) A new autosomal trisomy syndrome: multiple congenital anomalies caused by an extra chromosome. *J Pediatr* 57:338–345.

Steele MW & Breg WRJ. (1966) Chromosome analysis of human amniotic fluid cells. *Lancet* 1(7434):383–385

Stern A. (2012) *Telling Genes - The Story of Genetic Counseling in America*, Baltimore, MD: Johns Hopkins University Press.

Tips RL & Lynch HT. (1963) The impact of genetic counseling upon the family milieu. *JAMA* 184:183–186.

Tjio JH & Levan A. (1956) The chromosome number in man. *Hereditas* 42:1–6.

Trepanier A & Allain DC. (2020) Adapting genetic counseling practice to different models of service delivery. In: Bonnie S LeRoy, Patricia M Veach & Nancy P Callanan (Eds) *Genetic Counseling Practice: Advanced Concepts and Skills* 2nd edition, Hoboken, NJ: Wiley Blackwell. https://doi.org/10.1002/9781119529873.ch14

Uebergang E, Best S, De Silva MG, & Finlay K. (2021) Understanding genomic health information: how to meet the needs of the culturally and linguistically diverse community—a mixed methods study. *J Community Genet* 12(4):549–557.

Veach PM, Bartels DM, & Leroy BS. (2007) Coming full circle: a reciprocal-engagement model of genetic counseling practice. *J Genet Couns* 16:713–728.

Volk B, SM, A. & SM, S. (1964) Fructose -1- phosphate aldolase deficiency in Tay-Sachs disease. *American Journal of Medicine* 36:481.

Wailoo K. (2001) *Dying in the City of the Blues: Sickle Cell Anemia and the Politics of Race and Health*, Chapel Hill, NC: University of North Carolina Press.

Wang C, Paasche-Orlow MK, Bowen DJ, et al. (2021) Utility of a virtual counselor (VICKY) to collect family health histories among vulnerable patient populations: A randomized controlled trial. *Patient Educ Couns* 104:979–988.

Weatherall DJ. (1963) Abnormal haemoglobins in the neonatal period and their relationship to thalassemia. *Br J Haematol* 9:625–677.

Welch BM, Wiley K, Pflieger L, et al. (2018) Review and comparison of electronic patient-facing family health history tools. *J Genet Couns* 27:381–391.

Wilson RA. (2021) Dehumanization, disability, and eugenics. In: M Kronfeldner (ed) *The Routledge Handbook of Dehumanization*, Abingdon: Taylor & Francis Group.

Wray NR, Lin T, Austin J, et al. (2021) From basic science to clinical application of polygenic risk scores: a primer. *JAMA Psychiatry* 78:101–109.

Yip CH, Evans DG, Agarwal G, et al. (2019) Global disparities in breast cancer genetics testing, counselling and management. *World J Surg* 43:1264–1270.

Young JL, Mak J, Stanley T, et al. (2021) Genetic counseling and testing for Asian Americans: a systematic review. *Genet Med* 23:1424–1437.

2

Building a Working Alliance Through Culturally Conscious Interviewing

Gayun Chan-Smutko

INTRODUCTION

This chapter is a starting point for new learners to develop clinical interviewing skills. Clinical interviewing can be thought of as a dynamic process of inquiry and exchange of information. The genetic counselor uses clinical interviewing skills to gain necessary information to support their genetic risk assessment and provide appropriate recommendations and information to the patient. Importantly, the goal of clinical interviewing, as the origin of the word interview ("to see each other") suggests, allows providers and patients to gain an understanding of each other. This metaphor of approaching a relationship with the goal of reaching understanding is a powerful concept upon which to build a working alliance with the patient. The skills involved in the clinical interviewing process are multifold; the new learner will develop and practice skills around different ways of *questioning* to gain practical and experiential information as well as a sense of the patient's thoughts and feelings behind the topic in question. If *questioning* forms the backbone for interviewing, skills such as conveying *attentiveness* and *genuineness* and

A Guide to Genetic Counseling, Third Edition. Edited by Vivian Y. Pan, Jane L. Schuette, Karen E. Wain, and Beverly M. Yashar.

engendering *trustworthiness* are essential components in the anatomy of clinical interviewing. *Cultural humility* and *reflexivity* innervate the backbone and the essential components of clinical interviewing and are core to the mindset of a culturally conscious practitioner.

A culturally conscious practitioner recognizes that interactions are inherently culture bound and the essentialness of bringing together cultural awareness, knowledge of systems of power and oppression, and a variety of clinical interviewing techniques for building a safe and affirming environment for patients and families. New learners and seasoned practitioners and instructors alike must ground their skills with historical and present-day understanding of interlocking forms of oppression including racism, ableism, homophobia, transphobia, and xenophobia which structure the health care and educational systems in which we operate and create health inequities within the communities we serve. The culturally conscious practitioner is self-aware of their own cultural self and cultivates a reflective practice to understand how their beliefs, values, and perspectives impact their counseling interactions. Reflexivity in thought adds an element of critical inquiry to reflective practice, where the genetic counselor examines their feelings, reactions, and motives behind their thoughts and actions. This chapter will inform new learners of ways they can integrate inclusive practices into their interviewing skills. Although the content is focused on the initial genetic counseling encounter, clinical interviewing techniques are pertinent in follow-up care, post-test genetic counseling, and research genetic counseling encounters.

BUILDING AND MAINTAINING A WORKING ALLIANCE: KEY ATTRIBUTES

The working alliance (also known as therapeutic alliance (Horvath and Greenberg, 1994) refers to the relationship between patient and genetic counselor. This alliance is collaborative, reflecting the mutualism between provider and patient when defining and reaching the patient's genetic concerns. The Reciprocal Engagement Model, or REM, is a model that reflects genetic counseling practice and a core tenet of REM is that the *relationship* is integral to genetic counseling which reflects the value of human connection, particularly in times of distress (Veach et al., 2007; Murray et al., 2022). "The relationship serves as the *conduit*, providing an alliance in which the patient feels supported, cared about, connected, and validated" (Veach et al., 2007).

Carl Rogers and colleagues are credited with describing key attributes of the counselor, including respect, genuineness, and empathy, that correlate with successful counseling sessions that focus the session on the relationship and ensure that the patient's needs are being met (Jon Weil, 2000). Key attributes and assets that are interwoven into a genetic counselor's toolkit which facilitate the working alliance include cultural humility, trustworthiness, attentiveness, respect, genuineness, and empathy.

Cultural humility

Cultural humility is a cornerstone for building a working alliance with patients. Cultural humility in clinical practice "incorporates a lifelong commitment to self-evaluation and critique, to redressing the power imbalances in the physician–patient dynamic, and to developing mutually beneficial and non-paternalistic partnerships with communities on behalf of individuals and defined populations" (Tervalon and Murray-García, 1998). An essential step towards developing humility is to define one's cultural self: the customs, beliefs, and values that you hold; your racial identity (Tatum, 1992) and other social dimensions of identity. Then notice ways in which your cultural self has been shaped by, or shaped in opposition to, dominant norms and values. Pay attention particularly to ways of knowing (e.g., the coded language of "professionalism" (Zayhowski and Sheridan, 2022)) and ways of doing (e.g., the valuing/devaluing of specific linguistic styles and accents over others) (Box 2-1). Another step is to develop a learning mindset that fosters self-acceptance (see **Growing your clinical interviewing process**), normalize informed risk-taking and experimentation, and commit to self-evaluation.

BOX 2-1. CULTURAL HUMILITY REFLECTION EXERCISE

Go deeper into the marginalizing and oppressive impact of dominant normative thinking by listing social identities such as age, size, disability, gender identity, race, sexual orientation, socioeconomic status, religion, marriage status, etc. that make you uncomfortable and why. Is it because you don't know enough? Or is what you think you know a broad enough picture or is it a stereotype? Do you feel satisfied with this discomfort, or can you connect it with a facet of dominant culture? What first person narratives can you seek out to educate yourself and demystify the unknown "other"? Students, instructors, and practitioners can extend their learning by sharing and discussing what they learned about themselves from this activity, particularly if you are able to establish some ground rules to discuss these topics courageously and allow one another to challenge respectfully in order to keep yourself accountable. Perhaps you are not personally to blame for receiving misinformation (from the dominant culture) about another group of people different from you; however, once you learn that you are wrong, it is your job to get it right. Accountability partnership among peers helps to nudge you along the cultural humility journey, continuing a feedback loop of trust. In a racially and ethnically mixed and diverse setting, it's important that the instructors take on the responsibility to ensure that Black, Indigenous, and People of Color (BIPOC) and students with marginalized identities do not shoulder the burden of educating others (tokenization).

Understanding the multidimensional ways *power* exists within the patient/ genetic counselor relationship is essential when understanding and practicing cultural humility. Incorporating education, self-reflection, and dialogue around power, privilege, positionality, and intersectionality form an essential foundation to health professions education (Martinez and Truong, 2020, 2021; Cahn et al., 2022). Some examples of power analyses are included below; however, you are likely able to add many more items to the list and add depth to these items as you continue your learning journey.

- An inherent hierarchy or imbalance of medical genetics knowledge and genetic testing knowhow exists, with the genetic counselor generally being most knowledgeable in these areas.
- As a health care professional, a genetic counselor is part of the larger health care system within which their services exist, a system that has a track record of harming marginalized people (Washington, 2006).
- Patients hold power, strength, and agency, and have the most expertise on their lived experience, assets, culture, beliefs, and values. These have direct bearing on how they receive, understand, utilize, and cope with genetic risk information.
- Drawing from sociological concepts of power, we also recognize that each member of the dyad has identities that hold socially constructed dynamics of power and privilege as well as disadvantage and oppression (Jones, 2014; Woolsey and Narruhn, 2018).

Reflecting on various forms of power is a key steppingstone for genetic counseling students, practitioners, and instructors alike to recognize the dynamic ways in which power imbalances can impact the working alliance.

How, then, do you mitigate the potential effects of power imbalances? The mindset and practices of cultural humility and reflexivity provide limitless opportunities. How and when do you consider 'cultural' factors in the working relationship? The answer is: all the time, beginning with awareness of and defining and understanding your cultural self. "One must keep in mind that the perspective a health care professional brings to his or her work is neither neutral nor culture free" (Ota Wang, 2001). In her 2001 paper, Ota Wang discusses the consequences of limiting our cultural competence strategies to essentializing large heterogeneous groups of people into categories of characteristics (stereotypes) based on their individual/collectivist views, the role of family, systems of punishments/rewards, or other factors. This focus on generalizations about presumed cultural knowledge is an oppressive practice that centers dominant (white, cis-heteronormative, ableist) culture while holding other ways of knowing and living as cultural "others" This type of *othering* is still present today over 20 years after Ota Wang's publication. By not recognizing that communication between two people is culture-bound we only come to know the other person through our own cultural lens. This form of othering leads us to unknowingly and persistently keep oppressed groups at the margins, because it centers the genetic counseling practitioner as representative of a cultural backdrop or normative standard against which all other cultures are compared. A singular focus on acquiring cultural knowledge serves to systematically homogenize groups that are in fact heterogenous. The consequence of normativity is the inability to recognize the relevance of social identities and cultural lenses of both patient and provider in genetic counseling encounters, holding cultural "others" at the margins. Thus, cultural humility requires the intentional centering of marginalized patients and their voices on the part of the genetic counselor. This idea of centering marginalized patients' voices and lived experiences is to be distinguished from empowerment, which suggests that patients inherently lack power as opposed to recognizing social constructs such as race and the reality of racism which disempowers and disadvantages them. We also need to distinguish this from a patient-centered approach—not to the exclusion of it, but complementary to it. The intentional centering of marginalized patients is identity-conscious, a social-political awareness of the need to redress power imbalances caused by the systematic valuing and devaluing of individuals based on race, disability, gender, and other identity markers and their voices on the part of the genetic counselor.

Trustworthiness

Another cornerstone of the working relationship is *trustworthiness*. A genetic counselor who is practicing humility does not assume that their "do good" focus is enough to engender a patient's trust. Limited self-awareness of one's privilege without understanding systemic inequities leads to questions such as: "How do we get marginalized populations to trust us?" and "Will a patient who needs a medical interpreter trust me or the interpreter?" The first example is a deficit-oriented perspective common in the health professions which places the burden of trust (i.e., deficit orientation)[1] on patients and communities instead of addressing the *systems* that disempower them and are therefore unworthy of trust (i.e., systemic racism (Williams et al., 2019; Braveman et al., 2022). A starting point for addressing power imbalances and injustice is to ask, "What does trustworthiness mean? What actions and behaviors convey that I'm worthy of trust?" In the second example, the anxiety around building trust through

---

[1] Deficit orientation comes from the K-12 and higher education literature and sees people as problems. Community cultural wealth orientation which also comes from education and has been applied to STEM graduate education is an antidote to deficit thinking which pervades education and healthcare (Cuena, n.d.; Yosso, 2005; Patton Davis and Museus, 2019; Acevedo and Solorzano, 2021).

medical interpretation brings into question the genetic counselor or trainee's faith in their rapport-building skills. One way to overcome distrust and discomfort working with interpreters is to recognize where that fear is coming from and addressing it; for example, convening a brief huddle with a medical interpreter prior to initiating the encounter in order to foster collaboration with the interpreter as a partner is a great way to address this discomfort. And digging further, asking "What are the historical and present-day underpinnings of social injustice and health care inaccessibility that impact the people served at my institution? What questions do we need to ask, then listen, reflect, and act with equity as a guiding principle with multiple stakeholders from the communities we serve making decisions with us?" (See also Chapters 9 and 10.) At the time of this writing, the United States was amid two pandemics: the COVID-19 pandemic and the ongoing pandemic of racism which exposed the fractured public trust in health care, the stark and persistent health inequities by race, and the imperative to build trust. Trustworthiness, then, is founded on the genetic counselor's prioritization of the therapeutic relationship and ability to center the patient's interests and demonstrate honesty.

As part of the trusting relationship that you are building, your patient may disclose very personal information about past or recent loss, grief, trauma, or harm. Strategies to discuss these factors and offer support are further explored in Chapters 4 and 5 and are inherently inclusive as they increase a patient's sense of safety in the session, sense of trust, and, depending on the subject, can facilitate a sense of self-efficacy around decision-making and autonomy.

Respect

Respect is predicated on appreciating the humanity in every individual and upholding the dignity that each person deserves universally, without bias or preference. It forms a foundation for a relationship essential for establishing mutual goals. Agency and autonomy are culture-bound concepts that patients have that can range from exercising personal choice to soliciting input and opinions from partner and family members (Resta, 2020). The genetic counselor is responsible for seeking to understand the ways in which a patient wishes to exercise their agency, through clinical interviewing skills such as questioning and attentive listening. Foundational clinical interviewing skills including trustworthiness and cultural humility are essential for respecting patient values and agency. Further reading on the elements of informed consent and facilitating decision-making are strongly encouraged.

Agreeing with the patient's opinions and behaviors cannot be mistaken for respect, nor is it a necessary condition for respect. In fact, being consciously aware of your disagreement can help you recognize when this disagreement becomes a deterrent to providing genuine care. It may be helpful to try the exercise in Box 2-2 and list patient behaviors or opinions that you anticipate may challenge your ability to maintain respect.

BOX 2-2. RAISING YOUR AWARENESS OF BIAS AND RESPECT[2]

1. Make a list of patient behaviors and/or opinions that you anticipate may challenge your ability to maintain respect for the individual.

   a. Are there dominant norms that could be at play? The goal is to challenge yourself to examine biases that can be important to you in your clinical practice.

   b. Are there any past experiences or encounters that you have had that are tied to one or more of the items on your list?

   Example:

   Your adult patient states "I can't make a decision until I speak with my [spouse or parent]."

   Dominant norms and biases: What are your personal views on decision-making and autonomy, particularly in medical situations? Below are example questions for raising your awareness of *potential* oppressive attitudes and thinking:

   • "it's my patient's body"—could you have a set interpretation of autonomy? What can you do to expand your perspective?

   • "maybe it's cultural"—what generalizations could be leading to this bias?

   • "my patient should speak up"—is this based on a singular interpretation of one "right" way to make decisions?

   • "I hope they come to the obvious decision"—what biases might come into play, particularly when your assessment is that the situation is high risk?

2. Share this list with your classmates (perhaps in a small group).

3. Discuss your lists and probe one another on the sources or reasons for why the behaviors or opinions may be challenging. The goal isn't to agree with one another, but to gain greater understanding through dialogue and feedback.

4. Brainstorm ways to work *around* or *through* some of these challenges hypothetically. Pick a few to role play. The goal is to prepare and

---

[2] Note to instructor: If you ask the class to embark on steps 2, 3, and 4, ensure that the class has co-created class ground rules for effective dialogue, and mechanisms for the class to check in with you. Consider making your own list and share one item, to model vulnerability and the purpose of the exercise. The exercise can be adapted as a journal prompt though be thoughtful about grading if you make it into an assignment. Arao and Clemans provide guidance around framing brave spaces for dialogue around social identities and social justice in the classroom (Arao and Clemans, 2013). Listen for dominant narratives in the classroom and develop skills for responding; not all perspectives warrant equal weight nor should have equal footing, as whiteness is normalized and as such can emerge to regain center stage in discussions, even in spaces intended to decenter whiteness (Whiteness, n.d.).

> desensitize a potentially uncomfortable moment through practice by building language and comfort in potentially challenging situations.
>
> 5. Self-reflection: Take a moment to write/reflect on whether you can still provide care and meet a patient's informational goals, even if you don't like their particular behavior or if you disagree with their opinion or decision.

Attentiveness

Attentiveness refers to the quality of actively paying attention to the needs of the patient(s). Genetic counselors demonstrate attentiveness through verbal and nonverbal cues, which are discussed further in the section on *Attending behaviors*. Attentive listening involves tuning in to the speaker's words, tone, and nonverbal cues, noting potential patterns in their statements (e.g., struggle to accept the reality of a diagnosis) and deeper meaning behind emotions (e.g., grief or shame). The goal of attentiveness is to encourage patients to occupy the emotional space, to the extent that they wish to, and, as a result, can be a validating experience for them. It involves your energy and motivation to follow patients, rather than lead, offering up the space within the session to your patients, to the extent that they wish to share and occupy. Attentiveness shows your patients that they are in an authentic two-way relationship, that you are trying to understand their experiences, and that they are worthy of your care and attention.

Genuineness

Another key attribute of good counseling is *genuineness*. As it sounds, this means being yourself within your professional role. A genetic counselor needs to be honest about their role and the limits of their knowledge. For example, a student genetic counselor would introduce themself as a student and enlist the help of their supervisor as needed during a session. Another aspect of genuineness is the counselor's awareness and appreciation of their own feelings and attitudes during the counseling session. These feelings are usually not verbally conveyed to the patient but are used by the counselor to increase their understanding of the situation and increase empathy toward the patient. Allowing yourself to understand and feel the emotions associated with the patient's story enables you to empathically listen with a sense of appreciation for their experience. Thus, some counseling theorists think of genuineness and empathy as forming a feedback loop. Genuineness can be viewed as a way of being that underlies providing true empathy.

The match between the counselor's inner process and the response to it is called *congruence*. For example, if there is a difference between what is said and what is expressed nonverbally there is a lack of congruence. It may not be possible to understand the feelings of a patient if you cannot identify and understand your own inner responses (Kolden et al., 2018). Therefore, counselors need humility to be genuine. It might be more effective to tell a patient that you do not understand but that you would like to do so rather than to disingenuously state, "I understand" when your patient tells you about a difficult experience or something outside of your experience (Kolden et al., 2018).

Counselors draw on professional experience and personal experience to understand the circumstances of their patients. However, there are times when personal experience can interfere with genuineness and/or empathy (see Chapter 5). Generally, countertransference refers to your inner experience when listening to your patient and can distract your attention away from the patient. It is a normal and natural part of human interaction (see Chapter 4). Noticing that countertransference is occurring helps you interrupt the thoughts and set them and your feelings aside so that you can return your attention to the patient. Returning to these thoughts and feelings later is equally important as you may gain new insights into your experiences through self-reflection (Hyatt, 2012; Redlinger-Grosse, 2020) and the lenses in which you see the world. It is valuable to reflect on how your patient's experiences are the same as and different from your own. Personal reflection is one of the ongoing tasks of a counselor (Anonymous, 2008; Matloff, 2006; Bellcross, 2012; Vanneste, 2012). A counselor may also find deeper meaning behind feelings that arise during a session, particularly unexpected feelings that stay with them for longer than usual, by working with a social worker or psychologist (Hyatt, 2012).

Genuineness cannot be imitated. You will find that your genuine voice and sense of self will increase as you gain experience and confidence. It is easier to sound confident or reassuring when you are confident and reassured from having been down a similar path many times. Adopting the words or behaviors of a supervising genetic counselor can be a starting point but it will not be sufficient for growth. You must learn to find your own voice through observation of various styles, through self-assessment, feedback, and self-reflection.

Empathy

Empathy is the ability to accurately understand the patient's experience as if it were your own and to communicate this understanding to the patient. "Empathy requires a constant shifting between my experiencing 'as you' what you feel and my being able to think 'as me' about your experience" (Murphy and Dillon, 2007, p. 130).

Empathy is a feedback loop. The counselor's attempts to demonstrate understanding will increase or decrease the empathic connection with the patient. The patient's response to the counselor will indicate whether the counselor is on-target and should do more of the same or is off-target and should change direction. One of the simplest demonstrations of understanding is a technique called reflection.

Using reflection, the counselor restates what the patient has said. The trick of doing this well is to express the patient's sentiments without sounding like a parrot. As you gain counseling skills, the reflections often go to a deeper level, expressing unstated sentiments that you have "heard."

If you appropriately and accurately capture the patient's view, the patient will feel better understood. This has the dual effect of increasing the patient's self-esteem and encouraging the patient to say more about the topic. It also makes the patient more receptive to further interaction with the counselor. If you only approximately capture the patient's thoughts and feelings but do so in a genuine and respectful way, the patient will probably correct you and continue. You can even add, "I'm hearing this … can you tell me if I am misunderstanding you?" Missing the mark altogether or failing to respond could suggest to the patient that their comment was not relevant to genetic counseling. Because empathy is so central to the ethos of genetic counseling, the topic is explored in greater detail in Chapter 4.

Summary

Genetic counselors have the power to practice cultural responsiveness and build a working alliance by extending their genuineness, empathy, and attentiveness in relevant and impactful ways beyond the normative practices in which they may feel most familiar. The knowledge differential will favor the genetic counselor when it comes to clinical genetics; however, the patient is best served when you can build a relationship that is mutually respectful and centers the patient's needs (autonomy). We need not be afraid to notice and name the impact of discrimination on health and wellbeing. It is within our scope and abilities to create a psychologically safe space to explore how social and personal identities and lived experiences impact the patient's ability to cope with genetic information and health information. The next section continues the discussion of a working alliance by incorporating an inclusive approach to clinical interviewing.

CREATING A WELCOMING AND AFFIRMING ENVIRONMENT

Generally speaking, the *clinical setting is* the environment in which a patient receives medical advice, treatment, and other health care services. Genetic counseling services are provided through a variety of settings: primary care offices, hospitals, outpatient clinics, private practice, or through a private company. There are multiple modalities such as phone, video conferencing, in-person, or even intake through a website or app, and often a clinical service provides more than one service delivery option. The type of encounter can be pre-test, post-test, results disclosure, or other types of continuing care. In any modality and encounter type, taking a few moments to create a sense of welcome and convey interest in the wellbeing of the patient and support members in attendance helps you begin to foster trust. This section will provide foundational reasoning and practical guidance on inclusive approaches to initiating your session and on facilitating a welcoming and affirming environment.

Inclusive approaches to initiating a clinical interview

Inherent power dynamics exist within the provider/patient relationship due to several factors, including difference in knowledge about genetics, inheritance, testing options, etc. The patient is coming to you for your expertise. Equally important in this knowledge equation is the patient's own lived experience and expertise in their cultural values and beliefs. An important starting point is to illuminate the ways in which systemic norms of *whiteness* differentially empowers and disempowers and permeates our health care system, from the ways in which we deliver care to the accessibility/inaccessibility of care. Whiteness refers to the systematic privileging of educational, health care, economic, language, and linguistic access and power to white people, particularly cis-gender heterosexual males who are nondisabled and speak English. Whiteness is not held within white people alone as these normative elements are internalized systematically at an early age in formal education settings and informally within social groups, cultures, and communities, for example. The inclusive-minded genetic counselor recognizes that the inherent power dynamics within the provider/patient relationship can be mitigated by being attuned to the patient's life experiences and the myriad of ways in which systemic causes of marginalization—such as racism, transphobia, homophobia, ableism, economic factors (employment, housing, food insecurity), caste, and other intersecting forms of oppression—shape their own experiences and that of their patients. The less-often recognized facilitators of inclusion are: 1) historical and present-day understanding of the impact of intersecting systems of oppression on health, mental health, and access to care; 2) the genetic counselors' awareness of the harms that can stem from white, patriarchal, cisgender, heterosexual, Christian normative thinking imbedded in the dominant US culture;[3] 3) the genetic counselors' self-awareness around ways in which they participate in normative whiteness (reflexivity); and 4) the motivation to mitigate these differences on the interpersonal level with patients. Part of continued inclusive practice is for the genetic counselor to operate within their sphere of influence to enact change that redresses systemic inequity.

An example of inclusive care is addressing cisnormativity by introducing yourself along with your pronouns. Gender identity is often assumed through a

---

[3] Patriarchy, racism, colorism, ableism, sexism, gender bias, and the present-day consequences of imperialism, colonialism, settler colonialism, and forced migration all work to produce and sustain societal inequities and injustice in different ways around the world. Even so, commonalities exist, and all forms of oppression are connected as they assign value and therefore unearned privileges to some while devaluing and oppressing others. In other words, privilege does not exist without oppression and devaluing is universally inhumane.

binary lens of masculinity and femininity in styles of dress, hair, and other outward forms of expression. As you introduce yourself to your patient, consider sharing your pronouns if you feel comfortable doing so. Commonly, you might ask the patient to confirm their name and date of birth to verify identity and maintain patient privacy. After verifying their identity, you can also invite them to share their pronouns and normalize this process by saying that you invite all of your patients to do this because you do not want to make assumptions about gender. Another time you can ask for pronouns can be during the intake, after you have had a chance to establish rapport and discuss goals of the session, particularly if your initial conversation may not be influenced by knowing a patient's gender identity. Remember that this is by invitation and that some patients may not feel safe disclosing their gender identity, which harkens back to the importance of understanding the historical and present-day relevance of transphobia and gender binary bias in medical genetics (Berro et al., 2020; von Vaupel-Klein and Walsh, 2021; Rolle et al., 2022).

If your clinical service obtains demographic information such as race, ethnicity, religious affiliation, access needs, sexual orientation, and gender identity, you have important information in the medical record to use in your session. A clinical service that cares to collect demographic information purposefully puts effort into providing the reason behind each question, and this intentionality can be reinforced by the registration staff and by the providers. It may also be appropriate to verify information that is in the medical record:

Example: (GC to a teen patient) "The medical record shows you go by X name. It's important that I get it right. Is this the name you want me to use?"

BOX 2-3. A NOTE ON DOCUMENTING GENDER IDENTITY

It is imperative that genetic counselors know current federal and state laws that restrict their patient's freedoms[4] and how their home institutions interpret the laws. Many of the transphobic laws are aimed specifically at children, rendering gender-affirming care illegal, inserting parental control over public-school curriculum on gender identity and sexual orientation, forced removal of trans youth from their caregivers, and banning transgender youth from participating in sports aligned with their gender identity. These bills intentionally misuse sex chromosomes as the determining factor for sex and gender, pathologizing transgender, gender diverse, and intersex individuals. Genetic testing lab practices vary widely, and proactive discussion with patients should be considered. For example, learning which labs report gender on test reports, which require information such as name consistent with the medical record, sex assigned at

---

[4] Trans Legislation Tracker: https://translegislation.com/.

birth and why (Gioacchino et al., 2022). Clearly conveying this information to patients is important for informed decision-making. Discussion of practices and policies on documenting gender identity and protecting patient welfare within your department and institution are warranted (Resta, 2022). Genetic testing labs, genetics professionals, and genetic professional societies need to take a vocal stand on weaponizing genetics against transgender, gender diverse, and intersex communities (Zayhowski et al., 2023).

Introducing the practice of asking a patient about their access needs creates a session that is inclusive at the outset. For patients with disabilities, mental health concerns, sensory processing differences, history of medical trauma, and neurodiverse patients, the question can build trust and improve the quality of service. When your patient's access needs are being met, their energy and focus can be more readily mobilized towards meeting their goals for the session. If you are sure that a specific type of accommodation cannot be met, explain why and consider exploring alternatives. After implementing an accommodation(s), it may also be appropriate to check in on how the accommodation is meeting the need.

Each individual genetic counselor will develop their own approaches to opening a session and showing interest in their patient's wellbeing. Some may adopt a conversational tone and ask how the patient is feeling that day and whether the patient had any trouble finding the clinic, or pleasantries about the weather and other relatively neutral topics. Spending a little time to get to know a patient is often an investment in the working relationship. You can attempt this with pediatric patients by preparing a few easy topics ahead of the visit. You can even have a stack of index cards with prepared questions that fit within your personal boundaries that the young patient can choose, and you and the patient can then take turns posing questions. (Child: "What's your favorite color?" Counselor: "Red! But guess what? I'm actually color blind so it takes a really bright red for me to know for sure that it's red.") This rapport building activity can be adapted in various ways to meet communication styles and developmental needs of your patients. No matter the developmental stage of your patient, it's more important to show up as a human who also provides professional expertise rather than being very focused on appearing as a professional.

Physical space

Picture a "typical" hospital or outpatient clinic waiting room: the physical space, color palette, type of chairs and arrangement of furniture. What atmosphere does a typical medical office or hospital waiting room create? What feelings come up for you when you think of being in the physical space that your mind conjured up? What cues clue you in on how much time has passed while waiting? Does it feel welcoming, like the physical space was designed with a range of access needs in mind?

Now imagine a clinical environment that deviates from this common theme; what kind of cues welcome you in and reflect back that you belong, and that this is an affirming environment? Would meaningful cues include LGBTQIA+ (lesbian, gay, bisexual, transgender, queer, questioning, intersex, asexual, plus diverse gender and sexual identities) flags? Would you want to bring support people to your appointment and would you be able to sit together? Would you have large width chairs for larger patients, short furniture, and sit-to-stand aids? Would there be different sensory areas? Make a list of meaningful environmental cues and designs and discuss them with classmates. For practicing genetic counselors, discuss and share lists with colleagues with a wide variety of social identities and from different disciplines and perspectives. As you discuss the challenge of reimagining an inclusive physical space as a team, identify the communities your clinic serves and invite them into the conversation and decision-making. What ways can the communities served by your clinic or institution and the neighborhood in which it is situated be reflected in the clinical spaces? Perhaps through murals and artwork that reflect and represent communities served by your clinic; bulletins on local community and social services could be a start. You may not be able to change everything and may have space limitations; however, the process of brainstorming and imagining inclusive and accessible designs has the potential to simultaneously bring out creativity, engagement, collaboration, and innovation, and the benefit of thinking without limits so that reimagining inclusion prepares all staff to address a variety of needs as the arise. This strategy can open doors for more inclusive initiatives beyond the physical space, such as culturally tailored patient education materials, community-based participatory research, and more.

Language access

Language access is a key pillar in providing equitable patient care. The genetic counselor is responsible for developing their personal comfort level and competence around clinical interviewing through interpretation. A few basic principles for genetic counselors and trainees new to communicating through interpretation include breaking up your sentences into shorter segments and pausing after each segment for interpretation before restarting; remembering to ask questions that help draw out the patient's understanding of the information you are providing; making eye contact with the patient (as opposed to primarily looking at the interpreter). When possible, pre-brief with the interpreter to provide them with an overview of what the session will cover and help them gain a sense of the types of information you will be requesting from the patient, as well as providing to the patient. A debrief can also be useful so that both the interpreter and genetic counselor give and receive feedback, improving their skill set for future genetic counseling encounters through interpretation. Recommendations for working with patients through medical interpretation can be found in Chapter 8 and for assessing patient understanding can be found in Chapter 5.

It is also important to note that working through sign language and language interpreters requires practice and self-reflection so that the student and genetic counselor can increase their comfort level, identify and reflect on personal biases and assumptions, and improve and expand their clinical interviewing skills overall. A patient's level of education and health literacy should not be assumed in any clinical encounters, particularly through interpreters. It is a common misconception of health care providers to conflate low health literacy in patients with low English proficiency or those who are deaf or hard of hearing.

Summary

You may be drawn to the genetic counseling profession because you enjoy genetics, collaborating in a multidisciplinary team, working with patients, or because of the opportunities to apply communication skills and genetics expertise in a variety of settings. Although these are all important reasons and may have some ring of familiarity or truth for you, these attributes are not automatic precursors to being inclusive and anti-oppressive. Genetic counselors need to educate themselves and be familiar with a range of ways in which individuals will identify themselves and seek first person narratives about lived experiences through various forms of media (podcasts, blogs, books, etc.). Get comfortable with the range and variety of ways of knowing and being, and learn to think intersectionally.[5] It is outside the scope of this chapter to provide instruction on: 1) concepts that critically evaluate power such as intersectionality and positionality; and 2) ways to critically engage in dialogue around ableism, sexism, anti-LGBTQIA+ bias, and racism in clinical practice. Therefore, genetic counseling students, practitioners, and instructors are encouraged to seek more education on ways that interlocking systems of oppression are embedded in our medical culture and professional legacy, in order to become more effective anti-oppressive practitioners (see **Resources** at the end of this chapter for a partial list of learning material connected to concepts in this chapter). When developing your advocacy skills it will be important for you to understand where, when, and for whom you choose to advocate, and for what belief(s). A genetic counselor who can recognize bias, ask a curious question in a nonjudgmental way, introduce affirming terminology, listen with compassion, or apologize when needed, is well on their way to being an inclusive and identity-conscious, and therefore effective, practitioner.

DEVELOPING MUTUAL GOALS OF A SESSION

One of the responsibilities of a genetic counselor when forming a working alliance is to learn and attempt to understand the patient's *expectations* and *goals*. Patients may have prior assumptions about medical and genetic information on

---

[5] A Look at Positionalities, Identity, Intersectionality and Privilege of Self. https://online.umich.edu/collections/racism-antiracism/short/personality-id-privilege/.

which their expectations about genetic testing are founded. Concerns about privacy and confidentiality, cost and insurance coverage, test turnaround time, and visit length are examples of patient questions that often fall within both domains of expectations and goals. Patient goals may be broad and concrete (such as doing as much screening or testing as possible to avoid cancer), specific (such as genetic testing for Ehlers-Danlos syndrome in order to gain access to needed care), or unattainable (such as predictive certainty around onset and course of disease). Understanding the motivating factors and psychological factors behind expectations and goals can be key to tailoring the session to a patient's informational and psychosocial needs. Therein lies the responsibility of a genetic counselor to provide clear information about the limits of genetic information. In this sense, you and your patient begin to "see each other" through understanding the boundaries of actionable and meaningful information and develop mutual goals for the session. It's important for genetic counselors to learn to balance patient goals and expectations with what is attainable and possible, like two paths converging to form parallel paths on which both members of the dyad can engage in partnership.

Initiating the conversation on goals

By prioritizing the provider–patient relationship as discussed in the earlier section on the working alliance, the counselor and patient become partners in defining the goals of the session. After you have established introductions, it's important to develop shared goals of the session with the patient. This often begins with sharing a few sentences about what you do as a genetic counselor, since often patients are told very little about the reason for the referral or have not heard of genetic counseling before. Inform the patient whether or not a physical exam is needed and if so, what the exam will entail, and why. It can also be reassuring to many patients to know that you are not heading into your meeting with them uninformed.

> **Genetic Counselor:** *"I'm a genetic counselor and my background and training helps me talk to people who have questions about their personal and/or family medical history. I've done a little 'background reading' in your chart, but I'd love to understand from you what you are hoping to gain from today's session?"*

If you are in a situation where you received very little background information (e.g., unclear referral indication and/or no medical records), you can also be honest.

> **Genetic Counselor:** *"[Explain your role as above]. Prior to this meeting, I was looking to see if we had any genetic testing records or medical records from you or your doctor. I didn't see anything and so I'm wondering if you wouldn't mind sharing what brings you in to this visit today?"*

Managing expectations

Part of setting and maintaining expectations in a session includes managing the time to the best of your ability. This may mean redirecting or focusing the patient's comments to meet goals more effectively. It may also involve communicating how much time is left in the appointment and that there are a few more key points to cover as you work towards reaching their goals. In some cases, a patient may already feel decided about their next steps, and you can draw on that as a tailored approach to the session. For example, if a patient has settled on pursuing genetic testing before you have had a chance to adequately explain the limitations of genetic testing, you can validate their stance and ask a follow-up question to learn more in order to fulfill your teaching and psychosocial assessment duty to the best of your ability: "Thanks for letting me know. Can you share with me what helped you arrive at this decision?" or "Thanks for letting me know. So let me share a few key points about the possible test results and how each one would impact your care differently."

It will be essential to have a nonassumptive approach to establishing goals and managing expectations. For example, patients may have cost management goals and knowing which genetic testing labs provide insurance pre-authorization assistance, financial assistance, or payment plans may be important. Provide the information clearly and concisely while avoiding words that may suggest judgment (e.g., "The test will 'only' cost $100"). Then ask follow-up questions based on the patient's reactions, responses, or questions. For example, if a lab offers a maximum out-of-pocket cost and you do not see a reaction from the patient, or if you are unsure how to interpret their reaction, you can follow-up with "This lab offers payment plans with no interest or additional costs. In other words, you can break up the amount into smaller amounts that you can pay monthly. You can set the amount per month. Does this sound like an option that would work for you?"

Balancing needs of more than one person

Goal setting can be complicated when multiple people are involved in a session. If an individual patient has brought others to the appointment, then attending to the influence and concerns of these people is important, too. For example, a person considering presymptomatic testing for a familial *BRCA1* variant might be strongly influenced by an at-risk or affected family member in the room. If your "patient" is a couple or a family, then the goals should be collectively constructed. A family-centered strategy for communicating genetic information can also help to ensure that index patients have support in communicating information (e.g., about disease etiology, cascade testing), and that relatives can support one another (Darr et al., 2016; Ahmed et al., 2022).

Balancing the needs of family members can be challenging. A genetic counselor may want to consider the broader context of a patient's primary support individuals, future care givers, and at-risk family members when discussing genetic testing for early-onset Alzheimer's disease, for example. In most medical

---

BOX 2-4. DEFINING FAMILY

How does one define *family*? Many family examples in this chapter assume genetically related individuals. For the purposes of psychosocial assessment and support which are dynamic processes embedded throughout a session, try to take a nonassumptive approach to the concept of family to include the patient's own definition of family. Who does the patient consider family (chosen, found, adopted, or kin for example)? When assessing the patients support system, ask questions that are geared towards understanding who your patient identifies as being important in their lives and with whom they have built a mutual and/or nurturing connection.

---

systems following a Western perspective, the patient's individual autonomy is the primary consideration. However, in genetics, the family is sometimes your "patient." By involving other family members, we may get a broader perspective of issues, identify resources or barriers, and develop common and attainable goals (Box 2-4). The counselor may have to consider individual needs and balance them against the needs of other individuals or the family as a group. This may mean arranging time to speak to individuals apart from their family as well as in a group (Kjoelaas et al., 2022). When the group reforms, the genetic counselor can facilitate the process by either inviting each member to share their perspective (if that is what you have contracted with the members); or, you can share your understanding and appreciation of the breadth of perspectives at the table. Offering your rationale behind a recommendation to speak separately and to the group is important as it is part of establishing your trustworthiness with the family through transparency.

Establishing attainable goals

Attainable (or realistic) goals are about balancing the differences between a patient's objectives (e.g., "I need these results as soon as possible," or "I'm seeking anonymous testing") and what is attainable and possible within the boundaries of the current state of technology, typical practice, or institutional policies. Some patient goals cannot be met, and your collaboration and support will help patients revise their initial expectations. For example, a patient hoping to learn onset or severity of a genetic condition may be overestimating the predictive power of a given test. We can help a patient reframe expectations and ability to cope with genetic information with facts (patient education techniques) and support (psychosocial techniques).

At times during the clinical interview, you may notice biases or assumptions behind a patient's expectations (e.g., "I want to do everything I can to have a healthy baby," or "Does this sex chromosome difference mean my child will be gay?"). There may be assumptions and biases that are ableist and heteronorma-tive in nature and are most often a result of phobia, misinformation (and disinformation), and lack of information, and these are not an indicator that the patient is inherently a "good" or "bad" person/parent/partner. Your awareness of countertransference (see Chapter 4) helps you notice the thoughts and feel-ings that arise from detecting patient bias; techniques discussed later in this chapter on recovery can help you reground and consider potential next steps. As you develop your counseling skills and confidence, you may find it helpful to frame patient biases in some situations, such as those in the examples above, as potential opportunities to deepen the working alliance using your questioning skills and psychosocial counseling skills (such as primary and advanced empathy).

To continue with a prenatal example, the average person is inundated with stories, media, and advertisements of people who we are supposed to perceive as young, white, cisgender pregnant women and play into our ingrained ableist con-ditioning, desires, and fantasies of parenting. Labeling a patient's stated goal of "doing everything I can to have a healthy baby" as right or wrong potentially disrespects individual perspectives and experiences and produces barriers in the working alliance. At the same time, part of our duty as a genetic counselor is to understand the ableist nature of these concerns and open opportunities to work with patients more deeply so that they can also unwrap some layers of their own biases that inform their perceptions and choices. The journey with the preconcep-tion or pregnant patient has the potential to be enriched by exploring concepts of "normal" and "healthy" together.

With the example above, the idea of "doing everything" is suggestive of a need to establish a sense of control in the face of fear. You can tentatively probe by asking: "You mentioned that you want to do 'everything you can'. Can you tell me what this involves, and what it means to you?" To inquire further into the ableist tendency to equate "happy" children with "normal" and "unafflicted by disease" and "unhappy/unfortunate" children with genetic conditions and illness, a probing question can be "We know that today's tests cannot test for every con-dition or trait. Can you share with me what you think of as a healthy child?" Probing in this way with respect and compassion can help a patient reveal to themselves their underlying biases and assumptions about health; for example, health as a state of living free of illness/disability (a medical model of illness and disability (Gould et al., 2019)). Inviting genuine and thoughtful exploration with patients in a safe environment has the potential to bring the genetic counselor closer to the ethical ideals of the profession[6] while simultaneously prioritizing the genetic counselor/patient therapeutic relationship (Farrelly et al., 2012; Gould et al., 2019). In other words, an anti-oppressive strategy is to limit cre-dence to dominant hegemonic norms through the lenses of curiosity and

---

[6] National Society of Genetic Counselors Code of Ethics. https://www.nsgc.org/POLICY/Code-of-Ethics-Conflict-of-Interest/Code-of-Ethics.

thoughtful inquiry whenever possible (Box 2-5). These seemingly small, interpersonal actions are particularly important when systemic injustices appear too big to handle.

Setting attainable goals recognizes the responsibility of genetic counselors to adjust to patient needs and expectations while staying grounded in the reality of what is possible/not possible and keeping patient implicit biases in mind, as well as the genetic counselor's own biases. This section is intended to provide

---

BOX 2-5. CORE VALUES IN TENSION

What other examples can you think of where tensions between core values can arise? How might you hold and potentially harmonize seemingly conflicting values? Consider and discuss the following questions and try to resist the desire for resolution as the conversations necessarily shift in different contexts. Let's take for example tensions between values held between disability justice,[7] the genetic testing industry (capitalism), individual right to make an informed decision (autonomy), and innovations in genomic medicine. For example, autistic self-advocates raise important questions about autism genetic research and genetic testing for autism spectrum disorders.[8]

- What values are expressed when these questions are ignored or marginalized by genetics professionals?
- When parents or caregivers of children with autism are routinely offered genetic risk assessment and testing, what role can genetic counselors play in asking unexplored questions with the parent/caregiver(s)?
- Can a genetic diagnosis of autism challenge internalized ableism or perpetuate it?
- Can a genetic diagnosis meaningfully improve or negatively impact an autistic child's social situation, environmental supports, self-image, self-determination; and, if so, in what ways?
- What are your personal views on treatment and intervention for autism? Are there internalized ableist lenses that could be upholding these views?
- What first-person narratives have you sought from autistic self-advocates and what are they saying about rights and justice?
- What do you personally understand about ableism in society as it pertains to autism and neurodiversity?

---

[7] 10 Principles of Disability Justice. https://www.sinsinvalid.org/blog/10-principles-of-disability-justice

[8] Autistic Self Advocacy Network Statement on Genetic Research and Autism. https://autisticadvocacy.org/wp-content/uploads/2022/03/genetic-statement.pdf.

TABLE 2-1. **Contracting through the session. In this example the mutual goal is to understand the family's clinical and molecular diagnosis of Lynch syndrome and explore ways of using this information to improve/manage their health**

Initial	"Based on the goals you shared with me, I'm going to talk about …"
Checking in	"I know you wanted to learn about how testing could impact your medical management. What other questions about medical management do you have?"
Revising	"You mentioned just now that your father had his genetic test done last week. His results could change the risk numbers that I was explaining. Let me go over what I mean by that."
Closing	"Thanks for sharing how you arrived at this decision. I mentioned earlier that your test will be available in x–xx days. Would you like to arrange a specific time for me to call you to discuss the results, or would you like to make an appointment to meet again to discuss them?"

anticipatory guidance and not a compulsory list of imperatives; the new learner will benefit from reflecting, discussing, brainstorming, and role-playing these ideas posed here on their own and with peers and supervisors.

Contracting

Contracting occurs when the genetic counselor articulates how mutually agreed upon goals of the session will be met. Contracting is initiated after the goals have been agreed upon and continues throughout a session as the interview unfolds. You will want to keep in mind what the mutual goals are, why they are important to your patient, and how you will strive to meet them. To aid in patient understanding of what you will be covering, you can also include the relevance of the information (Table 2-1).

Goals may need to be revised as new information comes to light in a session. For example, if a family history reveals substantial new information that needs to be discussed, it may be necessary to suggest a second appointment or referral to another genetics clinic to cover all the important topics. This could come up when a patient/family in the prenatal or pediatric setting has a family history of cancer. Another problem that can arise is the realization that you will not be able to meet the goals as expected. For example, if accurate risk assessment, test ordering, and results interpretation is dependent upon a family member's test report, establishing patient understanding around the rationale will facilitate necessary steps towards the goals.

PROMOTING SHARED UNDERSTANDING THROUGH INQUIRY: SPECIFIC INTERVIEWING TECHNIQUES

Effective interviewing can get to the heart of the patient's concerns, can assess the patient's understanding of genetic risk and disease processes, and attend to their psychosocial needs in the face of new information and uncertainty inherent in the process of genetic evaluation (Austin et al., 2014; Redlinger-Grosse et al., 2017). Asking questions, paraphrasing, reflecting, redirecting, using silence, and promoting a shared language are techniques that invite a patient to elaborate and share relevant information, experiences, concerns, beliefs, and perspectives. You are also encouraged to use the strategies discussed in this section with other techniques discussed in Chapter 5 that tailor information to individual needs and assess patient understanding with methods such as teach back (Riddle et al., 2021). Using a combination of strategies when counseling creates a more dynamic conversational flow, helps to pace the session, and as a result can be less cognitively and emotionally taxing for the patient. Employing these techniques conveys genuine interest and care which can be particularly useful for telemedicine (when there are usually fewer physical cues for both counselor and counselee), and when counseling through medical interpretation.

Questioning

Genetic counselors need to have several strategies for gathering information and generating discussion. The method selected should match the type of information that is needed (Table 2-2). Asking questions is one of the primary tools. Students will sometimes tell supervisors that certain questions are difficult to ask because the student perceives the question as personal. Through practice, you will be increasingly comfortable asking personal questions in calm, nonjudgmental ways. It will help to remember that if the answer to the question will be useful in helping the patient, then it is a valid question. Counselors should have specific reasons for asking the questions they do and should ask questions in systematic and purposeful ways.

Closed-ended questions are questions that typically can be answered with one or two words (often yes or no). These questions are useful for obtaining specific information. They keep discussions to a minimum and do not encourage in-depth descriptions or expressing emotion. Open-ended questions invite a patient to say more about a subject and give a more nuanced response. These questions can be the starting point for discussion.

It might seem that open-ended questions are preferable. This is not always true. Sometimes a brief specific answer is desired ("How old are you?"). At other times,

TABLE 2-2. **Interviewing Techniques**

Questioning

    Open-ended: Invites broad responses

    Focused: Guides response toward specific circumstances

    Closed-ended: Asks for yes/no answers or for specific details; does not encourage elaboration

Rephrasing: Restate your understanding of what the client has said

Reflecting: Repeat the last phrase of a client's statement as a question

From Baker et al. (1998) p. 59, Table 3.1

patients may be confused, wary, or reluctant to participate, and you can use closed-ended questions as a starting point. The most important guidepost when questioning a patient is this: Avoid making assumptions. If you're unclear about an aspect of a patient's experience or perception, or if you perceive that a particular issue is significant to a patient, ask about it.

Closed-ended question: Have you heard about genes before?

Closed, but somewhat more inviting: Have you considered genetic testing before, and if so, what were your initial thoughts on it?

Open-ended question: You mentioned that your sister had genetic testing. Please tell me a little more about what you know of her experience. (Although this is worded as a command, it serves the function of a question.)

Closed-ended question: Do you understand the information I have just provided?

Open-ended question: What questions do you have about the information provided?

More inviting of discussion: What are you thinking about the information we just went over?

Most inviting: How are you feeling about the information that we just went over?

Teach back: What is one takeaway that you want to share with someone when you go home today?

The intent of focused questioning is to create opportunities for the patient to identify specific experiences or insights that may be related to the current circumstances or decision-making process. Focused questions can also be used as a prompt to continue a discussion the patient may have truncated because they had said enough or was unsure whether the counselor wanted to hear more. The simple question "Can you tell me more about that day/conversation/experience?" allows the patient to share more about their experiences and for you as the counselor to understand what is important to the patient.

As the counselor, it is important for you to evaluate the patient's responses. For many, it will be the first time that they have been invited to tell a story by a professional. Are they intrigued by your question but unsure if they believe that you really want to hear the response? Are they hesitant because they don't yet feel ready to discuss the topic at this time? Or perhaps they might wonder why you are interested? In these instances, you may want to provide a summary of your thoughts as a counselor ("I asked about this because it may be relevant to your current situation, and I want to understand more about what you think"). It may also help to preface your question, particularly if it is inviting the patient's personal reflection. For example, "I noticed a shift when we were talking about your grandmother's recent diagnosis, and again right now when we were talking about cancer risk. I'm wondering if you could share a little more about what she means to you, and how this diagnosis has impacted you?"

Generally, when a mutually respectful relationship has been established with the counselor, a patient not only will respond to questions but will welcome them as an opportunity to explore relevant experiences and consider how these experiences have shaped their views. However, if a patient provides a general unfocused reply to your query, assess the reasons for this reaction. Might you have been unclear? Is the patient trying to avoid the interaction, or did you as the counselor make a wrong turn—for example, by unwittingly acting on an incorrect assumption about the patient or misinterpreting certain cues or responses. If the counselor's line of questioning is unfounded, it is necessary to stop and correct the direction of the conversation. You can also keep in mind that after experimenting with a few open-ended questions, you might find that some patients communicate in short answers and don't tend to elaborate. This is also appropriate, as patients might choose to stay in their comfort zone and are not obligated to share their stories.

Paraphrasing

Paraphrasing involves stating in your own words what the patient has just told you to reflect content and meaning. It is a valuable tool for demonstrating attentiveness and ensuring that you have understood what the patient intended to convey. It reinforces for the patient that you have understood a part of their experience. It is especially valuable when you and your patient have different language styles (such as use of unfamiliar words or metaphors) or are communicating over the phone.

> **Patient:** I can't believe I'm in this situation again. I thought I was in the clear and now my cancer has come back. We just planned a cross-country road trip to see my kids and grandkids. What am I going to tell them? They are going to be so crushed.
>
> **[Paraphrasing content] Genetic Counselor:** You thought you were cleared and so you planned a trip to see your family.
>
> **Patient:** Yes, and now I don't know if I should just postpone it, or try and still see them before I start treatment. But I don't even know what my treatment plan will be, and that's making me anxious too. Will I need more surgery, chemo, both? I just don't know.

Paraphrasing demonstrates your understanding, or your attempt to understand, which is a characteristic of empathy. It keeps the conversation focused on the patient while the counselor is playing an active role in helping the patient. It helps to think about the main message or messages in the story that your patient is telling you. In the above example, the counselor restates in their own words the main message of the patient's hope of staying cancer-free and seeing family, and in the below example also adds the patient's sense of worry. Following up with a tentative question conveys that you are open to being corrected.

Sometimes a patient's story contains thoughts and emotions that you may want to reflect to help the patient reveal feelings they were unaware of or hesitant about articulating. In the example above, the genetic counselor could say:

> **[Paraphrasing content and reflecting feelings] Genetic Counselor:** It sounds like you were really hoping to stay in the clear. Just when you were feeling like you could "get past" your cancer and plan something wonderful, cancer showed up again. Now you are also worried about worrying everyone. (Optional follow-up inquiry) Does it sound like I'm on the right track? You can tell me if I'm off the mark.
>
> **Patient:** Exactly! I'm just crushed, I can't put them through this again. Seeing them was going to be a big treat for me … for everyone. My grandkids love cooking with me and walking the dog with me, we keep talking about it. I told them I was feeling great, because I am; how do I tell them that I'm "sick" again? It's so unfair to them. [pause] In fact, it feels unfair to me too.

Attending behaviors

Nonverbal attending behaviors can include nodding, changing your facial expression at key moments to demonstrate that you are following the patient's emotional state, making eye contact, or leaning a little forward or backwards for emphasis. It can also mean matching the tone of the moment. It demonstrates that you are listening with the desire to understand, and you are nonverbally conveying to the patient that the space you are in together is for them.

Verbal attending behaviors have a similar effect and often encourage the patient to continue with their story. Verbal communication conveying attentive listening is particularly helpful with telephone counseling and working with patients with low/no vision. *Minimal encouragers* include short interjections such as "mm-hmm," "ah," "wow," to indicate that you are listening and encourage them to continue. *Brief phrases* that repeat a portion of a patient's statement in the form of a question can also encourage further exploration of the topic. It is also used to maintain the direction of a conversation. The following exchanges use brief phrases:

> **Patient:** Well, since my nephew was diagnosed with muscular dystrophy, my partner just seems scared about another pregnancy.
>
> **Genetic Counselor:** Your partner seems scared?
>
> **Patient:** Well, I guess we're both a little scared, you know, that it might happen to us?

> **Patient:** So that's my decision—a mastectomy is better than cancer.
>
> **Genetic Counselor:** Better than cancer?
>
> **Patient:** Well sure, that way I don't have to worry any more.

Repeating brief or final phrases encourages the patient to amplify their thoughts and ideas in a way that more clearly identifies the significance of their feelings or observations. This also gives you more information regarding the basis for the patient's thoughts and beliefs, so that you can respond without making assumptions. In the second example, the patient's comments about a mastectomy may indicate that she believes surgery will permanently protect her from cancer. As with any of the techniques mentioned in this section, repeating the patient's words should be used in combination with other techniques to avoid unintentionally appearing as if you are not really listening.

The following examples attempt to illustrate the differences between repeating, paraphrasing, and summarizing (akin to a longer version of paraphrasing).

Patient: There is no good option. I can't believe we are faced with these decisions. This is difficult.
Genetic Counselor: Yes, this really is truly difficult to be facing these options. (Repeating)

Patient: I feel like I gave this disease to my son.
Genetic Counselor: It seems like you feel responsible for your son's condition. (Paraphrasing)

Patient: I can't begin to tell you how upsetting this is. I never expected to be in this position. I keep thinking I'll wake up and find out it was all a dream.
Genetic Counselor: Clearly this is very upsetting and almost out of the blue. It sounds like it's hard to accept the situation you're in right now. (Summarizing thoughts and feelings.)

Role playing with a peer or supervisor and receiving feedback can be helpful as you practice these techniques. For example, you can ask your role play partner if your *repeating* technique felt as if you were parroting them, which may not come off as attentive. Through practice you will also expand your attending behaviors by tying in a statement that a patient shares during the session back into the current topic, where appropriate. Remember that coming up with a response doesn't need to be immediate; pauses are a natural part of the cadence in an emotional or reflective moment.

Redirecting

Redirecting is used by the counselor to manage the rate of information exchange—to direct the introduction and flow of topics, or to refocus the discussion when the patient has digressed to a new topic. The following are examples of statements that can be employed to redirect the counseling interaction:

That's an important issue, but first I'd like to go back to …
We will get to that, but first I think it would be helpful to hear …

Before moving on, let me ask you a little more about …

How about that other matter you mentioned regarding …

I'd like to slow down here a bit. How are you using what you just said about … in making the decision you are facing today?

That's an important question, which is best answered by your cardiologist. So, could we come back to …

Silence

Silence is a particularly effective technique that is often difficult for beginning counselors. Many patients use silence as a time to reflect on what has been said, to formulate what to say next, or to gain composure (McCarthy Veach et al., 2018). A counselor who fills the silence too quickly does not allow for these processes and may communicate the message that the counselor will determine the direction of the session without input from the patient. At times, a counselor may offer their own thoughts too quickly rather than waiting for the patient; this is especially true of beginners who are trying to be helpful by sharing their knowledge, their assessment, or by having answers. We show respect for a patient's story by pausing to take it in rather than rushing to comment on it. Some studies indicate that patients often will *not* mention their most important concern first. A longer pause may allow them to get to their deeper concerns. You can try working on this skill with a partner by counting to 10 before speaking during a role play session.

Promoting shared language

In general, a good interviewing technique is to mirror a patient's language to promote understanding of terminology and complex concepts such as inheritance, risk information, or uncertainty. It conveys to the patient that they are being understood as an individual. The counselor might say, "Well, what I call the 'non-working' gene and you call the 'bad' gene are really the same thing," and from this point on you would use the patient's term. However, mirroring language has limitations, and when a genetic counselor picks up on misinformation or outdated terms, they need to strategize ways to correct the information. A new learner may debate whether correcting a patient might negatively impact the working alliance. Part of the purpose of showing your trustworthiness in the working alliance is to have a foundation upon which you build respect for their wellbeing by assisting a patient or caregiver adopt concepts, and language, that help them gain new clarity and are affirming. In some situations, you may wonder if a speaker's (patient/caregiver/partner/family member) use of terms, particularly outdated or offensive ones, inhibits specific goals of genetic counseling, such as the patient's sense of worthiness and ability to cope. This can be troubling for genetic counselors when the speaker is a primary caregiver in the patient's life such as a parent, as it may impact the patient's self-esteem. A few relevant situations are discussed below:

- Misinformation: Some informational aspects of a session are essential for decision-making. Misapplication of terminology or misunderstanding of key information may need to be corrected so that misunderstanding doesn't continue.

- Diagnostic journey: During stages of the diagnostic journey, patients or parent(s) may have been provided terms and outdated/harmful syndrome names and terminology from prior health care providers. Parents and caregivers generally want to do well by their loved one. Introducing new terms, why you use them, and then checking in with the family is a collaborative approach to developing shared understanding through shared vocabulary. Doing so demonstrates respect and can have a positive impact on the patient's sense of self-worth and dignity.

- Established diagnosis: Consider a parent or caregiver who uses the term "low-functioning autistic" several times in a session in reference to a 45-year-old patient who was diagnosed almost two decades ago with autism. What do you glean about the patient's sense of self-worth, and about the relationship between patient and parent? What additional information do you need to assess both the patient's self-worth/autonomy and the relationship, which are often intertwined? Try a holistic and collaborative approach to introducing new language which includes mutual sharing of ideas and information. Doing so demonstrates respect and honors the patient's dignity.

Mirroring language that reflects how a patient expresses their understanding of their clinical situation shows regard for them. Developing a shared language promotes learning and understanding. As genetic counselors weigh and balance multiple needs within a session, some may feel more challenged by specific scenarios not addressed here, such as addressing discriminatory language. At the time of this publication there is a paucity of research on ways to address patient bias in genetic counseling where a patient makes a derogatory remark; for example, a parent who uses a derogatory term in reference to their teen's nonbinary gender identity. Addressing patient bias is discussed in the counseling, nursing, and medical literature (Eliason et al., 2011; Whitgob et al., 2016; Wheeler et al., 2019), and more dialogue and scholarship in this area would greatly enrich our genetic counseling models of practice.

Summary

Genetic counselors have a responsibility to attend to the emotions of their patients and work with their patients to attend to concerns that may be triggering their emotions (Austin et al., 2014; Redlinger-Grosse et al., 2017). Oftentimes these concerns arise from patient's own beliefs and understanding around disease, illness, disability, mental health, and health. Ask 10 people what *health* means to them and you'll get 10 answers with commonalities, contrasts, and nuanced differences. If a genetic counselor provides information and recommendations that are incongruent to the patient's belief system, it is the counselors' duty to probe into the possible reasons or areas of missed information. The Explanatory Model of Illness or EM is an approach that elicits the patient's own story behind illnesses in their personal history and family medical history when applicable (Abad, 2012). Asking patients questions from the EM, such as "what do you think caused your problem/concern" and "why do you think it started when it did," promotes patient engagement and has the potential to validate their experience. From here, the genetic counselor can formulate a greater understanding of the patient's illness beliefs (i.e., what they believe to be true), provide support, and also tailor their communication. These elements are one example of the natural oscillation between teaching and counseling in genetic counseling sessions while promoting the working alliance. Developing and implementing these techniques constitute culturally tailored counseling, which is good counseling.

GROWING YOUR CLINICAL INTERVIEWING PROCESS

"I am a work in progress." This mindset can be a useful antidote to setting unrealistic expectations that results from a pull towards performing perfectly (perfectionism), and our yearning to meet all of the needs of a patient ("do-good" mentality). Earlier in the chapter we examined facilitators of inclusivity in the working alliance and cultivating a learning mindset around examining power. Perfectionism is one trait of white supremacy culture (WSC), and self-education and reflection around perfectionism is part of the pathway towards dismantling internalized racism and WSC (*Dismantling Racism Works Web Workbook*, n.d.). Building an understanding around WSC traits, integrating them into your self-awareness and practice, and resisting weaponization of these concepts is essential for personal growth and critical to a social justice-oriented genetic counseling curriculum.

Getting into the learning zone (and staying there)

An important place for a new trainee to start is to think about their "why"—*what is my "why?" Why am I doing what I'm doing?* It's the difference between over-focusing on *doing* (how to counsel or how to educate) and having an objective behind the doing. When our objective is defined, we can tap into that sense of purpose anytime we need it: when we feel a lack of focus; when we are struggling with a developing skill; when we sense we want to innovate but are hesitant to try. Tapping into our "why" as a trainee can help refocus on what is important in the learning role, so that we can focus on the process of learning the craft. The art and practice of genetic counseling is challenging and keeping ourselves in the learning zone helps us continue to hone our skills.

The learning "zone" is the edge at which we push a bit past what we are comfortable doing. It helps you make gradual and incremental progress over the course of your training and beyond. Even when mistakes happen, which are normal and expected, they are opportunities to learn. In fact, without mistakes, far less learning takes place.

> *Example: You may be getting comfortable taking a family cancer history and initiating rapport-building, but you know you need to add more inter-viewing skills beyond intake. You have been working with your supervisor to provide comprehensive assessment and discussion of risk. You have a care-ful outline prepared, have practiced verbalizing and diagramming your explanation with classmates, and you take a leap forward with your next patient. During the intake you forget to ask some of your routine intake questions.*

Reflect on how you felt going into the session and during the session (What did you feel? Where did you feel it?) Examine how these feelings could have masked your abilities or overtaken your focus.

Introducing flexibility, gradually

The flexibility of the session refers not only to the topics to be covered but also to the order and ways in which they will be discussed. Counselors usually have an outline in mind for a session to help think of the flow of questions and infor-mation. As a new counselor you can start by following this outline to develop your comfort with conducting a session with the aim of having a logical and consistent flow. Part of beginner practice is also learning to assess whether you are comfortable addressing a patient's question as it arises, or whether you are more comfortable redirecting and saying that it's an important question that you will be addressing a bit later. Practicing both methods is important to expanding your skill set, flexibility, and adaptability! It's also helpful to set mini-goals towards practicing both methods, and small steps help to reduce anxiety around feeling a little thrown off. In some cases, you will need to use your empathic judgment to discern how much a particular issue might be distressing to a patient. For example, at the start of a pre-amniocentesis session, your patient asks how big the needle is. If you don't address the question about the procedure now, it is quite possible that the patient's fear will prevent her from participating in the ses-sion in any meaningful way. If it seems more appropriate, you can give a brief answer at the time the question is asked, promise to say more later, and then resume with the session. Ideally, try to remember to ask if the patient is satisfied with the answer after coming back to this topic later in the session. It's also a good idea to periodically stop and check whether the goals are being met; for example, you might say, "I know you wanted to learn about your testing options today. Do you feel like your questions have been answered?" (McCarthy Veach et al., 2018).

Recovering yourself and your session

We often feel a rush of emotions when we realize a mistake or miscommunication has occurred and it's essential to take note of these feelings. The same sensations can happen when a person in the session says something unexpected or surprising. We may freeze, or we may experience a flood of emotions, either of which can take our attention away from the session and/or patient. Noticing the emotions in the moment, and taking a few deep breaths, slows down the heart rate and restores a bit of calm.

Mistakes in the genetic counseling session can fall into different categories and we address two types here: misunderstanding the patient and making an error.

Misunderstanding the patient Communication is bidirectional and is naturally imperfect, as we apply our own biases when interpreting a patient's intended meaning. This is much like applying a template of prior information (beliefs, values, and experiences) to interpret a person's meaning behind verbal and nonverbal cues. Once you realize that a misunderstanding has taken place, it's important to take a pause, and return to a curious stance. The curious stance helps you take the opportunity to "return to wonder" or zoom out a bit and ask clarifying and often open-ended questions to elicit engagement from the patient. In this way, the duo of counselor and counselee are on an exploratory journey to achieving better understanding. If a patient communicates to you that they are being misunderstood, it is appropriate to thank them for their openness as you proceed with taking a curious stance, thereby showing your humility and trustworthiness and maintaining the working alliance. Notice if you are feeling defensive; this response is information indicating countertransference and is worth reflection around the nature of the defensiveness as it may be tied to internalized white supremacist traits that are calling upon you to reflect and learn.

Making an error based on prejudgment No practitioner is immune to making errors of assumption. Prejudgment can lead a genetic counselor down a line of interviewing choices that are out of alignment with the patient's goals and inhibit the genetic counselor's ability to collect or convey information effectively. Downstream impact can include uninformed decision-making or inadequate assessment of understanding. An example of not being aware or not addressing a potential error is provided below:

> *Example: The genetic counselor is meeting with a patient who is 17 weeks pregnant and the indication for referral is ultrasound findings suggestive of Down syndrome. When the genetic counselor asks the patient what they know about Down syndrome, which is a typical question that the genetic counselor*

asks in these situations, the patient shrugs their shoulders, shakes their head a little, and doesn't make eye contact. The short answers and lack of eye contact leads the genetic counselor to assume the patient is in shock. The counselor proceeds with the session. The genetic counselor repeats at various points in the session that the patient doesn't have to make any decisions today and asks if the patient has any questions. The continued appearance of disengagement leaves the genetic counselor flustered and unsure of what to do next and they are considering pulling out the consent form to go over it with the patient.

In the moment, this genetic counselor detects cues from the patient's body language and short answers. The genetic counselor feels flustered and unsure—noticing these feelings but not following up on what is causing the discomfort may lead to poor decision-making (proceeding to review the consent form). If the genetic counselor can recognize that feeling unsure is their own feedback information, it can lead them to step back, and take a stance of curious inquiry: Why am I unsure? What assumptions could I be making right now? Could I be missing something? What can I ask my patient to gain a better understanding of their present state?

Such errors have the potential to disrupt the working alliance, and another example of apologizing and recovering from an error is provided below. In this case, the genetic counselor misgenders the patient which is a common form of gender identity microaggression.

Example: The genetic counselor misgenders an adolescent patient named Jai while answering the parent's question about the patient. The counselor notices their error and acknowledges it swiftly: "I'm sorry Jai, you told me you use they/them pronouns and I made a mistake just now. I'll get it right!" and proceeds with the rest of the session using the correct pronouns.

In the above example, the genetic counselor's feeling of self-consciousness may be very heightened the moment they realize their mistake. It is normal to feel embarrassed and upset at yourself for causing harm and a necessary step to recover yourself is to recall that it's not about your feelings at this moment, even if you are able to recognize the discomfort. Only then can you enter a path to redressing the harm, which begins with *naming* the harm (e.g., misgendering), apologizing, and verbalizing your commitment to doing better. To name a harm is to speak the truth. To speak the truth is to demonstrate trustworthiness. Your actions are not the final determinant of how a patient will respond to the apology, but most people recognize and are receptive to a sincere effort.

Another significance of the above example is that you cannot make assumptions about Jai's prior experiences disclosing their gender identity to family members, friends, teachers, or health care providers. Your awareness of discrimination and cis-normative bias in education and health care tells you that: 1) you don't know what the patient has gone through up until now; and 2) without doing better, you might not know how to support Jai's socioemotional development going forward, as misgendering risks severing their trust in you.

Committing to doing better continues after the session is over. This includes a retrospective exploration of what happened (reflexivity): how was your apology? If you were in the shoes of the recipient of the apology, would it feel genuine? How did the rest of the session go, and in what ways did you contribute to the working alliance overall? Looking back also provides you with insight to apply towards looking forward with greater self-awareness so that you are less likely to make a similar mistake again, and more likely to refocus the session on the patient rather than on how you feel about your mistake. Furthermore, reflect on the mistake itself for growth; for example, if you realize that the mistake came from unfamiliarity with using nonbinary pronouns in the clinical setting, additional practice outside of sessions would be warranted. In short, these recommendations are examples of using humility as your guide.

When an apology is warranted, keeping the apology succinct and genuine is part of maintaining the working alliance, as it does not compel the recipient to take care of your feelings. The goal is to find a way to reground yourself so that you can recover the session. In a supervised setting, it may also help to pre-brief with your supervisor about strategies for handling these situations in a collaborative manner. Strategies such as practicing simple scenarios in your head or with a friend can reduce anxieties surrounding making mistakes.

Recognizing one's mistakes and addressing them is important for ensuring that you and the patient have the right information. Additionally, working on recovery is important for building self-awareness. It can be habit-forming!

Microaggressions

Here we address a specific type of harm that can arise in a genetic counseling setting where its significance is often under-recognized in the genetic counseling literature. Microaggressions are the indignities and slights that invalidate the lived experience of a person who holds marginalized and often intersecting marginalized identities (Pierce, 1969; Pierce et al., 1977; Sue et al., 2007). Microaggressions are often unintended, but that has little bearing on the impact. The source of most microaggressions are unrecognized internalized normative whiteness and assumptions made of others based on social identities (race, religion, disability, parental status, age, etc.). Drawing on your skills such as attentiveness, trustworthiness, empathy, and respect, and practicing cultural humility, helps you maintain flexibility in your responsiveness towards a patient, peer, or colleague who shares their personal experience of microaggression with you. Skills around recovering yourself can help you in the moment should a microaggression be directed towards you.

What do you do if your patient shares an experience of a microaggression? First, believe them. Try to resist rationalizing or seeking reasons behind the incident, as the impact is more important than the intent.

Try also to resist the urge to fix, but attend closely first. These are crucial strategies towards validating the patient's experiences authentically. Invite your patient to elaborate if they wish. Continue employing silence and other attentive listening strategies. If the situation occurred within your clinic or hospital, it is within your zone of influence, and you may wish to explore the patient's feelings around incident reporting. If the situation occurred outside of your zone of influence, consider what reasonable help you can offer.

In the end, fixing is not the overall objective. You will benefit from the practice of setting aside your assumptions and biases and resisting the urge to fix. Most importantly, you will have reaffirmed a psychologically safe environment for your patient. You may also find these strategies useful if a peer confides in you. An important mindset that underpins all of these responses is genuineness and respect for the person, along with demonstrating attentive listening.

What do you do if your patient directs a microaggression towards you? Genetic counseling trainees and practitioners holding marginalized identities based on race, ethnicity, disability, and LGBTQIA+ identities are not immune to the effects of bias and discrimination from patients (Eliason et al., 2011; Whitgob et al., 2016; Wheeler et al., 2019). Students who hold multiple marginalized identities experience challenges that are intersectional and cannot be categorized within one axis of identity alone. I share a few strategies that are preparatory in nature, and aimed at recovery in the moment and recovery after a session. First, there is no one way to handle a microaggression and the way in which it impacts you and the extent of the impact will depend on how core the social identity or identities are to you.

1. Preparation won't prevent patient bias, but can help you recover in the moment and after the session.
   - Learn about your institution's provider rights and policies, also known as patient/family/visitor code of conduct (Chary et al., 2021).
   - For students: if you find it applicable, it may be helpful to ask your supervisors about suggestions for handling "hot moments" during a session. This is applicable to not only patient bias, but other strong emotions such as patient anger or intrusive behaviors. "As you know I use gender fluid pronouns and I'm comfortable introducing my pronouns in a session. I'm wondering if we can talk through what we could do together as a team if a patient were to say something inappropriate or discriminatory towards me?"
   - For supervisors: open a conversation early in the rotation with your students. Be consistent in doing this with all students so that you are not only having this conversation with students of color or those with other marginalized identities. If you work in a team, consider brainstorming

group strategies around identity-conscious supervision practice, build consensus, debrief incidences as they arise, and reassess your practices on a regular basis. These strategies build intentionality into inclusion. Importantly, if an incident occurs, resist minimizing your student's experience of discrimination and bigotry as this causes further harm (silence and complicity) and enforces your power by prioritizing your comfort.

2. During the session, there are a variety of ways to address patient bias depending on how it is impacting you.

   - For students, you always have the right to transfer the session to your supervisor. Your psychological safety is important, and you may need to sever the working alliance that was already fractured by the patient's actions. For practicing genetic counselors, handing the session to a colleague may be in you and your patient's best interest as the patient's session objectives might be more effectively achieved through a new working alliance with another provider.

   - You may feel the need to calm yourself with a few breaths. In these brief moments of collecting yourself you may need to ask yourself "Can I still provide quality care and information to my patient?"

   - Check your toolbox and ask: "Do I have one sentence I can say that draws a boundary to protect myself from further harm?"

3. After the session, debrief with a trusted peer, supervisor, and/or faculty member. You will feel the benefits of tapping into your web of support. Assess whether there is something you could do differently to recover in the moment; however, remember that you were not being too sensitive, this was not perpetrated by you, and the relationship was severed by your patient (not by your reaction, thoughts, or actions).

Even if the incident occurred some time ago, you can still debrief at a time that feels right, if you wish. "Can we talk sometime today? I had a rough experience with a patient last week. They frequently talked over me, tapped their foot when I answered a question, and at one point interrupted and said 'at least I can understand your accent, unlike Dr. K. You just can't find a *regular* doctor these days.'" In this scenario, it's important that the supervisor recognizes: 1) at least three identity-related aggressive behaviors (also known as exclusionary acts) perpetrated by the patient against their student; and 2) that these types of acts are commonly and not exclusively committed against international students of color.

This section is intended to render visible the experiences of students who are Black, Indigenous, and People of Color (BIPOC), gender diverse, intersex, queer, disabled, international, undocumented citizens, and more, that are often silenced or brushed aside by the white cis-heteronormativity of our profession. It is by no means a comprehensive look at microaggressions and bias and more research with intersectional approaches is needed around strategies that address microaggressions and outcomes in a variety of settings (educational, clinical, research, industry) when the microaggressor is a genetic counselor, instructor, trainee, peer, supervisor, manager, colleague, or patient/family member.

CONCLUDING GUIDANCE

There is no single best way to communicate, and when it comes to prioritizing human relationships, shedding the idea of a single "best practice" can be liberating. (The concept of best practice which focuses on form and policy has great merit in other contexts.) Certainly, it is good (and responsible) practice to collect and present information in an ordered fashion; it is better (and responsive) practice to develop different ways to assess and work towards mutual understanding. It is good to be culturally informed, but better to also strive to be culturally humble and culturally responsive in your practice. Furthermore, more research and scholarship from genetic counselors with disabilities and marginalized identities needs to be supported and uplifted, as the quality of their scholarship through the lenses of their experiences is likely to add more depth and breadth to our profession's understanding of what "good" clinical interviewing techniques entails.

Learning your craft, including clinical interviewing skills, takes practice and revision. Set small goals, in addition to large ones. Role play and brainstorm various ways to address clinical situations with peers while also practicing attentive listening, genuineness, cultural humility, respect, and trustworthiness as you engage with (and seek feedback from) each other in this manner. After a role play or clinical day, journal your reflections and/or debrief with an experienced colleague or peer. Trying new strategies expands your skill set, while reflexivity deepens your understanding of your impact. When you are struggling, zoom out a little on the situation and try to view it holistically; think about the strategies and skills that are most collaborative. The crux of the clinical interviewing and genetic counseling process is centering the patient's access needs, informational needs, and psychosocial needs.

Wherever you are in your development as a genetic counselor, the stage you are at right now is an excellent place to reflect on your inclusive practice strategies. As a student you may wonder what authority you have in your status a to go against the grain of dominant white cis-heteronormative practice. As a practicing genetic counselor, a genetic counseling educator, and/or a genetic counseling supervisor, parts of this chapter may bring up a range of emotions, challenges, and discomfort. As you sit in the discomfort, define a *purpose* around the discomfort; because, without defining a purpose, the tendency is to avoid discomfort, thereby avoiding growth. This growth mindset keeps you on your learning edge where challenge and conflict are neither inherently bad nor feelings or situations to be avoided.[9] The further along you are in your career, the more influence you have and the power and privileges that come along with it. We are members of a health care infrastructure that is structured to categorize, deny, and oppress as much as it is also meant to help, to treat, and to heal. Within your sphere or zone of influence, particularly within the one-on-one working alliance in clinical interviewing, you always have a choice: to be oppressive (by reasserting historical imbalances of power), to do nothing at all (complacency in our complicity), or to work towards transforming care for a more just society (Woolsey, Narruhn, 2018).

ACKNOWLEDGEMENTS

I wrote this chapter to amplify the lived experiences and cultural wealth of marginalized patients, students, and colleagues. I am grateful to countless individuals from whom I have learned so much. I am grateful to Vivian Ota Wang, MS, MPhil, PhD, Tala Berro, MS, CGC, and Kim Zayhowski, MS, CGC for their valuable insights and feedback on the chapter. I thank editors Vivian Pan, MS, CGC and Karen Wain, MS, CGC for their constructive feedback and for seeing value in an instructive chapter that attempts to reflect key strategies for culturally conscious genetic counseling interviewing. I also appreciate the work of Diane Baker, MS, CGC and Kathryn Spitzer Kim, MS, CGC who were authors of this chapter in the 1st and 2nd editions respectively, as portions on pages 12-15 and 34-39 were drawn from their written work.

RESOURCES

Demystifying Disability – What to Know, What to Say, and How to be an Ally
By Emily Ladau
https://www.penguinrandomhouse.com/books/646508/demystifying-disability-by-emily-ladau/

Medical Apartheid: The Dark History of Medical Experimentation on Black Americans from Colonial Times to the Present.
By Harriet A. Washington
https://www.penguinrandomhouse.com/books/185986/medical-apartheid-by-harriet-a-washington/

---

[9] Conflict avoidance is a white supremacy culture trait endemic to the daily interactions we have with one another and serves WSC by preventing authenticity and accountability in interactions and maintaining emotional distance between human beings. Again, no one is immune to WSC traits, and everyone has the capacity to learn and do better.

Talking About Race
From the National Museum of African American History and Culture
https://nmaahc.si.edu/learn/talking-about-race

The National LGBTQIA+ Health Education Center
https://www.lgbtqiahealtheducation.org/

The Principles of Trustworthiness
From the Association of American Medical Colleges (AAMC) Center for Health Justice
https://www.aamchealthjustice.org/resources/trustworthiness-toolkit

Systems of Oppression
From the UnLeading Project at York University
https://www.yorku.ca/edu/unleading/systems-of-oppression/

REFERENCES

Abad PJB. (2012) Explanatory models of illness may facilitate cultural competence in genetic counseling. *J Genet Couns* 21(4):612–614. https://doi.org/10.1007/s10897-012-9487-9

Acevedo N & Solorzano DG. (2021) An overview of community cultural wealth: toward a protective factor against racism. *Urban Educ* 00420859211016531. https://doi.org/10.1177/00420859211016531

Ahmed S, Jafri H, Faran M, et al. (2022) Cascade screening for beta-thalassaemia in Pakistan: Relatives' experiences of a decision support intervention in routine practice. *Eur J Hum Genet* 30(4):406–412. https://doi.org/10.1038/s41431-021-00974-y

Anonymous. (2008) A genetic counselor's journey from provider to patient: A mother's story. *J Genet Couns* 17(5):412–418; discussion 419–423. https://doi.org/10.1007/s10897-008-9171-2

Arao B & Clemens K. (2013). From safe spaces to brave spaces: A new way to frame dialogue around diversity and social justice. In: L Landreman (ed.), The Art of Effective Facilitation: Reflections from Social Justice Educators, Sterling, VA: Stylus.

Austin J, Semaka A, & Hadjipavlou G. (2014) Conceptualizing genetic counseling as psychotherapy in the era of genomic medicine. *J Genet Couns* 23(6):903–909. https://doi.org/10.1007/s10897-014-9728-1

Bellcross C. (2012) A genetic counselor's story of birth, grief, and survival. *J Genet Couns* 21(2):169–172. https://doi.org/10.1007/s10897-011-9430-5

Berro T, Zayhowski K, Field T, et al. (2020) Genetic counselors' comfort and knowledge of cancer risk assessment for transgender patients. *J Genet Couns* 29(3):342–351. https://doi.org/10.1002/jgc4.1172

Braveman PA, Arkin E, Proctor D, et al. (2022) Systemic and structural racism: definitions, examples, health damages, and approaches to dismantling. *Health Aff (Millwood)* 41(2):171–178. https://doi.org/10.1377/hlthaff.2021.01394

Cahn PS, Makosky A, Truong KA, et al. (2022) Introducing the language of antiracism during graduate school orientation. *J Divers High Educ* 15(1):1–6. https://doi.org/10.1037/dhe0000377

Chary AN, Fofana MO, & Kohli HS (2021) Racial discrimination from patients: institutional strategies to establish respectful emergency department environments. *West J Emerg Med* 22(4):898–902. https://doi.org/10.5811/westjem.2021.3.51582

Cuena R. (n.d.) *Cultural Capital and Rural Surgical Practice: A Female Surgical Oncologist's Perspective on Practicing in Rural America.* American College of Surgeons. https://www.facs.org/for-medical-professionals/news-publications/news-and-articles/bulletin-brief/032222/dei/ Accessed December 30, 2022.

Darr A, Small N, Ahmad WIU, et al. (2016) Addressing key issues in the consanguinity-related risk of autosomal recessive disorders in consanguineous communities: Lessons from a qualitative study of British Pakistanis. *J Community Genet* 7(1):65–79. https://doi.org/10.1007/s12687-015-0252-2

Dismantling Racism Works Web Workbook. (n.d.) DRworksBook. https://www.dismantlingracism.org/ Accessed July 2, 2023.

Eliason MJ, DeJoseph J, Dibble S, et al. (2011) Lesbian, gay, bisexual, transgender, and queer/questioning nurses' experiences in the workplace. *J Prof Nurs* 27(4):237–244. https://doi.org/10.1016/j.profnurs.2011.03.003

Farrelly E, Cho MK, Erby L, et al. (2012) Genetic counseling for prenatal testing: where is the discussion about disability? *J Genet Couns* 21(6):814–824. https://doi.org/10.1007/s10897-012-9484-z

Gioacchino VD, Essendrup CA, Galasinski CS, et al. (2022, April 7) *Gender Inclusivity in the Genetics Lab.* Nsgc-Perspectives. https://perspectives.nsgc.org/Article/TitleLink/Gender-Inclusivity-in-the-Genetics-Lab Accessed May 24, 2024.

Gould H, Hashmi SS, Wagner VF, et al. (2019) Examining genetic counselors' implicit attitudes toward disability. *J Genet Couns* 28(6):1098–1106. https://doi.org/10.1002/jgc4.1160

Horvath AO & Greenberg LS. (Eds) (1994) *The Working Alliance: Theory, Research, and Practice* (pp. xii, 304), Hoboken, NJ: John Wiley & Sons.

Hyatt J. (2012) Countertransference in the genetic counseling setting: one counselor's personal journey. *J Genet Couns* 21(2):197–198. https://doi.org/10.1007/s10897-011-9435-0

Jones CP. (2014) Systems of power, axes of inequity: parallels, intersections, braiding the strands. [Editorial]. *Med Care* 52(10 Suppl 3):S71–S75 https://doi.org/10.1097/MLR.0000000000000216

Kjoelaas S, Jensen TK, & Feragen KB. (2022) Dilemmas when talking about Huntington's disease: a qualitative study of offspring and caregiver experiences in Norway. *J Genet Couns* 31(6):1349–1362. https://doi.org/10.1002/jgc4.1610

Kolden GG, Wang C-C, Austin SB, et al. (2018) Congruence/genuineness: a meta-analysis. *Psychotherapy* 55(4):424–433. https://doi.org/10.1037/pst0000162

Martinez K & Truong KA. (2020, August 3) Online anti-oppressive orientation during COVID-19. *Diverse: Issues In Higher Education.* https://www.diverseeducation.com/students/article/15107463/online-anti-oppressive-orientation-during-covid-19 Accessed May 24, 2024.

Martinez K & Truong KA. (2021, April 9) From DEI to JEDI. *Diverse: Issues In Higher Education.* https://www.diverseeducation.com/opinion/article/15109001/from-dei-to-jedi Accessed May 24, 2024.

Matloff ET. (2006) Becoming a daughter. *J Genetic Couns* 15(3):139–143. https://doi.org/10.1007/s10897-005-9012-5

McCarthy Veach P, LeRoy BS, & Callanan NP. (2018) *Facilitating the Genetic Counseling Process: Practice-Based Skills* Second edition, Cham: Springer International Publishing. https://doi.org/10.1007/9783319747996

Murphy B & Dillon C. (2007) *Interviewing in Action in a Multicultural World* Third edition, Belmont, CA: Brookes Cole/Cengage Learning.

Murray B, Tichnell C, Burch AE, et al. (2022) Strength of the genetic counselor: patient relationship is associated with extent of increased empowerment in patients with arrhythmogenic cardiomyopathy. *J Genet Couns* 31(2):388–397. https://doi.org/10.1002/jgc4.1499

Ota Wang V. (2001) Multicultural genetic counseling: then, now, and in the 21st century. *Am J Med Genet* 106(3):208–215. https://doi.org/10.1002/ajmg.10009

Patton Davis L & Museus S. (2019, July 26). Identifying and disrupting deficit thinking. *Spark: Elevating Scholarship on Social Issues.* https://medium.com/national-center-for-institutional-diversity/identifying-and-disrupting-deficit-thinking-cbc6da326995

Pierce CM. (1969). Is bigotry the basis of the medical problems of the ghetto? In: JC Norman (Ed., *Medicine in the Ghetto* (pp. 301–312), New York, NY: Meredith Corporation.

Pierce CM, Carew JV, Pierce-Gonzalez D, & Wills D. (1977) An experiment in racism: tv commercials. *Educ Urban Soc* 10(1):61–87. https://doi.org/10.1177/001312457701000105

Redlinger-Grosse K. (2020) Countertransference. In: Bonnie S LeRoy, Patricia M Veach, & Nancy P Callanan (Eds.) Genetic Counseling Practice: Advanced Concepts and Skills *Second edition*, Hoboken, NJ: Wiley Blackwell. https://onlinelibrary.wiley.com/doi/abs/10.1002/9781119529873.ch8

Redlinger-Grosse K, Veach PM, LeRoy BS, & Zierhut H. (2017) Elaboration of the reciprocal-engagement model of genetic counseling practice: a qualitative investigation of goals and strategies. *J Genet Couns* 26(6):1372–1387. https://doi.org/10.1007/s10897-017-0114-7

Resta RG. (2020) Complicated shadows. In: Bonnie S LeRoy, Patricia M Veach, & Nancy P Callanan (Eds) Genetic Counseling Practice: Advanced Concepts and Skills Second edition, Hoboken, NJ: Wiley Blackwell. https://doi.org/10.1002/9781119529873.ch2

Resta RG. (2022, May 15) The power of symbols: the pedigree as a tool of conformity and oppression. *The DNA Exchange.* https://thednaexchange.com/2022/05/15/the-power-of-symbols-the-pedigree-as-a-tool-of-conformity-and-oppression/

Riddle L, Amendola LM, & Gilmore MJ. (2021) Development and early implementation of an Accessible, Relational, Inclusive and Actionable approach to genetic counseling: The ARIA model. *Patient Educ Couns* 104(5):969–978. https://doi.org/10.1016/j.pec.2020.12.017

Rolle L, Zayhowski K, Koeller D, et al. (2022) Transgender patients' perspectives on their cancer genetic counseling experiences. *J Genet Couns* 31(3):781–791. https://doi.org/10.1002/jgc4.1544

Sue DW, Capodilupo CM, Torino GC, et al. (2007) Racial microaggressions in everyday life: Implications for clinical practice. *Am Psychol* 62(4):271–286. https://doi.org/10.1037/0003-066X.62.4.271

Tatum BD. (1992). *Talking about Race, Learning about Racism: The Application of Racial Identity Development Theory in the Classroom.* https://equity.ucla.edu/wp-content/uploads/2017/01/Tatum-Talking-About-Race.pdf Accessed May 24, 2024.

Tervalon M & Murray-García J. (1998) Cultural humility versus cultural competence: A critical distinction in defining physician training outcomes in multicultural education. *J Health Care Poor Underserved* 9(2):117–125. https://doi.org/10.1353/hpu.2010.0233

Vanneste R. (2012) How I learned that one mistake does not define me. *J Genet Couns* 21(2):235–236. https://doi.org/10.1007/s10897-011-9458-6

Veach PM, Bartels DM, & LeRoy BS. (2007) Coming full circle: a reciprocal-engagement model of genetic counseling practice. *J Genet Couns* 16(6):713–728. https://doi.org/10.1007/s10897-007-9113-4

von Vaupel-Klein AM & Walsh RJ. (2021) Considerations in genetic counseling of transgender patients: cultural competencies and altered disease risk profiles. *J Genet Couns* 30(1):98–109. https://doi.org/10.1002/jgc4.1372

Washington HA. (2006) *Medical Apartheid: The Dark History of Medical Experimentation on Black Americans from Colonial Times to the Present*, New York, NY: Doubleday.

Weil J. (2000) *Psychosocial Genetic Counseling*, Oxford: Oxford University Press.

Wheeler M, de Bourmont S, Paul-Emile K, et al. (2019) Physician and trainee experiences with patient bias. *JAMA Intern Med* 179(12):1678–1685. https://doi.org/10.1001/jamainternmed.2019.4122

Whiteness. (n.d.). National Museum of African American History and Cultur https://nmaahc.si.edu/learn/talking-about-race/topics/whiteness Accessed June 2, 2024.

Whitgob EE, Blankenburg RL, & Bogetz AL. (2016) The discriminatory patient and family: strategies to address discrimination towards trainees. *Acad Med* 91(11 Association of American Medical Colleges Learn Serve Lead: Proceedings of the 55th Annual Research in Medical Education Sessions), S64–S69. https://doi.org/10.1097/ACM.0000000000001357

Williams DR, Lawrence JA, & Davis BA. (2019) Racism and health: evidence and needed research. *Annu Rev Public Health* 40(1):105–125. https://doi.org/10.1146/annurev-publhealth-040218-043750

Woolsey C & Narruhn RA. (2018) A pedagogy of social justice for resilient/vulnerable populations: structural competency and bio-power. *Public Health Nurs (Boston, Mass.)*, 35(6):587–597. https://doi.org/10.1111/phn.12545

Zayhowski K, Koeller D, Giannetti Sferrazza L, et al. (2023, June 14) An Urgent Call for Genetics Organizations to Support Transgender and Intersex Communities. NSGC Perspectives.https://perspectives.nsgc.org/Article/an-urgent-call-for-genetics-organizations-to-support-transgender-and-intersex-communities Accessed May 24, 2024.

Zayhowski K & Sheridan CN. (2022, June 27) *Queer Erasure in Standards of Professionalism*. NSGC Perspectives. https://perspectives.nsgc.org/Article/queer-erasure-in-standards-of-professionalism Accessed May 24, 2024.

Yosso TJ. (2005) Whose culture has capital? A critical race theory discussion of community cultural wealth. *Race Ethnic and Educ* 8(1):69–91. https://doi.org/10.1080/1361332052000341006

3

Family History: An Essential Tool

Jane L. Schuette and Diane R. Koeller

INTRODUCTION

… as so often happens in medicine, new developments do not eclipse the tried-and-true method; instead, they give it new meaning and power.

(Guttmacher et al., 2004)

Genetic counseling is dependent on the gathering of accurate, detailed, and relevant information. The family history, which is essentially a compilation of information about the physical and mental health of an individual's family, is a fundamental component of this process. Obtaining a family history provides a basis for making a diagnosis, determining risk, offering appropriate genetic testing, interpreting genetic testing results, recommending medical management, and assessing the needs for patient education and psychosocial support. The family health history (FHH) is an essential component to assessment of a patient's risk for a wide variety of conditions, from rare Mendelian disorders to common multifactorial diseases. These include such varied health concerns as cardiovascular disease (Moonesinghe et al., 2019; Wang et al. 2023), colorectal cancer (Kastrinos et al., 2020), breast cancer (Brewer et al., 2017; Osman et al., 2022), ovarian cancer (Bethea et al., 2021), osteoporosis

A Guide to Genetic Counseling, Third Edition. Edited by Vivian Y. Pan, Jane L. Schuette, Karen E. Wain, and Beverly M. Yashar.
© 2025 John Wiley & Sons Ltd. Published 2025 by John Wiley & Sons Ltd.

(Yang et al., 2020), asthma (Bao et al., 2017), type 2 diabetes (Lascar et al., 2018), glaucoma (McMonnies, 2017), clotting disorders (Tsai and Battinelli, 2021), bipolar disorder (Antypa and Serretti 2014; Birmaher et al., 2022), and many others. It is therefore of utmost importance that genetic counselors possess the skills necessary to gather and record an accurate and relevant family history.

The pedigree is the diagram that records the family history information, the tool for converting information provided by the client and/or obtained from the medical record into a standardized format. It demonstrates the biological relationships of the client to family members using symbols, vertical and horizontal lines, and the presence and/or absence of disorders or traits through shading, color, hatching, and abbreviations. When complete, the pedigree stands as a quick and accurate visual record that assists in providing genetic counseling and disease risk assessment. An analysis of the pedigree reveals the number of family members affected or unaffected with a particular disease, condition, or trait, ages of family members (including at diagnosis or at death, if relevant), and may suggest the pattern of inheritance of a disorder within a family. Information that aids in making a diagnosis and about the natural history of a disorder and its variable expression among family members may be revealed in the pedigree. It offers a means for identifying family members at risk for being affected with a disorder as well as estimating risks for recurrence in future offspring. The pedigree may also indicate a history of other conditions for which an evaluation and/or genetic counseling are recommended.

The process of obtaining a family history and constructing a pedigree may reveal the social relationships of the client to family members. Information about adoption, divorce, separation, and estranged relatives may be obtained. Pregnancy loss, infertility, or death of family members is also recorded. The family history may provide information that suggests the extent of the medical, emotional, and social impact of a disorder for a family. Beliefs developed by family members, explaining who in the family is at risk and why, may be shared. And finally, when obtained at the beginning of the genetic counseling process, the family history can be a critical instrument for establishing a productive relationship with the patient and family.

This chapter reviews the components of gathering a family history and constructing a pedigree. In addition, opportunities for psychosocial assessment and patient education that present themselves during the process of taking a history are explored.

THE EVOLUTION OF THE PEDIGREE

Interest in family origins has existed for thousands of years as evidenced in many historical texts, including religious texts from Christianity, Judaism, Islam, and others. The pedigree, as a diagram using lines to connect an individual to their offspring, was developed in the fifteenth century as one of several techniques for illustrating ancestry (Resta, 1993). However, the use of the pedigree to demonstrate inheritance of traits is a more recent convention, dating back to the mid-nineteenth century, when the inheritance of color blindness was documented in a publication by Pliny Earle utilizing symbols (circles and squares) to represent the members of a family (Resta, 1993).

Throughout the history of the pedigree, a variety in styles and symbols has been commonplace, reflecting differences in individual preferences, professional training, and national styles. The representation of men and women as squares and circles, respectively, by American geneticists, and as the astronomical symbols for Mars and Venus by English geneticists, was one major difference in the use of symbols evident in the early twentieth century (Resta, 1993). In the 1990s, surveys of pedigrees recorded in clinical practice and in professional publications demonstrated extensive variation in the use of pedigree symbols and nomenclature. A survey of genetic counselors published in 1993 showed discrepancies even in common symbols such as those used to indicate pregnancy and miscarriage (Bennett et al., 1993). A review of medical genetic textbooks and human genetics journals also identified inconsistencies in the use of symbols (Steinhaus et al., 1995). Since the value of the family history in establishing an accurate diagnosis and risk assessment is diminished if symbols and abbreviations cannot be interpreted accurately, a Pedigree Standardization Task Force (PSTF) was formed in 1991 through the National Society of Genetic Counselors in conjunction with the Pacific Northwest Regional Genetics Group (PacNoRGG) and the Washington State Department of Health. Recommendations for standardized human pedigree nomenclature were developed and peer reviewed. These recommendations, which have helped to set a more universal standard, were published in the *American Journal of Human Genetics* (Bennett et al., 1995a) and the *Journal of Genetic Counseling* (Bennett et al., 1995b), and have been adopted internationally (Bennett et al., 2008). The National Society of Genetic Counselors (NSGC) adopted the following Standard Pedigree Symbol Position Statement in 2003:

> Standardized pedigree symbols offer a consistent method of recording and interpreting family history, increasing uniformity of medical information and enhancing quality control in clinical genetics, medicine, genetic education and research (NSGC, 2003).

In 2008, the task force (now called the Pedigree Standardization Work Group [PSWG]) established that their recommended nomenclature had become the only consistently acknowledged standard for constructing a family medical history (Bennett et al., 2008). Only minor changes to pedigree symbols were proposed at the time, including some guidance for documentation of transgender individuals. However, other organizations (such as the National Comprehensive Cancer Network [NCCN]) included different nomenclature for gender diverse individuals in their guidelines. Studies of genetic counselors indicated discrepancies in how transgender and gender diverse (TGD) individuals were documented on pedigrees

(Berro et al., 2019; Zayhowski et al. 2019; Sheehan et al., 2020). Interviews of TGD individuals also showed that community members largely preferred different nomenclature than that recommended by NSGC and NCCN (Barnes et al., 2020). In 2022, NSGC published a standardized pedigree nomenclature update centered on sex- and gender-inclusivity, which was created with input from genetic counselors and members of the TGD community (Bennett et al., 2022).

As the FHH and pedigree have evolved, they have become invaluable tools in research, public health, and personalized medicine. Historically, the pedigree was used to provide evidence for the establishment of the inheritance pattern of disorders and then as an essential component of linkage analysis, assisting in the identification of disease loci. It remains important for gene discovery and in the validation of gene/disease associations. In public health, FHH has been touted as the penultimate tool for screening the population at large for many preventable, chronic conditions (Khoury et al., 2016; Duke et al. 2021). An FHH reveals individuals who may benefit from health promotion, disease prevention strategies, increased medical surveillance, and/or genetic counseling and testing referral (Duke et al., 2021).

National recognition of the utility of FHH was exemplified by the US Surgeon General's Family History Initiative, which resulted in a free web-based tool, My Family Health Portrait. This collaborative effort involving multiple agencies, including the National Institutes of Health (NIH) and the Centers for Disease Control (CDC), was launched in 2004 to remind health professionals and patients about the value of family history and to make the process of collecting and analyzing data easier for health professionals and individuals. The tool organizes family history information and generates a pedigree and a report, which people are encouraged to bring to their health care provider for further discussion and action. In the US, Thanksgiving has also been declared National Family History Day to encourage families to share health information with one another.

Despite the increased appreciation of the importance of FHH, it remains underutilized. The National Human Genome Research Institute (NHGRI) Family Health History Group, an open-membership community of professionals, scientists, and clinicians, was created to help identify implementation gaps in FHH collection and suggest solutions. Identified gaps included lack of patient knowledge and appreciation of family history value, lack of provider knowledge of family history collection and usage, lack of workforce optimization, limited effectiveness of digital tools and interoperability within and among electronic health records (EHRs), and limited health care administration policies that facilitate family history collection. Proposed strategies to address these gaps include education for patients and providers, modernized FHH tools that are compatible with modern smart devices and EHRs, and increased numbers of geneticists and genetic counselors in clinical care (Wildin et al., 2021).

According to the NSGC Position Statement on Family Health History:

> The National Society of Genetic Counselors (NSGC) recommends that patients and their healthcare practitioners jointly collect family health history (FHH) to facilitate comprehensive risk assessment for routine and specialty care. In addition, NSGC supports standards to integrate appropriate FHH information into the patient's electronic health record (EHR), including information about first-, second-, and third-degree relatives. EHRs must have the capacity to adapt to ongoing genetic and technological advancements as they relate to collecting FHH. Relatives' genetic test results and other pertinent medical records should be reviewed and documented in accordance with all relevant federal, state, and local privacy laws and guidelines (NSGC, 2023).

Clearly, the family history and pedigree are firmly established as vital for the evaluation, risk assessment, and genetic counseling of a patient in whom a genetic disease is suspected. Furthermore, FHH has remained indispensable as genomic testing has become standard practice, since results are interpreted in the context of clinical data. The collection and analysis of a comprehensive family history contributes to the complex analysis of genomic sequencing results and facilitates the identification of variants of interest. Inheritance from an affected versus unaffected parent and/or the recognition that similarly affected siblings (or other family members) share variant(s) of interest contribute to variant classification by providing segregation data, an important component of assessing the potential for a causal relationship between variant and disease. This essential tool has remained critically relevant, even as genomic sequencing technology has evolved.

FAMILY HISTORY BASICS

The family pedigree is one of the most powerful tools of a genetic counselor. It serves not only as a history-taking tool to record biological relationships and facts, but also as a sociological aid in counseling by serving as a record of family social relationships.

(Bennett et al., 1993)

A family history should be obtained from all clients seeking genetic evaluation and/or counseling to facilitate comprehensive risk assessment for routine and specialty care (NSGC, 2023). The information obtained, whether positive or negative, affects patient care; therefore, the quality and accuracy of the information is critical. Guidelines for obtaining a family history and constructing a pedigree were developed by experienced genetic counselors to prevent inaccurate interpretation of patient and family medical and genetic information and to improve the quality of patient care provided by genetic professionals (Bennett et al., 1995a, 2008, 2022). This includes the construction of at least a standard three-generation pedigree, containing information on the client, the client's first-degree relatives (children, siblings, and parents), second-degree relatives (half-siblings, aunts, uncles, nieces, nephews, grandparents, and grandchildren), and ideally third-degree relatives (first cousins).

The pedigree usually begins with the individual for whom an evaluation is being performed or for whom genetic counseling is being provided. The consultand (or client) is the individual(s) seeking genetic evaluation, counseling, or testing, usually due to the presence of a positive personal and/or family health history. "Proband" is the term that designates the family member who brings the family to medical attention (Bennett et al., 1995a, 1995c; Marazita, 1995). Consultand and proband may be the same person, and there may be more than one consultand seeking genetic services.

The nature of the referral or reason for the visit provides a focus for the process of obtaining a family history. Is this a referral for genetic counseling because of a family history of a particular disorder? Is this a diagnostic evaluation, and if so, for what reason? Or is this a reproductive genetics consultation, and if so, for what indication? During a diagnostic evaluation prompted by findings suggesting a diagnosis of a particular disorder, such as neurofibromatosis type I (NF1) for example, the counselor would obtain a three-generation pedigree that includes a series of focused questions about the presence of symptoms and signs of the disorder (in this case, NF1), especially in first-degree family members. This information is important to the patient's evaluation, because the presence of a first-degree family member is one of the criteria considered in establishing a diagnosis of NF1 (Gutmann et al., 1997). This example of a *targeted* family history includes questioning seeking evidence in support of and/or opposed to a particular diagnosis. Essentially all family histories are targeted, based on the indication for the genetics evaluation. A targeted family history relies on the specificity of the indication for the evaluation and the degree of confidence given to the diagnosis provided. For example, a referral for a family history of intellectual disability is relatively nonspecific, whereas a referral for a family history of tuberous sclerosis complex (TSC) is very definitive.

Inquiring about the presence of physical features associated with a particular diagnosis is important when obtaining a family history; this may help to establish a diagnosis and potentially affected family members may be identified. In the case of tuberous sclerosis, asking about a history of seizures and learning disabilities, problems associated with TSC, may indicate a family member who is also affected. Or, if the indication for the visit is a history of fetal loss, the counselor would not only inquire about a family history of fetal loss, but also about infant death, infertility, intellectual disability, and congenital disabilities in extended family members, seeking clues about the possibility of an inherited chromosome rearrangement, X-linked condition associated with male lethality, or other inherited conditions.

In many settings, general questions about FHH are asked regardless of indication, as this may help identify hereditary concerns beyond the presenting purpose for the appointment. During a preconception consultation for two carriers of cystic fibrosis (CF), for example, the counselor may obtain FHH that includes additional pertinent history requiring discussion and/or that may impact counseling and risk assessment. Typically, more general questions might include the following: Are there any individuals in your family with intellectual disability, congenital anomalies, inherited disorders, or chronic disease? Is there any history of stillbirth, multiple pregnancy loss, or infant death? These general questions should be asked when obtaining any FHH in the clinical genetics setting, while more specific and focused questions depend on the reason for genetic evaluation and counseling.

Traditionally, family history data is obtained and the pedigree is drawn in the presence of the client(s) whether virtually or in person, for example, telemedicine or in a clinic setting. The family history should be obtained in an environment that is comfortable and free of distractions. It should also be obtained in a setting that preserves confidentiality. The family history can be obtained at any point during the initial genetic counseling visit, although it is often acquired early in the visit as it can help inform risk assessment and counseling, while also establishing rapport with the client. In some instances, it may be deferred until the end of the visit or even until the time of a follow-up appointment. This may be the case when counseling issues are more emergent, such as in a newly established diagnosis in a newborn or abnormal ultrasound findings in an ongoing pregnancy.

Alternative methods to the traditional face-to-face collection of FHH are often used to save time and for enabling case preparation on the part of the genetic counselor as well as the client. Methods include a family history questionnaire sent to patients in advance of their appointment electronically or by mail, phone interview, and/or completion of a questionnaire on an electronic device handed to the patient immediately prior to the start of the in-clinic visit. Pedigrees are then drawn by hand or created using various software programs using the data submitted by the client. This may include the generation of a "pedigree skeleton," which may be completed at the time of the in person or virtual appointment. Clinical practices often employ genetic counselor assistants (GCAs) or train other staff members to assist with this task. For example, when there is a history of cancer in a close family member, it may be of particular importance to obtain medical records pertaining to the cancer diagnosis in order to provide the client with an accurate risk assessment. If done in advance, the initial appointment may be more productive.

The acquisition of family history during genetic counseling can be an opportunity for the counselor to make important observations, obtain psychosocial information from the client, and set the stage for a relationship of trust. Complex relationships, consanguinity, a history of multiple partners, pregnancy loss, or an unexpected death may not be accurately captured by a family history questionnaire and may more likely be revealed in person. In person discussion affords the opportunity to explain why such information may have relevance to the patient's evaluation. For example, patients may not be inclined toward, or even consider, including information about spontaneous pregnancy loss unless specifically prompted. Furthermore, the family history and pedigree are often more accurate when the client is present during its construction (McGrath and Edwards, 2009); in fact, the details of a family history obtained through a questionnaire or phone interview may need to be confirmed with the client in person (Conway-Pearson et al., 2016). A study comparing over 1,000 pedigrees pre-genetic counseling (completed online by patients) and post-genetic counseling (updated by genetic counselors during a visit) found that reviewing family history with the genetic counselor impacted eligibility for testing for 9% of clients (Vanderwall et al., 2022). Another study found that a family history of seizures is reasonably accurate for siblings and offspring, but is underreported in parents, and therefore careful questioning may be needed to facilitate recall (Ottman et al., 2011).

A pedigree is part of a client's medical record. Pedigrees can be drawn using paper or preprinted forms designated by the institution for inclusion in the medical record. Stencils for pedigree construction and symbols are available, although some genetic counselors find their use to be awkward, preferring instead to construct the pedigree freehand. Pedigrees can also be generated via software programs and either printed for scanning into the EHR or incorporated directly into the record digitally. Many EHRs also have embedded pedigree tools. If hand drawn pedigrees are scanned into the EHR, they should be drawn using dark ink to improve legibility. Taking a pedigree in pencil can sometimes be useful, especially for the novice, but it should then be redrawn in ink or in a pedigree software program.

GATHERING THE INFORMATION AND CONSTRUCTING A PEDIGREE

Gathering the family history and constructing a pedigree is a process best conducted in a step-by-step fashion. Standardized symbols and nomenclature should be used as they offer a consistent method of recording and interpreting family history information. NSGC endorses the use of standardized pedigree symbols and lines depicted in the Human Pedigree Nomenclature Practice Guidelines (Bennett et al., 2008, 2022), both in clinical practice and in medical/scientific publications.

Overview of Pedigree Construction and Standard Symbols

Some of the commonly used pedigree symbols are summarized in Table 3-1. It is important to distinguish between gender and sex when determining appropriate symbol use. Sex is a category assigned at birth based on biological attributes such as the appearance of external genitalia and/or sex chromosome status. Gender is a social construct of norms, roles, behaviors, and identities of men, women, boys,

TABLE 3-1. Common pedigree symbols

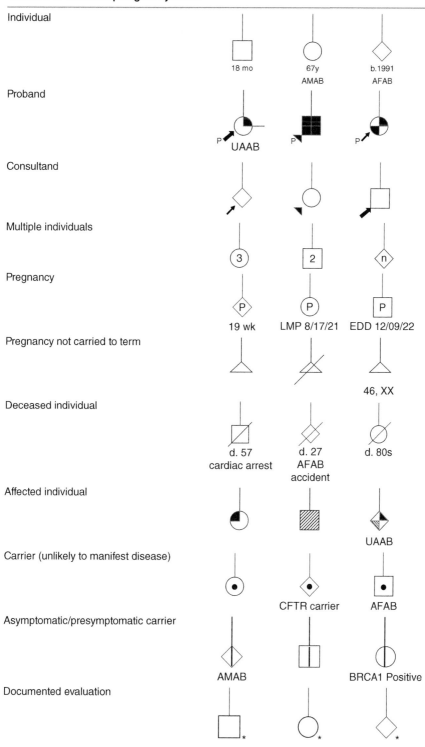

Individual	18 mo	67y AMAB	b.1991 AFAB
Proband	UAAB	P	P
Consultand			
Multiple individuals	3	2	n
Pregnancy	P 19 wk	P LMP 8/17/21	P EDD 12/09/22
Pregnancy not carried to term			46, XX
Deceased individual	d. 57 cardiac arrest	d. 27 AFAB accident	d. 80s
Affected individual			UAAB
Carrier (unlikely to manifest disease)		CFTR carrier	AFAB
Asymptomatic/presymptomatic carrier	AMAB		BRCA1 Positive
Documented evaluation	*	*	*

Adapted from Bennett et al., 2022.

girls, and gender diverse people. Both sex and gender exist on a spectrum and are not binary. Symbols on a pedigree are used to represent gender. A man is designated by a square, a woman is designated by a circle, and a nonbinary person or individual whose gender is not specified is designated by a diamond. For transgender or gender diverse individuals, the symbol used should represent their gender identity with their sex assigned at birth noted below the symbol. For example, a transgender man would be denoted as a square with "AFAB" for "assigned female at birth" noted underneath. For intersex individuals, "UAAB" for "unassigned at birth" can be used under their gender symbol. In cases where gender identity has not been expressed (i.e., children under age 2–3 years, pregnancies, and still-births) the symbol can be used to represent sex (square for male sex, circle for female sex, diamond for unassigned sex).

The proband or consultand is identified with an arrow (Table 3-1); the proband is distinguished from the consultand using the letter P next to the symbol. It is extremely important to identify the consultand; otherwise, someone looking at a large pedigree may be unable to determine to whom the pedigree pertains.

A number placed inside a symbol is an indication of how many people of a particular gender are in a sibship. For example, a square with a 5 inside means five men. An "n" can be used inside a symbol to indicate an unknown number of individuals (Table 3-1).

A pregnancy is symbolized by a "P" inside a square or a circle if fetal sex is known or inside a diamond if unknown or intersex. The "age" of the pregnancy is recorded by listing the first day of the last menstrual period (LMP), gestational age (e.g., 20 wk), or estimated date of delivery (EDD). Triangles represent pregnancies not carried to term; that is, miscarriages or elective terminations (a diagonal line may be drawn through the symbol to represent an elective termination). If the sex of a fetal demise is known, the chromosome complement (e.g., 46, XY) and/or the sex should be written below the symbol (Table 3-1).

A diagonal line drawn through a symbol indicates that the person represented is deceased (Table 3-1). This is a visual way of recording who is alive or deceased on a pedigree. It is worth noting that some clients may find it offensive or psychologically challenging to have a deceased relative crossed off when a genetic counselor is recording the pedigree in their presence, and therefore the diagonal line can easily be added when the client is not present or after the patient visit.

A shaded symbol indicates an individual affected with a condition that is known or suspected to be genetic (Table 3-1). More than one condition can be shown by partitioning the symbol into three or four sectors and filling in the sectors using different patterns or colors. Be careful if using different colors via a pedigree software tool and printing in black and white as some details may be lost. For colors and shading, aim to make them high contrast so they are accessible to those with diminished contrast sensitivity and use a color palette that is accessible to those with colorblindness. As long as shading, colors, and/or sectors are defined in a key, any designation can be used. Even when standardized pedigree symbols are used, it may be essential to include a key (also called a legend). The key provides information that is vital to interpreting the pedigree, including less commonly used symbols (e.g., adoption) as well as the unique symbols used to represent the presence of conditions and/or traits in family members.

A carrier who is unlikely to manifest a disease, such as a person who is heterozygous for a pathogenic variant in a gene associated with autosomal recessive disease, is denoted with a dot inside the individual symbol. A person who is currently unaffected but could later manifest disease, such as a cancer-free person who is heterozygous for a *BRCA2* pathogenic variant and has a risk of developing a *BRCA2*-related cancer in the future, is denoted with a vertical line through the individual symbol (Figure 3-1).

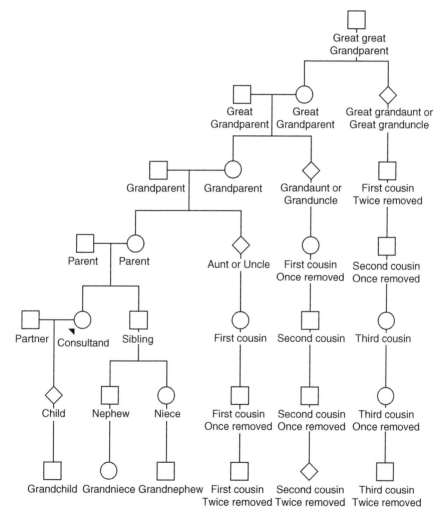

Relationships are all in relation to the Consultand (indicated with an arrow).

FIGURE 3-1. *Relationships*

When the pedigree is being constructed, information about affected status that has not been documented (e.g., diagnoses reported by the client) should be distinguished from a diagnosis that was established by an examination, laboratory study, and/or a review of medical records. A diagnosis documented by an evaluation is indicated by an asterisk (*) (Table 3-1).

There are four "line definitions" to orient generations within a pedigree (Table 3-2) (Bennett et al., 2008). A **relationship line** connects two partners. A break in the relationship line (a double slash) indicates the relationship no longer exists. The **line of descent** extends vertically (or sometimes diagonally if there are space constraints) from the relationship line (or an individual) and connects to an individual (who does not have siblings) or to the horizontal **sibship line**. Each sibling (including each pregnancy, whether or not it is carried to term or results in a live birth) is attached to the sibship line by an **individual's line**.

If a person has had children with multiple reproductive partners, it is not always necessary to show each partner, especially if such information is not relevant to the family history. For example, a line of descent can extend directly from a parent without including the partner (Table 3-2).

Twins share the same line of descent but have different individual lines. If twins are known to be monozygotic, a horizontal line is drawn above the symbols (not between the symbols, since that would indicate a relationship line) (Table 3-2).

When obtaining a family history from a client who is adopted out of their biological family, it is essential to distinguish between the adoptive (nonbiological family) and the biological or birth family. In either situation, brackets are placed around the symbol for the adopted individual. If the nonbiological parents are included, a dotted line of descent is used. Otherwise, a solid line of descent is used, just as for any other biological relationship (Table 3-2).

A line of descent with a single horizontal line at the bottom indicates that an individual or pair do not have children. If they do not have children due to elective sterilization, such as tubal ligation, this can be documented below the lines. A line of descent with double horizontal lines at the bottom indicates infertility. If the cause of the infertility is known (such as endometriosis), it can be documented below the lines (Table 3-2).

A double horizontal relationship line is drawn to represent a consanguineous (biologically related) couple. If the degree of relationship is not obvious from the pedigree (e.g., third cousins), it should be indicated above the relationship line (Table 3-2).

The need to represent pregnancies conceived through assisted reproductive technology (ART), such as artificial insemination by donor, is common. The conventions for symbolizing the biological and social relationships involved in ART within a pedigree are outlined in Table 3-3. Some general rules include placing a "D" inside the symbol for the egg or sperm donor. An "S" inside the gender symbol denotes a surrogate (gestational carrier). If this individual is both the ovum donor and a surrogate, they are referred to only as a donor (in the interest of genetic assessment). The pregnancy is placed directly below the individual

TABLE 3-2. **Common pedigree lines**

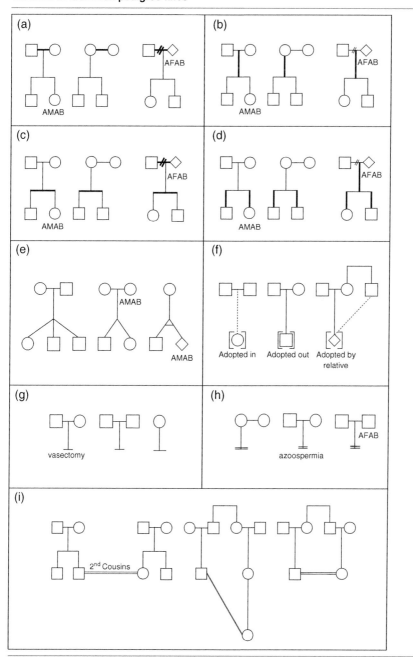

a) Relationship line; b) Line of descent; c) Sibship line; d) Individuals' line; e) Twins, triplets, etc.; f) Adoption; g) No children; h) Infertility; i) Consanguinity
Adapted from Bennett et al., 2008.

TABLE 3-3. Assisted reproductive technologies (ART): symbols and lines

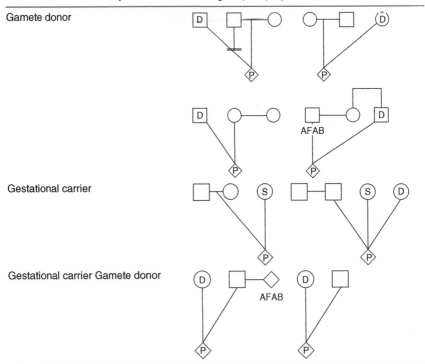

D = Gamete (sperm or egg) donor; S = Surrogate (gestational) carrier; P = Pregnancy (placed below pregnant person)
Adapted from Bennett et al., 2022.

carrying the pregnancy with a connecting line of descent. The relationship line is between the partners who will be parenting the future child (regardless of sexual orientation or gender). No relationship line is needed for individuals who will be parenting the future child without a partner. By using these rules, any method of ART can be clearly illustrated (Bennett et al., 2022) (Table 3-3). Documenting elective sterilization (e.g., tubal ligation or vasectomy) is useful as a factor when assessing risks for recurrence (Table 3-2).

The Standard Information Recorded on the Pedigree

The counselor should aim to record ages and/or year of birth of the client and family members (especially first-degree relatives) on the pedigree, below the symbol or to the right, if necessary, regardless of whether these individuals are reported to be affected or unaffected with a disorder. The age reached by an apparently unaffected family member may have important implications not only for that particular family member but for the client as well. For individuals reported to be affected with a particular disorder, the age of onset or age at diagnosis should be obtained. This is particularly important for many adult-onset conditions. For example, a client whose maternal grandmother and maternal aunt developed breast cancer before menopause may be at greater risk for breast cancer than the general population. A client whose mother was reported to be unaffected with cancer at age 65, however, may have a similar lifetime risk of breast cancer to that of the general population.

The units used to measure ages should be included after each number using standard abbreviations (e.g., 35 y (years), 4 mo (months), 20 wk (weeks), 3 dy (days)). It is important to note that the ability of clients to recall dates of birth or ages is variable, especially with respect to information on extended family members. Unless precise information is required, the counselor may wish to encourage the client to provide close estimates by asking, for instance, whether the family member is in their 50s, 60s, or 70s (although some pedigree drawing software tools do not allow input of ranges or imprecise ages). It also may not always be necessary to collect ages of all family members, if not useful for the risk assessment or counseling.

The health status of the client and each family member (or pregnancy) needs to be recorded succinctly. This includes information about the presence of congenital anomalies, developmental delay, intellectual disability, inherited disorders, mental health, cancer diagnoses, and chronic illness. Specific and accurate information is best. For example, if a family member is reported to be affected with "muscular dystrophy," the type of muscular dystrophy should be specified if possible. In most circumstances, if a family member at age 70 is reported to have had "heart problems requiring medication, multiple hospitalizations, and triple bypass surgery," it is adequate to record coronary artery disease or heart disease. The type of information recorded may differ depending on the reason for referral or specialty of the provider recording the pedigree. For instance, a genetic counselor in a cancer clinic may elect not to collect or record information about intellectual disability or heart disease, if it would not impact the cancer risk assessment.

Although information recorded on a pedigree should not be too wordy, the use of multiple abbreviations can be confusing. For example, "CP" may be an abbreviation for cleft palate or cerebral palsy, and "ASD" is used for autism spectrum disorder as well as atrial septal defect. If abbreviations are used, they may need to be defined in a key.

If a family member is deceased, the cause and age at death are recorded on the pedigree. It may also be important to inquire whether any family members, especially first-degree relatives, had pregnancies that resulted in miscarriages, stillbirths, or infant deaths. Often clients will omit information about unsuccessful pregnancies, as well as data on siblings and other relatives who are not living or who died at or around the time of birth. It is also important to distinguish whether individuals who have no children have remained childless by choice or because of a known biological reason (infertility).

It is helpful to include the name and professional background (e.g., MS, RN, MD) of the person who recorded the pedigree. It is also important to identify the historian, the person providing the family history information. Information about extended family may be subject to questions of accuracy if provided by someone other than a close biological relative. Recording the date the pedigree was obtained or updated is also relevant, particularly if the pedigree includes ages of family members instead of dates of birth.

The Pedigree Standardization Work Group has recommended that the indication for obtaining the family history be recorded on the pedigree; for example, "cancer risk assessment," abnormal ultrasound" (Bennett et al., 2008). This will serve to clarify the purpose, relation, and significance of the information reported.

The Step-by-Step Process

The counselor may wish to begin by providing a brief explanation to the client about the purpose and process of gathering the family history information. The counselor then asks sequential questions while, at the same time, drawing the pedigree. Usually, the counselor begins with drawing the client (the consultand) on the pedigree and obtaining the information described above (e.g., health status, age). If the client is an adult and has a partner, the partner may also be placed on the pedigree at this point, which helps with the positioning of the pedigree appropriately on the paper or form (usually in the center).

During questioning, use language and terms that are likely to be familiar to your patient or client and, in turn, listen to the language and terms that your client uses. This will help to assess an individual's ability to receive and communicate health information. It is appropriate to use medical terminology if it is clearly understood by your patient. However, be prepared to use plain, concise language or descriptive terms to facilitate comprehension; that is, ask about the presence of muscle weakness rather than a myopathy. Consider that your patient may not recall the medical history of all family members; asking about hospitalizations and/or surgery history for key family members may help to facilitate recall. Also consider the way your questions are formulated. Rather than leading your client with a question like, "Your siblings are in good health, right?" Ask instead, "Do your siblings have any health problems?" If obtaining a family history focused on a particular disease type, more specific questions can be asked, such as "Do your siblings have any history of heart disease?" It is also courteous and compassionate to acknowledge recent events such as miscarriage, the death of a close family member, or a recent serious diagnosis, if the acknowledgement is authentic and genuine (Bennett, 2010).

It may be easiest to obtain family history information beginning with the proband and proceeding through the family members, recording the standard information for each, in a systematic order that makes it easy for the patient to follow. The counselor guides the client by proceeding through each first-degree relative, usually by first asking whether the client has had children and/or pregnancies. When hand drawing a pedigree, it is easier to obtain information on the children before finding out about any siblings, simply because of the practical consideration that offspring are drawn on the pedigree on a line below the client. (If a child is the patient, it is usually easier to obtain information on their siblings before information is requested on the parents.) Whether all pregnancies were conceived with the same partner and whether all siblings within a sibship have the same biological parents should be ascertained consistently. Otherwise, such information may not be revealed or could be learned after the pedigree is complete, causing legibility concerns due to corrections. The counselor needs to indicate on the pedigree any pregnancies conceived with different partner(s) or any siblings who have a different biological parent, if relevant to the present indication.

The counselor may then ask whether the client has siblings and whether such siblings have had any children or pregnancies; if so, information about their ages and health is elicited. The counselor can next inquire about the client's biological parents (whether living or deceased; their physical and mental health status), continuing through each family member until a three-generation pedigree has been constructed. When constructing a pedigree for adult-onset disorders, two generations of ascent (parents and grandparents) and two generations of descent (children and grandchildren) should be included.

It is important to obtain both parents' sides of a family history, even if the visit is for risk assessment and counseling regarding a history of a particular disorder on one side of the family. A complete family history allows the counselor to determine whether there are additional factors that may influence risk assessment and avoids any unintentional assignment of blame by focusing on only one side of the family. Often, additional risks are identified while obtaining a family history, necessitating discussion and/or evaluation (Venne and Scheuner 2015; Orlando et al. 2020; Vance 2020). A question mark may be placed above the line of descent in instances in which little is known about the family history to indicate the appropriate inquiries were made.

A three-generation pedigree is usually adequate and is considered standard. Error rates in diagnosis, in age at diagnosis, even in the existence of relatives increase as the degree of relationship increases (Murff et al., 2004; Flint et al. 2021). For many common diseases, having an affected close relative is the strongest predictor of an individual's lifetime risk for developing disease (Walter and Emery, 2006). This is true for most single gene disorders as well, although at times, especially for conditions with reduced penetrance and variable expressivity, information on extended family members may be useful. For example, a family history obtained for a patient in whom physical findings suggest the diagnosis of Marfan syndrome may include pertinent information beyond three generations. A positive history of sudden death in early adulthood in one or more distant family members may contribute toward the establishment of a diagnosis.

When the pedigree appears complete, many counselors ask a series of general questions about the presence of congenital anomalies, intellectual disability, and inherited disorders. More specific questions about the existence of associated anomalies or specific signs and symptoms may be asked when warranted, as in a targeted family history. This effort may seem redundant, but often clients recall additional important information after the pedigree has been completed, especially if the counselor makes a final extra attempt to elicit such recollections.

Ancestry

Obtaining family history has traditionally included inquiring about ancestry for purposes of patient care, establishing a differential diagnosis and/or for risk assessment based on consideration of disorders known to occur at a higher frequency within a particular ancestral group. Such information may impact testing recommendations and test selection (Daly et al., 2020). In previous editions of this text, the term ethnic background, rather than ancestry, was used; however, ethnicity, like race, is a social, not biological, construct. Furthermore, self-reported race and ethnicity are often poor predictors of genetic ancestry, particularly in populations with high rates of admixture, such as African American and Latino populations (Lee et al. 2010; Mersha and Abebe 2015). Using self-reported ancestry information to make diagnostic or testing decisions can reduce the clinical sensitivity and specificity of tests for admixed populations and widen health disparities. Increasingly, pan-ethnic genetic tests (such as expanded carrier screening in prenatal/preconception genetics and multigene panel testing in cancer genetics) are used instead of smaller, more targeted tests. In cases where ancestry would not impact whether a person meets criteria for testing or what test is to be ordered, it may not need to be asked.

If ancestry information is needed, it may be necessary to briefly explain the purpose for making the inquiry as having potential implications for the diagnostic evaluation, testing recommendations, and/or risk assessment. For instance, information about Ashkenazi Jewish ancestry is often needed in cancer risk assessments to determine whether an individual meets testing and/or insurance coverage criteria for *BRCA1* and *BRCA2*. A counselor performing a risk assessment for *BRCA1* and *BRCA2* could say "Some inherited cancer risks are more common in individuals of Ashkenazi Jewish ancestry. Do you know if there is any Ashkenazi Jewish ancestry in your family?" The question about ancestry should be posed in a manner that is clear to the client(s). Consider using alternative words or phrases such as "country of origin" or ask specifically about a particular ancestral group to ensure that clients thoroughly understand what information is being sought.

Gender Inclusivity

Gender diversity should be acknowledged and respected while collecting a family history. When discussing a pedigree with a client, a counselor can explain how different symbols are used to depict different genders—squares for men, circles for women, and diamonds for nonbinary individuals. Genetic counselors should avoid the use of binary gender language when possible. For instance, rather than asking how many brothers and sisters a client has, a counselor can ask how many siblings they have and then ask about each of their genders.

Genetic counselors should also avoid making assumptions about what pronouns a person uses or what organs they were born with based on their gender. For instance, if a cancer genetic counselor asks whether any women in the family have had ovarian cancer, a client may not inform them of a transgender uncle who had ovarian cancer.

While all pedigrees should aim to accurately reflect gender for all family members, it is not always necessary to inquire about sex assigned at birth. Transgender and gender diverse individuals face significant disparities and threats to their safety within and outside of health care. If it is not clinically relevant, a counselor does not need to inquire about sex assigned at birth for all relatives. For instance, this information would be unlikely to impact a risk assessment for familial adenomatous polyposis and is therefore unnecessary.

To ensure that gender diverse individuals are accurately represented on the pedigree, counselors can either preface the pedigree with the information they're looking for or check in at the end of the pedigree. Suggested approaches for checking in include: "Is there anyone in your family who identifies as transgender?" or "Is there anyone in your family who has a different gender identity than the sex they were assigned at birth?" (Barnes et al., 2020).

Consanguinity

Reproduction between people who share a common ancestor(s) is more common in certain populations due to multiple factors including culture, geography, gamete donation, and religion. Globally, consanguineous couples (second cousins or closer in relation) and their offspring account for over 10% of the population, with the highest rates of consanguineous marriage occurring in north and sub-Saharan Africa, the Middle East, and West, Central, and South Asia, with the countries of Pakistan and India having the highest (Bittles and Black, 2010). Some highly consanguineous populations include successive generations of unions between relatives with complex consanguinity loops (Bhinder et al., 2019).

The presence of consanguinity in the family history may have relevance for the genetic evaluation, the differential diagnosis, or counseling visit. If the biological parents of a patient for whom an evaluation is being performed, or if parents of an ongoing pregnancy in which abnormal fetal findings are identified, share a common ancestor, then greater consideration may be given to the possibility of an autosomal recessive disorder. However, when inquiring about consanguinity the counselor may need to explain the reason for the question and use terms that are likely familiar to the patient: "Are your families related to one another? Do you share any common ancestors? Are you and your partner blood relatives? Is there any chance that you and your partner are related to one another other than by marriage?"

It is also important to note that clients sometimes describe biological relationships inaccurately, and therefore the counselor should carefully establish the exact nature of every relationship that is a potential source of ambiguity. For example, sometimes the term second cousin is used to describe a family member who is actually a first cousin-once removed (see Figure 3-1). Additionally, the concept of family may be more about social rather than biological relationships depending on the client's cultural practice as well as changes in the postmodern family, such as blended families, adoption, assisted reproductive technology. Clients' definitions of family and descriptions of their relationships may include nonbiological individuals due to their social ties (McGrath and Edwards, 2009). Tracing the exact nature of relatedness with the client will often clarify the degree of relationship.

Adoption

People who are separated from their birth parents, orphaned, and/or adopted may feel frustrated when entering the genetics realm, which often begins with the collection of family history information; some have even sought genetic counseling and testing because of their anxiety surrounding their lack of knowledge about their biological family's medical background. Increasingly, people with limited information about one or both sides of their biological family are seeking direct-to-consumer testing to connect with biological relatives and learn more about potential health risks. However, the availability of DNA testing does not obviate the usefulness of a family history, because testing is often performed and interpreted within the context of established risk factors.

Recognition of the importance of family history, including known medical history of the adoptee and their biological parents, has resulted in legislation to require the collection and disclosure of non-identifying social, medical, and psychological information in many states (Venne et al., 2003). As of 2019, all US states have provisions in statutes that allow access to nonidentifying information to adoptive parents or guardians of minors and almost all states allow access to nonidentifying information to adult adoptees. The benefits of genetic testing for adopted minors needs to be balanced against the risks of stigmatization and discrimination. The American Society of Human Genetics (ASHG) and the American College of Medical Genetics (ACMG) states that genetic testing in the adoption process should be "(1) consistent with preventive and diagnostic tests performed on all children of a similar age, (2) generally limited to testing for medical conditions that manifest themselves during childhood or for which preventive measures or therapies may be undertaken during childhood, and (3) not used to detect genetic variations within the normal range" (The American Society of Human Genetics Social Issues Committee and The American College of Medical Genetics Social Ethical and Legal Issues Committee 2000). There is no uniformity in the extent and type of medical and family history information collected at the time of adoption or mechanisms to confirm the validity of the information (Bennett, 2010). There may be little information of value known by the birth parent(s) and/or collected by the adoption intermediaries. The ages of biological parents may be such that later onset diseases in the birth parents and relatives may not be apparent, and there is often no mechanism for updating information on the health status of relatives. Genetic counselors should familiarize themselves with laws regarding the collection and disclosure of information in the states where they practice to assist their adopted clients and their families with obtaining family history information. Additional information can be found at childwelfare.gov.

Efficiency and Time Constraints

Obtaining FHH can be a lengthy undertaking, especially in instances of large, extended families, multiple affected individuals, or numerous disorders or health problems. If the client is an enthusiastic participant with an affinity for details or storytelling, the completion of this task could potentially occupy most of the time allotted for the clinic visit. Although no short-cut will be able to elicit equivalent information, there are several tips to consider for streamlining this process.

1. **Be prepared**. This refers to some of the first considerations when obtaining a family history: the who and what. The counselor needs to be prepared for each case.
2. **Prepare the client**. Explain the purpose of obtaining a family history to the client and clearly indicate the kind of information needed. This will assist the client in reporting relevant data.
3. **Control the process; keep the client focused**. The counselor may need to provide guidance to the client and refocus questioning as needed. The counselor should ask direct, clear, and specific questions.
4. **Be aware of time**. It can be helpful to communicate time constraints to a client at the start or throughout the visit if family history collection is taking more time than is available.
5. **Listen**. Listening is a complex skill, and it must be done efficiently in a multitasking environment: the counselor must listen attentively while simultaneously drawing an accurate pedigree, framing directed questions, sorting through family history data, and interpreting information. Listening requires attending to all communication, including spoken language and visual methods, such as sign language. Listening carefully is important for accuracy. Sometimes clients provide relevant family history information during contracting or other parts of the visit. Remembering these details during family history collection will help with efficiency and rapport building as the client will not have to repeat previously communicated information and may feel heard.
6. **Be aware of accuracy issues**. The counselor needs to develop the ability to quickly assess what information is relevant, what information is suspect, and what information is likely to be inaccurate. The more distant a family member, the more likely the medical information provided about them is

unreliable. For example, a report of a second cousin having intellectual disability as a result of birth trauma should not be taken as a definitive diagnosis. Refer to further accuracy concerns below.

7. **For the novice: Practice!** Many genetic counseling students acquire facility in obtaining family histories and constructing pedigrees by practicing with friends and fellow students.

8. **Know when to use shortcuts.** For large families that include little relevant history, use abbreviation symbols for drawing sibships and extended family members (Table 3-1). Consider when family members' ages may not be relevant and/or inaccurate, and therefore unnecessary.

Verification of Pedigree Information and Documentation of Affected Status

Documenting the family members known to be affected with a particular disorder in a pedigree is essential. This may require verifying family history information for ensuring an accurate diagnosis and for providing accurate counseling. Verification can be accomplished by obtaining the medical records of the proband or other affected family member(s), genetic tests or other laboratory results, pathology reports, autopsy results, and in some instances, by performing examinations of key individuals. For example, when a couple is counseled regarding a family history of a rare autosomal recessive disorder, it is important to not only obtain documentation of the diagnosis but also results of the genetic testing of the affected family member (if performed). The accuracy of risk assessment depends on confirmation of the diagnosis, and information regarding the sensitivity and specificity of targeted testing depends on whether the affected family member's variants are known. If the affected family member has had testing that revealed identifiable pathogenic variants, then negative carrier studies in the client would have greater predictive value. For a client who is concerned about a family history of cancer, pathology reports that document tumor types and medical records that confirm diagnoses are critical components of an accurate risk assessment. If the family member of interest is deceased and the medical records are not available, then sometimes a death certificate can provide useful information.

Accuracy

An inaccurate family history is a reality of genetic counseling. Possible errors include incorrect diagnoses, wrong ages at diagnosis and/or symptom onset, errors in maternity or paternity, lack of knowledge about the existence of certain relatives who do not have a disease (leading to overestimates of risk) and lack of knowledge about those who do have disease (leading to underestimates of risk). There is also variability in accuracy depending on the disease being reported. For example, patient-reported positive family histories of cancer for first-degree relatives are accurate and valuable for breast and ovarian cancer risk assessments, whereas underreporting has been noted to be a limitation for other types of cancer (Ottman et al., 2011; Vento, 2012; Augustinsson et al., 2018). Negative family history reports for ovarian and endometrial cancers are also less useful (Murff et al., 2004). Verification of information, particularly in more distant relatives, is often difficult or impossible.

There are many reasons a client may have limited or uninformative FHH information. Individuals who were not raised by, or who have limited contact with, one or both of their biological parents may not have as much knowledge about FHH as someone with a close relationship with both of their biological parents. Increasingly, same-sex partners are choosing to have children without learning which of them is the biological parent, which may limit knowledge about whose family history is relevant to the child(ren)'s health. Studies have also shown that LGBTQ+ individuals are more likely to have strained family relationships and reduced communication about FHH (Rolf et al., 2022). Other studies have shown racial and ethnic disparities in FHH reporting, with individuals of African American, Hispanic, and Asian ancestry reporting significantly less cancer family history information compared to White individuals (Rositch et al. 2019; Maves et al. 2020). Members of marginalized racial and ethnic groups in the US are also disproportionately affected by social determinants of health that impact life expectancy, including safe housing, job opportunities and income, access to nutritious foods, safe air and water, and gun violence. Factors limiting life expectancy can reduce FHH informativeness. For instance, if multiple family members died in their 50s due to environmentally induced respiratory disease, the ability to determine whether they would have developed cancer or dementia later in life had they lived longer is limited. This may inhibit a counselor's ability to perform a comprehensive cancer or dementia risk assessment for the patient.

Pedigree Updating

Updating the family history is an essential component of a follow-up evaluation for clients with or without an established diagnosis. Additional information may be obtained that provides further clues about a possible diagnosis; or, in the instance of an established diagnosis, the births of additional family members may indicate other at-risk individuals for whom evaluations are indicated. Additionally, the health status of family members may have changed, affecting the risk assessment provided to the patient. As Table 3-1 shows, the situation of a client who has an increased risk of developing a condition (e.g., a positive DNA test for an autosomal dominant adult-onset condition) but was asymptomatic at the time the family history was obtained, is represented by a vertical line down the center of the symbol. If the client later develops symptoms, the symbol is shaded when the pedigree is updated. When the pedigree is updated, the date and recorder should be noted, so that the most current version is readily identifiable.

Issues of Confidentiality

The pedigree is a record of sensitive information, including family relationships, the health status of family members, dates of birth, marriages and partnerships, gender identity, and pregnancies. Notably, data is usually gathered from an individual patient and recorded without family members' consent or knowledge. Confidentiality and privacy are issues warranting consideration because family members may not be aware that personal health information has been recorded and individuals may learn unwanted information about themselves or others if the pedigree is made available. For example, if the medical records, including the pedigree, of an individual are shared (with appropriate authorization), a relative could learn previously undisclosed information such as adoption, misattributed paternity or maternity, or disease risk. It could be argued that an implicit consent exists because the information has been shared within the family, and therefore written consent for documentation and inclusion in an individual's medical record is not required (Lucassen et al., 2006).

It is generally not advisable to record family members' names on the pedigree, although if necessary first names or initials can be included to make it possible for the counselor to refer by name to a family member when asking questions. Use of birth year or age, year of death or age at death, rather than complete birth dates or dates of death of relatives, are compliant with the Health Insurance Portability and Accountability Act (HIPAA) guidelines in which exact dates are considered private and protected information (Bennett et al., 2008). Some institutions record patient-reported names and ages of relatives in their pedigree software database but upload a redacted version without identifiers of relatives into the EMR.

Additional confidentiality concerns arise when it is necessary to release information (with a signed medical record release) to a third party, such as an extended family member or insurer. Not all the information recorded in a pedigree may be necessary or appropriate for other individuals or parties to obtain. Full names of family members should not be imaged into the patient's electronic medical record without obtaining consent from these individuals, because of the possibility that the information will be released. A pedigree may also contain information about pregnancy termination, pregnancies conceived through assisted reproductive techniques, or presymptomatic carrier status that is not relevant to the purpose of the request for information. Genetic counselors need to carefully limit what information is included on a pedigree or review its contents before sending to a third party, since it may be appropriate to omit information deemed irrelevant or potentially stigmatizing. One alternative, especially if the pedigree was not specifically included in the request for information, is to provide the clinic chart note and genetic counseling letter without the pedigree, as these documents generally contain a summary of the pertinent family history information. This, however, may not be an option that can be exercised by the counselor. If pedigrees are routinely imaged into a patient's electronic record or included in the hospital chart, the decision to include the document will be made according to the institution's policies. The safest course is to discuss potential areas of concern with one's institution and one's clients before releasing pedigrees to third parties.

An alternative method for tracking information, such as names and contact details, necessary to facilitate verification of family history information, is a number system in which each generation is recorded with a Roman numeral to the far left of the pedigree, and each individual within a particular generation is then assigned an Arabic number, from left to right, in ascending order (e.g., I-1, I-2). When this identification method is used, the names of family members for whom medical records have been requested can be recorded separately, allowing the pedigree number to serve as a means of identifying the family member on the pedigree. Spouses or partners may be given the same number with a different lowercase alphabetical letter (e.g., I-2a and I-2b). This method of identification is particularly useful for large research pedigrees and for pedigrees that will be published.

When publishing or presenting pedigrees, it is very important to protect confidentiality as much as possible. Pedigrees should only be included in publications or external presentations when they are necessary to convey key findings or to educate readers/listeners. Research participants should be made aware of whether their FHH or pedigree may be included in publications during the informed consent process. When publishing pedigrees of clients seen clinically, it is best practice to ask for their consent prior to publication. Some journals require documentation of consent of patients being presented in a publication. All protected health information should be removed from the pedigree prior to publication. Details of the pedigree that do not impact its interpretation can also be changed to further protect the privacy of the family. For instance, you may be able to change the number of people in sibships, their genders, or their ages without impacting what the pedigree is trying to convey. Grouping unaffected relatives together is another way to make a pedigree less recognizable. You can also remove diagnoses or health information that is not relevant to the indication being presented. You may add the disclaimer "details of this pedigree have been altered to protect anonymity" to the description of the pedigree figure in a publication.

INTERPRETING THE FAMILY HISTORY AND PEDIGREE ANALYSIS

The pedigree should be an accurate and easily interpretable diagram from which risk information can be derived. Diagnostic testing may define risk for patients and clients in absolute terms, but decisions to undertake testing are often based on an assessment of family history data (see Table 3-4 "Red flags"). In other instances, when testing is not feasible or informative, risk information is based solely on the analysis of the pedigree. It is therefore critical for the genetic counselor to carefully evaluate the data and to consider the possible modes of inheritance when providing risk information. See Table 3-5 "Tips for evaluating pedigrees."

Three important considerations in the interpretation of the family history data warrant discussion, including variable expressivity of inherited disorders, reduced penetrance, and the value of a negative family history.

TABLE 3-4. Red flags in a family history suggestive of a genetic condition

Multiple	• Multiple relatives with the same condition, particularly if it is rare
	• Multiple common disorders in related individuals, particularly if diagnosed at younger ages than is typical
	• Multiple pregnancy losses in an individual or couple
	• An individual with two or more medical conditions
	• A fetus or infant with multiple anomalies
	• Developmental delay and additional medical condition(s)
	• Dysmorphic features and additional medical condition(s)
Rare	• Rare disease, particularly if it is in multiple relatives
	• Bilateral disease in paired organs, such as eyes, kidneys, lungs, breasts
	• Unusual birthmarks
	• Hair anomalies
Congenital or early-onset	• Congenital heart disease
	• Congenital or juvenile deafness, blindness, or cataracts
	• Early-onset cancer diagnosis
Unexplained	• Unexplained sudden cardiac death, sudden cardiac arrest, or cardiomyopathy
	• Unexplained hypotonia
	• Unexplained ataxia
	• Unexplained seizures
Progressive	• Progressive cognitive impairment
	• Loss of developmental milestones
	• Progressive behavioral problems
	• Progressive neurological condition, movement disorder, and/or muscle weakness
	• Progressive loss of vision and/or hearing

Adapted from Bennett, 2010.

Variable Expressivity

The concept of variable expression of inherited conditions, especially those that are dominantly inherited, should always play a role in determining what questions to ask the client when obtaining a family history. Previously noted is the need to ask not only about the presence of a given disorder in relatives but also about the presence of associated physical features. For example, the proband in Figure 3-2 was referred for a diagnostic evaluation because of cleft palate and micrognathia. Also reported was a family history of cleft palate in two first-degree relatives, the mother and sibling. The differential diagnosis for these anomalies and family history includes a condition known as Stickler syndrome, an autosomal dominant disorder involving cleft palate, micrognathia, myopia, retinal detachment,

TABLE 3-5. Tips for evaluating pedigrees

Are individuals in more than one generation affected?	• Mostly likely dominant inheritance • If there is consanguinity in more than one generation or carrier frequency is high, also consider autosomal recessive inheritance
Are males and females affected?	• Most likely autosomal inheritance • Females can be affected with X-linked (generally with milder symptoms) if there is skewed X-inactivation or if they carry bi-allelic pathogenic variants
What are the most likely patterns of inheritance?	• Autosomal dominant, autosomal recessive, and X-linked conditions are more common than mitochondrial and Y-linked conditions
Are only males affected?	• Consider X-linked inheritance
Is there male-to-male transmission?	• Rules out X-linked and mitochondrial inheritance
Is transmission only through females?	• Consider X-linked or mitochondrial inheritance
Are there multiple pregnancy losses?	• Consider a chromosome rearrangement
Are there any additional factors to consider when interpreting the pedigree?	• Reduced or incomplete penetrance, variable expressivity, anticipation, heterogeneity, mosaicism, imprinting, sex-limited or sex-restricted disorders, the presence of more than one condition or disorder, misattributed paternity or maternity, small family size, or family members dying prior to expected age of onset of a condition can all limit/impact pedigree interpretation

Adapted from Uhlmann 2009, p. 108.

hypermobile joints, and degenerative arthritis. When obtaining the family history, the genetic counselor should inquire about the presence of physical features associated with this condition in other family members to collect data in support of a diagnosis and the inheritance pattern, while potentially identifying additional affected family members. The absence of supporting data in family members may weigh against a particular diagnosis and/or may suggest the patient has a condition as a result of a *de novo* variant. In this particular pedigree (see Figure 3-2), the patient's mother reported a history of bilateral retinal detachments and hypermobile joints in addition to the cleft palate. The patient's sibling was reported to have early onset myopia in addition to cleft palate. This information, along with the diagnostic evaluation, helped to confirm a clinical diagnosis of Stickler syndrome in the proband as well as in the mother and sibling.

It is important to remember that disorders may present diversely within a family, and in some instances the sum of varying manifestations among multiple family members will suggest the diagnosis of a particular disorder. Figure 3-3

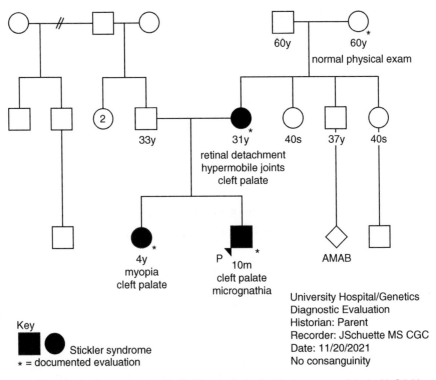

FIGURE 3-2. *Pedigree showing family history of physical features associated with Stickler syndrome*

illustrates such a family. The proband was initially referred at age 1 year for an evaluation due to U-shaped cleft palate, micrognathia, and several minor dysmorphic features. Multiple diagnostic studies including a chromosomal microarray, biochemical analyses, skeletal survey, renal ultrasound, and MRI were normal. At the time of a follow-up evaluation, global developmental delay was noted. When updating the family history, the proband's younger sister was reported to have a recent diagnosis of autism spectrum disorder, the mother was reported to have premature ovarian failure, and the maternal grandfather had been recently diagnosed with a Parkinsonian-type disorder with ataxia and tremor. This history strongly suggested the possibility of fragile X syndrome which was later confirmed. Fragile X syndrome had not initially been a consideration in view of the patient's presenting features of multiple congenital anomalies but became part of the differential diagnosis when the family history was updated.

Incomplete Penetrance

Many autosomal dominant disorders are associated with incomplete penetrance and a pedigree may reveal individuals who are likely carriers of pathogenic variants despite being asymptomatic. Evaluation and genetic counseling should be

Diagnostic Evaluation   Informant: Parent   Collected by: NP
Date: 12/5/2020, updated 10/1/2022   Proband: Jason Valentine   MRN: 77344221

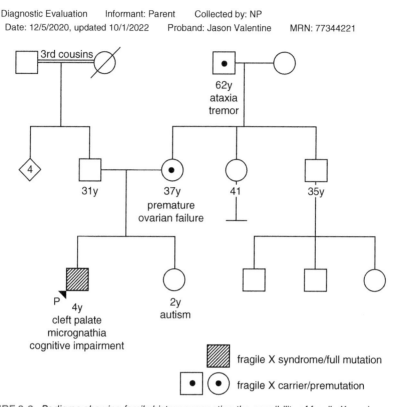

FIGURE 3-3. *Pedigree showing family history suggesting the possibility of fragile X syndrome*

recommended to such individuals due to the potential implications for health care management and surveillance. The pedigree in Figure 3-4 reveals a family history in which several individuals have breast cancer and are positive for a *BRCA2* pathogenic variant. Additionally, it is apparent that at least two reportedly unaffected family members are carriers of the pathogenic variant and others are at increased risk. The penetrance of some disorders is age dependent, as in the case of breast and ovarian cancer as well as many other conditions, and, therefore, the ages of family members are an important consideration for risk assessment.

Value of an Extended Negative History

An extended negative family history provides information that is often as important as a history of a genetic disorder in multiple relatives in several generations. Obtaining a negative history can be as straightforward as documenting the presence and ages of unaffected siblings of an individual with early-onset disease or more arduous due to the need for obtaining documentation of normal evaluations in family members at risk for colon cancer or inherited cardiomyopathy, such as negative colonoscopies or echocardiograms. For example, the pedigree in

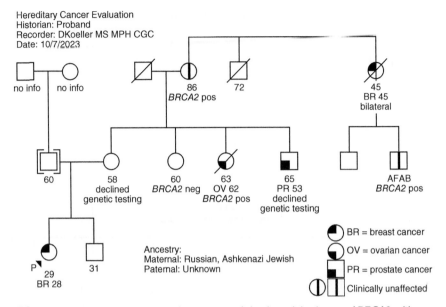

FIGURE 3-4. *Pedigree demonstrating autosomal dominant inheritance of* BRCA2 *with reduced penetrance*

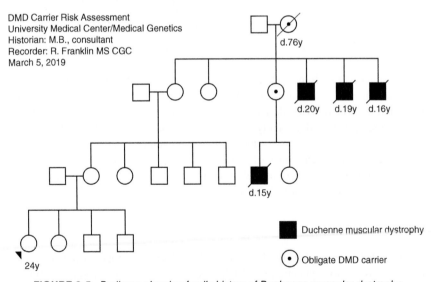

FIGURE 3-5. *Pedigree showing family history of Duchenne muscular dystrophy*

Figure 3-5 includes family history information for a client referred for genetic counseling because of a family history of Duchenne muscular dystrophy (DMD), an X-linked recessive disorder. Several of the client's distant relatives were reported to have died from complications of DMD. Of significant value is the presence of multiple unaffected males in the maternal family history. Such a history provides relevant information for assessing carrier risk; a Bayesian analysis reduces the client's *a priori* risk of 1/8 to 1/138. (See Chapter 8 for more information regarding Bayesian analysis.)

Complexity of Chronic Disorders

A positive family history of a common chronic disease is generally associated with relative risks ranging from two to five times those of the general population; an even greater increase in relative risk is associated with an increasing number of affected relatives and earlier ages of disease onset (Guttmacher, 2004; Bennett 2010). Examples of such common diseases include the following:

- Breast cancer occurring at less than age 45–50 years (premenopausal).
- Colon cancer occurring at less than age 45–50 years.
- Prostate cancer occurring at less than age 45–60 years.
- Vision loss occurring at less than age 55 years.
- Hearing loss occurring at less than age 50–60 years.
- Dementia at age 60 years or less.
- Heart disease at age 40–60 years or less.
- Stroke occurring at less than age 60 years.

(American Medical Association, 2004; Bennett, 2010)

Additionally, a strong family history of common chronic diseases may suggest a diagnosis of a Mendelian disorder. It is therefore critical to recognize different combinations of diseases within a pedigree, including the suggested pattern of inheritance, for facilitating a diagnosis in a potentially high-risk family. There are over 150 Mendelian disorders that include common conditions such as coronary artery disease, myocardial infarction, stroke, thrombosis, sudden death, arrhythmia, aneurysm, arteriovenous malformations, cardiomyopathy, and diabetes in adulthood (Scheuner, 2004).

PSYCHOSOCIAL ASPECTS OF OBTAINING A FAMILY HISTORY

Obtaining a family history involves communication, an exchange of verbal, nonverbal, and visual information. For the counselor, this exchange requires a conscious effort to hear, comprehend, and retain the objective and subjective information being relayed.

Since the counselor engages the client in an activity that requires participation of all parties—the client, the partner, the counselor, and perhaps extended family members or close friends if present—obtaining the family history can be an "ice breaker." It is an opportunity to create an ongoing dialogue with the family, and because many intimate family events and details are reported, the counselor can use this exchange to establish trust and to convey unqualified acceptance.

While gathering the family history, the counselor can benefit from the objective information contained in the pedigree itself. The composition of the client's nuclear family and significant relationships, experience with death, divorce, infertility, and/or adoption all contribute toward an emerging "picture" of the client that can be used in the consultation. However, a genetic counselor should carefully distinguish between objective data versus subjective impressions. This requires developing attuned attending skills, to note what is stated and to heed noteworthy statements, while simultaneously being cognizant of impressions and assumptions, and, importantly, their limitations.

Obtaining family history is also an opportunity to note the client's communication style. Is it open or closed? Are responses to questions detailed, succinct, brief, or even terse? What words are used when describing health? Do these words suggest a particular level of health literacy or knowledge? Does one family member provide most or all the information because they are the most knowledgeable, the primary coordinator of health care needs of the family, and/or the family historian? Does one family member consistently interrupt, correct, or contradict the other? Is there tension, stress, or does the exchange between family members appear relaxed and mutually supportive? Does the client and family appear anxious when identifying members of the family as affected with disease or are feelings suggesting guilt, distress, or discomfort apparent? What is the client doing when they are responding to questions? Is the client making eye contact?

A family's beliefs about the presence of a disorder in a family member may be shared while gathering the history. The emotional and psychological impact of living with an illness or disability in the family, particularly if sudden, premature, fatal, or lifelong and involving multiple complex medical and social needs, plus the nature of family relationships, can contribute toward a sense of emotional closeness and personal likeness with an affected relative (Walter and Emery, 2005). Sex and/or age of disease onset or death of the affected family member may also contribute to a patient's perception of disease imminence. Families may also have beliefs that serve to explain why certain members are affected with a disorder while others are not. Some may assume that sharing a family resemblance has predictive value in determining who will inherit a particular disorder. In other instances, a family may assume that only females or only males are at risk, even though the disorder is inherited in an autosomal dominant fashion. These beliefs are not necessarily overtly expressed and therefore the counselor must be attuned to these possibilities.

Some individuals and families recount an unsubstantiated cause for the presence of a disorder in a family member; this is not an uncommon occurrence when taking a family history. For example, the client may identify the cause of intellectual disability in a family member as "lack of oxygen" or the "cord was around the neck" during delivery. It is worth noting that such an explanation may be "the family story" and may have become the accepted cause. A sensitive counselor will understand that the suggestion of an alternative explanation for the disability could be disruptive, depending on when in the client/counselor relationship it is presented. The counselor should be cognizant of family assumptions and beliefs that present themselves while the history is being recorded, as these may impact the client's understanding of genetic principles and perception of risk.

A successful genetic counseling interaction involves a heightened sensitivity for anticipating and identifying potential issues that may present while obtaining the family history. However, beliefs, hunches, guesses, inferences, and/or speculations may interfere with what is being conveyed by the client. To be effective, the counselor needs finely tuned self-awareness to distinguish between what has been explicitly stated or demonstrated from what is illusory and perhaps requiring further exploration with the client.

SUMMARY

The family history and pedigree are the basis for providing clients referred for genetic evaluation and counseling with a diagnosis, risk assessment, education, and psychosocial support. Accuracy, detail, and relevance are paramount. The genetic counseling student should develop mastery of this fundamental task and employ standardized pedigree symbols and nomenclature that enhance the utility of the information obtained. An accurate and complete family history and pedigree are tools that lay the foundation for the highest standards of patient care and genetic counseling.

REFERENCES

American Medical Association. (2004) *Family Medical History in Disease Prevention.* https://www.ama-assn.org/sites/ama-assn.org/files/corp/media-browser/public/genetics/family_history02_0.pdf Accessed October 5, 2023.

Antypa N & Serretti A. (2014) Family history of a mood disorder indicates a more severe bipolar disorder. *J Affect Disord* 156:178–186. https://doi.org/10.1016/j.jad.2013.12.013

Augustinsson A, Ellberg C, Kristoffersson U., et al. (2018) Accuracy of self-reported family history of cancer, mutation status and tumor characteristics in patients with early onset breast cancer. *Acta Oncol* 57(5):595–603. https://doi.org/10.1080/0284186X.2017.1404635

Bao Y, Chen Z, Liu E, et al. (2017) Risk factors in preschool children for predicting asthma during the preschool age and the early school age: a systematic review and meta-analysis. *Curr Allergy Asthma Rep* 17(12):85. https://doi.org/10.1007/s11882-017-0753-7

Barnes H, Morris E, & Austin J. (2020) Trans-inclusive genetic counseling services: Recommendations from members of the transgender and non-binary community. *J Genet Couns* 29(3):423–434. https://doi.org/10.1002/jgc4.1187

Bennett RL. (2010) *The Practical Guide to the Genetic Family History* Second edition. Hoboken, NJ: Wiley-Blackwell.

Bennett RL, French KS, Resta RG, et al. (2022) Practice resource-focused revision: Standardized pedigree nomenclature update centered on sex and gender inclusivity: a practice resource of the National Society of Genetic Counselors. *J Genet Couns* 31(6):1238–1248. https://doi.org/10.1002/jgc4.1621

Bennett RL, French KS, Resta RG, et al. (2008) Standardized human pedigree nomenclature: Update and assessment of the recommendations of the National Society of Genetic Counselors. *J Genet Couns* 17(5):424–433. https://doi.org/10.1007/s10897-008-9169-9

Bennett RL, Steinhaus KA, Uhrich SB, et al. (1993) The need for developing standardized family pedigree nomenclature. *J Genet Couns* 2(4):261–273. https://doi.org/10.1007/BF00961575

Bennett RL, Steinhaus KA, Uhrich SB, et al. (1995a) Recommendations for standardized human pedigree nomenclature. *Am J Hum Genet* 56:745–752.

Bennett RL, Steinhaus KA, Uhrich SB, et al. (1995b) Recommendations for standardized human pedigree nomenclature. *J Genet Couns* 4(4):267–279.

Bennett RL, Steinhaus KA, Uhrich SB, et al. (1995c) Reply to Marazita and Curtis (Letters to the Editor). *Am J Hum Genet* 57:983–984.

Berro T, Zayhowski K, Field T, et al. (2019) Genetic counselors' comfort and knowledge of cancer risk assessment for transgender patients. *J Genet Couns* 29(3):342–351. https://doi.org/10.1002/jgc4.1172

Bethea TN, Ochs-Balcom HM, Bandera EV, et al. (2021. First- and second-degree family history of ovarian and breast cancer in relation to risk of invasive ovarian cancer in African American and white women. *Int J Cancer* 148(12):2964–2973. https://doi.org/10.1002/ijc.33493

Bhinder, M. A., Sadia, H., Mahmood, N, et al. (2019). Consanguinity: A blessing or menace at population level? *Annals of Hum Gen* 83(4): 214–219. https://doi.org/10.1111/ahg.12308

Birmaher B, Hafeman D, Merranko J, et al. (2022) Role of polygenic risk score in the familial transmission of bipolar disorder in youth. *JAMA Psychiatry* 79(2):160–168. https://doi.org/10.1001/jamapsychiatry.2021.3700

Bittles AH & Black ML. (2010) Consanguinity, human evolution, and complex diseases. *P Natl Acad Sci USA* 107(Suppl. 1):1779–1786. https://doi.org/10.1073/pnas.0906079106

Brewer HR, Jones, ME, Schoemaker MJ, et al. (2017) Family history and risk of breast cancer: an analysis accounting for family structure. *Breast Cancer Res Treat* 165(1):193–200. https://doi.org/10.1007/s10549-017-4325-2

Conway-Pearson LS, Christensen KD, Savage SK, et al. (2016) Family health history reporting is sensitive to small changes in wording. *Genet Med* 18(12):1308–1311. https://doi.org/10.1038/gim.2016.45

Daly MB, Pilarski R, Yurgelun MB, et al. (2020) Genetic/familial high-risk assessment: breast, ovarian, and pancreatic, version 1.2020: featured updates to the NCCN guidelines. *J Natl Compr Canc Netw* 18(4):380–391. https://doi.org/10.6004/jnccn.2020.0017

Duke NN, Jensen TM, Perreira KM, et al. (2021) The role of family health history in predicting midlife chronic disease outcomes. *Am J Prev Med* 61(4):509–517. https://doi.org/10.1016/j.amepre.2021.02.021

Flint ND, Bishop MD, Smart TC, et al. (2021) Low accuracy of self-reported family history of melanoma in high-risk patients. *Fam Cancer* 20(1):41–48. https://doi.org/10.1007/s10689-020-00187-0

Gutmann DH, Aylsworth A, Carey JC, et al. (1997) The diagnostic evaluation and multidisciplinary management of neurofibromatosis 1 and neurofibromatosis 2 NF2. *JAMA* 278(1):51–57.

Guttmacher AE, Collins FS, & Carmona RH. (2004) The family history - more important than ever. *The NEJM* 351(22):2333–2336.

Kastrinos F, Samadder, NJ, & Burt RW. (2020) Use of family history and genetic testing to determine risk of colorectal cancer. *Gastroenterology* 158(2):389–403. https://doi.org/10.1053/j.gastro.2019.11.029

Khoury MJ, Iademarco MF, & Riley WT (2016) Precision public health for the era of precision medicine. *Am J Prev Med* 50(3):398–401. https://doi.org/10.1016/j.amepre.2015.08.031

Lascar N, Brown J, Pattison H, et al. (2018) Type 2 diabetes in adolescents and young adults. *Lancet Diabetes Endocrinol* 6(1):69–80. https://doi.org/10.1016/S2213-8587(17)30186-9

Lee YL, Teitelbaum S, Wolff MS, et al. (2010) Comparing genetic ancestry and self-reported race/ethnicity in a multiethnic population in New York City. *J Genet* 89(4):417–423.

Lucassen A, Parker M, & Wheeler R. (2006) Implications of data protection legislation for family history. *Br Med J* 332:299–301.

Marazita ML. (1995) Defining 'Proband' (Letters to the Editor). *Am J Hum Genet* 57:981–982.

Maves H, Flodman P, Nathan D, et al. (2020) Ethnic disparities in the frequency of cancer reported in family histories. *J Genet Couns* 29(3):451–459. https://doi.org/10.1002/jgc4.1264

McGrath BB & Edwards KL. (2009) When family means more (or less) than genetics: the intersection of culture, family, and genomics. *J Transcult Nurs* 20(3):270–277. https://doi.org/10.1177/1043659609334931

McMonnies CW. (2017) Glaucoma history and risk factors. *J Optom* 10(2):71–78. https://doi.org/10.1016/j.optom.2016.02.003

Mersha TB & Abebe T. (2015) Self-reported race/ethnicity in the age of genomic research: Its potential impact on understanding health disparities. *Hum Genomics* 9(1):1. https://doi.org/10.1186/s40246-014-0023-x

Moonesinghe R, Yang Q, Zhang Z, et al. (2019) prevalence and cardiovascular health impact of family history of premature heart disease in the United States: analysis of the National Health and Nutrition Examination Survey, 2007–2014. *J Am Heart Assoc* 8(14). https://doi.org/10.1161/JAHA.119.012364

Murff HJ, Spigel DR, & Syngal S. (2004) Does This Patient Have a Family History of Cancer? An Evidence-Based Analysis of the Accuracy of Family Cancer History The Rational Clinical Examination Section Editors. *JAMA* 292(12):1480–1489.

National Society of Genetics Counselors (NSGC). (2003) Standardized Pedigree Symbol Position Statement. http://www.nsgc.org/about/position Accessed January 12, 2008.

National Society of Genetics Counselors (NSGC). (2023) Family Health History. https://www.nsgc.org/POLICY/Position-Statements/Position-Statements/Post/family-health-history Accessed June 9, 2023.

Orlando LA, Wu RR, Myers RA, et al. (2020) At the intersection of precision medicine and population health: an implementation-effectiveness study of family health history based systematic risk assessment in primary care. *BMC Health Services Research* 20(1015). https://doi.org/10.1186/s12913-020-05868-1

Osman K, Ahmet K, Hilmi T, et al. (2022) BRCA 1/BRCA 2 pathogenic/likely pathogenic variant patients with breast, ovarian, and other cancers. *Balk J Med Genet* 25(2):5–14. https://doi.org/10.2478/bjmg-2022-0023

Ottman R, Barker-Cummings C, Leibson DCL, et al. (2011) Accuracy of family history information on epilepsy and other seizure disorders. *Neurology* 76:390–396.

Resta RG. (1993) The crane's foot: the rise of the pedigree in human genetics. *J Genet Couns* 2(4):235–260. https://doi.org/10.1007/BF00961574

Rolf BA, Schneider JL, Amendola LM, et al. (2022) Barriers to family history knowledge and family communication among LGBTQ+ individuals in the context of hereditary cancer risk assessment. *J Genet Couns* 31(1):230–241. https://doi.org/10.1002/jgc4.1476

Rositch AF, Atnafou R, Krakow M, et al. (2019) A community-based qualitative assessment of knowledge, barriers, and promoters of communicating about family cancer history among African-Americans. *Health Commun* 34(10):1192–1201. https://doi.org/10.1080/10410236.2018.1471335

Scheuner MT. (2004) Clinical application of genetic risk assessment strategies for coronary artery disease: genotypes, phenotypes, and family history. *Prim Care* 31(3):711–737. https://doi.org/10.1016/j.pop.2004.04.001

Sheehan E, Bennett RL, Harris M, et al. (2020) Assessing transgender and gender nonconforming pedigree nomenclature in current genetic counselors' practice: the case for geometric inclusivity. *J Genet Couns* 29(6):1114–1125. https://doi.org/10.1002/jgc4.1256

Steinhaus KA, Bennett RL, Resta RG, et al. (1995) Inconsistencies in pedigree symbols in human genetics publications: a need for standardization. *Am J Med Genet* 56(3):291–295. https://doi.org/10.1002/ajmg.1320560314

The American Society of Human Genetics Social Issues Committee and The American College of Medical Genetics Social, Ethical, and Legal Issues Committee. (2000). *ASHG/ACMG statement: genetic testing in adoption. Am J Hum Genet* 66:761–767. https://doi.org/10.1086/302832

Tsai FD & Battinelli EM. (2021) Inherited platelet disorders. *Hematol Oncol Clin North Am* 35(6):1069–1084. https://doi.org/10.1016/j.hoc.2021.07.003.

Uhlmann WR. (2009) Thinking it all through: case preparation and management. In: WR Uhlmann, JL Schuette, & BM Yashar (Eds) *A Guide to Genetic Counseling* Second Edition, 93–131, Hoboken, NJ: Wiley.

Vance A. (2020) Family history risk assessment by a genetic counselor is a critical step in screening all patients in the ART clinic. *J Assist Reprod Genet* 37:2279–2281. https://doi.org/10.1007/s10815-020-01870-y

Vanderwall RA, Schwartz A, Kipnis L, et al. (2022) Impact of genetic counseling on patient-reported electronic cancer family history collection. *J Natl Compr Canc Netw* 20(8):898–905. https://doi.org/10.6004/jnccn.2022.7022

Venne VL, Botkin JR, & Buys SS. (2003) Professional opportunities and responsibilities in the provision of genetic information to children relinquished for adoption. *Am J Med Genet* 119A(1):41–46. https://doi.org/10.1002/ajmg.a.20071

Venne VL & Scheuner MT. (2015) Securing and documenting cancer family history in the age of the electronic medical record. *Surg Oncol Clin N Am* 24(4):639–652. https://doi.org/10.1016/j.soc.2015.06.001

Vento JM. (2012) Family history: a guide for neurologists in the age of genomic medicine. *Semin Pediatr Neurol* 19(4):160–166. https://doi.org/10.1016/j.spen.2012.09.002

Walter FM & Emery J. (2005) 'Coming down the line' - patients' understanding of their family history of common chronic disease. *Ann Fam Med* 3(5):405–414. https://doi.org/10.1370/afm.368

Walter FM & Emery J. (2006) Perceptions of family history across common diseases: A qualitative study in primary care. *Fam Pract* 23(4):472–480. https://doi.org/10.1093/fampra/cml006

Wang HP, Zhang N, Liu YJ, et al. (2023) Lipoprotein(a), family history of cardiovascular disease, and incidence of heart failure. *J Lipid Res* 64(7):100398. https://doi.org/10.1016/j.jlr.2023.100398

Wildin RS, Messersmith DJ, & Houwink EJF. (2021) Modernizing family health history: achievable strategies to reduce implementation gaps. *J Community Genet* 12(3):493–496. https://doi.org/10.1007/s12687-021-00531-6

Yang TL, Shen H, Liu A, et al. (2020) A road map for understanding molecular and genetic determinants of osteoporosis. *Nat Rev Endocrinol* 16(2):91–103. https://doi.org/10.1038/s41574-019-0282-7

Zayhowski K, Park J, Boehmer U, et al. (2019) Cancer genetic counselors' experiences with transgender patients: a qualitative study. *J Genet Couns* 28(3):641–653. https://doi.org/10.1002/jgc4.1092

4

Understanding the Counseling in Genetic Counseling Practice

Luba Djurdjinovic

INTRODUCTION

This chapter aims to consider the importance of fully appreciating psychosocial dynamics in the daily practice of genetic counseling and to identify opportunities that invite us to integrate psychological assessment and apply our counseling skills. I am committed to the belief that the vitality and longevity of the genetic counseling profession is very much tied to its psychological-based practice. I am not proposing that we should see ourselves as therapists, only that we remain committed to the earliest visions of our profession which support a relational-based process and honors psychological attunement as a tenet of the genetic counseling experience.

As the practice of genetic counseling has evolved, so has the commitment to assure that emotional and psychological needs of the counselee are recognized and met. Many have argued that the invitation to a counselee to share and begin a collaborative discussion is based in psychological principles and psychotherapy

A Guide to Genetic Counseling, Third Edition. Edited by Vivian Y. Pan, Jane L. Schuette, Karen E. Wain, and Beverly M. Yashar.
© 2025 John Wiley & Sons Ltd. Published 2025 by John Wiley & Sons Ltd.

theories that foster the counselee's awareness that their narrative will be "heard." When the counselee seems distracted and is responding to questions in a limited way, the counselor may default to "educating" the counselee, who may leave the appointment confused, uncertain, and possibly distressed.

As genetic counselors, we appreciate that it takes time and practice to refine counseling skills that reflect applied knowledge, willingness to understand through empathic listening, and thoughtful engagement to assure that disclosures and concerns are framed to help guide decisions. Genetic counselors appreciate that the practice of genetic counseling requires blending the medical, educational, and psychological considerations. How one frames a didactic discussion that is psychologically significant to the counselee involves application of counseling skills and conscious practice. Ongoing professional development requires appreciating current psychological theories, the value of self-awareness, and how both apply to individual genetic counseling appointments.

Four decades of publications by genetic counselors now offer insights into the interpersonal experiences of counselee and counselor during a genetic counseling session, document the range of complex considerations confronting the counselee, and explain how counseling approaches offer emotional support and guide decision making (Salema et al., 2019; Zimmermann and Shaw, 2020). Our profession, however, continues to experience an awkwardness in defining the "counseling" in genetic counseling, as it is less tangible than didactic information, and yet it distinguishes genetic counselors from most other health professionals. We aim to offer information as part of a collaborative process that invites the counselees to share their concerns, and in turn allows the counselees to invite us into their narrative and decision process. This collaborative process, also known in many counseling theories as the "working alliance," begins with a conscious commitment on the counselor's part to understand the counselee, beyond the indication for referral, that readies the counselor to become attuned to the counselee's narrative including their social, cultural, and religious milieu. As the counselor listens and learns, the counselee will become aware of the counselor's genuine regard. It is from this foundational step that a more psychologically based discussion begins, encouraging information sharing, understanding, and support for decision-making.

This chapter will not be inclusive of all published literature exploring the psychological dynamics and theories employed by genetic counselors. It aims to encourage you to observe, understand, and further explore the iterative psychodynamic aspects in your practice and consider its roots in the many established and emerging psychological theories.

The earliest definers of genetic counseling understood the need for psychologically based discussions of genetic concerns (Reed, 1955; Kessler, 1979) and urged active psychological discussion during a genetic counseling appointment. Dr. Seymour Kessler stated that genetic counseling is a "kind of psychotherapeutic encounter … that is concerned with human behavior" (Kesseler, 1979). Many have described psychologically rich discussions during the genetic counseling session (Weil, 2000; Biesecker and Peters, 2001;

Resta et al., 2006; Austin et al., 2014; Djurdjinovic and Peters, 2017; Biesecker, 2020). The nature of a psychotherapeutic encounter during a genetic counseling appointment has been debated, and multiple practice theories have emerged (McCarthy Veach et al., 2007; Biesecker et al., 2017; Biesecker, 2020). These contributions have supported the establishment of the counseling competencies that are used in graduate training programs, updated the definition of genetic counseling, and resulted in numerous calls to ensure that the genetic counseling experience continues to be psychologically rich (Resta et al., 2006). Regardless of the counseling theory one values most, we have a responsibility to commit to genuinely wanting to learn about the counselee, to limit assumptions about the counselee, and to set aside any overconfidence as to how the dialogue in a session will emerge. An appreciation for the verbal and nonverbal communication between counselee and genetic counselor is paramount (Weil, 2003). A psychodynamic matrix is present in all phases of a genetic counseling session and has the potential to influence discussions and decisions. It is this aspect of genetic counseling that is unique to our profession and will continue to distinguish the role of genetic counselor in various medical settings.

PSYCHOLOGICAL FRAMEWORK OF OUR PRACTICE

The genetic counseling session unfolds for the counselee and counselor through a willingness of all participants to join in a shared discussion that could have moments of unfamiliarity, awkwardness, and adjustment, as each person communicates information and gradually comes to a mutual acceptance of style. The emotional and psychological experience of a counselee is present throughout the session, and it often becomes evident in the early moments of an appointment. The tool most central to all genetic counseling sessions is the family history, where there is the opportunity to learn more about the counselee and family. The pedigree, in its simplest form, offers us clues to understand our counselee's existing relationships as well as absent relationships due to divorce, death, or adoption, and can be expanded to consider extra-familial relationships that influence individual and family dynamics (Eunpu, 1997; Peters et al., 2006). Sometimes counselees offer information about themselves and their concerns by statements such as "I need to know this for my children," presenting an opportunity to begin a conversation to better understand the worries that frame their statements. The patient's story and concerns need to be encouraged in all phases of the session.

The counselee's narrative is increasingly valued in the psychological community as practitioners seek to have the patient's voice be central to the process, as is the theoretical framework that may be applied to the counseling session (Gonçalves and Stiles, 2011; Fioretti et al., 2016; Spencer, 2016; MacLeod et al., 2021). It is the personal story and our attuned listening that allows for assessment of concerns, ethno-cultural perspectives, religious beliefs, and worry. Intergenerationally constructed beliefs and perceptions of risk ("I think I inherited that gene because I look like my mom") often shared by counselees invite further discussion and may reveal an emotional response that invites the counselor to learn more. As the counselee's story unfolds, the genetic counselor simultaneously understands that together they are entering into a dialogue that aims to support the counselee's use of genetic information in "a personally meaningful way that minimizes psychological distress and increases personal control" (Biesecker and Peters, 2001). If this initial implied collaboration is nurtured by the genetic counselor's genuine wish to know the counselee's circumstances and experiences, it will drive the genetic counseling process towards a "working alliance." The following case example aims to introduce the unfolding of a working alliance in the early phase of a genetic counseling appointment.

Kelly is 39 years old and was referred by her primary care provider to help her understand her lifetime cardiac risk. Kelly's brother died while watching a college football game with his housemates. Kelly's father had a cardiac arrest at work. He was 52 years old. One of her paternal aunts died at 43 years of age doing the family laundry.

Kelly has been experiencing fatigue and is concerned that she will have a sudden death. She is a 9th grade teacher and describes her profession as very stressful. She has two children, 9 and 10 years old, and worries about them all the time.

Counselor: Can you tell me what you hope I can help you with today?

Kelly: I just need to be prepared. Everyone in my family dies before 43 years of age and I know it will happen to me.

Counselor: Have you been evaluated by a cardiologist?

Kelly: Yes, but he did not understand.

Counselor: How have you dealt with this worry?

Kelly: Not well. I worry and feel like no one understands.

Counselor: Do you believe we have information to help you with this concern?

Kelly: Not sure.

Counselor: Can we start today by learning more about your family medical history and how your family has dealt with sudden death?

Kelly (while providing the family history in response to questioning about her brother): He was just sitting there having a good time.

Kelly: (in response to questioning about her aunt): They found her next to the washing machine. Everyone in the family is worried and we try not to talk about it.

Counselor: It sounds like you are trying to talk about it.

Kelly: Yes.

Counselor: I agree that your family medical history raises a question about a possible hereditary predisposition. Sometimes a genetic test can be helpful to identify a shared risk but not always. Do you think a genetic test would offer you information that would be helpful for you to feel more prepared?

Kelly: Not sure. Maybe you can tell me about it.

Working Alliance

Developing a working alliance is an iterative process of observation, understanding the counselee statements, prompting discussion, considering word choices, and at times appreciating nonverbal clues that help the counselee to "feel" understood and enhance the counselee's engagement in the objectives of the session. This concept of a working alliance has its origin in early psychodynamic theory. Bordin (1979) argued that counseling practice needs an alliance to reach a mutually agreed goal or hoped for change. He further argued that the strength of the alliance was key to change. It is the relational milieu that emerges in the working alliance that assures the counselee is "heard" and the "hopes" for the session are most likely to be achieved. In the practice of genetic counseling, a working alliance needs to be framed quickly in contrast to other counseling or psychotherapy practices. How we invite the counselee to describe their concerns and encourage a discussion is supported by these foundational elements throughout the session.

1. **Listening** is the "mortar" of a working alliance (Graybar and Leonard, 2005). The first step is a willingness by the counselor to understand what brings the counselee to the appointment and reflects a desire to learn more about the counselee's experience and beliefs. The counselor's invitation to understand more about the counselee aims to support the counselee to act in a personally congruent manner. Much has been written to inform the genetic counselor of the complexity and challenges that individuals and families with genetic risk face. Learning from published personal and family stories of impact of a genetic diagnosis can help to limit assumptions and biases that can disrupt attunement to the lived experience of the counselee and disrupt the integrity of the emerging work alliance (Sexton et al., 2008; Brown, 2012; Godino et al., 2016).

2. **Empathy** on the part of the genetic counselor assures that the need of the counselee is central to the process and invites an interpersonal dynamic that assists in entering into a more in-depth discussion of the meaning of genetic risk. Empathy can be difficult to define, and many authors have attempted to capture the complex nature of this specific form of connection. For example, Bellet and Maloney (1991) define empathy as "the capacity to understand what another person is experiencing from within the other person's frame of reference." The role of empathy in a genetic counseling encounter has been strongly supported as a central element in a client-centered approach to genetic counseling (Weil, 2000; Evans, 2006; McCarthy Veach et al., 2018). Empathy is thought of as having both affective and cognitive functions that provide the ability to deeply appreciate the counselee's experience and simultaneously consider how this concern and/or experience must be understood. The counselor's emotional attunement is simultaneously understood through a cognitive process that allows the counselor to imagine and fully appreciate the

counselee in that moment. This empathic attunement can be achieved through spoken and unspoken content (Kohut, 1984; Wolf, 1988) and evolves through three phases. The first phase attempts to integrate the content of the patient's story, identifying the patient's affective state and appreciating our own response to the story. The second phase requires careful consideration of the significance of the patient's story and the messages within. The final phase involves a decision on the part of the genetic counselor of how to effectively acknowledge the counselor's experience of "knowing." It is the genetic counselor's goal to foster empathic connection, to maintain a working alliance, to invite personal reflection, and to foster trust in the genetic counselor and the genetic counseling process (Bovee, 2007). It is through the counselor's empathic stance that a counselee begins to feel understood. Being understood by the counselor provides a platform for the formation of self-empathy and, in so doing, enhances the counselee's ability to personally appreciate the complexity of presented information, available choices, and the clinical course of a condition. Self-empathy is believed to be central to one's ability to make decisions or take actions (Jordan, 1997). A genetic counseling appointment that lacks empathic discussion, where the counselor has not been able to understand or respond to the counselee's experience, may result in the counselor transitioning to an educator role and running the risk of missing the opportunity to support the counselee, leaving the counselee feeling less able to apply the information offered or come to a decision.

We begin to experience empathy within our own life experiences and relationships and bring that skill into the counseling appointment. It is essential that a genetic counselor be aware of how one's own feelings, intuition and personal experiences support or hinder the emergence of empathic attunement with a counselee. A common challenge in maintaining empathic attunement is to "not take on" the counselee's feeling. This can be very difficult at times. In cases where empathic attunement is prematurely disrupted by a sympathetic response such as "I am sorry that happened," it may signal to the counselee that they should limit further discussion as though the counselor was made uncomfortable with the shared information. This moment of sympathy, which is not always inappropriate, requires the counselor to have the personal psychological agility to return to an empathic position with awareness that one's personal response may influence the genetic counseling discourse. It is crucial that a counselor is able to differentiate feelings of sympathy from feelings of empathy. The counselor's sympathetic response to an experience of a counselee involves an emotional response based in the counselor's personal life, as illustrated in the example below.

Jane was referred to learn about cancer predisposition genetic testing. During the introduction, she became teary and said, "I am not sure that I should have kept this appointment today. My father died last month and ..." Jane begins to weep, and the genetic counselor starts to tear up. The counselor is reminded of a deep personal loss, and to recover composure turns the discussion to another topic.

The sympathetic response on the part of the genetic counselor is real, yet it needs to be put aside and attention refocused on the counselee's narrative that triggered the response in the counselor. Later in the chapter, a discussion about transference and countertransference aims to distinguish between feelings of sympathy from having and/or responding to an implied or expressed belief.

3. **Trust** is achieved through respect, instilling confidence, and promoting feelings of safety. The working relationship can be influenced by issues of confidentiality and respect for physical and emotional boundaries. The ability to fully share personal and family information requires an understood agreement that the information will not be disclosed beyond the clinical genetics experience without permission from the counselee. This includes a clinical setting that limits what can be overheard, and recognition that for some patients, note-taking during the session can be unsettling if the content and purpose is not disclosed in advance. How we assure a counselee that any information they share will be held in confidence may influence whether a counselee is willing to disclose difficult issues, emotions, issues of paternity, and previous pregnancy terminations, matters commonly kept secret within families. Even with assurances about privacy, some counselees may still be tentative in sharing a personal narrative or concerns. This can be due to generalized anxiety about possible outcomes of the appointment, or it may be in response to the genetic counselor's eagerness and enthusiasm in forming a working alliance. Sometimes it is "too much, too fast." This can also be influenced by cultural perspectives, previous personal experiences, and/or disappointing medical encounters. Identifying the counselee's need to maintain physical or psychological boundaries does not necessarily dampen the emotional content, it assures that there is "safety" in its expression.

An additional consideration is respecting physical boundaries. We may feel drawn to comfort a patient during a moment of intense grief or despair, but how we offer understanding or support should be carefully considered. Physical comforting of the patient, such as hugging and touching, is generally discouraged and may even be considered disrespectful to the counselee. On a final note, it is also important to remember that the issues of boundaries are central to the counselor as well. Unless the counselor can feel safe, the process they direct will be fragmented and may not serve the needs of the counselee. It is appropriate for the counselor to create and, at times, define the boundaries that will allow for their full participation.

THEORIES THAT SUPPORT PSYCHOLOGICAL-BASED DISCUSSIONS

The psychological framework of a genetic counseling appointment is enhanced when we can more fully appreciate the dynamics through theoretical perspectives. There are many psychological theories that range from psychodynamic to family systems. Each of them can inform a genetic counselor's practice. Selecting a preferred counseling theory comes with learning, discussions with practitioners of a specific counseling model, and identifying the counseling approach that fits and supports the kind of discussions and dynamics that occur in genetic counseling.

Several psychological theories have been applied to the genetic counseling experience. Not every template will fit every situation or work for the duration of the counseling relationship. Our choice of theory will be influenced by the case, our skill level, and the constraint of available time.

Central to genetic counseling are the principles defined by Carl Rogers, who pioneered a form of psychotherapy that is described as "nondirective," "client-centered," or a "person-centered approach." The central hypothesis is that "a climate of facilitative psychological attitudes" promotes self-understanding and changes in attitude and behavior (Kirschenbaum and Henderson, 1989). Carl Rogers argued that for change to occur, three attitudes need to exist in any therapeutic relationship: genuineness, empathic understanding, and unconditional regard of the counselee. In addition to stressing the critical role of facilitative experience, he also argued for the centrality of a "nondirective" approach. Rogers (1942) wrote that "The non-directive viewpoint places a high value on the right of every individual to be psychologically independent and to maintain his psychological integrity." He went on to add, "In the field of applied science, value judgments have a part, and often an important part, in determining the choice of technique" (Rogers, 1942).

The historical influences of the eugenics movement and other sociopolitical events led to a quick acceptance of the nondirective tenet in the Rogerian client-centered theoretical framework. There have been many papers attempting to remind us of the origin and true meaning of nondirectiveness within the genetic counseling context (Kessler, 1992b; Weil, 2003; Resta et al., 2006; Weil et al., 2006). The three client-centered elements of genuineness, empathic understanding, and unconditional regard must be developed and maintained in the genetic counseling practice model. "When any of these three is missing, a message is given that emotional issues are not relevant to the counseling process" (Weil, 2003).

Several efforts to appreciate the dynamics within the genetic counseling session led to a call to define and describe the genetic counseling process. A consensus conference to consider the elements of the genetic counseling process resulted in the establishment of the Reciprocal-Engagement Model (REM) (Box 4-1), a distinct model of genetic counseling that guides practice and seeks to assure that a psychological milieu is achieved (McCarthy Veach et al., 2007). The model includes why and how genetic counseling is delivered to patients as described in its elements of tenets, including goals, strategies, and behaviors. It offers a framework for the practice of genetic counseling and acknowledges the centrality of the working relationship. REM will likely evolve with genomic advances and professional commitment to addressing the wide range of psychological experiences and responses in relation to risk and information (Biesecker, 2020).

BOX 4-1. TENETS OF THE RECIPROCAL-ENGAGEMENT MODEL

Genetic information is key
Counselees are seeking information and genetic counselors seek to offer information to enhance an understanding about risk and support any decisions related to managing a risk.

The relationship is integral to genetic counseling
The genetic counseling encounter is a relational-based experience that relies on a vibrant working relationship.

Patient autonomy must be supported
The genetic counselor has a role to support "self-directed" decisions and honor "the patient knows best."

Patients are resilient
Genetic counselors encourage counselees to draw on their personal abilities with the support of family and community resources to address challenging and painful events.

Patient emotions make a difference
Emotions are evident in the genetic counseling appointment and are invited as part of discussions of meaning, decision and "perceived resilience."

McCarthy Veach et al. (2007)

Each genetic counselor should decide the degree to which they choose to employ a theoretical framework to engage the counselee in discussions that may shift a psychological barrier or tension and support a decision-making process. With whatever counseling model a genetic counselor finds affinity with, there are always dynamics during the session that require the counselor to be agile in seeing, responding, and more fully understanding the counselee so as to maintain the working relationship.

APPRECIATING DYNAMICS THAT CAN ENHANCE AND/OR DISRUPT A SESSION

Disruptions to the working relationship are common and are not necessarily a failure but an observational moment that asks the genetic counselor to be nimble, adjust, and refocus on the counselee. Disruptions offer us avenues to more fully understand the impact of the information we provide, the decisions that may need to be made, and the value of creating meaning by the counselee.

Empathic break

Disruption to empathic listening is called an empathic break. This term describes a shift or a change in the interpersonal dynamics or what can feel like a loss of focus that signals a loss of an empathic connection. Such a break can result from many factors: conscious and unconscious perceptions that are not addressed—including issues of boundaries, autonomy, confidentiality—lack of cross-cultural sensitivity, or simple interruptions in the counseling session (phone calls, a knock on the door, hallway noises). The recognition of an empathic break can sometimes be difficult as it is often a momentary experience. It can result from the actions of the counselor as well as the counselee. The counselor may suddenly remember an issue that has not been explored and conversationally thrust it into the session. The counselee may feel that the counselor has minimized the counselee's concern, or an emphasis has been placed on some information, giving it greater significance than intended by the counselor. This may result in feeling confused, prompting the need to create distance. At this point, the counselee may not be psychologically available to continue with the session. It is essential to recognize a disruption or anticipate the impact of a counselor's inattention, or such action in the session may shift a focus. The shift could be brought to the attention of the counselor by a change in topic, body language, and/or the counselor feeling that something is different. This then requires a quick assessment by the counselor and an effort to move back into empathic attunement.

> *Krystal requested genetic testing to understand risks to her future children. One of her brothers has an undiagnosed intellectual disability and lives with her parents. "I have no communication with my parents, I left home when I was 17 years old." The counselor asked if Krystal could contact her parents to ask if her brother was seen in a genetic clinic or had genetic testing. Krystal looks down and says, "I guess you cannot help me. I am afraid that I will have a baby like my brother."*

At times a counselor may trigger an unexpected or angry response. To prevent the counselee from ending the appointment prematurely requires a conscious effort on the part of the genetic counselor to understand the counselee's perspective.

For example, in the above scenario it is critical that the counselor acknowledge to the counselee that they did not appreciate the counselee's family dilemma. This act of refocusing on the counselee is the first step to acknowledging disruption and "raising" empathy (Wolf, 1988). Recognizing that the genetic counselor did not fully appreciate Krystal's worry and family situation may have implied to the counselee that she was judged for a lack of connection to her family of origin. For many counseling professionals, one's ability to recognize disruptions in empathic attunement comes with postgraduate training and supervision.

Sometimes the counselee will, in the telling of their story, share some information that may be challenging to the values or perspective of the counselor. The counselor's need to reassess their perspective (even if it takes only a few moments) could signal disapproval or confusion to the counselee. This perception could lead to an empathic break, precluding a psychologically driven discussion. The counselor's ability to return to the empathically attuned position following an empathic break is an important skill. Sometimes the counselor finds it difficult to reconnect at the point at which the disconnection occurred. It is here that the counselor should attempt to "raise their empathy," in other words, to make a genuine effort to understand that helps the counselor return to the patient and the narrative. It is important to address an empathic break in a session. Sometimes acknowledging that a shift has occurred can reassure the counselees that their vulnerabilities are being attended to and that a sincere effort to understand is being offered.

Transference/countertransference

A more complex disruption to the working relationship is the experience of transference and countertransference that imposes an invalid understanding and a response to someone through an unconscious template that is superimposed on a person. Consider the basis of our first impressions about others: "I like them" or "there is something odd about them." Usually, this can be attributed to a historical experience, and it can sometimes be difficult to sort out what has stimulated our assumptions or beliefs. This imprint can happen on the part of the counselee or the genetic counselor. We all can have an unconscious response to another. The counselor's responsibility to make themself aware of such psychodynamic events can be essential to maintaining a working alliance. Furthermore, the value of this knowledge is not to provide a therapeutic intervention but to appreciate that it can be disruptive. Depending on the time frame of a genetic counseling session(s), it may be possible in some cases to invite a discussion that may allow for the unconscious to become conscious (McCarthy Veach et al., 2018; Redlinger-Grosse, 2020). This takes additional training and an intentional effort to recognize such a dynamic during any genetic counseling encounter.

The term transference has its roots in psychoanalytic theory, and it describes patterns of expectations that interfere with relationship building. These expectations are often unconscious and are not easily observable to the counselee or counselor. Transference is a ubiquitous phenomenon where one brings old patterns of expectations to new situations in attempts to create familiar structure to the event (Basch, 1980). This psychoanalytic concept can be generalized to all counseling experiences. Most genetic counseling sessions do not trigger unconscious psychodynamically driven transference responses as seen in psychoanalysis. Yet it does occur, in a more conscious way, where the counselee becomes aware of an assumption that triggers discomfort, possibly anger. When the counselee superimposes a belief, expectation, or feeling and it is recognized by the counselor as possibly transferential, one should not be quick to correct this transferred imprint. A hasty decision to correct can be disruptive to the working relationship, as the counselee may be unaware of the distortion and the resulting confusion may elicit an emotional response from the counselee. The challenge for the genetic counselor is not to unconsciously respond to the counselee's transference but to consider this imprint in how the counselee is experiencing the genetic counseling session or an emerging worry. Often this is an opportunity to return to a discussion about a hoped for expectation or concerns related to the appointment.

Countertransference is commonly defined as the reaction or response to a counselee's transference. It is generally the counselor's reaction to the counselee's story or assumption (Weil, 2000). The countertransference reactions in genetic counseling practice are most often of two types: associative and projective (Kessler, 1992c). Associative countertransference can arise when a counselee shares a belief or an experience that carries the counselor (usually momentarily) into their inner self. This introspection is often accompanied by a review of mental images and a recall of conversations. These remembered emotions may rise to the surface and the counselor may no longer be attending to what the counselee is saying and feeling. This distraction may impede or interfere with the full understanding of the counselee (Kessler, 1992a). In addition, the counselee may detect the counselor's distractedness or recognize the counselor's comments are about themselves and not the counselee. It is here that the empathic connection fails and fractures a discussion, often shifting focus back to didactic content of the session. Projection is a type of countertransference where a counselee has made assumptions about the experience of the counselor and the counselor feels challenged. In the face of feeling challenged, the counselor can become defensive and or challenge the counselee on their assumption. A familiar example is when a counselee will inquire whether a decision has angered the genetic counselor. In such cases of projection, the counselee's question may be because they are angry about their decision or with the necessity of having to decide.

Unconscious and conscious processes occur in the counselor as well as the counselee. The challenge is to appreciate psychodynamic clues to reduce the risk of disrupting the working relationship. Genetic counselors have a professional obligation to continue to attend to their own psychological emotional wellbeing; this will help to identify and limit bias and assumptions.

Questioning in the genetic counseling session may be a vehicle for expression of feelings. By asking "Why me?" or just "Why?" the counselee is attempting to share an emotional reaction and discover the meaning of the event. If emotion is what drives the question, the counselor's efforts to provide information rather than addressing the emotion behind the question will disrupt the "holding environment," and a facilitative moment for appreciating the patient's experience will be lost.

On occasion, questioning is an attempt to temporally distance oneself from the psychologically painful moment. A psychologically painful moment is not always visible to the counselor. This may occur when the "self" feels challenged and experiences feelings of shame, guilt, and, not too infrequently, anger. The question may be a request to repeat some information, "Tell me again what will happen," or it may be directed at the counselor "Do you have time to explain this to me?" Multiple questions may be asked, one immediately after another, without allowing time for a complete answer. Questioning can also seem confrontational, challenging the expertise of the counselor by inquiring about the certainty of the diagnosis and/or accuracy of testing. It is necessary to respect such expressions of the counselee's need to reduce the psychological tension and/or the release of intense feelings of anger and frustration.

In rare cases, questions may become barriers between the counselor and counselee. It is useful to attempt to understand what stimulated the barrier: was it an empathic break, or is the counselee tired and needing to end the discussion? It is natural for the counselor, recognizing the emerging barrier and resulting disruption in the working relationship, to try to limit a flow of disruptive questions. The counselor needs to rely on their evolving understanding of the counselee and the emotional content of the session to determine what to do next. There must be a balance; an open acknowledgement of the barrier may need to be accompanied by an offer of assistance to explore the emotional tensions that led to the questions. The ability to achieve this balance comes primarily from experience. One frequently employed intervention is to directly ask the counselee to elaborate on the present experience. One can generally assume that an attempt to describe the emotion is permission for the counselor's assistance. When a counselee appears to be inarticulate or says, "I can't put it into words," the counselor should refrain from giving information and instead consider support options. For example, the counselor may perceive a need to allow adequate time for the counselee to choose the next step. The counselee could be invited to return and continue the discussion. It is important for the genetic counselor to assess any risk factors (lack of support, suicide ideation) and to contract for continuation of the discussion (Peters, 1994).

DISCUSSING DIFFICULT ISSUES AND GIVING BAD NEWS

One of our most important roles as genetic counselors is to sit with a person or family and reveal that a genetic evaluation has identified a risk and that this risk carries implications that can change their understanding of themselves or a loved one, as well as their future. These conversations are frequently experienced as bad news. The psychological response to difficult news varies from person to person. It is, in part, influenced by the gap between what the counselee believes and what is now being presented (Buckman, 1992; Witt and Jankowska, 2018). One of the most critical steps for genetic counselors to manage is the assessment of what counselees believe and understand about the risks they face. This insight allows for structuring a discussion that honors the "gap" and provides adequate time to assist each counselee in their recognition of the issues surrounding the assumed and the real risks. During a disclosure discussion, two reactions are set in motion: the counselee awaits the news, and the counselor anticipates a response. The counselor needs to appreciate that the counselee may need to defend against a feeling (i.e., sadness) to the information provided. Whatever style of coping is presented by the counselee, it should be understood that the counselee's coping style is an effort to emerge intact from the discussion and experience. The genetic counselor can strive to achieve empathic attunement to support the counselee as they begin to integrate the information provided. This may not always be easy for the counselor, since it may prompt a feeling of sympathy. A quick recovery and return to attending to the feelings and comments of our counselees is critical. There are always situations where the news we are presenting will bring forth emotion, alarm, and disbelief. We need to practice caution in these moments and not prematurely disrupt the emotional tension to relieve our own discomfort. Most often, the counselee will seek to regain emotional equilibrium as they create meaning in the face of difficult news and signal to you to continue your explanation. Proceed cautiously with the explanation and stop periodically to seek what is needed from the counselee: "Tell me what you are feeling?," "Should we take a short break?," "What is most important for you to know now?" The goal is to find a balance between information giving and witnessing the impact of the news. Achieving this balance is part intuition, part experience, and mostly driven by taking direction from the counselee. Giving bad news is not easy, but genetic counselors have a unique opportunity to introduce troubling information in a manner that will be viewed over time as caring and supportive.

Reactions and Psychologically Challenging Experiences

The information that counselees learn in the genetic counseling process has the potential to be psychologically overwhelming and to result in an emotional response. Among the many responses to unexpected news, the most common are denial, anger, fear, despair, guilt, shame, sadness, and grief. These responses elicit in the counselee an emotional rather than a cognitive understanding of the implications of the information. The role of the genetic counselor is to provide what can be called "a holding environment," where there is appropriate support, empathy, and time for a response to be expressed and understood. Most people are psychologically resilient, in that they will bring their individual coping styles to adapt.

Denial   Denial is the inability to acknowledge to oneself certain information or news, is a common response when the information elicits shock and fear. This defensive psychological position emerges when other defenses no longer work.

The reaction of denial is usually short term and is part of a coping strategy applied to significant disappointment and impending or actual loss (Kubler-Ross, 1969). The counselee's failure to acknowledge some aspect of external reality that is apparent to others has been further delineated into the constellation of disbelief, deferral, and dismissal (Lubinsky, 1994). The careful delineation of these denial experiences can assist the counselor in choosing more appropriate interventions. To allow for a process that is respectful of any such defense, interventions should be considered only after the counselee has had adequate time to assimilate the news.

Andrew is 54 years old and was referred to learn about testing for Noonan syndrome. He was given this diagnosis in the newborn period based on several features, including growth restriction, webbed neck, and protruding ears, and placed for adoption. Individuals who have a diagnosis of Noonan syndrome are at risk of hypertrophic cardiomyopathy, renal anomalies, and bleeding disorders.

Andrew: I am here to learn if I really have Noonan syndrome. I have been reading about it and I see that as I get older, I may have to watch out for heart and kidney problems,

Counselor: Can you tell me who diagnosed you with Noonan syndrome?

Andrew: When I was a baby, I was given up by my mother. My new family adopted me when I was almost a year old. The doctors told my parents that I might grow up with problems because I have Noonan syndrome. My parents told me it was my webbed neck and funny ears that had them decide that I have Noonan syndrome. My parents thought I was special but worried that I would be slow. Guess that was not true. I am an electrician—a short electrician. I like telling everyone I have a rare genetic disease and I am not like the textbooks say. I like being different.

Andrew: All the doctors I ever saw said they never heard of it. It must be very rare. My new primary care nurse practitioner told me about you and genetic testing.

Counselor: Have you tried to learn about Noonan syndrome testing before?

Andrew: My wife and I tried to have a baby and her doctor said I should get tested. We never had any children—it is ok.

Counselor: Let me tell you about how a diagnosis of Noonan syndrome is made and how a genetic test can help. A genetic test does not always confirm a diagnosis. Some who have a diagnosis will not show a problem in a gene linked to Noonan syndrome. How would that make you feel?

Andrew: I am sure it will show that I have Noonan syndrome. If not, I guess that will be weird.

Counselor: Tell me more about how a negative test would make you feel weird.

Andrew: I guess, I liked having an explanation for why I am short and why I have this funny neck. I know you said I can still have Noonan syndrome and the test comes back fine.

Counselor: I have your genetic test result that examined the genes that have been linked to Noonan syndrome. The laboratory did not find a problem in a gene,

Andrew: I am really surprised. Do you think I should repeat the test? My parents picked me because I had Noonan syndrome.

Andrew's response lets the genetic counselor understand that the diagnosis of Noonan's syndrome has special meaning. It offers a unique opportunity to more fully explore how his clinical diagnosis of Noonan syndrome has shaped his self-perception and his understanding of value to his parents. Such an exploration would aim to support the counselee's effort to begin to modify a narrative of self (Helm, 2015).

Anger Anger is a complex and universal emotion that seeks to blame; in its most extreme form, there can be a wish to achieve revenge. Anger can be directed at others or at oneself (Lazarus and Folkman, 1984; Lazarus 1991). It can be subtle or overt. The counselee with an angry response to information is probably also experiencing fear, powerlessness, guilt, shame, or extreme anxiety. Anger can also be a critical step in the resolution of loss, as the counselee seeks meaning in the need to abandon the hope of a wanted or expected outcome (Kubler-Ross, 1969; Bowlby, 1980). Counselees need the opportunity to express and understand their anger. Assisting the counselee in an exploration of anger will invariably reveal other feelings, usually sadness. For some, anger is a "safer" emotional expression than sadness or grief. Providing the counselee with an opportunity to share the anger is the first step in transforming a feeling into deeper understanding.

A useful intervention is to invite the patient to discuss the anger. "You sound angry. Can you tell me more?" It is very important that the counselor remains non-defensive and it is especially crucial not to trivialize the anger (Peters, 1997). Anger can appear in the form of blame and may be focused on objects (e.g., a lab test), on someone in the past or future, or on the counselor—who represents the medical community. Anger can sometimes take other forms; a common one is crying. The inability to shift anger in the genetic counseling session can impede counseling goals or decisions that are being made (Smith and Antley, 1979; Schema, 2020). Interventions could include witnessing the feeling, honoring its role, and providing a working relationship that through empathic attunement lifts anger (usually for a short time), making it possible to address immediate issues (Mathiesen, 2012).

Joan has been experiencing memory loss and her neurologist referred her for genetic counseling for Alzheimer disease testing. Joan explained that her memory loss is being minimized by her family and she feels alone. After collecting an extensive family medical history that revealed a family member who had a diagnosis of dementia in her 70s, and describing to Joan the limited testing options, Joan expressed surprise and anger that there was no test that would diagnose her with dementia.

Joan: "I am not sure why I am here. I wasted my time and yours."

Counselor: "I know it is disappointing to learn about current genetic testing options. I can imagine that this is a scary experience, and you feel alone."

Joan: "Yes, I am alone."

Working with an angry counselee frequently evokes our own reactions to anger that need to be temporarily quelled. It is not uncommon to find oneself doubting how to manage anger in a session, and this can feel perplexing (Keppers et al., 2022). It can be helpful to speak with a colleague to understand the meaning of the interaction for the counselor and the counselee.

Guilt and Shame   Parents of children with genetic conditions frequently report feelings of guilt and shame (Kessler et al., 1984; Chapple et al., 1995; James et al., 2006). The emotions of guilt and shame have different origins and can provide the counselor with information about the counselee and possible approaches for discussing the issue. Counselees who hold themselves responsible for what they perceive as a negative outcome will frequently attempt to correct their guilt through self-blame, rationalization, or other intellectualization. Counselees who express shame are offering you an opportunity to appreciate that events have placed "a burden of the self" (Kessler et al., 1984). Patients experiencing shame will often attempt to reduce the psychological challenges to the self by means of denial and withdrawal. The counselor's ability to witness the guilt and shame response of the patient provides the first step in offering an intervention that shifts the patient from guilt and shame to a position of self-empathic understanding (Kessler et al., 1984). Genetic counselors should be cautious to not rapidly offer reassurances and instead should consider this an opportunity for exploration (Weil, 2000). It is the process of exploration that can offer some relief.

Loss, Grief, and Despair   Grief and despair are common responses to loss or anticipated loss. Families who learn that their child has a genetic disorder or who receive abnormal prenatal test results can experience a grief process like that of families in which a neonatal death has occurred (Munson and Leuthner, 2007; Rogers et al., 2008). The unexpected loss often results in feelings of shock, anger, yearning, and sadness that may be experienced in phases or concurrently (Kubler-Ross, 1969). Over time, several weeks and sometimes several months, resolution takes the form of gradual acceptance during which personal meaning is created. It is useful to appreciate that sadness or sorrow may be revisited at critical life cycle junctures. This does not necessarily suggest that the grief is unresolved (Hobdell and Deatrick, 1996). Yet, if the process is interrupted or blocked by disenfranchising the emotion, individual and families retreat, lose resiliency, and depression, anxiety, fear, and anger may result in protracted grief.

The genetic counseling experience brings into focus many personal perspectives on loss, a range of responses, and the diverse needs of our counselees. Psychological interventions can be beneficial for some (Leon, 1990). For the majority, resolution of grief takes the form of being "able to make the loss seem meaningful and to gain a renewed sense of purpose and personal identity" (Douglas, 2014; Ali and Bellcross, 2020). Our role as genetic counselors is to be open to listening to the counselee's experience. This act of witnessing the telling of their personal loss, even for a short time, offers emotional comfort to the counselee (Greenspan, 2003). Grief resolution is a process and the genetic counselor's invitation to understand the loss is a step (in some cases, the only steps available to the counselee) to move through the phases of grief and loss. On a self-care note, witnessing your counselee's sadness may trigger your own recall of a loss experience. It is important to take a few minutes and have some self-empathy for your personal experiences.

COPING STYLES

Psychologists have studied coping patterns and styles from different perspectives: psychodynamic, cognitive-behavioral, and neurophysiological. They have observed that most people have one or two primary coping styles which they rely on throughout their lives. Coping strategies are employed for problem solving or to change the meaning of what has been experienced (Pargament, 1997). A set of coping styles identified by Lazarus (1991) is summarized as follows:

Confronting: trying to change the opinion of the person in charge
Distancing: going on as if nothing happened
Self-Controlling: keeping feelings to oneself
Seeking Social Support: engaging in conversation in the hope of learning more
Accepting Responsibility: criticizing oneself
Escape-Avoidance: hoping for a miracle
Plan: identifying and following an action plan
Positive Reappraisal: identifying existing or potential positive outcomes

A coping strategy is not defined by a specific emotion but is an adaptive response to a psychologically challenging situation. Recognizing a coping reaction is helpful in guiding the genetics counseling session and identifying how best to assist the counselee in seeking support regarding a decision or adjusting to information provided in a genetic counseling session (McConkie-Rosell and Sullivan, 1999; Di Mattei et al., 2018).

Psychologically based interventions may be required when a counselee's coping strategy does not work and is disruptive to the counselee and their family. A simple and often effective intervention is asking the counselee to describe how the counselee managed other difficult situations. This may increase your awareness, allowing you to validate the personal experience and the current challenge that is now eliciting this coping strategy. Importantly, the objective in this process is to bring some awareness, but not to eliminate the coping strategy, since the coping strategy may be required for assisting the counselee in adjustment to or resolution of the experience that triggered the response.

SUPERVISION: AN OPPORTUNITY TO FURTHER EXPLORE AND UNDERSTAND OURSELVES AND SELF-CARE

The ability of counselors to master the psychological issues that can emerge in a genetic counseling session can often benefit from an organized analysis of content and experience. All professionals experience an evolution in their skill base and set standards that sometimes cannot be immediately achieved. We all want to feel competent and comfortable. To achieve this goal there needs to be a process by which we confront any awkwardness we may have or anxiety we may feel. "I want to say just the right thing; what is the right thing?"

Genetic counselors are witnesses to complex difficult decisions and a wide range of emotions, all of which can trigger personal reminders, anxiety, disappointment, or strong feelings. Our roles require us to be able to be aware of our own vulnerabilities and abilities to take in the experience of others (Weil, 2000). Periodic self-reflection allows us to see how we have changed in our professional role and what continues to be uncomfortable or puzzling in a genetic counseling session. Discussion with colleagues, formal genetic counseling supervision, or personal counseling are important resources for a practicing genetic counselor.

Genetic counselors who are drawn to the psychological aspects of our practice are invited to seek additional reading and training. One learning method that is underutilized in our profession is postgraduate case supervision. The supervision process ensures a continuing education experience, as well as an ongoing dialogue of self-awareness about vulnerabilities, tensions, and frustrations that may impact the counselee (Kennedy, 2000; Middleton et al., 2007) These discussions can occur on an individual basis with a clinician recognized to have more experience than the counselor, with a colleague, or under group supervision (leader or peer). The aim of such a discussion is to guide the counselor to a deeper and more complex understanding of the issues that were presented by the counselee and the personal meaning of the issues to the counselor. It will enhance appreciation of questions raised and responses to them, the conscious or unconscious interpersonal or family dynamics, and finally allow counselors to acknowledge themselves as part of the psychological milieu that stimulates a response from the counselee (Runyon et al., 2010).

Ideally, participation in postgraduate supervision case discussions allows for extended analysis of a case presentation as well as an opportunity for the counselor to fully appreciate how one's own psychological needs and tensions impact the cognitive tasks of the genetic counseling session. As our profession continues to mature, and as we seek to offer exemplary psychologically attuned genetic counseling, we need to continue to learn from each other and other psychologically trained professionals. Seeking a supervision group outside of our community of genetic counselors is another way to broaden our perspectives and skills. We could look at other professions that utilize postgraduate supervision with an experienced practitioner to support professional growth through guidance in a climate of trust. Genetic counselors who are concerned or are experiencing "compassion fatigue" as a byproduct of empathic connection may find that through supervision, they can limit the personal impact of the empathic demands and be able to fine tune a skill to achieve a delicate balance between empathic connection and detachment (Benoit et al., 2007; Lee et al., 2015).

CONCLUSION

Understanding the importance of the working relationship to the integrity of the genetic counseling appointment is essential. As genetic counselors, we have a responsibility to be observant, thoughtful, skilled, and committed to the psychological experiences in an appointment. The degree to which a counselor and counselee choose to explore the psychological content within the session will depend on the goals that are mutually set and the skills of the counselor. It is a disservice to the counselee to not be fully cognizant of the psychological framework that surrounds genetic counseling discussions. In a medical climate where other professionals are seeking roles with families facing genetic testing and diagnosis, it becomes more imperative that genetic counselors demonstrate and remain committed to the full scope of genetic counseling. Time constraints and the role expectations set in the definition of genetic counseling force some counselors to attend to the psychological aspects as the "last step," if time is remaining. To see genetic counseling as linear steps in a process inaccurately deconstructs the interactive dynamic aspect through the discussions in the appointment. In settings where counselors have the opportunity to meet families with social workers and psychologists, genetic counselors must still continue attending to the psychological dynamic. Our mental health colleagues can bring a special richness to the genetic counseling session, but it is only the genetic counselor who provides the unique knowledge base that allows for the unfolding of genetic and medical information in a psychologically attentive way. To distance ourselves from psychological skills is to lose the core of our professional role. I invite you to explore the psychological dynamics in our practice and commit to professional development that strengthens counseling skills and deepens your understanding of self in relation to your role as genetic counselor.

REFERENCES

Ali N & Bellcross C. (2020) A genetic counselor's guide to understanding grief. In: B LeRoy, P McCarthy Veach, & P Callanan (eds.) *Genetic Counseling Practice: Advanced Concepts and Skills* Second Edition. Hoboken, NJ: Wiley, pp. 79–108.

Austin J, Semaka A, & Hadjipavlou G. (2014) Conceptualizing genetic counseling as psychotherapy in the era of genomic medicine. *J Genet Couns* 23(6):903–909.

Basch MF. (1980) *Doing Psychotherapy*. New York, NY: Basic Books.

Bellet PS & Maloney MJ (1991) The importance of empathy as an interviewing skill in medicine. *JAMA* 266(13):1831–1832.

Benoit LG, Veach PM, & LeRoy BS. (2007) When you care enough to do your very best: genetic counselor experiences of compassion fatigue. *J Genet Couns* 16(3):299–312.

Biesecker BB. (2020) Genetic counseling and the central tenets of practice. *Cold Spring Harb Perspect Med* 10(3):a038968.

Biesecker BB & Peters KF. (2001) Process studies in genetic counseling: peering into the black box. *Am J Med Genet* 106(3):191–198.

Biesecker B, Austin J, & Caleshu C. (2017) Theories for psychotherapeutic genetic counseling: fuzzy trace theory and cognitive behavior theory. *J Genet Couns* 26(2):322–330.

Bordin ES. (1979) The generalizability of the psychoanalytic concept of the working alliance. *Psychother: Theory Res* Pract 16:252–260.

Bovee A. (2007, personal communication) Board certified genetic counselor.

Bowlby J. (1980) *Loss, Sadness and Depression*. New York, NY: Basic Books.

Brown I. (2012) *The Boy in the Moon: A Father's Journey to Understand his Extraordinary Son*. New York, NY: St. Martin's Griffin.

Buckman R. (1992) *How to Break Bad News*. Baltimore, MD: Johns Hopkins University Press.

Chapple A, May C, & Campion P. (1995) Parental guilt: the part played by the clinical geneticist. *J Genet Couns* 4(3):179–192.

Di Mattei VE, Carnelli L, Bernardi M, et al. (2018) Coping mechanisms, psychological distress, and quality of life prior to cancer genetic counseling. *Front Psychol* 16(9):1218.

Djurdjinovic L & Peters J. (2017) Special issue introduction: dealing with psychological and social complexity in genetic counseling. *J Genet Counsel* 26(2):1–4.

Douglas HA. (2014) Promoting meaning-making to help our patients grieve: an exemplar for genetic counselors and other health care professionals. *J Genet Couns* 23(5): 695–700.

Eunpu DL. (1997) Systemically-based psychotherapeutic techniques in genetic counseling. *J Genet Couns* 6(1):1–20.

Evans C. (2006). *Genetic Counseling: A Psychological Approach*. Cambridge: Cambridge University Press.

Fioretti C, Mazzocco K, Riva S, et al. (2016) Research studies on patients' illness experience using the narrative medicine approach: a systematic review. *BMJ Open* 6(7):e011220. doi: 10.1136/bmjopen-2016-011220.

Godino L, Turchetti D, Jackson L, et al. (2016) Impact of presymptomatic genetic testing on young adults: a systematic review. *Eur J Hum Genet* 24(4):496–503.

Gonçalves MM & Stiles WB. (2011) Narrative and psychotherapy: introduction to the special section. *Psychother Res* 21(1):1–3.

Graybar SR & Leonard LM. (2005) In defense of listening. *Am J Psychother* 59(1):1–18.

Greenspan M. (2003) *Healing Through the Dark Emotions: The Wisdom of Grief, Fear and Despair*. Boston, MA: Shabhala Publications.

Helm B. (2015) Exploring the genetic counselor's role in facilitating meaning-making: rare disease diagnoses. *J Genet Couns* 24(2):205–212.

Hobdell E & Deatrick JA. (1996) Chronic sorrow: a content analysis of parental differences. *J Genet Couns* 5(2):57–68.

James CA, Hadley DW, Holtzman NA, and Winkelstein JA. (2006) How does the mode of inheritance of a genetic condition influence families? A study of guilt, blame, stigma, and understanding of inheritance and reproductive risks in families with X-linked and autosomal recessive diseases. *Genet Med* 8(4):234–242.

Jordan JV. (1997) Relational development through mutual empathy. In: AC Bohart & LS Greenberg (eds.) *Empathy Reconsidered: New Directions in Psychotherapy.* Washington, DC: American Psychological Association, pp. 343–351.

Kennedy AL. (2000) Supervision for practicing genetic counselors: an overview of models. *J Genet Couns* 9(5):379–390.

Keppers R, McCarthy Veach P, Schema L, et al. (2022) Differences in genetic counseling student responses to intense patient affect: a study of students in North American programs. *Journal of Genet Couns* 31:398–410.

Kessler S. (1979) The genetic counselor as psychotherapist. *Birth Defects Orig Artic Ser* 15(2):187–200.

Kessler S. (1992a) Process issues in genetic counseling. *Birth Defects Orig Artic Ser* 28(1):1–10.

Kessler S. (1992b) Psychological aspects of genetic counseling. VII. Thoughts of directiveness. *J Genet Couns* 1:9–17.

Kessler S. (1992c) Psychological aspects of genetic counseling. VIII. Suffering and counter-transference. *J Genet Couns* 1(4):303–308.

Kessler S, Kessler H, & Ward P. (1984) Psychological aspects of genetic counseling. III. Management of guilt and shame. *Am J Med Genet* 17(3):673–697.

Kirschenbaum H & Henderson VL. (eds.) (1989) *The Carl Rogers Reader.* Boston, MA: Houghton Mifflin.

Kohut, H. (1984) *How Does Psychoanalysis Cure?* Chicago, IL: University of Chicago Press.

Kubler-Ross E. (1969) *On Death and Dying.* New York, NY: Macmillan.

Lazarus RS & Folkman S. (1984) *Stress, Appraisal, and Coping.* New York, NY: Springer.

Lazarus RS. (1991) *Emotion and Adaptation.* New York, NY: Oxford University Press.

Lee W, Veach PM, MacFarlane IM, & LeRoy BS. (2015) Who is at risk for compassion fatigue? An investigation of genetic counselor demographics, anxiety, compassion, satisfaction, and burnout. *J Genet Couns* 24:358–370.

Leon IG. (1990) *When a Baby Dies.* New Haven, CT: Yale University Press.

Lubinsky MS. (1994) Bearing bad news: dealing with mimics of denial. *J Genet Couns* 3(1):5–12.

MacLeod R, Metcalfe A, & Ferrer-Duch M. (2021) A family systems approach to genetic counseling: Development of narrative interventions. *J Genet Couns* 30(1):22–29.

Mathiesen AM. (2012) Counseling the "angry patient": a defining moment of changing focus from myself to the patient. *J Genet Couns* 21:209–210.

McCarthy Veach P, LeRoy BS, & Callanan NP. (2018) Genetic counseling dynamics: transference, countertransference, distress, burnout, and compassion fatigue. In: P McCarthy Veach, BS LeRoy, & NP Callanan (eds.) *Facilitating the Genetic Counseling Process.* New York, NY: Springer.

McCarthy Veach PM, Bartels DM, & Leroy BS. (2007) Coming full circle: a reciprocal-engagement model of genetic counseling practice. *J Genet Couns* 16(6):713–728.

McConkie-Rosell A & Sullivan JA. (1999) Genetic counseling - stress, coping, and the empowerment perspective. *J Genet Couns* 8(6):345–357.

Middleton A, Wiles V, Kershaw A, et al. (2007) Reflections on the experience of counseling supervision by a team of genetic counselors from the UK. *J Genet Couns* 16(2):143–155.

Munson D & Leuthner SR. (2007) Palliative care for the family carrying a fetus with a life-limiting diagnosis. *Pediatr Clin North Am* 54(5):787–798.

Pargament KI. (1997) *The Psychology of Religion and Coping: Theory, Research, and Practice*. New York, NY: Guilford Press.

Peters J. (1997, personal communication). Genetic Counselor.

Peters J, Hoskins L, Prindiville S, et al. (2006) Evolution of the colored eco-genetic relationship map (CEGRM) for assessing social functioning in women in hereditary breast-ovarian (HBOC) families. *J Genet Couns* 15(6):477–489.

Peters JA. (1994) Suicide prevention in the genetic counseling context. *J Genet Couns* 3(3):199–213.

Reed SC. (1955) *Counseling in Medical Genetics*. Philadelphia PA: WB Saunders.

Redlinger-Grosse K. (2020) Countertransference: making the unconscious conscious. In: BD LeRoy, P McCarthy Veach, & NP Callanan (eds.) *Genetic Counseling Practice: Advanced Concepts and Skills* Second Edition. Hoboken, NJ: Wiley, pp. 153–176.

Resta R, Biesecker BB, Bennett RL, et al. (2006) A new definition of genetic counseling: National Society of Genetic Counselors' Task Force report. *J Genet Couns* 15(2):77–83.

Rogers CH, Floyd FJ, Seltzer MM, et al. (2008) Long-term effects of the death of a child on parents' adjustment in midlife. *J Fam Psychol* 22(2):203–211.

Rogers CR. (1942) *Counseling and Psychotherapy: New Concepts in Practice*. Boston, MA: Houghton Mifflin.

Runyon M, Zahm, KW, Veach PM, et al. (2010) What do genetic counselors learn on the job? A qualitative assessment of professional development outcomes. *J Genet Couns* 19:371–386.

Salema D, Townsend A, & Austin J. (2019) Patient decision-making and the role of the prenatal genetic counselor: an exploratory study. *J Genet Couns* 28(1):155–163.

Schema L. (2020). Patient anger: insights and strategies. In: BD LeRoy, P McCarthy Veach, & NP Callanan (eds.) *Genetic Counseling Practice: Advanced Concepts and Skills* Second Edition. Hoboken, NJ: Wiley, pp. 109–130.

Sexton AC, Sahhar M, Thorburn DR, & Metcalfe SA. (2008) Impact of a genetic diagnosis of a mitochondrial disorder 5–17 years after the death of an affected child. *J Genet Couns* 17:261–273.

Smith RW & Antley RM. (1979) Anger: a significant obstacle to informed decision making in genetic counseling. *Birth Defects Orig Artic Ser* 15(5C):257–260.

Spencer AC. (2016) Stories as gift: patient narratives and the development of empathy. *J Genet Couns* 25:687–690.

Weil J. (2000) *Psychosocial Genetic Counseling*. New York, NY: Oxford University Press.

Weil J. (2003) Psychosocial genetic counseling in the post-nondirective era: a point of view. *J Genet Couns* 12(3):199–211.

Weil J, Ormond K, Peters J, et al. (2006) The relationship of nondirectiveness to genetic counseling: report of a workshop at the 2003 NSGC Annual Education Conference. *J Genet Couns* 15(2):85–93.

Witt MM & Jankowska KA. (2018) Breaking bad news in genetic counseling-problems and communication tools. *J Appl Genet* 59(4):449–452.

Wolf ES. (1988) *Treating the Self*. New York, NY: Guilford Press.

Zimmermann BM & Shaw D. (2020) How the "control-fate continuum" helps explain the genetic testing decision-making process: a grounded theory study. *Eur J Hum Genet* 28(8):1010–1019.

5

Patient-Centered Communication and Providing Information in Genetic Counseling

Jehannine (J9) Austin

INTRODUCTION

Patient-centered communication is the most fundamentally crucial, enshrined foundation of genetic counseling. The central element of genetic counseling practice is the relationship between counselor and patient/client (Veach et al., 2007).[1] This relationship is constructed and dependent on patient-centered communication. The challenge, of course, lies in determining how to operationalize this concept: what exactly does patient-centered communication look like in practice? To answer this

---

[1] For an excellent discussion of the different terms that we might use to refer to those we work with in genetic counseling practice (counselee, client, consumer, patient), please refer to "Advanced genetic counseling: theory and practice" (Biesecker et al., 2019). In this chapter, I will use "patient" for consistency with the literature in other areas of medicine around "patient-centered care."

A Guide to Genetic Counseling, Third Edition. Edited by Vivian Y. Pan, Jane L. Schuette, Karen E. Wain, and Beverly M. Yashar.
© 2025 John Wiley & Sons Ltd. Published 2025 by John Wiley & Sons Ltd.

question, we first need to establish the range of circumstances in which we practice.

Genetic counseling occurs in many different contexts and circumstances. In some contexts—for example, in prenatal, pediatric, and cancer settings— genetic counseling is often about facilitating testing and helping patients to navigate its implications. In other contexts—for example, psychiatric genetic counseling—there may be no immediate or obvious decision for a patient to make, and no genetic testing options; rather, the counseling may be about using genetic information to help the patient—at an existential level—to meaning- fully understand the answers to questions like "Why me? Why do I have mental illness? Is there anything I can do to prevent future relapses?" Though neither decision making, nor genetic testing, is always explicitly front and center of the genetic counseling interaction, there are commonalities that are shared between all genetic counseling contexts. Regardless of the specifics of the context and circumstance, at a higher level, genetic counseling can be defined as shown in Box 5-1:

BOX 5-1. DEFINITION OF GENETIC COUNSELING (RESTA ET AL., 2006)

Genetic counseling is:

"the process of helping people to understand and adapt to the medical, familial and psychological implications of genetic contributions to disease"

Note: Although genetic counseling is often conflated with genetic testing and/or risk communication, this definition of genetic counseling does not mention, necessitate, or rely on the provision of genetic testing or estimates for chance of recurrence of a condi- tion in the family, and does not focus on decision making.

To help people to *understand*, genetic counseling embraces the maxim of "knowledge is power," and seeks to provide patients with the most accurate and understandable information possible. However, it is important to make explicit that genetic *counseling* does (or at least should) not involve *only* providing genetic education (or genetic information). Genetic information—like genetic test result information—is a tool that genetic counselors use in the context of a psychothera- peutically oriented interaction (Austin et al., 2014) that focuses on helping the patient to *adapt*; for this, the patient–counselor relationship and patient-centered communication is foundational. It is a counseling interaction, rather than simply an educational or informational one.

Though, historically, genetic counseling was regarded as encompassing a spectrum of individual styles—ranging from purely education-based, to psychotherapeutic (Kessler, 1997)—over time, research evidence has accumulated to indicate that the best outcomes of genetic counseling are achieved for patients when counselors engage in a more counseling-oriented approach to their practice (Kessler and Antley, 1981; Edwards et al., 2008; Meiser et al., 2008). This holds true across multiple patient outcomes (e.g., satisfaction, empowerment)—even knowledge-based outcomes are facilitated by the use of more counseling-oriented approaches. Indeed, while genetic *information*, on its own, does not seem to reliably produce the outcome of helping people change behavior to protect their health (Hollands et al., 2016), there is some emerging evidence suggesting that the use of genetic information in the context of psychotherapeutically oriented genetic *counseling* may be able to deliver this kind of outcome (Semaka and Austin, 2019).

WHAT IS PATIENT-CENTERED COMMUNICATION?

Conceptually, "patient-centered communication" suggests a distinction from provider-centric communication, or illness-centered communication (Bardes, 2012). Indeed, genetic counseling originates in a Rogerian person-centered practice, whereby both patient and counselor bring valuable perspectives and expertise to the relationship that they build together: the counselor is an expert in the science of the condition that forms the indication for the visit, and the patient is the expert on their own experiences, values, and perspectives. The patient-centered approach to interactions seeks a more equal valuing of both types of expertise (Smets et al., 2007), where a patient's rights and autonomy are respected. Patient participation and involvement, and the quality of the relationship between the patient and health care professional, are key elements of patient-centered care that transcend health disciplines (Kitson et al., 2013), but the more nuanced ways in which patient-centered care is operationalized varies between disciplines (Kitson et al., 2013). In genetic counseling, attempts to operationalize the process of respecting patients' rights and autonomy—which are central to patient-centered care—often relate to, or intersect with, the concept of nondirectiveness.

As a term, "nondirectiveness" is deeply familiar to genetic counselors, and yet poorly understood and variously defined over time (refer to Jamal et al. (2020) for a summary). It can be helpful to understand the term in its historical context: the concept originated when genetic counseling was emerging as a profession, was primarily concerned with prenatal counseling, and was seeking to distance itself from the practice of eugenics (Stern, 2012). In this context, describing genetic counseling as "nondirective" indicated that practitioners would not "direct" their patients to terminate pregnancies with genetic conditions (Resta, 1997). Rather, genetic counseling sought to privilege patient autonomy in reproductive decision-making.

Since the early days, however, genetic counseling has evolved to expand into many different specialties, in some of which genetic counselors regularly give directions or advice to their patients (Resnicow et al., 2022) For example, "take folic acid prenatally," "participate in annual screening to detect and treat cancer early." Such advice giving, when we know that there is evidence that objectively supports better health outcomes for our patients, is morally the right thing to do—supporting autonomy is not enough on its own. Truly patient-centered communication involves a responsibility to ensure that when our patients are making health care decisions, these are not just autonomous, but both autonomous *and informed*.

It is worthwhile to define *autonomy* more specifically in terms of how it is typically considered in genetic counseling. Though in Western culture, "autonomy" is typically implicitly thought of as meaning *individual* autonomy, genetic counseling has its foundations in feminist ethics and in practice, and we tend to take a more relational view to understanding autonomy. In practice, genetic counselors tend to also value an individual's family and other relationships and recognize that people are embedded in a social and historical context (Mackenzie et al., 2000). Fundamentally, genetic counseling is about supporting and promoting people in exercising their rights to bodily autonomy in making health decisions. So, while as genetic counselors we may exercise our *own* rights to bodily autonomy in a range of different ways—for example, by choosing to have, or not have, genetic testing, prophylactic mastectomy, hormonal suppression of puberty, or an abortion (and in other ways: wearing a hijab or getting a tattoo)—our role with our patients is to help support and promote their rights to their own bodily autonomy in health decisions.

Though, in genetic counseling, our discourse tends to focus on the bioethical principle of autonomy, the practice of ensuring patients are *informed* relates to other ethical principles of beneficence (the responsibility to keep patient welfare at the heart of what we do; with regard to information, this might involve respecting their right to accurate information), non-maleficence (the responsibility to ensure that our actions do not cause harm; in regard to information, this might mean ensuring that patients are informed of potential consequences of decisions) in particular, but also justice (e.g., to ensure that everyone we work with is provided the information they need in a way that they can understand, and that we facilitate their use of that information in an equitable way). Indeed, ethical concepts beyond these four basic principles of bioethics are deeply relevant to genetic counseling practice: refer to Chapter 12 for more discussions on ethical genetic counseling.

Importantly, while we have a responsibility to ensure that patients are informed, this should *not* be taken to imply an expectation that the information we provide is used in a manner that is purely logical or rational, or that people make decisions that are objectively "right" in some way. The beauty of the patient-centered approach is that it embraces the whole human. Whole humans are complex and not governed entirely by logic and rationality—this is not a flaw to be corrected or overcome, but a feature to be appreciated and addressed. Our purpose in engaging in patient-centered communication in genetic counseling is to support our patients' autonomy in using the information that we provide in a manner that aligns best with their values, principles, and goals.

DECIDING WHAT INFORMATION TO PROVIDE IN THE CONTEXT OF PATIENT-CENTERED GENETIC COUNSELING

We cannot possibly give people all the information we have access to that pertains to a patient's indicated condition in the time that we have available to spend with them. And, indeed, that's not what patients want or need. Too much information can be overwhelming for anyone, it can impede our ability to process, and can actually reduce how much we take away from an interaction. So, how do genetic counselors decide and prioritize what particular pieces of information to give patients?

In some contexts, there will be protocols, policies, or guidelines that we can refer to, which will detail the specific informational content that we need to provide in a genetic counseling session. In other situations where such guidance does not exist, one of the issues that arises is the fear of litigation, which may drive genetic counselors, and their institutions, to err towards providing more information. It is important to explicitly acknowledge the bias towards providing more information, as it can—theoretically at least—result in a tension with engaging in truly patient-centered communication. In fact, research shows that in medical settings, patient-centered communication relates to a *decreased* frequency of lawsuits. (Levinson et al., 1997; Huntington and Kuhn, 2003). Further, some data shows that patient-centered care results in improvement in patient outcomes and higher satisfaction (which is a strong motivator to many health organizations, especially in the (USA) (Anderson et al., 1995; Stewart, 1995; Kinmonth et al., 1998; Stewart et al., 2000; Stewart, 2001). We need to actively attend to the patients' actual informational needs and tailor our information-giving accordingly.

When we are driven by our own agendas (i.e., thinking only from our own frame of reference, about the information we feel we need to convey), we can find ourselves providing information that patients do *not* want, or failing to provide information that they *do* want. For example, research shows that when a genetic diagnosis is being made in a pediatric setting, spending session time providing information about future pregnancies when the parents are—at least in that moment—only interested in understanding the impact of the condition on their existing child, can be experienced by patients as callous/damaging (Ashtiani et al., 2014). On the other hand, other studies reveal that if the genetic condition in question has manifestations (e.g., psychiatric) which are *not* disclosed to the family, this too can be damaging to rapport and trust (Cohen et al., 2017; Goodwin et al., 2017; Carrion et al., 2022).

So, when there are no policy or guideline documents to indicate which specific pieces of information we need to provide, how do we decide what to share? If we look to the National Society of Genetic Counselors' Code of Ethics for help in this matter, we find it states that genetic counselors should: "enable their clients to make informed decisions, free of coercion, by providing or illuminating the necessary facts, and clarifying the alternatives and anticipated consequences" (NSGC, n.d.). This helps—to a point—but the struggle then becomes determining what the "necessary facts" are, in a given situation. There are no agreed upon rules for this,

---

BOX 5-2. PRIORITIZING INFORMATION TO DISCUSS IN THE GENETIC COUNSELING SESSION

There are no agreed rules to define what information is "necessary" to provide in genetic counseling. But, as a guide, we can consider prioritizing spending time on topics that:

1. directly relate to the indication for the referral
2. are time sensitive in managing their current situation, or that may have a lasting impact for the patient (e.g., anticipatory guidance)
3. align with what the patient expresses a need to know about.*

* We need to use our communication and empathic skills to explore and understand the patient's informational needs and understanding.

---

but the criteria in Box 5-2 aim to help genetic counselors think through how to prioritize information discussed during a genetic counseling session.

When a particular topic addresses multiple of the criteria outlined in Box 5-2, the more important it is to address. Information that we feel is good for a patient to have, but that does not fall into at least one of these categories, could be provided in the context of a follow-up visit, and/or information provided to take home.

If we apply these principles to the situation introduced above, in which a new genetic diagnosis has been made in a pediatric setting, if the patient does not spontaneously express a need to know about the chance for recurrence in subsequent children (it is not as immediately or directly the reason for the referral, which is about the existing child, and it is not immediately time sensitive), we might offer this as a topic for discussion (e.g., "I know this might not be what you are thinking about right now, but if you are interested in knowing about the chances for future children you might have to have the same condition, we can talk about that") and if declined, simply provide them with information to take home about this and/or offer a follow-up appointment. If the new diagnosis confers an increased chance for psychiatric illness for the child, this could be argued to be directly related to the reason for referral (prognosis for the diagnosed condition), and could have a lasting impact for the patient (anticipatory guidance in terms of monitoring/managing emerging symptoms), and therefore could be prioritized for discussion.

PRINCIPLES OF PROVIDING PATIENT-CENTERED INFORMATION

Once we have decided *what* information to provide in the context of genetic counseling, we can now consider principles that we can use to guide us in how to best deliver the information. The genetic counseling community has spent a lot of time and energy on these kinds of questions—considering whether information can be delivered in a "balanced" or "neutral" way, what nondirectiveness looks like in practice, and how we use language, counseling aids, and written documents when delivering information to accommodate different levels of health literacy. These concepts will be discussed briefly below, before we consider what the *process* of providing information looks like in genetic counseling.

Can Information be Provided "Neutrally" or in a "Balanced" Way?

The reality is that the value of information (i.e., whether it is "neutral," or "balanced" or not) is not objectively classifiable. Rather, information that we provide—and the manner in which we provide it (e.g., nonverbal communication: our body positioning, gestures, eye contact)—is subjectively assessed by the patient in a manner influenced by their values, culture, experience, and so on. Additionally, factors beyond the *content* of the information that we provide can influence how information is perceived; for example, the tone of voice in which it is delivered, and the *sequence* in which we present different components of information. Even the structures that exist in which we present the information to patients influence how it is perceived (e.g., if there is a system set up by society to offer this test, it suggests that I should take it).

In the context of prenatal genetic counseling when a diagnosis of Down syndrome is made, patients have reported feeling that the information they were provided about the condition tended towards the medicalized and more negative (Sheets et al., 2011). As a result, efforts have—appropriately—been made to increase attention to disability rights in genetic counseling training, to avoid overt ableism and medicalization of Down syndrome and other conditions. We also need to ensure that we do not veer too far in the other direction and provide idealized pictures that suggest that families all experience having a child with Down syndrome as an exclusively bonding and positive experience; this does not reflect the reality of families' experiences. Thus, the goal is to ensure that families understand that all children with Down syndrome are different, in the same way that all children who do not have Down syndrome are different, and that families' experiences vary widely (Hippman et al., 2012). Just as we need to avoid ableism, it is absolutely critical that we should strive to ensure that any information we provide is not is tinged with any other kind of bigotry (racism, sexism, etc.). And certainly, more remains to be done in terms of how we address some related issues in practice; especially, for example, with regard to neurodiversity.

At a deeper level, it is worth considering what providing "balanced information" might look like in practice, other than simply avoiding bigotry or idealism—and whether it is achievable, given its subjective nature. In at least one study, what people meant when they said they wanted "balanced information" was an idea of what the future would look like in their specific situation (Hippman et al., 2012). This is of course deeply understandable, but also unachievable (because no one can predict the future). Often, articulating this for a patient could potentially be helpful, for example: "In situations like this, we can powerfully want to know exactly how this diagnosis will affect us personally, and our family circumstances—whether it will bring us closer together, or whether there will be difficulties that drive us apart—and we can't know that sort of thing for sure, which is frustrating. And living with and managing that kind of uncertainty is really hard."

Communicating Directly and "Nondirectiveness"

Many thought leaders within the genetic counseling profession have critiqued the concept of "nondirectiveness" for a variety of reasons, over several decades (Oduncu, 2002; Weil et al., 2006; Rehmann-Sutter, 2009; Jamal et al., 2020). For myself, one of my primary reasons for harboring a deep desire to consign the term to history emerges from the ambiguity regarding the definition of "nondirectiveness", which—together with a general, nebulous sense that "directive = bad"—has real and negative effects on genetic counselors' patient-centeredness in practice. Specifically, genetic counselors can be left feeling a need to avoid communicating in any way that could be construed as advice, suggestion, or even simply direct speech. With regard to the latter, for example, it has been my experience that genetic counselors often try to encourage parents to arrive at their own conclusion that their child's genetic condition is not their fault, instead of indicating this through direct speech. In this situation, rather than saying—directly—"it's not your fault," we tend towards simply providing information about inheritance—for example, "you can't control the genetic information you pass on"—and hope that the patient correctly derives the conclusion for themselves. In some situations, simply telling someone directly that it's not their fault can be hugely powerful—cathartic and healing—for the patient, and absolutely in alignment with patient-centered communication practices. These words are within our power but we sometimes withhold them to avoid the potential for being somehow construed as "direct*ive*", rather than simply direct. As you develop your own communication style, I encourage you to consider moving away from centering the concept of "nondirectiveness" and practice clear and direct patient-centered communication. For examples of how to practically do this, refer to the section below about facilitating decision-making.

Language

It is important to explicitly acknowledge and to be aware that the language in which we are trained tends to be fairly technical, complex, and jargon-laden. Our task is to make these technical, complex words and concepts understandable, meaningful, and useful to those we are counseling—who will range widely in their health literacy.[2] For example, even referring to a test result as being "positive"—something

---

[2] Please note that the strategies woven throughout in this chapter, but especially directly in this section and the subsequent one (about written information counseling aids etc.), all reflect health literacy best practices. The health literacy literature is a rich resource that has direct relevance to our practice and may be useful to interested readers.

genetic counselors do constantly and intuitively amongst ourselves—is jargon. To our patients, "a positive test result" might sound like something good, or that we "passed" something. To address this potential problem, the first step is awareness; challenge yourself to think about words that you now use routinely but that may be experienced by others as complex (e.g., "gene"), or words that might be understood to mean something different in genetics than in the rest of the world (e.g., "a positive test result"). Once we are aware of these words, we can think about and practice different ways of presenting this information; for example, by talking about how "the test result shows that you have [condition X]."

Mirroring language used by the patient can help with centering them in the communication process. Special care should be taken when communicating with patients around issues such as disability and neurodiversity. Specifically, while training often privileges "person first" language (e.g., "person with a disability," "person with autism"), some members of these communities prefer to use, and to be referred to with, identity first language (e.g., "I am/Alex is disabled," "I am/ Casey is Autistic"). If in doubt, check in with patients about their preferences. Similarly, for members of the LGBTQIA2S+ community, it is important to be mindful about language used in relation to partnerships, childbearing, and bodily organs (Ruderman et al., 2021; Rolle et al., 2022). It is important to recognize that preferred language around these issues is evolving, and remaining current is part of our duties with regard to lifelong learning as members of our profession. Of course, mirroring language may not always be appropriate; if a patient is using a slur, for example.[3] In these situations, simply modeling use of non-bigoted language may be the most appropriate response; but in some situations, challenging a patient's use of a slur could be considered (e.g., "That's right, yes—and just to point out, the term that we use now is intellectual disability," "When you say that your relative is 'crazy'—can you tell me what you mean by that?").

Metaphors and analogies can be another useful tool to facilitate patients' connection with the matter when describing complex concepts, such as how genes and environment interact together in contributing to the development of complex conditions. It is important to consider the way in which we use these, though, as they have limitations. For example, wrapping up a session with a metaphor like: "I'll leave the ball in your court then" when we mean "Contact me if you'd like to come back in" may not be optimal, as it may not be immediately clear to everyone. Similarly, while using analogies (e.g., our genome as a blueprint or a recipe book, proteins as building blocks etc.) can be useful, in some circumstances they can also potentially act as barriers. Using sports analogies with people who don't follow sports, or musical analogies with people who are not musicians, can create distance or barriers in the relationship. Analogies that use simple concepts, and that are as accessible to as many

---

[3] Of course, a slur that is directed at us should not be tolerated. Patient-centered counseling relies on mutual respect. A counselor whose patient is directing slurs at them has a responsibility to take care of their own safety first.

people as possible, are likely to be the most useful. In the context of psychiatric conditions, one of the analogies that we have developed and that patients/families have found to be helpful is the "Jar model" (Austin et al., 2014; Carrion et al., 2022). In this simple visual analogy, the central concept is that everyone has a mental illness jar, and that in order to be actively experiencing an episode of illness, the jar has to be filled to the top. We discuss with patients how there are two different kinds of vulnerability/predisposition/susceptibility factors that can be used to fill the jar—genetic factors are represented by balls, and environmental (or experiential) factors are represented by pyramids. We can use this concept to discuss how the amount of genetic factors we each have: 1) is constant over time; and 2) is nothing we can control. The amount of environmental/experiential vulnerability may change over time, and we may have some degree of influence over some of these elements, we do not have absolute control. For more information on this analogy refer to Austin (2019).

Written Information, Counseling Aids, and Educational Material

Communicating in different modalities provides opportunity for information to be taken in or understood in different ways. Although we tend to think of the primary mode of provision of information in genetic counseling as being speech/listening, other modalities, including counseling aids, pre-session educational materials, and post-session patient letters, are often used, and can in fact be very important.

Visual aids like graphics/pictures/drawings or even models/physical props, are used in genetic counseling to aid in conveying complex abstract concepts in more tangible formats. Intuitively, it would seem that such aids could have utility—being able to hear and see information seems like it should be reinforcing, especially in situations where there are language-based communication barriers, where a patient has low health literacy, and/or is young. However, the impact of these kinds of aids on the process and/or patient outcomes of genetic counseling interventions has not been extensively studied. Though patients may find great utility in counselors' use of a visual aid, in certain circumstances the use of some types of counseling aids may negatively impact patient-centered communication (Zikmund-Fisher et al., 2011).

The *manner* in which counseling aids are used is crucial. In some circumstances, a counselor using visual aids could become more didactic/educational in their style, which would be counter to a patient-centered approach. Rather than using a particular selection of visual aids in a standardized or rote way for everyone (or everyone with a particular indication), the selection and use of visual aids should be carefully considered and chosen to convey information that directly addresses the needs of each patient. For example, in the context of a psychiatric genetic counseling session (where the information provided is often geared towards helping patients understand that psychiatric conditions are no one's fault—and that combinations of various genes act together with the effects of our experiences to contribute to the development of these heterogeneous, complex conditions), there is typically no need for visual aids explaining chromosomes and DNA.

Any web-based or hard copy information provided to the patient or used during the session (counseling aids, videos, chatbots, etc.) needs to be considered through a lens of accessibility and health literacy (e.g., closed captions on videos, descriptive video for people with low vision or are blind, color schemes chosen to ensure accessibility for those who are color blind, attention to readability in text— aiming for grade 8 or lower) and attention to trust building, especially with marginalized groups. For resources on how to think about ensuring the services we provide are accessible to people of all literacy levels, please refer to reference: (AHRQ, n.d.).

Thoughtfully developed and delivered educational materials (e.g., materials developed through a process that involved the target group for which it was created), may—when provided in advance of a genetic counseling session—support a more patient-centric approach within the session itself. Specifically, providing information in advance of the session can potentially allow for the genetic counselor to operate more fully towards the top of their scope of practice; that is, providing counseling to help patients make personalized meaning of the information, rather than simply providing the information itself.

Patient letters deserve particular mention, as they can be especially important (Hunt Brendish et al., 2021). Taking in and accurately recalling the content of a genetic counseling session can be challenging, particularly when the patient is experiencing heightened emotions. Patient letters typically involve a narrative summary of the information provided, including important aspects of the patient's medical and family history, mechanisms of inheritance, chances for recurrence, and recommended follow-up. Letters of this nature can be valuable to patients as they can be used to prompt recall of information and/or can be used to share information with other family members. Copies of any laboratory results could be included with the letter, together with hard-copy pamphlets and/or links to electronic resources.

While it is common practice for genetic counselors to invite patients to get in touch if they have any questions, the patient experience is often that it isn't obvious what sorts of questions they might have that would be reasons to get back in touch in the future. Providing tangible examples—both verbally and in patient letters—of the sorts of questions or issues that might prompt a patient to get back in touch after their encounter might be helpful.

THE PROCESS OF PROVIDING INFORMATION IN PATIENT-CENTERED GENETIC COUNSELING

When thinking about the *process* of how to provide information in the context of genetic counseling, consider first that information should not be simply provided in a didactic or one-directional manner. A patient-centered process involves a dialogue: a bidirectional exchange of information. I consider it as a process comprised of three components (refer to Box 5-3), that ideally occur in an interwoven

> **BOX 5-3. THE THREE PROCESS ELEMENTS OF PROVIDING INFORMATION IN PATIENT-CENTERED GENETIC COUNSELING**
>
> 1. Exploring the patient's existing understanding of/experience with/explanations for the indicated condition/risk/situation.
> 2. Providing evidence-based information about the indicated condition/risk/situation (refer to "deciding what information to provide").
> 3. Exploring the patient's understanding of, and emotional reaction to, the information (including correcting misconceptions, and providing support).
>
> In the following sections, we will explore how to apply these elements in different genetic counseling settings.

manner rather than in linear, sequential steps. However, the process of seamless integration of these components is an advanced skill. Novice genetic counselors will usually start out by separating them into distinct components, and should work towards integrating them over time (for guidance about how to develop these skills refer to the section entitled: "The process of developing patient-centered communication skills" at the end of this chapter).

Helping Patients Understand the Etiology of the Indicated Condition

Establishing a clear understanding of the patient's explanation of the cause(s) of the personal or familial condition is foundational for any genetic counseling encounter, and is typically part of the contracting process. Without this step, research suggests that patients may not apply any new information that you provide them to themselves, or integrate it in any useful or meaningful way (Skirton and Eiser, 2003). Asking simple questions like the following can help:

"Can you tell me what you understand to be the cause of [your condition/the condition in your family]?"

"What have you heard from others about the cause of [your condition/the condition in your family]?"

The family history can often be used to reflect on perceptions of causation of, and experiences with, the indicated condition; even the absence of the indicated condition in a family can be informative to establishing a shared understanding of the patient's perceptions. More in-depth discussion of using family history as a tool can be found in Chapter 3.

Once we have a clear understanding of the patient's experiences and perceptions, the provision of evidence-based information about the indicated condition can be tailored to their specific context. For example, we can reinforce and validate components of their understanding of the facts about etiology that are accurate, and correct pieces that are less accurate. For example: "You said you thought that genetics was an important contributor to the cancer in your family—and that's absolutely correct—but there's other things that can contribute, too, and we can talk about all of that."

How we use language (e.g., avoiding jargon), and counseling aids, as described above, can facilitate making the information we provide accessible and allow for conversation rather than lecturing.

Throughout this process, the counselor's role is to be attuned to the patient's reactions to the discussion, noticing body language, facial expressions, and verbal reactions that indicate reactions. Any cues the counselor notices can be explicitly explored. Questions like the following can be effective: "I see you frowning—I can try explaining a different way if that might help?"

If visual cues are unclear (e.g., if counseling is being provided by telephone), simple direct questions about reactions to the information can be used, such as "teach back," which can look like this:

"This is a lot of information, I know. I want to make sure that our conversation is as useful for you as possible, so can you tell me what you're understanding and what questions you have?"

It is important to consider what to do if, in response to these sorts of questions, it becomes clear that a patient has not understood issues that are fundamentally important to allowing them to effectively navigate their situation. It is not necessary for a patient to have a perfect understanding of everything we have said, but addressing misunderstandings that have an impact on their ability to navigate their situation is important. In these situations, trying a different strategy for providing the information could help (e.g., different visual aids or using analogies). Directly addressing a misunderstanding might look like this:

"Oh ok, I can understand how you would think that because your child's condition is genetic, they must have inherited it from you, but actually that's not what happened here. In your child, although this condition is genetic, it wasn't inherited. The genetic difference they have just happened in them—by chance, new, for the first time—you didn't pass it on. I know that's an odd idea, but this can happen. I want you to know this because this means that you don't need to worry about whether you will develop [medical condition x] like they have. Let me try a different way of explaining this ..."

Body language, facial expressions, and verbal reactions can also indicate emotional reactions. Emotional reactions can act as a barrier to our ability to process information we are receiving, so it is important to help our patients to identify them, and to address them when we can. Emotions that often come up in relation to discussions about conditions that have a genetic contribution can include (combinations of), for example, guilt, blame, shame, fear, relief, grief. Naming and addressing these emotions can be some of the most powerful work involved in genetic counseling, for example:

> *"I know that in situations like this, people can often feel guilty. I am not sure if this is something you are feeling, but just in case, I need you to know that this is absolutely not your fault."*

If it is not clear what emotions someone is feeling, simple questions like the following can be really helpful:

> *"I feel like I lost you there for a moment—can you tell me what you are feeling about this right now?"*
>
> *"It's hard to tell over the phone sometimes, so I just thought I would ask: I'm wondering how you're feeling about all this at the moment?"*

Breaking "Bad News" and Heightened Emotional States

As humans, in situations where we are consumed with emotions like shock, denial, grief, and/or anger we are often unable to take in information in a useful or meaningful way (Ashtiani et al., 2014). A genetic counselor's role in these situations is usually to go slowly and provide space and support for patients' emotions. After exploring the patient's understanding of their situation as described above, summarize the main message of the information you are providing as simply and directly—and as compassionately—as possible; for example:

> *"The test results came back, and they show that you have the same genetic variant as your mom, which means that you have an increased risk of developing breast or ovarian cancer."*

Rather than just continuing to talk after providing this summary, allow space and time for the patient to respond, feel, and express emotion. You may want to actively invite their reaction; for example:

> *"I know that this is not news that you wanted to hear. I'm sorry. What can I do to best support you?"*
>
> *"Would it be helpful for me to talk with you about how confident we can be in this test result? Or perhaps I could tell you about what options are available to you next? Or if you need a minute just to process, and you'd like me to step out, I can do that too."*

Often, a very human reaction to hearing something we perceive to be bad news is needing to understand: "Are you sure? How do we know? Could there be a mistake? How could this [bad thing] happen?" While the temptation here might be to dive into, for example, a detailed explanation of the accuracy of amniocentesis results, and the technicalities of nondisjunction events, that's often not the sort of answer to the question that people need, or can process when they are in the immediate moment of freshly trying to process bad news. The kind of answer to the question that they need in the moment might be along the lines of a brief confirmation of the certainty of the result and then acknowledging the unfairness of the event, and how it's not their fault. And then you can tell them that when they're ready, you can help them understand more about exactly how this happened; you can tell them that there are options for this—you can start talking about it today, or you can make another appointment with them, and either way, you will give them some information about it to take home to look at later when they are ready. Providing people with information to take home in this situation is very important, because of the way in which heightened emotion impairs our ability to engage with and recall information.

Risk Communication

In the same way that genetic counseling is often conflated with genetic testing (refer to Box 5-1), it can also be conflated with the process of simply having a conversation with people about the chance for the recurrence within a family of a condition with a genetic contribution. Note that while discussion about recurrence risk is within a genetic counselor's scope of practice, the scope of practice describes what we *can* do, not what we *must* do for every patient. In fact, review of the definition of genetic counseling and our code of ethics reveals that genetic counseling neither requires, nor relies on, the provision of estimates of chances for illness recurrence within a family. Nevertheless, the ability to communicate about risk is an important component of many genetic counseling encounters and an important skill for genetic counselors to have.

Risk communication can take many forms in genetic counseling, such as discussion of chances for occurrence or recurrence and in the context of weighing treatment or management options in a given situation. It is worth exploring some fundamental concepts about risk as a foundation for ensuring that our communications about this topic are patient-centered.

What is "risk"?   Although we often conflate the concepts in medicine, risk is not a synonym for probability. "Risk" involves probability, but incorporates more than that; it implies a probability of a particular *undesirable* type of outcome. Therefore, how people experience and perceive risk is not governed only by rational cognitive appraisal of a numeric probability, it also involves an emotional subjective appraisal of that probability and its outcomes—and this incorporates contextual factors (e.g., family history, worry), and perceptions of the severity of the outcome associated with the probability (for more discussion of this, refer to Austin (2010)). When we are discussing risk, we are inherently discussing uncertainty; we are not talking about definitive yes or no outcomes, we are talking about *probability* of an outcome. In discussing probabilities of outcomes, we are essentially quantifying our uncertainty. While we may feel there is more or less certainty about estimates of probability in different situations (e.g., more certainty in a situation where we are discussing the chance for an autosomal recessive condition occurring in a child of carrier parents, and less when probabilities are derived from empiric data), uncertainty is attendant to all discussion of risk because, by definition, there is no certain outcome. In some situations, risk communication may involve discussion about how a greater degree of certainty may be achievable (e.g., further testing like amniocentesis after prenatal screening indicating increased chance of the fetus having Down syndrome). In other situations—for example, in the context of chances for developing a complex disorder—the uncertainty may be unresolvable. Uncertainty is uncomfortable for many people, and therefore discussing risk can be challenging—especially when unresolvable—and it is important to address this.

One of the things that counselors tend to notice is that the way in which our patients appear to appraise risks does not seem to always and necessarily reflect how we think about the numbers we have told them. While it might be tempting to interpret this to mean that patients don't understand probabilities, an alternate interpretation is that patients are making meaning out of the numbers we provided them in terms of their own subjective perceptions of context and severity of the outcome. This alternate interpretation raises questions about what matters most: correct recall of the objective probability that was provided, or an understanding of the risk in terms of one's experience and values? A decision-making theory called "fuzzy trace" theory refers to detailed representations (e.g., recall of the objective probability that was provided) as "verbatim," and to "bottom-line meanings" (e.g., an understanding of the risk in terms of one's experience and values) as "gist" (for more about this, refer to Biesecker et al. (2017)). As mentioned above, the goal of genetic counseling is not to guide patients to a certain kind of "objectively logical" decision based on accurate verbatim recall of the information we provide them. Rather, gist understandings of the information are valuable, and research shows that people tend to reason using gist rather than verbatim understanding in making decisions (Reyna, 2008). Our role in communicating risk is to provide the best, most accurate information about numbers that we can (when people want this), to ensure that we are making risk as understandable and as accessible as possible, and to accept that accurate verbatim recall is not a measure of the utility of our efforts.

Patient-centered risk communication in genetic counseling   The fact that the word "risk" connotes an undesirable outcome as well as probability has important ramifications for our choice of language when discussing probabilities with patients in genetic counseling. For example, when discussing probabilities for a Deaf couple to have a Deaf child, the use of the word "risk" is inappropriate (if having a Deaf child is not an undesirable outcome for the family, using a word that implies undesirability is ableist and damaging) and using the less loaded "chance" is a good option.

When communicating about risk, contracting is important. Not everyone attending a genetic counseling session may want to know exact numeric chances for a given outcome (Borle et al., 2018), and in patient-centered communications, such wishes are respected. In some contexts, risk can be meaningfully discussed without specific numbers. For example, for some people it is enough for them to understand that: a particular outcome that they fear is not 100% guaranteed; that everyone has some chance for the outcome in question; and that there are things that they can do to mitigate (though not eliminate) the chance of that outcome. Importantly, whether or not a person wishes to hear exact numeric chances for a given outcome may change over the course of a genetic counseling session too (in one study, almost 20% of patients changed their minds about whether they wanted to discuss specific numeric chances for illness recurrence during the course of a genetic counseling session (Borle et al., 2018))—and this is one of the reasons why contracting is something that should be considered a process rather than a single event.

In practice, when engaging in risk communication with patients who have indicated that they do wish to know a specific number, the three-elements of providing information (Box 5-3) can be applied as follows.

To explore a patient's existing perceptions of chance for a particular outcome, the counselor can ask questions like: "what is your sense of what the chance might be?," "have you read/heard anything about what the chances might be?" This can also be an opportunity to explore whether they have thought about if there are chances that for them would cross a threshold of being "too high" to choose a particular course of action. The patient's perceptions of the nature of the indicated outcome—their perceptions of the "severity" of the outcome—and what it means to them are also valuable topics to explore.

Once that baseline shared understanding has been established, information about the probability for the indicated condition can be presented. The nature of the type of information provided about risk matters. For example, because risk perception is such a subjective experience, qualitative appraisals of risk (e.g., "quite low") should never be used without also providing numbers—essentially, our own subjective appraisal of the number provided matters a lot less than the appraisal of the patient. Also—and importantly—people typically understand and make meaning from absolute risks (20% chance for outcome X) more readily than they do relative risks (chance for outcome X is 50 times higher). Indeed, relative risks can be quite misleading, and absolute risks should be used wherever possible.

Another important strategy to consider in communicating about risk is framing. Framing can apply in different ways. First, for example, we can frame probabilities in terms of chance to develop the outcome, and chance to NOT develop the outcome. This is very important, because although—objectively—they convey the same information, these two framings can be perceived very differently.

> *"Given that you have [autosomal dominant condition X], we know that any child you have will have a 50%, or 1 in 2 chance to have the same condition. Another way of saying the same thing is that any child you have will have a 50%, or a 1 in 2 chance NOT to have the condition that you have."*

Second, especially in the context of complex (or multifactorial) conditions, we can and should frame probabilities for a particular outcome in the patient's specific circumstance by providing contextual information about population-based data wherever possible. For example, in talking with a patient about the chance for their child to develop schizophrenia based on empiric data and their family history (where there is no evidence of an underlying syndrome like 22q11 deletion syndrome), I might explain that their child has a chance of about 10–30% (or 1–3 in 10) to develop the condition (which is the same as a chance of about 70–90% to NOT develop schizophrenia), and that in the general population, everyone has a chance of about 1% (or 1 in 100) to develop schizophrenia. When discussing probabilities for different outcomes, it can be helpful to explain where the numbers come from; for example, using the above situation:

> *"We know the chance for your child to develop schizophrenia is about 10% (or 1 in 10) from studies that have looked at how often a child of a parent with schizophrenia develops the same condition—this number reflects what these studies found."*

Visual aids can be particularly useful for risk communication: icon arrays (i.e., a set number—usually 100—of icons, like human figures, being visually presented with a proportion shaded in to represent the probability of a particular event) in particular have been shown to help people to understand chances, even when they may have lower numeracy (Galesic et al., 2009). Icon arrays can be used to represent both population-based risk (for context), and to represent the patient's own specific risk.

With regard to understanding of risk and probabilities, while we might like to aim for our patients having a perfect understanding of the probabilities, and being able to repeat the messages we provided, this is not always possible. After asking a patient what they heard and what they understood about the chances you discussed with them, and attempting to correct any misconceptions around recall of numeric probabilities (e.g., using different visual aids), ultimately, it is less important that the patient is able to repeat the probability that was provided, than it is for them to make meaning of that number—for them to understand the "gist" (Biesecker et al., 2017). For example, it's less important that a patient recall that the chance to have a child with schizophrenia (based on empiric data and family history information) is specifically in the range of 10–30%, and more important that they understand: 1) the child will have a higher chance to develop the condition than someone with no family history of the condition; but 2) it is *not* a foregone conclusion that their child will have the condition; and 3) the chance for their child *not to have* the condition is larger than their chance to have it.

Finally, exploring emotional reactions to the numbers provided is crucial (e.g., "Can you tell me how that number feels to you?"). This can provide an opportunity to validate any feelings of, for example, discomfort with uncertainty, or relief at the understanding that the outcome they were concerned about is not guaranteed. It can also provide an opportunity to provide support around beginning to process feelings of denial, or anger or sadness.

Facilitating Decision-Making (and Addressing the Question: "What Should I Do?")

Risk communication is often intimately interconnected with facilitating decisions in genetic counseling. As discussed above, a genetic counselor's role in facilitating decisions is to support patients in making informed and (relationally) autonomous decisions. In some situations, a patient/family will find making a decision to be fairly straightforward, but in other circumstances it can be more challenging.

The three elements of providing information in patient-centered genetic counseling described in Box 5-3, and the principles for deciding what information to provide described above, are key to facilitating decision-making. However, as humans do not make purely rational decisions, information alone is often not enough to satisfactorily facilitate decision-making. As humans, to make a decision, information needs to be understood, and *evaluated in the context of our needs and values.* Therefore, an additional key element in facilitating informed and autonomous decisions involves helping patients/families to appraise the information and potential outcomes of the decision at hand in terms of their needs and values.

Explicit conversation about values and needs can be opened by asking patients questions like:

> *"What are the factors you are balancing/considering in making this decision?"*

Asking patients about how making a decision in either direction would influence their actions going forward can help illuminate a values-aligned decision; for example:

> *"If you chose to have the amniocentesis and it showed the fetus has Down syndrome, how would you use that information?"*

In thinking about responding, a patient/couple might realize, for example, that they wouldn't choose to terminate a pregnancy based on a diagnosis Down syndrome, but the information would help them feel more prepared for the birth. Similarly, asking questions about what would be best- and worst-case outcome scenarios can be useful:

> *"What might be a worst-case scenario or best-case scenario for you here? Is it more important for you to avoid the worst-case scenario or have the hope for a best-case scenario?"*

This kind of question could lead a patient to realize that, for them, the worst-case scenario might be, for example, losing a pregnancy as a complication of amniocentesis. And for others, the worst-case scenario might be dealing with uncertainty for the remaining duration of the pregnancy and being unprepared for the birth of their child. This can help in turn to shed light on the decision at hand.

Prompting patients to reflect on how they make other kinds of decisions for themselves that they later feel good about (e.g., what process they go through, whose opinions or perspectives do they seek out) can illuminate whether there are other people with whom it would be helpful for them to consult (time permitting), or whether there are character traits or values they need to uphold.

When it is a couple or a family that is engaged in a decision-making process—for example, a couple making a joint decision regarding prenatal testing—this can add a layer of complexity, especially if the different individuals are not in agreement about the decision, or do not have close alignment of values. In these situations, helping each individual to express and articulate their values and positions, and think about how they have successfully made decisions together in other contexts, can be helpful.

Sometimes, after we have provided all of the necessary, available information to the best of our ability, and guided patients through trying to consider the decision at hand in light of their own needs and values, we might still get asked: "Yes, but what would you do/what should I do?" Some may attempt to embody a (supposedly) "nondirective" stance by providing responses along the lines of "I can't tell you what I would do/what you should do, that is up to you. Sorry." Viewed through the lens of patient-centered communication—intuitively and instinctively—this is not a satisfactory response. It is too easy to imagine, as a patient, feeling abandoned in this scenario, and indeed research shows that information only in these situations is not enough for some people (Salema et al., 2019). For a profession founded on the relationship between counselor and patient, a response that leaves your patient feeling abandoned is not only inadequate, but can actually be damaging.

So, what should we do when confronted with a patient asking us what to do? First, we need to ensure that we have done our best to provide the most understandable, comprehensive, and accurate information, and—if possible—to understand the factors driving the patient to ask this question. A patient-centered response to this kind of plea for help might look something like this:

"Well, I have heard you talk a lot about A and B, and how C matters deeply to you. So— given that—it sounds like perhaps D might be the right option because it would best allow you to meet those needs/values. How does that feel to you?"

In the same vein, in response to a question about "what would you do?" a more patient-centered response than "I can't tell you that, it's your decision" would be something along the lines of:

"Of course, you and I are different people with different circumstances and values and so on, and I need you to know that regardless of how I might approach this, I will support you in whatever decision aligns best for you given your values and circumstances. But for me, in this situation, I think my values of X and Y would be driving me towards thinking about making the decision this way—to prioritize outcome [A] over [B]. And in my situation, I have Z history/support/context that is affecting me. So, I think I would maybe choose C. Does that make sense to you? Does it help you to see how your own values and circumstances could inform your own decision here?"

Or alternatively:

"I am not sure what I would do. But I have seen many patients struggle with making this decision, so you're not alone. I've seen patients use pro/con lists, compare the worst vs best-case scenarios, take some time and talk it through with a loved one, or journal about their thoughts to help them make their decision in this sort of situation. Everyone is different in what works best for them in approaching it. Would any of those strategies help you, do you think?"

THE PROCESS OF DEVELOPING PATIENT-CENTERED COMMUNICATION SKILLS

Developing a counseling-based, patient-centered communication approach to genetic counseling is a developmental process for practitioners. Individuals selected for entry into genetic counseling programs are often people who have excellent interpersonal skills—they are great communicators, who are good at listening and empathizing. However, on entering a genetic counseling training program, trainees typically experience a sense of realization that there is lots of *information* that they need to learn in order to feel confident in communicating with patients. After all, the role of the genetic counselor is to help patients, not just by providing compassionate support, but by helping them to understand the complex information that they might need to know as relevant to their particular situation. As a result, the focus for trainees often initially becomes about learning and storing knowledge about the etiologies of genetic conditions, their medical manifestations, the associated testing options, the management strategies that are available, and so on. Acquiring this sort of knowledge is necessary in order for the genetic counseling trainee (and indeed for practitioners throughout their careers) to feel confident and competent in their role as expert in the science of the condition that constitutes the reason for a patient's visit.

Alongside the acquisition of this knowledge, the genetic counseling trainee enters a phase in clinical encounters where we focus on the delivery of *accurate* information to our patients. This reflects where our focus is during this phase of training, and we are often being evaluated on our ability to be comprehensive in covering topics and our accuracy in our explanations of concepts. The natural consequence of this is that during this phase of development as genetic counseling practitioners, we tend to pay less attention to the counseling—or human— elements of the interaction. This phase of development is more about establishing and consolidating our confidence in our role as expert in the science of the condition in the clinical encounter.

Our role is not just to provide *accurate* information, however; it is also to ensure that the information we provide is *understandable*—explicitly acknowledging the tension inherent to balancing the accurate and the understandable is important. To be accurate, we tend to feel the need to be complex and technical and use jargon—the opposite of understandable. So, as we progress in our development towards being both accurate *and* understandable, we refine our craft through deepening our understanding (the quote often attributed to Einstein about how, if you can't explain something simply, you don't understand it well enough, is true) and by practicing different strategies for explaining, such as: reflecting on jargon and using clear language strategies for communicating this, integrating analogies, trying different visual aids, role playing, or talking with colleagues about the approaches they use to convey concepts.

While providing information to patients that is both accurate and understandable is an excellent skill to have developed, this is not (or—at least—should not be) the end of the growth trajectory. Even if we are diligently providing the best, most understandable and accurate information to everyone, we may actually still be centering ourselves in our interactions; for example, our need to teach the patient a concept. This can be a comfortable place to be: information provision is controllable, we have the power, and there's no unsettling need to address unpredictable and messy emotions. Some counselors, despite valuing engaging with patients in a deeper way, might experience *institutional* pressure to cover so much information that they feel there is no time for anything else. However, the practice of truly patient-centered communication requires—as the term suggests— centering the *patient*; it requires that we center ourselves and our own agendas less. Specifically, we need to return to where we started—to interpersonal skills—and combine these with our newly acquired expertise in explaining complex concepts in a way that is both accurate and understandable. We need to re-engage with—or cultivate—our ability to communicate empathically, and to truly listen.

It is reconnecting with/developing these skills that facilitates our transition from mere providers of information, to genetic counselors: to earn this title, we need to combine our ability to provide accurate and understandable information about very complex concepts with skills in truly engaging, listening, and empathizing. It is truly *listening* to our patients, hearing their fears, needs, and wants, and empathizing with their situations, that allows us to figure out which specific elements of our expert knowledge of the condition we can offer, and how to frame it to address those needs. This is lifelong work.

Ultimately, the goals for us as skilled practitioners in the art of genetic counseling are that:

1. we have confidence that all the specialized technical knowledge we have accumulated is there, in our brains, waiting to be called upon if needed by the patient we are interacting with (or, of course, that we know where to find it!); and

2. we have confidence in our interpersonal skills—listening and empathy—to identify what pieces of information to draw on and when.

By way of a specific example, in my area of practice (psychiatric conditions), patients might present for a genetic counseling session because they have questions about the chance for their child to develop a psychiatric condition. I have learned over time that though they are—on the surface—asking for information, a simple number, that's not *really* what the question is about. This question is almost never asked out of pure intellectual curiosity, or as some sort of cognitive enterprise. I have come to understand—by trying hard to really listen to what is said (and to what is *not* said), and by empathizing with those that I am interacting with—that questions about recurrence estimates are almost always borne out of emotional needs. People asking questions like this tend to:

1. worry (that something "bad"—mental illness—will happen to their child); and/or

2. want a sense of control (to know if there is anything they can do to influence whether this bad thing happens or not); and/or

3. feel guilty because of pre-emptive anticipation that if their child develops mental illness, it would be their fault.

I cannot address these emotions in any meaningful way simply by providing a number. And if I only provide a number in this situation, I have come to feel that

I am providing a disservice—even though, superficially, I would have given them exactly what they asked for. That is not to say that one should not provide any numbers or specifically answer their questions. Rather, we should listen to what the questions are really about and address those concerns.

So, when a patient opens a session with the question "what is the chance that my child will develop a psychiatric condition?," although the easiest and most straightforward response might be to just tell them a number, the patient-centered response might look a bit different. My approach might involve offering immediate reassurance/confirmation that we can absolutely talk about what those chances are, and why they are what they are. But I might also then try to help the person who is asking me this question to dig a bit deeper, to try to articulate whatever they can about what is motivating them to ask me this question, and why the answer matters. It's only through this conversation that I am able to address the real, deeper reasons for their visit, to talk about their fear, what they may or may not be able to do to reduce risk, the difficulty of living with uncertainty, and any guilt. These kinds of attempts to understand the patient in a deeper way are—to me—the core of truly patient-centered communication.

The lifelong process of building and honing patient-centered communication skills requires self-reflection. This can be a practice that we engage in independently, and/or with support; for example, through role playing and/or peer supervision (Clarke et al., 2007; Middleton et al., 2007; Sexton et al., 2012). The following types of question might be good starting points for reflecting on one's practice approaches independently or in peer supervision:

- What questions didn't I ask? Why?
- What cues did I not respond to? Why?
- What niggling doubts or worries do I have about that session?
- What steps can I take so that I can address these things more consistently in the future?

In answering these questions, think beyond simply answering the question by saying "I didn't have enough time." If you find yourself wanting to answer these questions with responses along these lines, challenge yourself to think about what you *really* mean. I inevitably find that what I really mean when I say I don't have enough time for something, is "I am choosing not to prioritize [X]." Sometimes this subtle re-framing can help us to consider things differently. And, if time is truly a barrier, consider ways to "hack" the communication process, such as scheduling a follow-up appointment (creating more time) or providing written information before or after the visit (communicating without using up appointment time).

How we prioritize our time should relate to our values—the things we value should be the things we spend time on. This is as true in genetic counseling interactions as it is in life in general. Really try to move beyond the superficial answers and get to the very bottom of understanding why you didn't engage with the things you missed; for example, identify things you didn't say for fear of not knowing how to handle the patient's emotions that might be provoked as a consequence.

SUMMARY

Fundamentally, genetic counseling helps people to make meaning of genetic information, and therapeutically supports people in exercising their (relational) autonomy to use this information—in alignment with their values—to manage their health in the context of uncertainty. Genetic counseling is, therefore, both founded and dependent on patient-centered communication. The relationship-building between the counselor and patient is central to the beneficial outcomes of the interaction. In this era in which genetic counseling is increasingly being conceptualized within health care as a specialty that exists simply to facilitate and deliver genetic testing (Chanouha et al., 2023), it is imperative that we ensure that we retain focus on the true source of the value that we provide—and that relates to our counseling skills. Information—like genetic test results—is best thought of as a tool we use in the patient-centered communication practice that is genetic counseling.

In many ways, genetic counseling training can be considered an "extreme sports" version of communication training: we communicate incredibly complex information to people who are often in states of distress or heightened emotion. The skills required to do this well can be learned, and honed over time, and are enormously transferrable beyond the direct patient care setting. It is these skills that allow us to not only provide exemplary patient care, but also underlie our being sought after by industry and labs, and that contribute to our potential for success as entrepreneurs. Essentially, no matter where our genetic counseling training ultimately takes us, the patient (person)-centered communication skills we develop will facilitate our success.

REFERENCES

Agency for Healthcare Research and Quality (AHRQ). (n.d) Index of resources. Available at https://www.ahrq.gov/health-literacy/research/index.html Accessed June 14, 2024.

Anderson RM, Funnell MM, Butler PM, et al. (1995) Patient empowerment. Results of a randomized controlled trial. *Diabetes Care* 18:943–949.

Ashtiani S, Makela N, Carrion P, & Austin J. (2014) Parents' experiences of receiving their child's genetic diagnosis: a qualitative study to inform clinical genetics practice. *Am J Med Genet A* 164A(6):1496–1502.

Austin J, Semaka A, & Hadjipavlou G. (2014) Conceptualizing genetic counseling as psychotherapy in the era of genomic medicine. *J Genet Couns* 23(6):903–909.

Austin JC. (2010) Re-conceptualizing risk in genetic counseling: implications for clinical practice. *J Genet Couns* 19:228–234.

Austin JC. (2019) Evidence-based genetic counseling for psychiatric disorders: a road map. *Cold Spring Harb Perspect Med* 10(6):a036608.

Bardes CL. (2012). Defining "patient-centered medicine." *N Engl J Med* 366:782–783.

Biesecker B, Austin J, & Caleshu C. (2017) Theories for psychotherapeutic genetic counseling: fuzzy trace theory and cognitive behavior theory. *J Genet Couns* 26:322–330.

Biesecker B, Peters K, & Resta R. (2019) *Advanced Genetic Counseling: Theory and Practice*, New York: Oxford Academic.

Borle K, Morris E, Inglis A, & Austin J. (2018) Risk communication in genetic counseling: Exploring uptake and perception of recurrence numbers, and their impact on patient outcomes. *Clin Genet* 94:239–245.

Carrion P, Semaka A, Batallones R, et al. (2022) Reflections of parents of children with 22q11.2 Deletion Syndrome on the experience of receiving psychiatric genetic counseling: Awareness to Ac'. *J Genet Couns* 31:140–152.

Chanouha N, Cragun DL, Pan VY, et al. (2023) Healthcare decision makers' perspectives on the creation of new genetic counselor positions in North America: exploring the case for psychiatric genetic counseling. *J Genet Couns* 32:514–525.

Clarke A, Middleton A, Cowley L, & Guilbert P (2007) Report from the UK and Eire Association of Genetic Nurses and Counsellors (AGNC) Supervision Working Group on Genetic Counselling Supervision. *J Genet Couns* 16:127–142

Cohen W, McCartney E, & Crampin L. (2017) 22q11 deletion syndrome: parents' and children's experiences of educational and healthcare provision in the United Kingdom. *J Child Health Care* 21:142–152.

Edwards A, Gray J, Clarke AJ, et al. (2008) Interventions to improve risk communication in clinical genetics: systematic review. *Patient Educ Couns* 71(1):4–25.

Galesic M, Garcia-Retamero R, & Gigerenzer G. (2009) Using icon arrays to communicate medical risks: overcoming low numeracy. *Health Psychol* 28:210–216.

Goodwin J, McCormack L, & Campbell LE. (2017). "You don't know until you get there": the positive and negative "lived" experience of parenting an adult child with 22q11.2 deletion syndrome. *Health Psychol* 36:45–54.

Hippman C, Inglis A, & Austin J. (2012) What is a "balanced" description? Insight from parents of individuals with down syndrome. *J Genet Couns* 21:35–44.

Hollands GJ, French DP, Griffin SJ, et al. (2016) The impact of communicating genetic risks of disease on risk-reducing health behaviour: systematic review with meta-analysis. *Brit Med J* 15:352:i1102.

Hunt Brendish K, Patel D, Yu K, et al. (2021) Genetic counseling clinical documentation: Practice Resource of the National Society of Genetic Counselors. *J Genet Couns* 30:1336–1353.

Huntington B & Kuhn N. (2003) Communication gaffes: a root cause of malpractice claims. *Proc Bayl Univ Med Cent* 16:157–161; discussion 161.

Jamal L, Schupmann W, & Berkman BE. (2020) An ethical framework for genetic counseling in the genomic era. *J Genet Couns* 29:718–727.

Kessler S. (1997) Psychological aspects of genetic counseling. IX. Teaching and counseling. *J Genet Couns* 6:287–295.

Kessler S & Antley RM. (1981) Psychological aspects of genetic counseling: analysis of a transcript. *Am J Med Genet* 8:137–153.

Kinmonth AL, Woodcock A, Griffin S, et al. (1998) Randomised controlled trial of patient centred care of diabetes in general practice: impact on current wellbeing and future disease risk. The Diabetes Care From Diagnosis Research Team. *Brit Med J* 317:1202–1208.

Kitson A, Marshall A, Bassett K, & Zeitz K. (2013) What are the core elements of patient-centred care? A narrative review and synthesis of the literature from health policy, medicine and nursing. *J Adv Nurs* 69:4–15.

Levinson W, Roter DL, Mullooly JP, et al. (1997) Physician-patient communication. The relationship with malpractice claims among primary care physicians and surgeons. *JAMA* 277:553–559.

MacKenzie C, Stoljar N, & Ebrary I. (2000) Relational *Autonomy: Feminist Perspectives on Autonomy, Agency, and the Social Self.* New York, NY: Oxford University Press.

Meiser B, Irle J, Lobb E, & Barlow-Stewart K. (2008) Assessment of the content and process of genetic counseling: a critical review of empirical studies. *J Genet Couns* 17:434–451.

Middleton A, Wiles V, Kershaw A, & Everest S. (2007) Reflections on the experience of counseling supervision by a team of genetic counselors from the UK. *Genet Couns* 16(2):143–155.

National Society of Genetics Counselors (NSOG). (n.d.) Code of Ethics. Available at: https://www.nsgc.org/POLICY/Code-of-Ethics-Conflict-of-Interest/Code-of-Ethics Accessed June 14, 2024.

Oduncu FS. (2002) The role of non-directiveness in genetic counseling. *Med Health Care Philos* 5:53–63.

Rehmann-Sutter C. (2009) Why non-directiveness is insufficient: ethics of genetic decision making and a model of agency. *Med Stus* 1L 113–129.

Resnicow K, Delacroix E, Chen G, et al. (2022) Motivational interviewing for genetic counseling: A unified framework for persuasive and equipoise conversations. *J Genet Couns* 31:1020–1031.

Resta R, Biesecker BB, Bennett RL, et al. 2006. A new definition of genetic counseling: National Society of Genetic Counselors' task force report. *J Genet Couns* 15:77–83.

Resta RG. (1997) The historical perspective: Sheldon Reed and 50 years of genetic counseling. *J Genet Couns* 6:375–377.

Reyna VF. (2008) A theory of medical decision making and health: fuzzy trace theory. *Med Decis Making* 28:850–865.

Rolle L, ZayhowskiK, Koeller D, et al. (2022) Transgender patients' perspectives on their cancer genetic counseling experiences. *J Genet Couns* 31:781–791.

Ruderman M, Berro T, Torrey Sosa L, & Zayhowski K. (2021) Genetic counselors' experiences with transgender individuals in prenatal and preconception settings. *J Genet Couns* 30:1105–1118.

Salema D, Townsend A, & Austin J. (2019) Patient decision-making and the role of the prenatal genetic counselor: an exploratory study. *J Genet Couns* 28:155–163.

Semaka A & Austin J. (2019) Patient perspectives on the process and outcomes of psychiatric genetic counseling: An 'empowering encounter' *J Genet Couns* 28(4):856–868.

Sexton A, Hodgkin L, Bogwitz M, et al. (2012) A model for Peer Experiential and Reciprocal Supervision (PEERS) for genetic counselors: development and preliminary evaluation within clinical practice. *J Genet Couns* 22:175–187.

Sheets K, Best R, & Brasington C. (2011) Balanced information about Down syndrome: What is essential? *Am J Med Genet* 155A(6):1246–1257.

Skirton H & Eiser C. (2003) Discovering and addressing the client's lay construct of genetic disease: an important aspect of genetic healthcare? *Res Theory Nurs Pract* 17:339–352.

Smets E, Van Zwieten M, & Michie S. (2007) Comparing genetic counseling with non-genetic health care interactions: Two of a kind? *Patient Educ Couns* 68(3):225–234.

Stern AM. (2012) *Telling Genes*. Baltimore, MD: Johns Hopkins University Press.

Stewart M. (2001) Towards a global definition of patient centred care. *Brit Med J* 322:444–445.

Stewart M, Brown JB, Donner A, et al. (2000) The impact of patient-centered care on outcomes. *J Fam Pract* 49:796–804.

Stewart MA. (1995) Effective physician-patient communication and health outcomes: a review. *CMAJ* 152:1423–1433.

Veach P, Bartels DM, & Leroy BS. (2007) Coming full circle: a reciprocal-engagement model of genetic counseling practice. *J Genet Couns* 16:713–728.

Weil J, Ormond K, Peters J, et al. (2006) The relationship of nondirectiveness to genetic counseling: report of a workshop at the 2003 NSGC Annual Education Conference. *J Genet Couns* 15:85–93.

Zikmund-Fisher BJ, Dickson M, & Witteman HO. (2011) Cool but counterproductive: interactive, Web-based risk communications can backfire. *J Med Internet Res* 13:e60.

6

Evaluating and Using Genetic Testing

Natasha Strande and Karen E. Wain

INTRODUCTION

The landscape of clinical testing for genetic disorders and risk factors has evolved dramatically over the past 40–50 years. Genetic testing was originally available within niche areas of expertise based on test methods or gene-specific expertise. Laboratories were categorized by the methodologies performed. Cytogeneticists performed karyotypes, fluorescence *in situ* hybridization (FISH), and other cell-based techniques used to identify large structural genomic variation, while molecular genetics laboratories focused on Sanger sequencing and related methods for single-gene analysis. Laboratories developed reputations for expertise with certain genes or specific syndromic disorders often linked to research projects at a university or academic center. However, since the early/mid-2000s, with the advent of more comprehensive, high-resolution testing methods, declining costs, and recognition of more effective population-based approaches, the paradigm of clinical genetic testing has shifted away from boutique laboratories with niche specialties toward broad testing approaches, like exome and genome sequencing and universal carrier screening panels, that are not targeted to specific ethnic backgrounds (Gregg et al., 2021; Manickam et al., 2021). This paradigm

A Guide to Genetic Counseling, Third Edition. Edited by Vivian Y. Pan, Jane L. Schuette, Karen E. Wain, and Beverly M. Yashar.
© 2025 John Wiley & Sons Ltd. Published 2025 by John Wiley & Sons Ltd.

shift required improvements and standardization in gene and variant curation, more comprehensive variant classification guidelines, and revised perspectives on how to determine the right test, for the right person, at the right time.

Genetic testing has the potential to offer dramatic benefits, both clinically and psychologically, for patients and their families. Genetic testing can confirm a suspected diagnosis, inform accurate assessment and management of health and reproductive risks, and provide prognostic insight for decision-making about clinical care. High-quality testing now has clinical utility for patients across most major clinical specialties throughout the lifespan, including preconception, prenatal, pediatrics, and through adulthood. In addition, genetic testing may now be included in some general wellness programs or offered to the public regardless of personal or family history through population-based screening models and commercial direct-to-consumer products (Buchanan et al., 2020; Fernandes Martins et al., 2022). These exciting changes to the fields of clinical and laboratory genetics bring the hopeful promise of improved patient care through better access to testing, more efficient testing options, and test development that ensures quality test results for all patient populations. But these goals are not yet fulfilled and genetic counselors play an important role in this ever-evolving space.

Genetic counselors must have an understanding of the movement toward broad, genomic approaches to clinical genetic testing and how to appropriately select and critically assess genetic test results for incorporation into clinical care based on a given scenario. Understanding the capabilities and limitations of various test methods allows genetic counselors to make informed test selections and follow-up recommendations. An awareness of the ongoing growth of clinically relevant scientific knowledge, including gene and variant curation efforts, improved variant interpretation processes, and the available resources that inform this work will support the genetic counselor's critical roles as a patient advocate and expert within multidisciplinary teams.

This chapter provides an overview of genetic testing methodologies, laboratory processes, and the incorporation of genetic tests into clinical care across a variety of clinical settings. We will also provide an introduction to the resources and processes used for genomic variant interpretation and give practical examples to illustrate real-life scenarios that may arise when considering test selection and making follow-up recommendations based on the results.

CLINICAL GENETIC TESTING

Common Clinical Purposes for Genetic Testing

Genetic testing is incorporated across multiple clinical disciplines, including reproductive medicine/prenatal, general pediatric or adult genetics, hereditary cancer, cardiovascular, neurology, and immunology. Genetic counselors are important to the testing process because they provide critical expertise, ensuring the most appropriate test is ordered for the patient and that results are understood. Regardless of the clinical setting, genetic testing can be categorized based on a variety of purposes. For simplicity we have categorized these purposes into the following general categories, though we acknowledge that some overlap can occur in some testing situations (e.g., somatic testing can provide both diagnostic and prognostic value).

Diagnostic genetic testing   Diagnostic genetic tests are typically prompted by the presence of a patient's clinical features or symptoms with the goal of identifying an underlying genetic etiology and making or confirming a genetic diagnosis (Wise et al., 2019). The patient's features, relevant clinical history, and/or specific clinical diagnoses directly inform the test selected. A genetic diagnosis can provide prognostic information and allow for personalized clinical management and gene-specific patient support resources that may not be possible with only a general clinical diagnosis. Obtaining a genetic diagnosis may also enable known variant testing (cascade testing) for family members. While most diagnostic testing can be performed on blood specimens, if there is suspicion that the genetic change occurred after conception (i.e., mosaicism), it is critical to perform testing on the tissue type suspected to be involved in disease (e.g., skin biopsy) (Wallace et al., 2022).

Clinical example: Genome sequencing is ordered for a 3-year old child with clinically diagnosed global developmental delays and epilepsy, to identify a genetic cause and potentially drive seizure treatment.

Genetic screening   The purpose of genetic screening is to identify individuals at increased risk, agnostic of clinical symptoms or family history, for a particular disease or condition. The main goal is to more effectively identify those who would most benefit from relevant diagnostic testing or clinical management changes while minimizing exposure to unnecessary clinical tests or procedures. Screening tests must balance test sensitivity and specificity parameters (described below) to optimize detection of true positive and true negative results while minimizing false positive and false negative results. These tests are typically offered to all individuals of a given population (e.g., all pregnant patients) and assess for defined genetic risk variants or biochemical evidence of disease. Screening tests may involve identifying individuals who are heterozygous carriers of pathogenic variants for recessive disorders, metabolites indicative of disease in a newborn (newborn screening), testing all tumor samples of a given type to screen for individuals with hereditary cancer syndromes, and screening for fetal or tumor DNA fragments that are circulating in a person's bloodstream (Giardiello et al., 2014; Fabie et al., 2019; Samura 2020; Sagaser et al. 2023).

Clinical example: Prospective parents are offered a carrier screening panel to identify heterozygous, pathogenic genetic variants associated with an increased risk for an autosomal recessive disorder in future pregnancies.

Known variant testing In contrast to broad testing approaches, there are several clinical situations that warrant targeted genetic testing for a known genetic variant previously identified in a patient's family member, including: 1) presymptomatic testing for patients with a known family history and a known variant for risk assessment; 2) testing a symptomatic patient when a causative variant was previously identified in a family member; and 3) to aid in variant interpretation. When testing for known pathogenic variants, the outcomes are often more straightforward, with clear positive and negative reports that can directly inform clinical decision-making. On the other hand, segregation studies, where testing of family members is pursued for a variant of uncertain significance (VUS) found in a proband, are often done to aid in variant interpretation (Richards et al., 2015; Tsai et al., 2019). Variant-specific testing may require some coordination with the testing laboratory to ensure the lab has positive controls available, if needed, and to confirm the optimal test methodology. Notably, depending on results, such testing may yield a diagnostic result, or, alternatively, result in dismissal of the variant as causative.

> *Clinical example: A patient's mother tested positive for a pathogenic variant in BRCA1 and the patient would like to know whether the variant was inherited to inform clinical care.*

Somatic genetic testing While classic genetic testing has focused on identifying germline variants (i.e., variants that were present at conception and are expected to be found in all cells of the body), there are clinical scenarios and specific specialties where tests for somatic (or acquired) variants are especially important. Somatic variants are those that are only present in a subset of a patient's cells, because they were acquired sometime after conception, and may be tissue-specific. Somatic variants can arise very soon after conception or much later in life. Somatic testing has become an important part of oncology care through tumor-specific genetic tests that can identify acquired tumor-specific genetic variants (Giardiello et al., 2014). These results can inform cancer diagnosis, prognosis, and treatment choice and efficacy.

> *Clinical example: A colorectal tumor is removed from a 50-year old patient and sent to pathology for microsatellite instability (MSI), immunohistochemistry (IHC), acquired MLH1 gene promoter methylation, and BRAF targeted gene testing to assess for Lynch syndrome and to drive selection of cancer therapeutics.*

Personalized genomic risk stratification efforts There are increasing efforts to develop tests and clinical implementation guidelines that can be used to provide personalized risk profiles across larger segments of the population, allowing genomic medicine to reach beyond the rarer genetic disorders. Two examples include pharmacogenomic tests and polygenic risk scores (PRS). Pharmacogenomics is the study of how genetic variants influence drug metabolism, which has been characterized for several gene–drug pairs. For some medications, pharmacogenomic results can help to optimize medication dosing to improve efficacy and minimize side-effects (Roden et al., 2019). Polygenic risk scores provide an individual's risk assessment for a specific disease based on the coinheritance of hundreds to thousands of common genetic variants that individually may only contribute a very small increase or decrease in risk, but in combination could significantly alter a patient's risk for disease (Abu-El-Jaija et al., 2023). For example, PRS may help to identify individuals at moderately increased risks for common diseases, like cancer or cardiovascular disease, or provide prognostic information about severity of symptoms if combined with high-impact genetic variants. At this time, increased diversity in genomic data resources and clear medical actionability guidance are needed to ensure equitable test benefits and the clinical adoption of PRS.

> *Clinical example: A neurologist may consider CYP2C9 and HLA-B genotyping prior to prescribing phenytoin to treat seizures due to the narrow therapeutic index and risk for Stevens-Johnson syndrome.*

TESTING METHODOLOGIES

Regardless of the clinical context for which genetic testing was ordered, the basic goal is to evaluate an individual's chromosomes, genes, or proteins to identify deviations from the accepted reference state that may inform disease or carrier status. Reference standards have been developed for each type of test using data from unaffected individuals to establish expected normal ranges/ values for the given test. In the context of genomic sequence data, the human reference genome, generated through the Human Genome Project, serves as that standard, and continues to be updated and maintained by the Genome Reference Consortium (GRC). Historically, genetic tests have been broadly categorized based on the biological target under evaluation; for example, cytogenetic testing describes the analysis of chromosomes, molecular testing describes analysis of the DNA or RNA sequence, and biochemical tests evaluate enzymatic activity, metabolites, and protein levels (Table 6-1) (Gersen and Keagle, 2013; Durmaz et al., 2015; Buckingham, 2019; Goswami and Harada, 2020). Typically cytogenetic tests detect larger scale genomic changes at the chromosome level, such as changes in chromosome number, structure, and arrangement. Conversely, molecular tests typically have much higher resolution and look more closely at the DNA or RNA sequence for base pairs that differ from the reference sequence at the nucleotide level or for changes in DNA methylation status (epigenetic). Biochemical tests detect changes in the levels of gene products (i.e., proteins and enzymes) and often have a quantitative output. While these broad categorizations continue to be useful, rapid advancements in technologies have narrowed the gap between these fields. This is

TABLE 6-1. Overview of common genetic testing techniques with limitations and clinical application

Category	Test type	What does it detect?	Smallest variant detected	Example of clinical use	Considerations
Cytogenetics	Karyotype	Large chromosome changes (large deletions, duplications); structural changes (translocations, inversions, marker chromosomes)	5–10 Mb	Suspicion of balanced translocation in family with recurrent miscarriages	Requires intact cells to be cultured for analysis in metaphase. Can identify balanced structural changes not detectable by array
	FISH	CNVs; structural rearrangements (translocations, inversions, marker chromosomes)	50 kb –1 Mb	Familial follow-up testing to test for CNV observed in proband on array. Identify specific translocations or CNVs in tumors to guide treatment	Metaphase analysis requires cultured cells, but interphase analysis can be done on fixed tissue. Probes must be designed for specific CNV. Small duplications (<500 kb) can be difficult to detect.
	Microarray	Unbalanced CNVs; regions of homozygosity (if SNP probes are used)	Variable— based on probe coverage	Proband with syndromic clinical features suggestive of large CNV	Cannot detect sequence variants, very small CNVs, or balanced rearrangements. Frequently used for GWAS and PRS in research and for DTC ancestry testing (SNP-based).
Molecular	Genotyping	Targeted, specific genotypes of interest (usually common variants)	Variable	Evaluation for common founder variants in specific populations	Rare, nearby variants can disrupt accurate detection of targeted variants.
	Sanger sequencing	Sequence variants; small insertions and deletions	1 bp	Targeted testing for a sequence variant identified in an affected relative	A single assay can only target small regions of DNA (300–1000 bp max size). Multiple assays are typically required to sequence an entire gene.

RT-PCR	Quantitative analysis for known variant (particularly for somatic variants)	Exon level	Detection and monitoring of cancer-specific variant before and after treatment (e.g. *BCR-ABL1* translocation in CML)	Quantitative assay that can be useful in monitoring minimal residual disease after cancer treatment. Assays must be designed for specific regions of interest (specific SNV or CNV).
MLPA, MS-MLPA	CNVs; Differentiate methylated vs unmethylated DNA (MS-MLPA)	Exon level	Clinical suspicion for an imprinting disorder such as Prader-Willi Syndrome	High throughput and cost effective, but does not provide comprehensive CNV analysis, since the assay is gene/region specific.
NGS/MPS	Most approaches can easily detect SNVs and small insertions/deletions targeted by the assay. Depending on the gene coverage and depth of sequencing CNVs may be detected. Typically only genome sequencing can accurately detect structural variants (e.g., inversions, translocations) and deep intronic variants	1 bp	*NGS gene panel:* clinical suspicion for specific, genetically heterogeneous condition, such as hereditary cancer *Exome/genome:* clinical presentation of non-specific phenotype(s) with wide differential, such as neurodevelopmental disorders	Large NGS panels are often run off of exome/genome backbones with the data analysis limited to predefined genes (e.g., exome-based data could be used for separate cardiovascular and neurodevelopmental panels). At this time, short-read sequencing is often most accurate at the sequence level, but long-read sequencing can provide better detection of large genomic rearrangements and is becoming more accessible.
RNA sequencing	Amount of normal and aberrant RNA transcripts, providing information about gene splicing and expression	1 bp	Follow-up testing to determine splicing impact of a previously identified DNA variant near an exon–intron boundary	RNA is less stable than DNA and therefore samples must be properly and quickly sent to the testing laboratory.

(continued)

TABLE 6-1. (Continued)

	Mitochondrial sequencing	Sequence variants; small insertions and deletions; large CNVs within the mitochondrial genome	1 bp	Clinical suspicion for a mitochondrial disorder with prior negative testing for nuclear genetic causes	Variant detection is contingent on methodology used, but is often NGS testing.
Biochemical	Mass Spectrometry	Metabolites and/or disease-relevant analytes based on size and charge	N/A	Screen for panel of metabolites (such as phenylalanine) as part of routine NBS in newborn	Can be used for screening, diagnosis and monitoring of biochemical conditions. Does not provide sequence information. Multiple methods (GC, LC, etc.) can be used to separate metabolites for analysis.
	Enzyme activity	Activity levels for specific enzymes	N/A	Follow-up testing for a child with suspected Mucopolysaccharidosis, Type III after inconclusive genetic testing	Multiple methods can be employed depending on the enzyme. Often provides information about disease severity or for phenotype correlation.

Abbreviations: CML: chronic myelogenous leukemia; CNV: copy number variant; DTC: direct to consumer; FISH: fluorescent in situ hybridization; GC: gas chromatography; GWAS: genome-wide association studies; HPLC: high-performance liquid chromatography; kb: kilobases; Mb: megabases; MLPA: multiplex ligation-dependent probe amplification; MPS: massively parallel sequencing; MS-MLPA: methylation specific-MLPA; MS: mass spectrometry; N/A: not applicable; NBS: newborn screening; NGS: next generation sequencing; PRS: polygenic risk score; RT-PCR: real time polymerase chain reaction; SNP: single nucleotide polymorphism; SNV: single nucleotide variant; UPD: uniparental disomy particularly true for cytogenetic and molecular testing, as molecular technologies evolve to detect large chromosomal changes and cytogenetic techniques incorporate higher resolution testing (Goswami and Harada, 2020). A basic understanding of the evolving landscape of genetic testing is helpful to contextualize current approaches and appreciate the necessity of keeping abreast of the latest advances in testing.

Cytogenetic Tests

Classic cytogenetic techniques (e.g., karyotype) provide low resolution chromosome analysis (limit of resolution ~3–5 megabases) and are still often used to detect balanced rearrangements and fully characterize structural chromosomal rearrangements. Fluorescent labeling of DNA probes led to the ability to perform higher resolution testing such as FISH (100–500 kilobases) in the 1980s and later chromosomal microarray analysis (CMA), which can detect copy number variants (CNV) in the range of 50–100 kilobases in size. Further advancements in microarray techniques that incorporate probes with single nucleotide polymorphisms (SNPs) allow detection of regions of homozygosity that can be important if an imprinting disorder is suspected (Durmaz et al., 2015).

Molecular Tests

Sanger sequencing has been the longstanding gold standard technique for detecting small DNA changes (substitutions and small deletions/insertions) at the nucleotide level, while techniques such as multiplex ligation-dependent probe amplification (MLPA) and real-time polymerase chain reaction (rt-PCR) have been the standard techniques for detecting gene level gains and losses. While these techniques still remain useful (particularly when orthogonal confirmation is needed), they have limitations with respect to scope (region targeted by the assay) and throughput. Completion of the Human Genome Project and the development of more comprehensive genetic testing techniques, such as massively parallel sequencing (or next generation sequencing (NGS)), which allows simultaneous sequencing of multiple gene targets or even an entire genome and detection of both small and larger DNA changes, has revolutionized the field of genetics. The declining costs of these technologies has facilitated the move away from single target testing, using techniques such as Sanger sequencing, towards large-scale, high-resolution testing as a first tier approach for genetic testing in many scenarios (Durmaz et al., 2015; Goswami and Harada, 2020; Lalonde et al., 2020).

Furthermore, significant improvements in the bioinformatics needed to process and analyze the extensive data generated by these methods now make large CNVs detectable with NGS data, again blurring the delineation between cytogenetic and molecular testing. These advancements allow laboratories to assess many different variant types and targeted genes using a single comprehensive testing approach, such as exome or genome sequencing, and to bioinformatically filter the sequence data to only reveal variants in the genes of interest (Goswami and Harada, 2020). For example, a laboratory might offer separate diagnostic gene panel tests for epilepsy and hereditary cancer using an exome or genome sequencing platform in both scenarios to generate data, and then apply bioinformatic filtering to limit analysis to only the relevant genes that correlate with the patient's phenotype. This offers several advantages to the laboratory and patient, including consistency in testing across panels, cost and time efficiency, the ability to reflex to exome or genome analysis, and perform reanalysis based on advances in gene discovery and/or the emergence of additional clinical features.

Biochemical Tests

In the context of metabolic diseases, it is often more important to determine a patient's levels of a specific protein or their overall enzymatic activity levels to establish a metabolic diagnosis and/or the severity of disease. These tests are typically performed by a biochemical laboratory using different methodologies such as tandem mass spectrometry, high-performance liquid chromatography (HPLC), and gas chromatography–mass spectrometry (GCMS) (Murphy et al., 2018). In addition to providing quantitative outputs, these techniques are often very sensitive and highly cost effective, which is why most newborn screening programs implement biochemical testing to screen for inborn errors of metabolism. Additional genetic testing may be warranted to elucidate the underlying molecular mechanism for an inborn error of metabolism, but it is not always necessary if the biochemical diagnosis is definitive.

TEST PARAMETERS

Regardless of what testing methodology is used, the quality of all clinical testing can be evaluated using the same basic test parameters to understand the limitations of each test. These test parameters include analytical and clinical validity, clinical utility, and predictive value and typically vary based on lab and technology utilized (Burke, 2014; Trevethan, 2017). Each test parameter is defined below within the context of genetic testing, with their relationships to one another depicted in Figure 6-1. While these test parameters can be useful when comparing test offerings across laboratories, it is worth noting they were originally developed for clinical chemistry tests and do not have universally accepted definitions for genetic tests. The ACCE (analytical validity, clinical validity, clinical utility, and ethical, social, legal implications) framework developed by the Center for Disease Control's (CDC) Office of Public Health Genomics is often cited in the literature when defining these parameters with respect to genetic tests, but is not universally implemented across laboratories (Pitini et al., 2021). Therefore, it may be useful to ask the laboratory to explain any discrepancies noted between laboratories, if not apparent from their test listings.

Analytical validity is the ability of a test to accurately measure the targeted analyte. The analyte is defined as the substance being measured by the test, which can

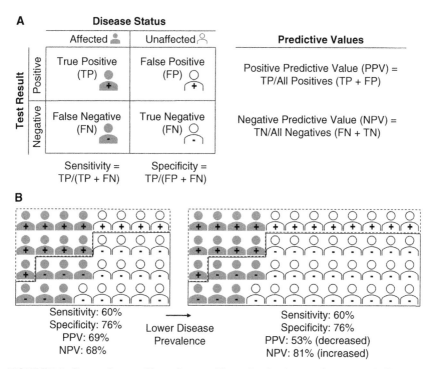

FIGURE 6-1. Parameters and formulas used in evaluating test performance. A. *Formulas to calculate each test parameter are shown.* **B.** *Examples of hypothetical test performance demonstrated using visuals for the calculation of each parameter. Sensitivity and specificity decrease as the proportion of false test results (FN and FP respectively) increases. Panel on the right shows how PPV and NPV are impacted by reducing disease prevalence but maintaining test sensitivity and specificity*

be a specific protein, genomic region targeted for sequencing, genotype of interest, or enzymatic activity. The analyte is often easy to define in biochemical testing, but can be defined differently across molecular testing laboratories depending on how the test is designed. For example, the biochemical test for Tay-Sachs disease evaluates the enzymatic activity of hexosaminidase A; however, the molecular analyte may be the entire gene, coding regions only (exons), or only specific known causative genetic variants (Toro et al., 2020). As previously noted, the move towards larger genomic analyses (i.e., large gene panels, exome, genome) presents greater variability across laboratories with respect to the included molecular analytes when testing for heterogeneous conditions (e.g., hearing loss, neurodevelopmental disorders). Analytical validity is based on several components which are critically evaluated and continually monitored for each test offered by clinical laboratories:

Analytic accuracy is the degree of agreement of the test result to the "true value" of the analyte. Ideally this is based upon a "gold standard" or reference analyte. In the context of molecular testing, this refers to the ability of the test to detect the correct genomic sequence present in the tested individual. It is particularly important to understand this parameter when testing for genes that contain highly repetitive sequences, such as pseudogenes (e.g., *PMS2* and *PMS2CL* pseudogene).

Analytic precision is the agreement between measurements, or the "reproducibility" of the test result. Test reproducibility should be shown by testing the same set of samples multiple times at varying time points across instruments and across laboratories if possible. This parameter is particularly important to consider when a quantitative value is informative, such as with inborn errors of metabolism where analyte levels can dictate the severity of disease.

Analytic sensitivity is not only the ability of the test to accurately detect an analyte, but includes a sense of the lower limit of detection of the analyte (in other words: what is the lowest level of analyte that the test can accurately detect consistently). Analytic sensitivity is particularly important in situations where detecting a low level of analyte is clinically relevant, such as with biochemical testing for metabolites or when mosaicism might be suspected, where only a small number of cells might harbor the genetic variant of interest.

Analytic specificity is the ability of the test to detect only the analyte of interest as opposed to also detecting off-target analytes, thereby limiting the number of false positive results. Achieving high analytic specificity in molecular testing can be particularly challenging if the target sequence has high homology (similarity) to a different region of the genome that is not of interest. This can sometimes be an issue with FISH probes that may use highly repetitive sequences and therefore hybridize to multiple different chromosomes.

Clinical validity refers to the accuracy of a test in detecting the presence of the associated disorder or phenotype. Unlike analytic validity that pertains to the ability of a test to detect a specific *analyte* of interest, clinical validity refers to the ability of a test to accurately detect the *disease* of interest (Burke, 2014; Trevethan, 2017). In some cases, presence of the analyte will be synonymous with presence of the disease, but this will vary for conditions with lower disease penetrance. A test with high clinical validity assumes a tight correlation between the tested analyte and disease, in other words there is substantial evidence that a positive test result is indicative of the presence of disease. In the context of molecular testing, clinical validity refers to the correlation of the analyzed variant(s)/gene(s) to the presence, absence, or risk for the disease of interest. This concept, while still beneficial, has required some re-framing in the context of broad testing techniques, such as exome/genome sequencing and CMA, that will identify genomic variation involving genes that may not have substantial evidence for disease causality. In a later section, we describe efforts to standardize ways to evaluate the clinical validity of a gene–disease relationship. Similar to analytic validity, clinical validity can be measured through a test's clinical sensitivity, clinical specificity and clinical predictive value and can be calculated using the formulas shown in Figure 6-1.

Clinical sensitivity refers to the ability of the test to detect disease (as opposed to the analyte) when disease is present. A test with high clinical sensitivity will reliably detect disease in affected individuals. Because clinical sensitivity is a measure of how accurately a test can detect disease, this parameter can be impacted by disease penetrance and genetic heterogeneity. A test can be 100% analytically valid, but if the disease of interest has reduced penetrance then the test may have very low clinical sensitivity. If a test can reliably detect the analyte of interest (e.g., all known disease-causing genetic variants) and the genetic disorder is 100% penetrant, the estimate of clinical sensitivity may approach that of the analytical sensitivity, with a large enough sample population. Additionally, high clinical sensitivity may be difficult to achieve for conditions that are highly heterogeneous, such as neurodevelopmental disorders, if not all possible causative genes are included in the selected test. Clinical sensitivity/utility and analytic sensitivity are often confused.

Clinical specificity is the ability of the test to discriminate between those with and without the suspected phenotype or disease. A test with high clinical specificity can accurately identify all patients without disease, in other words all unaffected individuals will have a negative test result. Without a high degree of analytic specificity, a test, by definition, cannot have a high degree of clinical specificity. One challenge in accurately determining the clinical validity of NGS based sequencing tests is the detection of VUSs, which cannot be categorized as negative results, thereby resulting in reduced clinical specificity. Limiting broad comprehensive testing to highly heterogeneous conditions, such as neurodevelopmental disorders, and using more focused approaches for less heterogeneous conditions can help maximize clinical specificity.

Clinical utility is the ability of the test to affect positive patient outcomes, which can be defined in different ways. As a result there is significant variability in how clinical utility is defined with respect to genetic testing, with narrow definitions focusing on the ability to improve treatment effectiveness and prognosis and broad definitions including diagnostic value and improvements in quality of life of affected individuals (including psychological impact). Clinical utility generally requires balancing clinical, economic, and psychological measures of possible benefit as well as possible harm (Burke et al., 2010). Clinical utility is important for informing test utilization guidelines and decisions by third-party payers (insurers) about whether to reimburse for a test. Evidence of clinical utility is usually not collected during the research or test development phases and may be difficult to document or measure.

Predictive value is also a measure of clinical validity and pertains to the ability of the test to identify the presence (or absence) of the disease. This is an important measurement for clinical interpretation and epidemiological studies and endeavors such as disease screening. The predictive power of any clinical test is directly related to the tested population and likelihood of disease in that population (Trevethan, 2017).

Clinical positive predictive value (PPV) is the proportion of positive results amongst all the individuals who have the disease. In other words, the PPV of a test indicates the likelihood that a positive result correlates with presence of disease. This parameter is measured at the population level and therefore is heavily influenced by the disease prevalence in the evaluated population (Figure 6-1B). Thus, when disease prevalence is high in a particular population, the predictive value can also be very high. Importantly, the positive predictive power of a test may differ greatly in the general population if the disease prevalence is significantly different from the original tested population. Conversely, when disease prevalence is low, such as in rare diseases, the PPV is likely to be low also. The PPV improves when the clinical sensitivity and specificity are high, but is most influenced by specificity.

Clinical negative predictive value (NPV) is the proportion of negative test results amongst all of the individuals that are unaffected. In other words, the NPV of a test indicates the likelihood that a negative result correlates with absence of disease. The NPV is inversely related to the disease prevalence of the tested population, meaning that when disease prevalence is low, NPV is high.

All of the above test parameters are directly related to whether a given test outcome is consistent with what is expected. In other words, does a positive test result truly reflect the presence of the tested disease or analyte (this scenario is defined as a true positive)? Alternatively, does a negative test result reliably indicate the absence of the tested disease or analyte (this scenario is defined as a true negative)? Or, are there situations in which a test result is falsely positive or falsely negative? In an ideal situation, a test would never produce a false positive or false negative result, but in practice these do sometimes occur and it is important to understand why a test result may not be consistent with the expected outcome. Inconsistencies can occur at the analytical level as a result of inaccuracies in the testing method or at the clinical level for a variety of reasons, including reduced penetrance or misclassified disease. Examples of possible reasons for false negative and false positive results are listed below:

False negative results (individual has disease, but tests negative) can occur as a result of:

- Analytical reasons:
  - insufficient analytic sensitivity (defined above) due to limitations of the testing method (e.g., testing only covers certain regions of the genes of interest)
  - sample mix-up or other pre-analytical (prior to analysis) error.
- Clinical reasons:
  - the patient's clinical features may not be fully apparent or appreciated, leading to inappropriate/incomplete testing (e.g., a negative epilepsy gene

panel for a newborn with seizures may not comprehensively evaluate for larger copy number variants such as the recurrent 15q13.3 microdeletion known to be associated with epilepsy and other syndromic features that may not be present at birth) (van Bon et al., 2022);

○ the genotype is not present in the tissue tested (e.g., blood sample negative by testing, but mosaicism is present in a neurofibroma that was not tested).

False positives (individual does NOT have disease, but receives a positive test result) can occur due to:

- Analytic reasons:
  ○ insufficient analytic specificity (defined above), which could be due to cross reactivity of the test (e.g., testing method cannot accurately discriminate between a variant in the pseudogene versus the gene of interest).
- Clinical reasons:
  ○ accurate test result but the phenotype has not manifested, possibly due to reduced penetrance or late age of onset;
  ○ the patient may have been considered clinically unaffected due to unappreciated variable expressivity, mild features, or incomplete clinical assessment.

The goal with any clinical testing is to limit the frequency of false positive and false negative results to optimize the accuracy of the test. Irrespective of the testing scenario, when an inaccurate result is suspected, it is important to consider why this may have occurred and follow-up with the testing laboratory to further evaluate the validity of the result. In some cases, it may be necessary to repeat testing using a newly collected sample and/or perform testing using a different method (orthogonal) that is more sensitive. Much of this process is part of standard laboratory practices and workflows that are initiated when an inaccurate result is identified within the lab to ensure quality testing, but sometimes the inaccurate result does not come to attention until after the result has been reported to the provider. In these situations, the provider (often a genetic counselor) can serve a critical role in test quality by communicating the potential error to the laboratory. It is important for genetic counselors to acknowledge the potential for inaccurate results and be prepared to discuss concerns with the laboratory and patient.

GENETIC TEST QUALITY AND DEVELOPMENT

Ensuring Quality in Clinical Genetic Testing

Most countries require some level of oversight of laboratories that perform clinical testing. In the US, all clinical laboratories are regulated by the Centers for Medicare & Medicaid Services (CMS) through the Clinical Laboratory Improvement Amendments (CLIA), which dictates the minimal laboratory requirements needed to ensure test results are accurate, reliable, timely, confidential, and with limited risk of harm to patients. All laboratories providing results to US clinicians or patients that will inform patient care must obtain CLIA certification, with the exception of laboratories in New York and Washington states where CLIA-certification is superseded by state regulatory agencies that have added requirements. For this reason, New York state approval for a given laboratory's test typically indicates high quality. Depending on what type of CLIA certificate the testing laboratory obtained, they are required to be inspected by the state CMS agency or one of several accredited organizations approved by CMS. The latter route typically encompasses participating in the organization's accreditation program, which must meet the minimal CLIA requirements, though many programs exceed these requirements. Many laboratories subscribe to programs provided by the Joint Commission on Accreditation of Healthcare Organizations (JCAHO) and the College of American Pathologists (CAP), but other approved voluntary organizations exist.

These accreditation programs ensure that laboratories are accountable for the quality of their testing by routinely assessing the laboratory's compliance to CLIA regulations (Clinical Laboratory Improvement Amendments of 1988), including:

- Ensuring laboratory staff have proper qualifications and maintain technical competency.
- Maintaining valid, accurate, and appropriate test methods.
- Implementing quality assurance programs to calibrate and monitor test quality using appropriate standards.
- Traceability of measurements and calibrations to national standards.
- Ensuring suitability, calibration, and maintenance of test equipment.
- Safety and appropriateness of the testing environment.
- Proper sampling, handling, and transportation of test items, including patient samples.

Laboratories outside the US are eligible for CLIA-certification, with over 50 international laboratories holding active CLIA certification as of 2023 (Centers for Disease Control and Prevention 2023). CLIA-certified laboratories outside the US are subject to the same accreditation programs as in the US, as CMS does not recognize non-US laboratory accreditation programs. While other organizations exist that accredit and certify laboratories in other countries, such as the International Laboratory Accreditation Cooperation (ILAC), any testing that will be used in the US to inform clinical decisions and patient care must be performed in a CLIA-certified laboratory, with the exceptions of New York and Washington as noted above.

Beyond the mandated regulations mentioned above, most quality laboratories also follow guidelines provided by professional and other certification organizations pertaining to genetic testing. In the US, professional guidelines for many types of biochemical/molecular/cytogenetic tests are provided by the American College of Medical Genetics and Genomics (ACMG), the Association of Molecular Pathologists (AMP), and CAP. One such example includes ACMG's "Standards and Guidelines for Clinical Genetics Laboratories" publications accessible on the ACMG website, which include requirements, considerations, and standards for validating cytogenetic, biochemical, and molecular genetics tests (American College of Medical Genetics and Genomics, 2021).

Professional Qualifications of Laboratory Personnel In most countries, laboratory personnel must meet some minimum qualifications and maintain technical competency, which varies by their role in the lab, with the most significant requirements needed at the director level. Under CLIA regulations, qualifications of laboratory personnel vary depending on the complexity of the testing performed by the laboratory, with those performing "high complexity" testing required to have laboratory directors with a PhD or MD/DO degree and be certified in an approved specialty by the appropriate board, such as the American Board of Medical Genetics and Genomics (ABMGG), American Board of Clinical Chemistry (ABCC), and others (Clinical Laboratory Improvement Amendments of 1988). While most molecular genetic testing is considered high complexity, it is worth noting that CLIA requirements for personnel (including directors and clinical consultants) in laboratories performing lower complexity testing are less stringent and may not include specialty training (e.g., human genetics). Other professional organizations, such as ACMG and CAP, do provide guidance that require genetic expertise and certification in various laboratory roles (American College of Medical Genetics and Genomics, 2021). There is more variability as to what level of education and expertise is needed for other laboratory roles, including laboratory supervisors, technologists, technical and clinical consultants, and other supporting roles. Many laboratories now employ certified genetic counselors to leverage their clinical expertise in many roles, including clinical result interpretation, assessing appropriateness of test orders, and serving as a liaison between the laboratory and ordering clinicians and patients. Laboratory genetic counselors serve an integral role in the laboratory by providing their expertise at every step of the test development and ordering processes, from selection to interpretation (Christian et al., 2012). Ultimately, it is beneficial to be aware of the numerous types of laboratory personnel, their roles and qualifications, and what accreditation program a given laboratory uses to ensure quality of the laboratory staff and testing procedures.

Regulation of Genetic Tests In the United States, and many European countries, the clinical laboratory director is responsible for developing and establishing the validity and accuracy of all testing performed in the lab. This includes selecting the most appropriate testing method and considering the strength of evidence supporting a gene-disease relationship to determine if there is sufficient evidence to include a particular gene on a testing panel or to report variation in that gene. Most genetic tests are categorized as laboratory developed tests (LDTs), previously known as "home brew tests," due to the limited number of commercially available standardized genetic tests. The Food and Drug Administration (FDA) is a US federal agency that reviews and approves commercially available test kits, known as *in vitro* diagnostic devices (IVDs) and analyte specific reagents (ASRs) which may be used in LDTs. While the FDA claimed oversight of LDTs in 1992 under the Medical Device Amendments (MDA) initiated in 1976, it was not until 2010 that they expressed interest in exerting regulatory oversight over LDTs. Since that time there have been several drafts of guidance and proposed legislation to develop an oversight framework, with the most recent one being the Verifying Accurate Leading-edge IVCT (*in vitro* clinical test) Development (VALID) Act (VALID Act 2023). Although the details of this ongoing debate are beyond the scope of this chapter, as a genetic counselor it is important to be aware of the dynamic and changing landscape of genetic testing oversight and related policies.

The Importance and Value of Proficiency Testing   Errors in laboratory testing are inevitable, but high-quality laboratories have measures in place to quickly identify and correct errors when they occur and then modify their testing processes to prevent future errors. There is limited data published regarding genetic testing laboratory errors due to the educational nature of quality monitoring programs, but what has been reported indicates most laboratory errors occur in the pre-analytical (prior to analysis) and the post-analytical (after analysis has been completed) phases and fewer errors occur in the analytical phase (during testing/analysis) of testing (Bonini et al., 2002). Pre-analytical errors occur during sample submission and accessioning (when samples are being received by the lab) and examples include mislabeled samples, inappropriately collected specimens, and improper handling and transport of samples. Post-analytical errors occur after analytical testing has been performed and may involve clerical errors in reporting, such as mislabeling a report with the wrong patient information, but may also occur if test results are not communicated in a manner that is clearly understood by the ordering clinician, resulting in misinterpretation of the results.

Analytical errors can often be avoided or mitigated when laboratories partici-pate in ongoing proficiency testing (PT) programs that externally validate the laboratory's ability to accurately assess a set of standard samples for a specific result. While CLIA laboratories are required to have quality assurance programs in place, PT is only required for established regulated analytes, which are rarely used in genetic tests. However, laboratories voluntarily following ACMG or AMP guidelines are required to perform PT and some accreditation programs, such as CAP, provide PT opportunities for a number of tests. PT is an important way to ensure quality laboratory performance and should be considered a quality indicator when selecting a laboratory for testing.

Assessing Quality of Non-Clinical Grade Testing Thus far, this chapter has focused on the quality of clinical-grade testing, but genetic counselors need to be aware of other types of test results that patients may receive and how they differ from clinical-grade testing. The number of commercial testing companies that market direct-to-consumer (DTC) genetic testing has drastically increased over time with more than 26 million consumers reported, as of 2019, to have purchased these services from four major companies (Regalado, 2019). There is great variability in the testing offered by each company and whether health professionals are involved in the ordering process (Fernandes Martins et al., 2022). Some of the DTC tests offered are regulated by the FDA while others are not. When helping a patient understand their results, it is critical to understand the limitations of DTC testing. DTC laboratories that are CLIA-certified and CAP-accredited must follow the same standards as outlined above for clinical testing and therefore may be more reliable, however it is important to understand the methodology used to detect the variants assessed. Many DTC testing companies prefer to utilize SNP genotyping arrays, which may have high accuracy for common variants, but have limited ability to accurately detect rare variants. Ultimately, it may be necessary to evaluate whether a patient needs confirmatory testing from a clinical laboratory and/or additional clinical testing to confirm or rule out suspected disease.

In addition to DTC results, patients may participate in a research program that provides genetic test results to patients. Given the lack of oversight regarding research genetic test results, it is even more important to understand the limitations of testing performed in a research setting. If test results will be used to inform clinical care, they should be confirmed in an appropriately certified clinical laboratory under the necessary regulatory oversight to ensure accuracy. This may involve providing a new clinical sample, depending on how the research sample is stored. It is worth noting that CLIA-certified laboratories may also perform research testing and most CLIA-certified laboratories have a research and development arm for validating new clinical tests.

Clinical Genetic Test Development

Many of the concepts addressed in the previous sections are critical to understanding how clinical genetic tests are developed. Before any new tests can be offered to clinicians and patients in the US, under CLIA regulations, laboratories must validate the test's analytical performance by evaluating its accuracy, precision, sensitivity, and specificity. It is important to note that CLIA regulations with respect to test development focus on the analytical validity of the test and do not assess clinical validity or clinical utility of a test. In the past, clinical genetic test development was often very gene-centric and driven by research interests requiring at least some evidence supporting the gene's role in disease, thus ensuring that some level of clinical validity was met. With the paradigm shift towards more comprehensive and inclusive gene panels and exome/genome tests, laboratories may include genes in their analyses with variable levels of evidence supporting disease causality, though laboratory guidelines from professional societies continue to be developed to adapt to the changing landscape (Strande et al., 2017; Bean et al., 2020).

Test Validation   Beyond understanding what genes and regions are covered by a particular test, it is also useful to know how a test is validated, what testing methodology is employed and its limitations, and other knowns and unknowns of the test. While there is no global standard for validating a clinical genetic test, the ACCE framework noted above is most widely cited with respect to evaluating genetic tests (Centers for Disease Control and Prevention, 2010). This framework is not intended as a prescriptive model for laboratories when validating a test; however, it does provide 44 questions, encompassing concepts such as clinical and analytical validity, utility, economics, and ethics, as a basis to scientifically evaluate the validity of a genetic test (Pitini et al., 2021). Unfortunately, in most countries, there is no regulatory agency or professional organization that reviews or approves the introduction of new tests (Organisation for Economic Co-operation and Development, 2007). However, many professional societies provide practice guidelines to aid laboratories in best practices when developing and maintaining new tests. This guidance can be broadly applicable to test validation or specifically address the validation of a targeted technique or clinical application of a method. Countries with universal health care and/or strong public health systems will only reimburse tests that have been reviewed by government-appointed experts or a governmental health care funding agency, thereby serving as a *de facto* test approval system. Furthermore, many laboratories have found it necessary and helpful to collaborate with clinicians and/or clinical researchers when developing new genetic tests to help decide which are most clinically useful and valid.

Despite the lack of standard recommendations for test validation, achieving high analytical validity is a basic element of test validation for all laboratories. Establishing analytical validity requires the use of appropriate reference standards, typically patient samples known to be positive or negative by "gold standard" techniques (Umemneku Chikere et al., 2019). Ideally these standards would be well characterized and used across laboratories; however, that is often not possible due to the rarity of most Mendelian diseases and the limited number of samples available. Fortunately, laboratories may work together to exchange de-identified patient samples for use during the validation process of a new test, though this practice is self-governed and not required. Large collaborative efforts—such as the Genome In A Bottle (GIAB) consortium, The Personal Genome Project (PGP), and the Global Alliance for Genomics and Health (GA4GH)—have led to the development of a small number of benchmark samples and tools (Global Alliance for Genomics & Health, 2023; National Institute of Standards and Technology, 2023; Open Humans Foundation, 2023). Samples tested during validation are often limited in terms of the scope of the patient population and types of variants tested, which may bias the reported test parameters, including detection rate. Any known limitations of the test and testing technology observed during validation should be disclosed. Limitations of the test might include specific types of variants that cannot be detected, regions of genes that are not adequately targeted, and classes of variants that are not reported.

Policies for Interpreting and Reporting Test Results In addition to technical considerations in test development, laboratories must also develop policies and protocols that describe how variants will be interpreted and reported. It is important to be aware that not all laboratories report out all observed variants depending on the type of testing ordered, especially for exome and genome tests, and therefore it may be necessary to contact the laboratory for clarification as to their policy. In the case of VUSs identified through exome and genome tests, laboratories may report only VUSs that correlate with the patient's clinical features and any other VUSs may not be mentioned (Rehm et al., 2023). Laboratories should also have policies in place to govern how often they will reassess their gene panel offerings and add newly described disease-causing genes that are clinically relevant, as well as how often variants will be reassessed (Deignan et al., 2019).

The Clinician's Role in Implementing Newly Developed Tests While it is up to the laboratory to decide when to provide new test offerings, genetic counselors and other health care providers should independently decide when a new test has sufficient evidence to warrant offering it to a patient. This can often be challenging for newer types of tests that may not yet have a gold standard comparison but have shown promise in a research setting or limited population cohorts, such as polygenic risk scores (PRS) or epigenetic signature tests. Unfortunately, there is often a substantial time gap between when new tests become available and when clinical guidelines are released by professional societies, requiring clinicians to use their best judgment regarding the utility of new tests and rely on standards of clinical care to critically evaluate the published claims of the test. Genetic counselors are encouraged to consult with their clinical team members and other local medical specialists to establish standards of practice for offering genetic tests in the absence of existing professional guidelines or consensus statements. Furthermore, genetic counselors and other health care providers must consider when their patients with negative testing may benefit from additional tests using newer, more comprehensive and/or sensitive technologies. Fortunately, most laboratories define their test parameters and often consider the clinical utility and validity of the test as it is developed. While this information may not always be readily available to the public, it should be available upon request by contacting the laboratory.

GENOMIC VARIANT INTERPRETATION

Key Genomic Resources

A variety of evidence types and information resources are considered for clinical genetic test development and for the interpretation of test results (Richards et al., 2015). Historically, laboratories relied solely on their internal databases of affected and unaffected individuals, the available published literature, and research connections to establish and interpret genetic testing. These siloed approaches prevented most individual laboratories from observing most rare variants, leading to higher VUS rates and a lack of collaboration. To address these issues, large-scale data-sharing and other collaborative efforts became a major milestone of the last two decades (Firth et al., 2009; Landrum et al., 2016). These efforts led to the development of more powerful, globally representative population-based genomic datasets (which help us appreciate the range of normal variation), the normalization of laboratory and patient data-sharing, and the advent of well-funded consortia which engage clinicians, laboratories, researchers, and patients to develop curated databases containing clinically relevant genes and variants (Chen et al., 2022; Rehm et al., 2015). While laboratories utilize internal data, both publicly available and licensed resources have become standard in bioinformatic pipelines and variant interpretation protocols. Understanding how these resources were developed and are maintained will help the user appreciate their unique strengths and weaknesses and how they can be encountered and employed across work settings (Table 6-2).

Curated Scientific Literature Resources   Expertly curated resources that collate scientific literature pertaining to the clinical implications of a particular gene or variant are essential for interpreting genetic test results and help identify the strongest literature. A major strength of these resources is expert-level input and the summary of pertinent evidence across sources into a single resource. However, maintenance of these resources can require significant effort and the information presented is limited to the time the resource was last updated. These databases may be publicly available or licensed products and often are used as proxies for manual literature searches that can be implemented in bioinformatic variant filtering for large NGS-based tests (Richards et al., 2015). In a single individual's exome data, thousands of variants are identified and stored in a variant call file (VCF), far too many for a laboratory to manually assess. Cross-referencing a patient's data, bioinformatically, with gene-lists, phenotype-lists, and variant-lists from curated literature resources provides a mechanism for focusing on the variants that are most likely to be clinically relevant, based on current literature.

One in-depth curation effort, funded by the National Human Genome Research Institute (NHGRI), is the Clinical Genome Resource (ClinGen) which includes well-defined algorithms focusing on four key concepts: 1) gene–disease validity; 2) variant pathogenicity; 3) dosage sensitivity; and 4) clinical actionability (Rehm et al., 2015). These are expert-led efforts across multiple institutions and countries to develop and apply evidence-based criteria to promote accurate and consistent

TABLE 6-2. **Genomic databases and resources**

Curated scientific literature	
Clinical Genome Resource (ClinGen) Curation Projects (https://www.clinicalgenome.org/)	• ClinGen Curation Activities include: gene-disease validity; variant pathogenicity; clinical actionability; dosage sensitivity. • Created and curated by experts across multiple institutions and subspecialties according to predefined criteria which have been vetted by peer-reviewed processes. • Since these are ongoing projects, not all genes have been evaluated. If a gene or region entry has not been updated recently it may not reflect new literature.
GeneReviews (www.genereviews.org)	• Provides summaries of literature necessary for multiple components of patient care, including pathogenesis, medical management, genetic testing, and risk estimation. High quality, in-depth reviews written by clinical experts. • This resource does not cover all genetic syndromes and a review may not exist for newly discovered genes or chromosomal regions. Publication dates may not be recent and new literature may not be captured.
Human Genetic Mutation Database (HGMD) (http://www.biobase-international.com/product/hgmd)	• A database of genomic variants that have been published in the medical literature. It is a helpful resource for finding specific variants that are in the literature and is easily searchable in its catalog format. This can be a helpful tool to augment literature searches. • The publicly available HGMD database is not frequently updated, compared to the licensed version. The variant classifications assigned in HGMD may not reflect clinical grade laboratory interpretation standards and may be the opinion of authors. Thus, each submitted paper should be evaluated independently.
Online Mendelian Inheritance in Man (OMIM) (www.omim.org)	• Provides concise literature summaries related to gene function, reported genetic variants, genotype–phenotype relationships, and clinical synopses. • There is not an entry for every gene and existing entries may not be updated consistently. There can be inconsistencies in the depth of information provided and outdated or refuted information may not be removed. Key literature should be reviewed directly. • Note that OMIM submissions to ClinVar typically list variants as "pathogenic." These assertions are based on the assertions of the authors of the relevant publication and may not represent recent interpretation using current resources or guidelines.

(continued)

TABLE 6-2. *(Continued)*

Population databases

Genome Aggregation Database (gnomAD) (http://gnomad.broadinstitute.org/)	• Largest population database to date with multiple ethnic groups represented and includes the majority of data from previous population databases. • Provides statistical analyses of the overall variation observed in a gene compared to expectations based on size (constraint metrics). These constraint metrics are available for different types of variants and can be useful for assessing the potential impact of a particular type of variant in a known disease gene or a variant in a gene of uncertain clinical significance.
Database of Genomic Variants (DGV) (http://dgv.tcag.ca/dgv/app/home)	• Includes copy number variants from various types of control populations, often from published studies. Studies vary in size, quality, and participant characteristics. • Entries may not include many details related to the study participants or provide clinical interpretations. • The Gold Standard dataset available on the site aggregates high confidence calls to provide frequency information.
Catalogue of Somatic Mutations in Cancer (COSMIC) (http://cancer.sanger.ac.uk/cosmic)	• Largest database of expert-curated somatic variants relating to human cancers.

Patient/Clinical databases

ClinVar (https://www.ncbi.nlm.nih.gov/clinvar)	• A comprehensive database which accepts submissions from clinical laboratories, clinicians, literature, patient registries, and research studies. • Contains a growing number of actively curated variants for which expert panel submissions or interlaboratory interpretation discrepancy resolutions are available. Variants which have been reviewed by a ClinGen expert panel have now been given FDA approval. • Contains both sequence and copy number variant submissions.
DatabasE of genomiC variation and Phenotype in Humans using Ensembl Resources (DECIPHER) (https://decipher.sanger.ac.uk/)	• A comprehensive database that accepts individual case submissions from clinician-partners and can include phenotype and inheritance data. • Contains both sequence and copy number variant submissions. • May also display all variants identified for an individual, including benign variants.
Leiden Open Variation Database (LOVD) (http://www.lovd.nl/3.0/home)	• Gene-specific databases can be rich resources when they are actively used and curated by invested researchers. Some are affiliated with an expert group and/or clinical testing laboratories. • Entries may be out of date and/or incomplete. Phenotype data and a clinical interpretation may not be present. The interpretations may not have utilized current clinical interpretation guidelines.

TABLE 6-2. (*Continued*)

Browsers and other tools	
NCBI Variation Viewer (http://www.ncbi.nlm.nih.gov/variation/view/)	• View a variant within the genomic context and link to publicly available databases and literature resources. • Aligned with ClinVar and other NCBI efforts.
UCSC Genome Browser (https://genome.ucsc.edu/)	• View a variant within the genomic context and link to publicly available databases and literature resources.
ClinGen Allele Registry (https://clinicalgenome.org/tools/educational-resources/materials/the-clingen-allele-registry/)	• Assigns a unique identifier for each genomic variant. • Catalogs varying nomenclature across transcripts and other variant details.
Variant Effect Predictor (http://www.ensembl.org/info/docs/tools/vep/index.html)	• Useful for pulling data from multiple sources, including computational models, population allele frequencies, and evolutionary conservation.
MARRVEL (http://marrvel.org)	• Compile data at the gene level or the variant level from multiple sources, including OMIM and population databases. • Will convert cDNA nomenclature to genomic coordinates if the transcript is provided.

standards for sequence and copy number variant assessment and to inform evidence-based decisions for medical management and genomics program development. This resource can help a genetic counselor understand to what extent a variant in a gene might be associated with (potentially causative for) a defined phenotype and help define the manner in which the gene causes disease (i.e., disease mechanism), such as haploinsufficiency (disease caused by loss of one functional gene copy). This foundational knowledge then supports variant specific curation to clarify the particular phenotypes caused by or associated with specific sequence variants or categories of variant type. The clinical actionability curation can help to operationalize decisions about which genes to include for broad screening programs or prioritize for payer-based utilization programs.

Clinical and Case Databases　The acceptance of genomic data-sharing as a critical strategy to improve our genomic knowledge base has fostered the development of several powerful resources which provide laboratories and clinicians with more immediate access to information about patients with similar genotypes and phenotypes that are clinically identified around the world. These efforts, in part driven by limitations due to historical gene patents, began as publicly available laboratory-specific databases and locus-specific, research-oriented gene databases that provided de-identified clinical data and often included relevant literature citations. Nationally funded efforts to support broader data sharing followed in the United States with case-based

CNV data made available in dbVar and eventually the development of ClinVar, a universal database of genomic variants spanning all phenotypes, which includes submissions from research groups and clinical laboratories worldwide (Landrum et al., 2016). In a parallel timeline, similar efforts in the United Kingdom culminated in the DECIPHER database which links laboratories and clinical genomics providers to provide tiered levels of data access based on an institution's position within the National Health Service (Firth et al., 2009). De-identified data from DECIPHER is publicly available and, because submissions are typically clinician driven, may include more detailed clinical histories. Related efforts, such as the Human Gene Mutation Database, continue to arise globally (Stenson et al., 2020). While these databases provide an important data-sharing mechanism, the entries can represent a range of submitter types (including literature reports or data from large research studies) with varying degrees of clinical expertise and may be incomplete. Any submitted variant classifications should be considered in light of the submission type and date, and whether parameters for classification were provided.

General Population and Control Databases One of the assumptions used in variant interpretation is that genetic variants that cause rare disease are expected to be ultra rare or absent in the general population or control dataset. Therefore, large population-based genomic data resources and high-quality genomic control datasets have been critical to inform clinical testing and have grown exponentially in recent years. The previous standard for research studies assessing the potential pathogenicity of a variant was to test about 100–200 control chromosomes from unaffected individuals with racial or ethnic backgrounds (based on physical appearance, geographical location, or patient report) that matched the reported cases (affected individuals). This soon changed as large genomic datasets representing either well-phenotyped control individuals, such as the Exome Sequencing Project, or aggregated datasets that approximate the general population, illuminated the impressive genomic variation across humans (Chen et al., 2022; Exome Variant Server, n.d.). One such important resource is the Genome Aggregation Database (gnomAD) which evolved from the Exome Aggregation Consortium (ExAC) (Chen et al., 2022). Historically, the saturation of genomic research with White/European participants has contributed to higher VUS rates amongst non-White patients and has exacerbated inequities in the clinical utility of various genetic tests across populations (Popejoy et al., 2018). Without more diverse and global population data, one might conclude that a variant is more likely to be pathogenic based on rarity in a single subgroup; however, knowing that it is prevalent (depending on disease prevalence) in individuals from another subgroup would prevent this erroneous conclusion. Making our large-scale data resources fully representative will improve the quality of genetic testing for all.

These data resources are now critical for NGS-based genetic analysis by allowing for variant-filtering based on overall and subpopulation allele frequencies.

Allele frequency refers to the number of times a variant (an allele) is observed in a population out of all the variants at that particular genetic locus. For example, an autosomal variant in a heterozygous state observed once in a group of 100 individuals, or 200 total alleles, equates to an allele frequency of 0.005 or 0.5%. Laboratories typically rely heavily on minor allele frequency (MAF), the frequency of the rare allele, when filtering a patient's variant data to identify the variants most likely to be disease-causing, based on the premise that pathogenic variants for rare disease should be rare themselves (Richards et al., 2015). Population databases, like gnomAD, may have the greatest utility for variant assessment in rare disease, often in pediatric settings and for individuals with more severe phenotypes such as epileptic encephalopathies. This is because individuals with these phenotypes are less likely to be included in population-based genetic datasets. Genetic counselors should consider age of onset, disease variability, and penetrance associated with the clinical phenotypes they are working with to gauge whether the presence of a pathogenic variant in population data is plausible. For example, many pathogenic *BRCA1* variants are present in gnomAD because these variants do not cause very early lethality or disability and are often undiagnosed because a person has not yet presented with disease. Use of gnomAD phenotype-specific data subsets can help with this.

The development of large-scale genomic resources now also includes considerations for ease of use and interoperability. Most major genomic data resources provide links to related resources and have often created user-friendly visual genomic browsers that can be customized to display desired data tracks across resources. For example, one could view data from ClinVar, gnomAD, OMIM, and ClinGen within the DECIPHER browser to facilitate data comparisons. These genomic resources are expected to continue to grow and increase in utility as additional large genomic research efforts and the inclusion of more diverse and broadly representative cohorts are incorporated.

Evaluating Gene–Disease Relationships

To interpret genetic tests, it is critical to consider the strength of evidence supporting a potential gene–disease relationship, before one begins to consider the potential pathogenicity of any given variant in that gene. All variants in a gene of uncertain clinical significance should be considered a VUS (Richards et al., 2015). Prior to 2017, no standardized approaches existed for evaluating the strength of a gene–disease relationship, leading to vast variability in the inclusion of genes on testing panels. While resources such as OMIM were and continue to be helpful in aggregating publications proposing gene–disease relationships, this resource does not assess the claims made about the evidence supporting that relationship. To meet this need, the ClinGen Consortium developed a standardized framework to evaluate the validity of gene–disease relationships, which has been widely adopted (Strande et al., 2017). Curation of all disease-associated genes is the ultimate goal but, given the time-intensive nature of this process, will likely be ongoing for many years.

It is important to note that although this framework exists, it is not required that a laboratory implement this particular method for curating genes. Genes that have not yet been curated by ClinGen may be evaluated in different ways across laboratories; therefore, general familiarity with this framework can help genetic counselors critically evaluate test results. This framework provides a qualitative descriptor for the strength of evidence supporting a gene–disease relationship, coupled with a semi-quantitative approach to calculate scores that would be equivalent to each level of classification. Classifications supporting a disease relationship range from "Definitive" to "Limited," and "Contradictory" classifications are used to describe situations where a gene–disease relationship is unlikely based on direct evidence. Lastly, there is a category for "No Known Disease Relationship" to be applied in situations where no evidence has emerged to suggest a role in disease. Each curated classification is with respect to a specific disease entity and specific mode of inheritance; therefore, a single gene could be curated for more than one disease entity (Strande et al,. 2017). For example, the *SMAD4* gene is associated with both Myhre syndrome and juvenile polyposis/hereditary hemorrhagic telangiectasia due to gain of function and loss of function disease mechanisms, respectively (McDonald and Stevenson, 2021; Lin et al., 2022). Gene-disease classifications represent the strength of evidence reported at the time of data collection and are expected to change over time (with the exception of the definitive category). Thus, a reported variant in a gene of uncertain significance (a VUS) may be reclassified if emerging literature indicates a newly appreciated gene–disease relationship. A genetic counselor's awareness of this potential and ability to identify the need for re-analysis or an updated literature search can have direct impacts on patient care (Wain, 2018; Wain et al., 2020).

Since this framework was published, there have been efforts to synergize across laboratories, research groups, and other genetics institutes that have been actively curating gene–disease relationships for their own endeavors. The Gene Curation Coalition (GenCC) was formed to facilitate public sharing of curated gene–disease relationships and provide a mechanism to harmonize approaches and to resolve identified discrepancies when appropriate (DiStefano et al., 2022). Given the time-intensive nature of the ClinGen gene curation efforts, the GenCC provides another avenue to assess gene–disease validity and facilitates transparency for laboratories that submit their data. It is important to note that, similar to other public databases, the methods of curation vary and some discretion is needed when comparing across submitters. Despite this variability, there is immense value in this data to inform gene panel selection and test development, with recent guidance from ACMG suggesting laboratories limit diagnostic panels to genes with moderate or above evidence for disease causality (Bean et al., 2020). The value of gene–disease validity data also extends to variant interpretation by providing critical information about the types of variants that cause a given disease, as will be described below (Richards et al., 2015).

Clinical Variant Interpretation

Once a gene–disease relationship is established, it is then necessary to determine what variants in that gene cause disease versus represent normal variation. Significant effort has gone into standardizing variant interpretation processes to aid in consistency and transparency across laboratories. Variant interpretation guidelines exist for the two major types of germline genetic variation: CNVs that encompass one or more genes and sequence variants (Richards et al., 2015; Riggs et al., 2020). Separate guidelines have been developed for the evaluation of somatic cancer variants (Li et al., 2017; Horak et al., 2022). Many of the key elements necessary for clinical variant interpretation are present in each of these frameworks, but this section will predominantly focus on germline sequence variant interpretation guidelines.

The most widely cited guidelines for germline sequence variant interpretation were published in 2015 as a joint consensus between ACMG and AMP and have since been adopted in Europe by the Association for Clinical Genomic Science (ACGS) as well as by many clinical laboratories (Richards et al., 2015). These guidelines were developed with Mendelian conditions in mind and were intended to be somewhat generalizable to allow broad application across different disease domains. Sequence variant interpretation has evolved over time from a fairly subjective description of a variant classification process to a more structured qualitative framework that uses the major types of evidence (described below) to assess the likelihood that a variant is pathogenic (disease-causing). The five classifications used in the current guidelines describe the gradient of confidence in the classification with "pathogenic (P)" being highly likely to cause disease and "benign (B)" being highly unlikely to cause disease. Variants with less certainty regarding disease causality are classified as "likely pathogenic (LP)" or "likely benign (LB)" as appropriate. Variants that do not have sufficient evidence in one direction or the other are classified as "variants of uncertain significance" (VUS). It is worth noting, that the threshold for "likely" is somewhat arbitrarily defined in these guidelines as having 90% certainty that a variant is benign or pathogenic.

These classifications are determined by assessing specific criteria that are weighted based on their strength of evidence in the following categories: 1) population data; 2) co-segregation, phenotypic, and allelic evidence; and 3) computational/predictive and functional data. Each criterion is categorized on a spectrum from benign to pathogenic and given a weight ranging from "supporting" to "very strong" which can be adjusted depending on the amount of data available for a given criterion. Extensive review of each criterion is outside the scope of this chapter, but understanding the types of evidence that inform variant classification (often drawn from the key resources described above) and how they are weighted and aggregated to form a final classification is fundamental to critically evaluate any patient's laboratory report.

Population Data   Population data provides the opportunity to calculate the frequency or number of times a variant is observed in a given population. If the variant is observed predominantly in disease-affected populations that will be evidence in favor of pathogenicity. In contrast, a variant that is only observed in healthy or unaffected individuals is evidence suggesting it is benign. The more times a variant is seen in an affected or unaffected population, the stronger the weight of evidence. Setting a threshold for the frequency of variant observations is contingent on disease prevalence, penetrance, and heterogeneity and, therefore, can vary by gene. Laboratories may set a generic allele frequency cutoff for genes that do not have robust prevalence estimates and may use more specific frequency cutoffs when such knowledge exists or for ultra-rare conditions. As noted in the genomic resources section, databases like gnomAD are fundamental in helping assess the population data criteria.

Cosegregation, Phenotypic, and Allelic Data   A genetic variant shown to cosegregate with disease status in one or more families provides evidence in support of pathogenicity. The larger the family and the more times the variant cosegregates with disease, the stronger the evidence. Conversely, if a variant does not cosegregate with disease (e.g., only seen in one of ten affected individuals in a family and also seen in unaffected individuals), that might be evidence against pathogenicity. Variants arising at or after the time of conception are referred to as *de novo* and support pathogenicity when the patient has a phenotype consistent with the gene affected. There is an additional criterion that can be applied when a patient has a phenotype that is highly specific and strongly correlated with the gene of interest. This should be used with caution since genetic testing is often ordered for patients with phenotypes that have high genetic heterogeneity, and are therefore not highly specific, such as neurodevelopmental disorders. Lastly, observing a variant in combination with another clearly established pathogenic variant in the same gene may be evidence for or against pathogenicity, depending on the expected disease inheritance pattern.

Computational/Predictive and Functional Data   A significant number of criteria fall into the computational/predictive category, which heavily relies on information about the variant's predicted impact on the protein (e.g., the variant is expected to result in a truncated protein versus it only alters a single amino acid). Application of these criteria requires knowledge of disease mechanisms (e.g., gain or loss of function). Variants that are predicted to truncate a protein (e.g., nonsense, frameshift) are typically expected to lead to absent protein or to have a more severe effect on the protein and, therefore, are weighted strongly in favor of pathogenicity, if the disease mechanism is loss of function. Similarly, the location of a variant within an important region of the protein (e.g., a DNA binding domain) or in regions where recurrent pathogenic variants occur can be evidence in support of pathogenicity. Finally, *in silico* predictors that use computational modeling of DNA sequence conservation, protein sequence, and structure to predict pathogenicity of missense variants have gained more traction and can provide supporting evidence for or against pathogenicity, but these have not been fully evaluated across all genes and diseases. In some cases, additional functional data may exist that experimentally demonstrates an altered impact on the protein function. However, it can often be challenging to determine whether this sort of data is relevant to the expected phenotype. Additional guidance has been published to help groups critically evaluate functional data in the context of variant interpretation (Brnich et al., 2019).

A major goal of the ACMG/AMP guidelines is to provide consistency in application across labs which, despite remaining challenges, has improved since 2015 based on variant concordance data across laboratories piloting the framework in 2016 and again in 2020 (Amendola et al., 2016; Amendola et al., 2020). Continued evolution of the framework as more groups implement it and make further specifications to the rules and criteria will hopefully aid in consistency. Notably, many gene/disease specific variant interpretation guidelines have been published through efforts within ClinGen (Clinical Genome Resource, 2023a). Other key modifications to these guidelines are leading to more quantitative approaches that leverage a Bayesian framework to convert each strength level to a probability of pathogenicity. A key challenge with the current guidelines is the ability to assess variants with lower penetrance and other non-Mendelian disease variants, but there is ongoing work in that area. Many of the basic principles outlined above for germline sequence variant interpretation are also applicable to the assessment of CNVs and somatic variants. Population data, allelic evidence, and phenotypic data are all critical for the evaluation of CNVs and somatic variants. Additionally, CNV interpretation must take into account the size, number, and types of genes involved in the chromosomal gain or loss (Riggs et al., 2020). Somatic variant interpretation utilizes a different classification system that categorizes variants into tiers based on whether therapeutics can effectively target the variant in question, but again several of the same evidence criteria are helpful in assessing variants (Li et al. 2017; Horak et al., 2022).

Laboratories are not required to follow any of these guidelines and even those that do are free to make modifications, therefore it is important to understand that some variability in variant interpretation is expected across laboratories. As a genetic counselor, this means you could encounter scenarios where two different patients (even within the same family) receive different classifications for the same variant. In these scenarios, contacting the testing laboratories can be extremely beneficial to help understand discrepancies, and in some cases these conversations may result in a laboratory reassessing and reclassifying the variant. This may be especially true if significant time has passed since the laboratory reported the variant, as both gene–disease validity classifications and variant interpretations are time sensitive and subject to change as more evidence becomes available. Variant reanalysis is another area where lack of standardization, despite recent guidance from ACMG, has resulted in dramatically different policies across laboratories.

The ability to independently assess a reported variant and provide accurate information to patients is a critical skill set for genetic counselors, given that laboratories are not perfect and available evidence is continually changing. In fact, surveys of variant interpretation activities across practicing genetic counselors highlight the importance of this skill set (Reuter et al., 2018; Zirkelbach et al., 2018; Wain et al., 2020). Furthermore, as the patient's provider you will have more detailed information about the patient than the laboratory and may learn additional information that can contribute to the overall classification of a variant over time. For example, follow-up cascade testing may show that your patient's variant cosegregates with disease in several distant relatives, which may be sufficient evidence to shift a variant from uncertain to likely pathogenic. Lastly, it is important to realize the distinction between a pathogenic variant or positive genetic test result and the overall case level interpretation for the patient. The latter requires consideration of the patient's phenotype and level of concordance with the genetic test result. Depending on the clinical picture, the case-level result could be uncertain even if genetic testing reveals a pathogenic variant. For example, if the phenotype associated with the pathogenic variant only partially overlaps with the patient's phenotype.

PUTTING IT INTO PRACTICE

Selecting the Right Test

Genetic counselors are frequently directly involved in determining the most appropriate genetic testing options based on each patient's unique circumstances. Several factors are likely to be considered in these decisions, including: 1) clarity on the purpose of the genetic testing in each clinical context; 2) understanding of the limitations of test methodologies; 3) current practice guidelines and accepted clinical recommendations; 4) patient-specific factors, such as clinical and family history, personal motivations, and concerns; and 5) financial circumstances. As described above, genetic testing can be used to establish a genetic diagnosis, screen for genetic risks, determine individual risk based on known familial variant testing, and inform treatment. The exact situation will determine whether the best test is broad in scope (exome/genome sequencing) or focused (single variant testing). Yet, even newer, broad test options have technical limitations and older techniques, such as karyotype or FISH, are still highly relevant depending on the clinical need (e.g., to identify balanced chromosomal rearrangements).

Relying on up-to-date clinical practice guidelines developed by professional organizations with specific expertise is most ideal for informing test selection. These guidelines may represent expert consensus, especially in circumstances of more limited research, or can be the product of a systematic evidence review and subsequent formal evaluation of existing evidence. These can provide clear support for the use of specific genetic testing in defined populations or clinical situations (e.g., ACMG recommending exome or genome sequencing as a first-tier test for patients with congenital anomalies, global developmental delay, or intellectual disability) (Manickam et al., 2021). However, these valuable guidelines are not available for all clinical situations and genetic counselors may need to decide between various clinically-relevant test options that vary in scope, cost, potential diagnostic yield, likelihood of a VUS, or other factors.

Patient-specific factors are an important consideration and warrant exploration to assess how important obtaining a genetic diagnosis is to the patient, particularly in understanding how it could impact care, and what a preferred timeline and tolerance for ambiguous information might be. Some clinicians may make assumptions that patients will struggle with ambiguity or complexity and may choose testing strategies that lengthen the diagnostic process in an attempt to minimize uncertainty. This, however, may not be consistent with the patient's priorities. For known variant testing, the test selection hinges on accurate knowledge of the genetic variant of interest. The specific variant type will determine the necessary test method to ensure reliable and informative results. For example, a CNV might require targeted CMA or FISH, whereas a missense sequence variant would likely require Sanger sequencing.

Finally, financial concerns remain a necessary consideration for many patients. Whether a patient has commercial insurance, Medicare or Medicaid coverage, or would have to pay for testing out of pocket, unfortunately continues to impact testing decisions. At times, these considerations may even lead to the intentional use of a test with a suboptimal diagnostic yield because it is a required step in an approved testing algorithm set forth by an insurance policy. In these circumstances, the clinician must remain aware of test limitations in order to supplement or build upon the testing strategy over time to maximize diagnostic opportunities. Genetic counselors should also be aware of and advocate for patient access to financial assistance programs to minimize how financial impacts can limit equitable access to testing. In the sections below, we will discuss how some of these factors can guide post-test clinical considerations.

Interpreting Genetic Test Reports

A "Negative" Test Report—No Variants Reported: Clinical Considerations   A negative test report simply means that no variants were included on the report. How informative this is, or how it will be received by the patient, is another matter. For known variant testing where the laboratory had a positive control sample, a negative test is typically considered a "true negative" and a highly reliable result that effectively rules out a diagnosis or elevated risk. But for diagnostic or screening tests, a negative result must be interpreted in light of specific test methodology limitations. For example, a 23-variant cystic fibrosis carrier panel has significant limitations compared to a pan-ethnic carrier screening panel because it focuses on a limited number of specific variants within a single gene that have variable clinical relevance across ethnically diverse populations. Thus, the focused panel is likely to be negative for many patients because it does not include all of the potentially clinically relevant genetic content (Westemeyer et al., 2020).

Similarly, many clinical disorders are genetically heterogeneous and can be caused by a wide variety of variant types, including sequence variants, copy number variants, methylation abnormalities, and repeat expansions. Understanding how and when a test was performed will help determine if additional tests are needed or if reanalysis might be useful, especially for tests that use an exome or genome-based platform. Many genetic tests are frequently updated as the genomic knowledge base continues to improve. This leads to revisions to gene panel content, changes to bioinformatic analysis pipelines to improve variant calling and annotation, and laboratory reporting policy changes that could impact which variants are ultimately included on a report. These scenarios represent the complexities of analytical and clinical sensitivity for NGS-based tests, since a variant may be sequenced and available within a patient's data yet be missed by tertiary analysis steps (e.g., bioinformatic filtering). This is in contrast to analytical false negatives due to sample mix-up or other assay-specific problems.

A "Positive" Test Report—Variant(s) Reported: Clinical Considerations

The term "positive" can refer to a test report that includes any type of reported variant (including VUSs) or reports that only include diagnostic variants, so it can be important to clarify the intended meaning. A report with a "positive test" heading that only included VUSs could easily be misinterpreted by patients or clinicians with limited genetics experience. Furthermore, even a reported variant that is classified as likely pathogenic or pathogenic may or may not be diagnostic for a patient. For example, a single, heterozygous, pathogenic variant in an autosomal recessive gene could be called "positive." Therefore, when receiving a positive test report, one should consider several details to inform clinical interpretation and decision-making. Variant-specific details to consider include how the variant was classified and the level of evidence that supports that classification as well as the zygosity of the observed variant(s) and how this relates to the associated disorder. When the variant was classified is also important, since variant classification guidelines and available data-resources have changed over time. For example, if a patient comes to the clinic with a test report from several years ago it may be important to determine if newly available evidence exists that would impact classification of previously reported variants.

Assessing the level of clinical correlation between the patient and/or family history and the associated disorder is a critical step after receiving a positive test result, for both pathogenic variants and for VUSs. This is an opportunity to ask "Does this result make sense?" given what is known about a patient's history. This is an important role that clinical geneticists may play on a health care team if dysmorphology or other physical exams are needed (Baldridge et al., 2017). Sometimes additional clinical assessments are needed for this, such as an ophthalmology exam, a skeletal survey, or a brain MRI. Newly acquired clinical information should be provided to the laboratory because it may aid in reclassifying a variant. Our appreciation for the variable expressivity, including subtle or mild symptoms, penetrance estimates, and the synergistic impacts of multiple variants on clinically described phenotypes, especially for classical genetic syndromes, continues to improve. This has particularly been noted through the use of exome and genome sequencing and population-based genomic studies offered to patients irrespective of disease, which have illuminated the milder ends of phenotypic spectrums, by identifying patients who otherwise would not have been referred for a genetics evaluation in the past (Buchanan et al., 2020; Martin et al., 2020).

In addition to reported variants that may be directly related to the clinical indication for testing, when exome or genome testing is ordered some positive reports may include variants that are unrelated to a patient's current clinical situation but may be clinically relevant. Two broad types of these results are *secondary findings* and *incidental findings*. Secondary findings are highly penetrant genomic variants with potential medical actionability which the laboratory should purposefully seek to identify in a patient's exome/genome sample when possible, regardless of whether they relate to the purpose of testing, unless the patient opts-out of receiving such results. The ACMG maintains a list of genes recommended for reporting of pathogenic and/or likely pathogenic variants as secondary findings for exome and genome tests (Miller et al., 2023). Incidental findings are genetic variants that are unavoidably observed during testing, appear to be unrelated to the reason for testing, but may be clinically relevant for patient care. One example of an incidental finding would be a 200 kilobase deletion that includes the *ENG* gene observed by CMA ordered for a patient with developmental delay. This deletion is above laboratory reporting size thresholds and is clinically relevant because heterozygous loss of *ENG* (haploinsufficiency) is associated with hereditary hemorrhagic telangiectasia type 1, but there is no evidence that the deletion is causative for the patient's developmental delays (McDonald and Stevenson, 2021). Laboratories have discretion to provide patients with various opt-in or opt-out opportunities for both secondary and incidental findings; however, some decisions to report incidental findings are made on a case-by-case basis with variability across laboratories.

For the most part, variants detailed on positive clinical genetic test reports will be true analytical positives because laboratory standards require data quality thresholds and/or the use of orthogonal (independent) methods for variant confirmation. However, the possibility of false-positive results is very important in some clinical situations, such as prenatal *screening* tests (e.g., NIPS, quad screen) and newborn screening, which assesses for metabolic abnormalities via blood spot. These types of positive screening tests should be followed-up with appropriate diagnostic testing. Genetic tests that are marketed direct-to-consumer may also report variants to consumers with accompanying descriptions of clinical implications. While some of these tests have FDA-approval for very specific variants that are more commonly observed in affected individuals, the methodologies employed can produce inaccurate results depending on adjacent variation that interferes with accurate detection. For this reason, it is often best to have these findings confirmed and interpreted by a clinical diagnostic laboratory before clinical actions are taken.

Illustrative Cases

Positive newborn screening result—understanding next steps The following example has been adapted from an exemplary published case example; however, some details have been modified or fictionalized to help illustrate key teaching points (Wang, 2020). A premature female infant, born at 32 weeks with normal prenatal ultrasounds and first trimester screening, was found to have reduced acid α-glucosidase enzyme activity (GAA) by newborn screening. Additional follow-up testing (including molecular testing for variants in *GAA*) was ordered while the baby was in the NICU, along with a genetics consult to evaluate the patient for Pompe disease (GAA deficiency). Pompe disease is an autosomal recessive glycogen storage disorder with two distinct presentations: 1) infantile onset characterized by muscle weakness, failure to thrive, hypertrophic cardiomyopathy, and death by two years if untreated; and 2) adult onset with a much milder presentation characterized by proximal muscle weakness and respiratory insufficiency. Elevated blood creatine phosphokinase and urinary hexose tetrasaccharide (uHex4) levels can be seen in patients with Pompe disease, but are nonspecific features (Leslie and Bailey, 2017).

When the patient's parents were notified of the positive NBS result, their pediatrician was somewhat dismissive of the result, suggested that follow-up testing would likely determine that it was a false positive result, and told the parents not to worry or look up information online. However, the patient's mother did search online for Pompe disease and found outdated information describing the disease as fatal. She then discussed the information with her mother, who responded that it sounded similar to the cause of death for one of her previous children who died of a lysosomal storage disease. Prior to conception of their baby, the couple had informed their provider about this history and were comforted by negative prenatal carrier screening results performed for the mother. The patient's mother brings these concerns back to her daughter's pediatrician, who documents the information in the baby's chart and reassures her that these concerns will be addressed during her genetics consultation. The baby's parents are confused, frightened, and angry.

The baby's echocardiogram was normal and follow-up testing showed normal blood creatine phosphokinase levels but elevated uHex4 levels. Molecular testing for variants in the *GAA* gene revealed two pathogenic variants, including the common splice variant that is known to cause late onset disease and a second novel truncating variant likely associated with infantile onset disease. In preparing to meet with the family, the pediatric genetic counselor reviewed both variants and considered whether it is possible to accurately predict age of disease onset, since infantile disease requires urgent treatment to improve motor outcomes. Acknowledging that elevated uHex4 is a nonspecific feature seen in Pompe patients and that it can also be elevated in premature infants, it is critical to get repeat uHex4 testing to ensure an accurate reading.

In reviewing the patient's chart, the pediatrician's note regarding family history and negative prenatal testing should raise concerns and warrant further follow-up to understand what prenatal testing was performed and why it was negative. It is important to understand that carrier screening has lower sensitivity than diagnostic testing since VUSs are intentionally not reported for carrier panels, which could increase clinical false negative results. Additionally, some carrier testing may not comprehensively sequence the genes of interest, but instead only assess specific common pathogenic variants. In this particular case the mother's testing was a limited, common variant panel that did not assess for novel pathogenic variants, and no testing had been ordered for the father.

The genetic counselor prepared to help the family navigate the difference between screening tests and diagnostic tests, anticipating their current emotional state and reactions to their daughter's diagnosis after they likely considered themselves at low risk. She also prepared to coordinate parental testing to determine the inheritance of each variant for potential future family planning. Parental cascade testing showed that the severe, truncating variant was maternally inherited and the known splice variant was paternally inherited. Because the maternal variant was not included on the carrier panel, her report was issued as negative. This complete information helped the parents understand their current situation, despite their attempts to identify genetic risks prenatally. While the pediatric genetic counselor cannot change how their prenatal care was approached, she can facilitate adaptation to their current situation and help them understand why their daughter's results indicate some uncertainty in potential symptom severity, age of onset, and that symptom monitoring and long-term follow-up will be indicated.

This case illustrates the importance of understanding sensitivity and specificity of diagnostic versus screening tests. These concepts may not be obvious to patients, but are critical to understanding why results may appear discrepant and in this particular case could help alleviate some of the frustration and confusion felt by the family after learning their child had Pompe disease. Additionally, this case highlights the value of confirmatory testing and the utilization of multiple test types to fully characterize a patient's disease. The limited specificity and predictive ability of the biochemical tests to distinguish between infantile and late onset disease highlight the utility of molecular testing in this case.

Which gene panel is right for my patient? A 38-year-old woman is referred for genetic counseling and testing due to a recent diagnosis of Brugada syndrome which was identified after repeated episodes of syncope (fainting) and heart palpitations. She attends the appointment with her wife and you learn that the couple has been exploring options to start a family, including discussions about pregnancy for either of them versus adoption. The patient's family history is largely uninformative, with the exception of a maternal cousin who died at age 50 of a heart attack. Receiving the diagnosis was very scary for the patient and she shared that she is having a hard time processing all the new information involved. Her wife is very vocal during the appointment and has a folder full of printed information she found online about Brugada syndrome. She remarks that they want the "best" testing available to make sure they can find the genetic cause. The patient indicates agreement by nodding but looks down at the table while doing so. When prompted, she replies that she just wants clear information that will help her to be healthy.

Genetic testing in cardiovascular settings often utilizes gene sequencing panels that vary in size and phenotypic scope. Several laboratories offer these panels and most likely a genetic counselor in this setting has one or two preferred laboratories based on their experience with test report clarity, the soundness of the variant interpretation, and possibly customer service aspects such as ease of communication and billing processes. Panels provide a comprehensive approach to obtaining a genetic etiology that is more or less phenotype-specific depending on the panel. Brugada syndrome is one type of cardiac arrhythmia disorder that can be caused by multiple genes (Brugada et al., 2022). As such, laboratories could offer both Brugada-specific gene panels and larger arrhythmia panels that include genes for Brugada and other types of arrhythmia disorders. The level of confidence in a clinical diagnosis is often a factor in deciding between these approaches. For this patient, the genetic counselor may want to consider the ability of a particular test to meet both the patient's and the clinical team's goals while avoiding unhelpful outcomes.

While exploring the couple's goals and helping them appreciate one another's different perspectives, the genetic counselor also provided information to help them share in the decision about test approaches. He described how larger panels assess more genes, which can be helpful if there is phenotypic overlap between arrhythmias, but this also leads to the potential for more VUSs which may be challenging to interpret, especially if they are not specific to Brugada syndrome. The smaller panel would be more specific to Brugada syndrome. The genetic counselor also utilized understanding of gene curation efforts, which have highlighted genes on arrhythmia panels that were historically included despite insufficient evidence for association with Brugada (Hosseini et al., 2018).

After discussing the balance between one comprehensive test that maximizes efficiency versus a focused test that minimizes uncertainty, the patient was clearly favoring a focused panel. Her wife shared that her style of coping with perceived threats or uncertainty was to take action to feel more control, while the patient stated that she wanted to avoid unnecessary stressors that wouldn't clearly help them figure out how to live with this diagnosis. They both wanted to be able to return their attention to family planning and understood that the patient would be followed by cardiology regardless of the outcome of her genetic test. They also understood that they could meet with the genetic counselor in the future to learn of relevant updates or if there were changes in the patient's health. In the end, they agreed to pursue the smaller, focused Brugada panel.

This case illustrates how a genetic counselor can help a patient navigate the menu of possible genetic testing options while ensuring clinical utility and alignment with patient needs. The right test option may not be the same for all patients with the same clinical indication and the genetic counselor does not necessarily need to subscribe to the same approach every time. Even if a comprehensive panel is used for the majority of patients in a given clinic, there may be times when an alternative should be considered based on the patient's unique goals and perspectives. In this situation, the couple reacted to a new diagnosis in different ways. In addition to utilizing psychosocial skills, the genetic counselor's understanding of evidence-based gene curation, and the ability to relay aspects of this in lay terms, helped the couple align the need for a quality test with the desire to minimize uncertainty.

My patient's exome report includes variants of uncertain significance—now what? A 2-year-old boy was referred to genetics to discuss the results of trio exome sequencing that was ordered by his neurologist due to a recent diagnosis of epilepsy. His development, prior to his seizure onset, had been mildly delayed with some specific concerns about fine motor skills and expressive language development, but his pediatrician had been taking a "wait and see" approach. He was born premature at 34 weeks gestation and had mild hypotonia with feeding difficulties. No family history of neurodevelopmental disorders had been shared with the neurologist. The exome report included two VUS: a *de novo* missense variant in the *SYNGAP1* gene and a maternally inherited nonsense variant in the *AGTR2* gene.

To prepare for the family's appointment to review results, a genetic counselor would likely consider the types of evidence used for variant classification and should think critically about whether one or both of these variants is likely to be contributing to the child's seizures and delays. This is important to ensure the clinical care team thoroughly understands the potential implications and degree of uncertainty of the findings and to prepare to meet the family's needs. Families vary in the depth of information they need when digesting their child's genetic test results; some individuals are information-seekers and others are not. Some individuals may view an uncertain result as an indication that genetic information is generally not useful and could disengage. Furthermore, receiving more than one finding from a genetic test can be overwhelming and confusing so it is the genetic counselor's responsibility to help the family adapt to the information and manage any uncertainty. This may include helping the family to prioritize their decisions if they are interested in connecting with support or research organizations, especially when several variants are reported.

In addition, the genetic counselor will consider the technical limitations of the exome performed for this patient. Many laboratories include CNV-calling via exome sequencing so it would be important for the genetic counselor to understand if this was completed, which may require contacting the laboratory, if the patient had not had previous CMA testing. Additional tests to assess for methylation abnormalities or repeat expansion disorders may be indicated after clinical evaluation, so anticipating how to raise this with the family is relevant.

Haploinsufficiency (loss of one functional copy) of *SYNGAP1* is known to cause neurodevelopmental disorders, including developmental delay, intellectual disability, and seizures (Holder et al., 2019). However, the identified variant has never been reported in the literature or observed by the testing laboratory, and has not been submitted to ClinVar or other genetic databases. It is also absent from population databases. Predicting the impact of a missense variant on protein function is challenging and, without other reported cases or functional studies, we are limited to predictions from computational algorithms (e.g., CADD, Poly-Phen, SIFT), which have limited sensitivity and specificity. The *AGTR2* gene is not definitively associated with a disorder or clear phenotype, though there has been some literature suggesting a possible association with neurodevelopmental disorders. The gene was curated by the ClinGen Gene-Disease Validity and Dosage Sensitivity Workgroups, though not recently (Clinical Genome Resource, 2023b). Because the lab considers *AGTR2* a gene of uncertain significance, all variants observed in the gene are classified as VUS, even a nonsense variant that would lead to loss of gene expression and is absent from population databases.

A *de novo* variant, when parentage is confirmed, in a gene that fits the child's clinical history is a strong piece of evidence. Seizures are well-documented in patients with pathogenic *SYNGAP1* variants. While this patient's developmental milestones have only been mildly delayed, his age should also be considered as he is young and his cognitive abilities will become more apparent with age. However, a novel missense variant may or may not be impacting protein function. In contrast, a nonsense variant that introduces a new stop codon and is predicted to lead to nonsense-mediated decay and loss of gene function is a frequent finding in patients with neurodevelopmental disorders. Since the *AGTR2* gene is on the X chromosome and the patient is male, the maternal inheritance does not rule this out as a possible cause and this could be purposely explored while taking the family history. While expert curation was appropriately cautious about a potential gene–disease relationship for *AGTR2*, additional literature may have become available since the time of that curation or could be published in the near future. The genetic counselor could perform a focused literature search related to *AGTR2* for more recent reports and to more clearly understand the proposed phenotypes described in the literature to date.

In this case, the two variants may both be of clinical interest, though the *SYNGAP1* variant is likely to be more compelling as a possible diagnostic finding initially since it is *de novo* and *SYNGAP1* is a well-described gene that is highly associated with seizures. The genetic counselor will need to assess how the family understands and reacts to these findings and help them to discuss what actions, if any, they might find helpful. They could connect with gene-specific or general patient support organizations or they may be interested in seeking out research opportunities that could clarify the meaning of the child's results. They may also simply want to follow up with the genetic counselor over time to remain informed of new literature, variant reclassifications, or other updates. A genetic counselor who has a foundational understanding of variant classification and available resources, who will help ensure that all clinical team members remain updated, may be more likely to establish trust on the part of the patient and family, so that they remain engaged in optimal care even in the face of uncertainty and change.

CONCLUSION

Genetic testing is now widely available for broad diagnostic purposes, screening for disease status and risk, focused assessment for known genetic variants, and to inform disease management and prognosis. Genetic counselors play crucial roles in evaluating the clinical usefulness of these tests, determining how they should be implemented in care, and ensuring that test results are correctly understood by both patients and nongenetics colleagues. Genetic counselors must be knowledgeable about test methodologies, gene curation, and variant interpretation, and they can apply their critical thinking and assessment skills to increase the value of genomic medicine throughout health care specialties. These considerations are particularly important prior to the utilization of new technologies, which may have a higher likelihood of inconclusive test results. As broad-scope genetic tests, like exome and genome sequencing, are further implemented across clinical care, genetic counselors will continue to be essential members of clinical care teams whose genomics expertise helps them facilitate evidence-based clinical recommendations and patient-focused decision-making, communicate with laboratories about testing strategies and results, and ensure that updated genomic knowledge is incorporated into clinical care through data re-analyses or variant re-interpretation over time.

REFERENCES

Abu-El-Jaija A, Reddi HV, Wand H, et al. (2023) The clinical application of polygenic risk scores: a points to consider statement of the American College of Medical Genetics and Genomics (ACMG). *Genet Med* 25(5):100803. doi: 10.1016/j.gim.2023.100803.

Amendola LM, Jarvik GP, Leo MC, et al. (2016) Performance of ACMG-AMP Variant-Interpretation Guidelines among nine laboratories in the Clinical Sequencing Exploratory Research Consortium. *Am J Hum Genet* 98(6):1067–1076. doi: 10.1016/j.ajhg.2016.03.024.

Amendola LM, Muenzen K, Biesecker LG, et al. (2020) Variant Classification Concordance using the ACMG-AMP Variant Interpretation Guidelines across Nine Genomic Implementation Research Studies. *Am J Hum Genet.* 107(5):932–941. doi: 10.1016/j.ajhg.2020.09.011.

American College of Medical Genetics and Genomics (2021). ACMG Technical Standards for Clinical Genetics Laboratories (2021 Revision). https://www.acmg.net/ACMG/Medical-Genetics-Practice-Resources/Genetics_Lab_Standards/ACMG/Medical-Genetics-Practice-Resources/Genetics_Lab_Standards.aspx?hkey=0e473683-3910-420c-9efb-958707c59589 Accessed August 4, 2023.

Baldridge D, Heeley J, Vineyard M, et al. (2017) The Exome Clinic and the role of medical genetics expertise in interpretation of exome sequencing results. *Genet Med* 19(9): 1040–1048. doi: 10.1038/gim.2016.224.

Bean LJH, Funke B, Carlston CM, et al. (2020) Diagnostic gene sequencing panels: from design to report - a technical standard of the American College of Medica Genetics and Genomics (ACMG). *Genet Med* 22(3):453–461. doi: 10.1038/s41436-019-066-z.

Bonini P, Plebani M, Ceriotti F, et al. (2002) Errors in laboratory medicine. *Clin Chem* 48(5):691–698.

Brnich SE, Abou Tayoun AN, Couch FJ, et al. (2019). Recommendations for application of the functional evidence PS3/BS3 criterion using the ACMG/AMP sequence variant interpretation framework. *Genome Med* 12(1):3. doi: 10.1186/s13073-019-0690-2.

Brugada R, Campuzano O, Sarquella-Brugada G, et al. (2005, Updated 2022) Brugada Syndrome. In: GeneReviews® [Internet]. MP Adam, GM Mirzaa, RA Pagon, et al. (eds), Seattle, WA: University of Washington. https://www.ncbi.nlm.nih.gov/books/NBK1517/ Accessed May 28, 2024

Buchanan AH, Kirchner HL, Schwartz MLB, et al. (2020) Clinical outcomes of a genomic screening program for actionable genetic conditions. *Genet Med* 22(11):1874–1882. doi: 10.1038/s41436-020-0876-4.

Buckingham L. (2019) *Molecular Diagnostics: Fundamentals, Methods, and Clinical Applications* Third edition, Philadelphia, PA: FA Davis Company.

Burke W, Laberge A-M, & Press N. (2010) Debating clinical utility. *Pub Health Genomics* 13(4):215–223. doi: 10.1159/000279623.

Burke W. (2014) Genetic tests: clinical validity and clinical utility. *Curr Protoc Hum Genet* 81(1):9151–9158. Doi: 10.1002/0471142905.hg0915s81.

Centers for Disease Control and Prevention (2010) ACCE Model Process for Evaluating Genetic Tests. https://www.cdc.gov/genomics/gtesting/acce/index.htm#print Accessed April 14, 2023.

Centers for Disease Control and Prevention (2023) Clinical Laboratory Improvement Amendments (CLIA) Laboratory Search. https://www.cdc.gov/clia/LabSearch.html# Accessed June 21, 2023.

Chen S, Francioli LC, Goodrich JK, et al. (2022) A genome-wide mutational constraint map quantified from variation in 76,156 human genomes. *bioRxiv*. doi: 10.1101/2022.03.20.485034.

Christian S, Lilley M, Hume S, et al. (2012) Defining the role of laboratory genetic counselor. *J Genet Couns* 21(4):605–611. doi: 10.1007/s10897-011-9419-0.

Clinical Genome Resource (2023a) Sequence Variant Interpretation. https://www.clinicalgenome.org/working-groups/sequence-variant-interpretation/ Accessed August 25, 2023.

Clinical Genome Resource (2023b). AGTR2 Gene-Disease Validity. https://www.search.clinicalgenome.org/kb/genes/HGNC:338. Accessed August 25, 2023.

Clinical Laboratory Improvement Amendments of 1988, 102 Stat. 2903, Public Law 100–578.

Deignan JL, Chung WK, Kearney HM, et al. (2019) Points to consider in the reevaluation and reanalysis of genomic test results: a statement of the American College of Medical Genetics and Genomics (ACMG). *Genet Med* 21(6):1267–1270. doi: 10.1038/s41436-019-0478-1.

DiStefano MT, Goehringer S, Babb L, et al. (2022) The Gene Curation Coalition: a global effort to harmonize gene-disease evidence resources. *Genet Med* 24(8):1732–1742. doi: 10.1016/j.gim.2022.04.017.

Durmaz AA, Karaca E, Demkow U, et al. (2015) Evolution of genetic techniques: past, present, and beyond. *Biomed Res Int* 2015:461524. doi: 10.1155/2015/461524.

Exome Variant Server. (n.d.) NHLBI GO Exome Sequencing Project (ESP), Seattle, WA. https://evs.gs.washington.edu/EVS/ Accessed August 14, 2023.

Fabie NAV, Pappas KB, & Feldman GL. (2019) The current state of newborn screening in the United States. *Pediatr Clin North Am* 66(2):369–386. doi: 10.1016/j.pcl.2018.12.007.

Fernandes Martins M, Murray LT, Telford L, et al. (2022) Direct-to-consumer genetic testing: an updated systematic review of healthcare professionals' knowledge and views, and ethical and legal concerns. *Eur J Hum Genet* 30(12):1331–1343. doi: 10.1038/s41431-022-01205-8.

Firth HV, Richards SM, Bevan AP, et al. (2009) DECIPHER: Database of Chromosomal Imbalance and Phenotype in Humans Using Ensembl Resources. *Am J Hum Genet* 84(4):524–33. doi: 10.1016/j.ajhg.2009.03.010.

Gersen SL & Keagle MB. (2013) *The Principles of Clinical Cytogenetics*, New York, NY: Springer.

Giardiello FM, Allen JI, Axilbund JE, et al. (2014) Guidelines on genetic evaluation and management of Lynch syndrome: a consensus statement the US Multi-Society Task Force on colorectal cancer. *Gastroenterology* 147(2):502–526. doi: 10.1053/j.gastro.2014.04.001.

Global Alliance for Genomics & Health (2023) https://www.ga4gh.org/ Accessed August 14, 2023.

Gregg AR, Aarabi M, Klugman S, et al. (2021) Screening for autosomal recessive and X-linked conditions during pregnancy and preconception: a practice resource of the American College of Medical Genetics and Genomics (ACMG). *Genet Med* 23(10):1793–1806. doi: 10.1038/s41436-021-01203-z.

Goswami RS & Harada S. (2020) An overview of molecular genetic diagnosis techniques. *Curr Protoc Hum Genet* 105(1):e97. doi: 10.1002/cphg.97.

Holder JL, Hamdan FF, & Michaud JL. (2019) *SYNGAP1*-Related Intellectual Disability. In: GeneReviews® [Internet]. MP Adam, GM Mirzaa, RA Pagon, et al. (eds), Seattle, WA: University of Washington. https://www.ncbi.nlm.nih.gov/books/NBK537721/ Accessed May 28, 2024.

Horak P, Griffith M, Danos AM, et al. (2022) Standards for the classification of pathogenicity of somatic variants in cancer (oncogenicity): Joint recommendations of Clinical Genome Resource (ClinGen), Cancer Genomics Consortium (CGC), and Variant Interpretation for Cancer Consortium (VICC). *Genet Med* 24(5):986–998. doi: 10.1016/j.gim.2022.01.001.

Hosseini SM, Kim R, Udupa S, et al. (2018) Reappraisal of reported genes for sudden arrhythmic death: evidence-based evaluation of gene validity for Brugada Syndrome. *Circulation* 138(12):1195–1205. doi: 10.1161/CIRCULATIONAHA.118.035070.

Lalonde E, Rentas S, Lin F, et al. (2020) Genomic diagnosis for pediatric disorders: revolution and evolution. *Front Pediatr* 8:373. doi: 10.3389/fped.2020.00373.

Landrum MJ, Lee JM, Benson M, et al. (2016) ClinVar: public archive of interpretations of clinically relevant variants. *Nucleic Acids Res* 44(D1):D862–868. doi: 10.1093/nar/gkv1222.

Leslie N & Bailey L. (2007, Updated 2017) Pompe Disease. In: GeneReviews® [Internet]. MP Adam, GM Mirzaa, RA Pagon, et al. (eds), Seattle, WA: University of Washington. https://www.ncbi.nlm.nih.gov/books/NBK1261/ Accessed May 28, 2024.

Li MM, Datto M, Duncavage EJ, et al. (2017) Standards and guidelines for the interpretation and reporting of sequence variants in cancer: a joint consensus recommendation of the Association for Molecular Pathology, American Society of Clinical Oncology, and College of American Pathologists. *J Mol Diagn* 19(1):4–23. doi: 10.1016.j.jmoldx.2016.10.002.

Lin AE, Brunetti-Pierri N, Lindsay ME, et al. (2017, Updated 2022) Myhre Syndrome. In: GeneReviews® [Internet]. MP Adam, GM Mirzaa, RA Pagon, et al. (eds), Seattle, WA: University of Washington. https://www.ncbi.nlm.nih.gov/books/NBK425723/ Accessed May 28, 2024.

Manickam K, McClain MR, Demmer LA, et al. (2021) Exome and genome sequencing for pediatric patients with congenital anomalies or intellectual disability: an evidence-based clinical guideline of the American College of Medical Genetics and Genomics (ACMG). *Genet Med* 23(11):2029–2037. doi: 10.1038/s41436-021-01242-6.

Martin CL, Wain KE, Oetjens MT, et al. (2020) Identification of neuropsychiatric copy number variants in a health care system population. *JAMA Psychiatry* 77(12):1276–1285. doi: 10.1001/jamapsychiatry.2020.2159.

McDonald J & Stevenson DA. (2000, Updated 2021) Hereditary hemorrhagic telangiectasia. In: GeneReviews® [Internet]. MP Adam, GM Mirzaa, RA Pagon et al. (eds), Seattle, WA: University of Washington. https://www.ncbi.nlm.nih.gov/books/NBK1351/. Accessed May 28, 2024.

Miller DT, Lee K, Abul-Husn NS, et al. (2023) ACMG SF v3.2 list for reporting of secondary findings in clinical exome and genome sequencing: a policy statement of the American College of Medical Genetics and Genomics (ACMG). *Genet Med* 25(8):100866. doi: 10.1016/j.gim.2023.100866.

Murphy M, Srivastava R, & Deans K. (2018) *Clinical Biochemistry: An Illustrated Colour Text.* Edinburgh: Elsevier.

National Institute of Standards and Technology. (2023). Genome in a Bottle Consortium. https://www.nist.gov/programs-projects/genome-bottle Accessed August 14, 2023.

Open Humans Foundation. (2023). The Personal Genome Project. https://www.personalgenomes.org/# Accessed August 14, 2023.

Organisation for Economic Cooperation and Development (2007). OECD Guidelines for Quality Assurance in Molecular Genetic Testing. https://www.oecd.org/health/biotech/38839788.pdf Accessed May 28, 2024

Pitini E, Baccolini V, Migliara G, et al. (2021) Time to align: a call for consensus on the assessment of genetic testing. *Front Public Health* 9:807695. doi: 10.3389/fpubh.2021.807695.

Popejoy AB, Ritter DI, Crooks K, et al. (2018) The clinical imperative for inclusivity: race, ethnicity, and ancestry (REA) in genomics. *Hum Mutat* 39(11):1713–1720. doi: 10.1002/humu.23644.

Regalado A. (2019) More than 26 million people have taken an at-home ancestry test. *MIT Technology Review* (11 February). https://www.technologyreview.com/2019/02/11/103446/more-than-26-million-people-have-taken-an-at-home-ancestry-test/ Accessed May 28, 2024.

Rehm H, Berg JS, Brooks LD, et al. (2015) ClinGen - The clinical genome resource. *N Engl J Med* 372:2235–2242. doi: 10.1056/NEJMsr1406261.

Rehm H, Alaimo JT, Aradhya S, et al. (2023) The landscape of reported VUS in multi-gene panel and genomic testing: time for a change. *Genet Med* 100947. doi: 10.1016/j.gim.2023.100947.

Reuter C, Grove ME, Orland K, et al. (2018) Clinical cardiovascular genetic counselors take a leading role in team-based variant classification. *J Genet Couns* 27(4):751–760. doi: 10.1007/s10897-017-0175-7.

Richards S, Aziz N, Bale S, et al. (2015) Standards and guidelines for the interpretation of sequence variants: a joint consensus recommendation of the American College of Medical Genetics and Genomics and the Association for Molecular Pathology. *Genet Med* 17(5):405–24. doi: 10.1038/gim.2015.30.

Riggs ER, Andersen EF, Cherry AM, et al. (2020) Technical standards for the interpretation and reporting of constitutional copy-number variants: a joint consensus recommendation of the American College of Medical Genetics and Genomics (ACMG) and the Clinical Genome Resource (ClinGen). *Genet Med* 22(2):245–257. doi: 10.0138/s41436-019-0686-8.

Roden DM, McLeod HL, Relling MV, et al. (2019) Pharmacogenomics. *Lancet.* 394(10197):521–532. doi: 10.1016/S0140-6736(19)31276-0.

Sagaser KG, Malinowski J, Westerfield L, et al. (2023) Expanded carrier screening for reproductive risk assessment: An evidence-based practice guideline from the National Society of Genetic Counselors. *J Genet Couns* 32(3):540–557. doi: 10.1002/jgc4.1676.

Samura O. (2020) Update on noninvasive prenatal testing: a review based on current worldwide research. *J Obstet Gynaecol Res* 46(8):1246–1254. doi: 10.1111/jog.14268.

Stenson PD, Mort M, Ball EV, et al. (2020) The Human Gene Mutation Database (HGMD®): optimizing its use in a clinical diagnostic or research setting. *Hum Genet* 139(10):1197–1207. doi: 10.1007/s00439-020-02199-3.

Strande NT, Riggs ER, Buchanan AH, et al. (2017) Evaluating the clinical validity of gene-disease associations: an evidence-based framework developed by the Clinical Genome Resource. *Am J Hum Genet* 100(6):895–906. doi: 10.1016/j.ajhg.2017.04.015.

Toro C, Shirvan L, & Tifft C. (1999, Updated 2020) HEXA Disorders. In: GeneReviews® [Internet]. MP Adam, GM Mirzaa, RA Pagon, et al. (eds), Seattle, WA: University of Washington. https://www.ncbi.nlm.nih.gov/books/NBK1218/ Accessed May 28, 2024.

Trevethan R. (2017) Sensitivity, specificity, and predictive values: foundations, pliabilities, and pitfalls in research and practice. *Front Public Health* 5:307. doi: 10.3389/fpubh.2017.00307.

Tsai GJ, Ranola JMO, Smith C, et al. (2019) Outcomes of 92 patient-driven family studies for reclassification of variants of uncertain significance. *Genet Med* 21(6):1435–1442. doi: 10.1038/s41436-018-0335-7.

Umemneku Chikere CM, Wilson K, Graziadio S, et al. (2019). Diagnostic test evaluation methodology: a systematic review of methods employed to evaluate diagnostic tests in the absence of gold standard - An update. *PLoS One* 14(10):e0223832. doi: 10.1371/journal.pone.0223832.

van Bon BWM, Mefford HC, de Vries BBA, et al. (2010, Updated 2022) 15q13.3 Recurrent Deletion. In: GeneReviews® [Internet]. MP Adam, GM Mirzaa, RA Pagon et al. (eds).

Seattle, WA: University of Washington. https://www.ncbi.nlm.nih.gov/books/NBK50780/ Accessed May 28, 2024.

Verifying Accurate Leading-edge IVCT (*in vitro* clinical test) Development (VALID) Act of 2023. H.R.2369.

Wain K. (2018) A commentary on opportunities for the genetic counseling profession through genomic variant interpretation: reflections from an ex-lab rat. *J Genet Couns* 27(4):747–750. doi: 10.1007/s10897-018-0247-3.

Wain KE, Azzariti DR, Goldstein JL, et al. (2020) Variant interpretation is a component of clinical practice among genetic counselors in multiple specialties. *Genet Med* 22(4):785–792. doi: 10.1038/s41436-019-0705-9.

Wallace SE, Amemiya A, & Mirzaa GM. (2022) Resources for genetics professionals — Mosaicism. In: GeneReviews® [Internet]. MP Adam, GM Mirzaa, RA Pagon, et al. (eds). Seattle, WA: University of Washington. https://www.ncbi.nlm.nih.gov/books/NBK585455/ Accessed May 28, 2024.

Wang RY. (2020) A newborn screening, presymptomatically identified infant with late-onset Pompe disease: case report, parental experience, and recommendations. *Int J Neonatal Screen* 6(1):22. doi: 10.3390/ijns6010022.

Westemeyer M, Saucier J, Wallace J, et al. (2020) Clinical experience with carrier screening in a general population: support for a comprehensive pan-ethnic approach. *Genet Med.* 22(8):1320–1328. doi: 10.1038/s41436-020-0807-4.

Wise AL, Manolio TA, Mensah GA, et al. (2019) Genomic medicine for undiagnosed diseases. *Lancet.* 394(10197):533–540. doi: 10.1016/S0140-6736(19)31274-7.

Zirkelbach E, Hashmi S, Ramdaney A, et al. (2018) Managing variant interpretation discrepancies in hereditary cancer: clinical practice, concerns, and desired resources. *J Genet Couns* 27(4):761–769. doi: 10.1007/s10897-017-0184-6.

7

The Medical Genetics Evaluation

Shane C. Quinonez

The patient evaluation is an invaluable aspect of a genetics clinic visit. With increasing access to genetic testing it is tempting to consider the possibility of only needing genotypic data with little need for phenotypic information. Confirming a genetic diagnosis, however, relies on a positive genetic test result and an overlapping phenotype. Furthermore, the medical genetics evaluation is useful in both deciding on an appropriate testing strategy and providing support (or lack thereof) for a specific genetic clinical diagnosis, especially if the results of testing are uncertain.

Genetic counselors often have a primary role in the collection of the patient's history, a fundamental component of the evaluation process. This information along with the physical examination is utilized to establish a differential diagnosis and to make an initial recommendation for genetic testing and/or other diagnostic testing, such as radiographic studies and biochemical testing. Follow-up counseling sessions to review results, diagnoses, and medical management recommendations also utilize information gathered in the initial history, such as the family and social history, for tailoring the delivered information and counseling to the individual patient's family.

A Guide to Genetic Counseling, Third Edition. Edited by Vivian Y. Pan, Jane L. Schuette, Karen E. Wain, and Beverly M. Yashar.
© 2025 John Wiley & Sons Ltd. Published 2025 by John Wiley & Sons Ltd.

Historically, medical genetics was almost exclusively practiced at large academic health care institutions with most clinics staffed by genetic counselors and board-certified medical geneticists. However, increased demand for clinical genetic testing and increased throughput enabled by next-generation sequencing (NGS) technologies, have contributed to a changed clinical landscape. Patients are likely to encounter genetic testing in specialty-specific clinics, such as cardiovascular and cancer genetics clinics, which are typically staffed by genetic counselors, cardiologists, and oncologists, respectively, and not by board-certified medical geneticists. Thus, the clinical evaluation in these clinics is typically not as comprehensive as that performed in a medical genetics clinic and is more targeted to the specific specialty and/or organ-system.

In addition to the varied types of clinics performing genetic evaluations, the availability of NGS in the form of panel-based testing, exome sequencing (ES), and genome sequencing (GS) has allowed a single test to be used for multiple genetic conditions. As a result, it has become easier for providers to order comprehensive genetic testing for patients, and in certain situations this has diminished the need for extensive differential diagnoses and tiered testing strategies. These comprehensive genetic tests are standard of care, first-tier tests that are increasingly ordered by nongenetic providers, including pediatric neurologists, developmental pediatricians, and oncologists and, in many instances, have resulted in medical genetics clinic referrals of patients with test results in hand (Lionel et al., 2018).

This chapter describes the components of a medical genetics evaluation including the history of the present illness, medical history, social history, and general physical and dysmorphology examinations. While the availability and efficacy of NGS has the potential to alter when a medical genetics evaluation might occur, it is essential for genetic counselors to understand its process to be able to provide comprehensive and/or effective interdisciplinary care. The elements are performed to ensure the medical genetics team has all of the necessary information to generate a differential diagnosis, select appropriate genetic test(s) if indicated, deliver accurate recurrence risk counseling, make disease medical management recommendations and provide patient-specific pre- and post-test genetic counseling.

COMPONENTS OF THE MEDICAL GENETICS EVALUATION

The primary components of the genetics evaluation are the medical history and physical examination. The totality of the information collected is synthesized in a way that weights the presence of unique and/or rare findings, allowing for the generation of a differential diagnosis, a list of genetic and nongenetic conditions that could be the cause for a patient's history, signs (observable patient findings such as a skin rash or broken bone), and symptoms (subjective experiences of the patient which are reported to the provider such as a headache or muscle cramps).

The differential diagnosis is used to determine a plan for recommended testing and/or additional evaluations with the ultimate goal of establishing a specific and accurate diagnosis. Patients may receive a clinical diagnosis, a molecular diagnosis, or both. A clinical diagnosis is made based on a patient's signs, symptoms, past medical history, and physical examination findings. A molecular diagnosis is made based on a genetic test result which has identified a disease-causing, or pathogenic, variant in a patient. Some diagnoses have established clinical diagnostic criteria which make a clinical diagnosis definitive, while other diagnoses require genetic testing for confirmation. Some diagnoses will be "syndromic" and relate to a likely or suspected syndrome, a constellation of major and minor anomalies seen together frequently enough to be reproducibly identifiable. Trisomy 21, Smith Lemli Opitz syndrome (SLOS), and DiGeorge syndrome (22q11.2 deletion syndrome) are examples of common genetic syndromes. While all three syndromes include some degree of intellectual disability, each has specific findings that distinguish them from other syndromes. Patients with trisomy 21 have a recognizable pattern of dysmorphic features, such as downslanting palpebral fissures, epicanthal folds, and single palmar creases; while SLOS is typically associated with microcephaly and 2,3 toe syndactyly (Devlin and Morrison, 2004; Nowaczyk and Wassif, 2020). DiGeorge syndrome may include unique findings such as thymic aplasia and characteristic congenital heart malformations (McDonald-McGinn et al., 2020).

Collecting a Patient's Medical History

The elements of a medical history and order of when they are typically obtained are listed in Table 7-1. The primary reason a patient is undergoing a genetic evaluation and their past medical history are almost always identified first as this information sets the stage for the entire visit. This can be collected from multiple sources, including clinical notes from the referring provider, medical records, and the patient and family interview. Since the medical evaluation in a specialty-specific genetics setting is often targeted, collecting the medical history may also require distinguishing what information is useful versus less important. There may be specialty-specific modifications to the medical evaluation which contribute to more streamlined clinic visits and these may impact which components of the medical history are gathered, as discussed below.

History of the Present Illness

The history of the present illness (HPI), or chief complaint, represents the aspects of the medical history primarily driving the medical genetics evaluation. In almost every case, the patient is being seen to address a specific question or questions, and this is often related to determining whether there is a genetic cause for a personal or family history of a medical problem or problems. For example, the visit for a patient referred to an adult medical genetics clinic for evaluation of a dilated aorta would focus on identifying the potential genetic cause for this finding. The question being asked has usually been raised by a member of a patient's health care team, such as the primary care physician (PCP) or a subspecialist such as a cardiologist or neurologist; although at times, the question has been raised by the patient or patient's family. A patient may ask their PCP if they are at an

TABLE 7-1. Basic components of a medical history

Identify the chief complaint or reason for visit	
Determine main questions/concerns of patient, family, and health care providers when possible Record the patient's own words when possible	Important questions include: • What is your primary reason for this visit? • What do you hope to learn from this visit?

Ascertain the history of present illness (HPI)	
Describe patient's problems related to visit	Identify nature of problem(s) • onset • duration of symptoms • changes in symptoms • previous medical or surgical management

Obtain past medical history	
Some elements may be included in the HPI depending on the age of patient and reason for visit. Some elements (i.e., prenatal and neonatal history) may be excluded in adult patients who do not have a history of congenital anomalies or intellectual disability.	

Elements in a prenatal history	• Age of parents
	• Prenatal exposures and timing
	  • maternal illness
	  • medication use
	  • alcohol, tobacco, recreational drugs
	  • environmental exposures
	  • major trauma

Elements in a neonatal history	• Birth history
	  • delivery type, complications
	  • gestational age, size
	• Initial newborn exam
	  • Apgar scores
	  • length, weight, head circumference
	• Nursery course
	  • ICU stay, treatments

Elements in an infancy/early childhood history	• Development
	  • social, motor, adaptive milestones
	• hearing/speech assessments
	• vision assessment
	• childhood illnesses
	  • type and age of onset

Chronic or major medical problems Surgeries Major trauma Hospitalizations	list and indicate age of onset indication, surgery type, date resulting complications reason, date

TABLE 7-1. (*Continued*)

Current medications	• type, dose • nontraditional treatments/alternative supplements
Medication allergies	type, reaction
Describe the social history	
Habits Diet, exercise	alcohol, tobacco, drug use
Education	• level achieved • academic strengths/weaknesses • special programming/classes
Living situation	• people in home including caretakers and dependents • socioeconomic status
Employment Religious beliefs Support system(s)	occupation, unemployment, disability

Adapted from Petty (2009).

increased risk for breast cancer because their mother and maternal grandmother both had the condition. To answer this question, the PCP may refer the patient to a cancer genetics clinic for evaluation.

It is not only important to assess the HPI provided by the referring physician as described above, but also from the patient's perspective. It is useful to begin with asking about the patient's understanding of the reasons for the genetic evaluation. Often this will provide some insight regarding the patient's understanding, hopes, feelings, and expectations for the visit. When asking this question, it is worthwhile mentioning that you have reviewed their records and have an understanding of the reason for referral but hope to get their perspective as well. Otherwise the patient may feel as if the provider is not prepared for their clinic visit. Knowing that a provider has reviewed their medical history will often put patients at ease and may build rapport early in the visit.

It is not uncommon for a patient or the patient's parents to be uncertain about the reasons for referral or to have an alternative purpose in mind other than the provider's reason for referral. If there is uncertainty or a misunderstanding on the part of the patient, it is usually necessary to have a discussion to resolve any confusion. If not resolved at the beginning of the visit, this may result in difficulties with all subsequent aspects of the evaluation, especially the genetic testing and counseling. If the patient is clear about the purpose of the genetic evaluation, collecting the HPI may be as simple as combining the data provided by the referring clinician with the information presented by the patient. While there is never a "perfect" amount of information to gather, its relevance to the diagnostic process and to medical decision-making should be balanced with the time allotted for the visit. This process may require guiding patients by direct questioning in order to collect data as efficiently as possible.

Pre-clinic preparation may enable the creation of a differential diagnosis for the HPI-related medical condition. With a differential diagnosis in mind, counselors can ask targeted questions regarding the conditions on the differential. In the example of a patient referred to an adult medical genetics clinic for evaluation of a dilated aortic root, the associated differential diagnosis is relatively broad and includes a number of connective tissue disorders, including Marfan syndrome (Legius et al., 2021). Knowing this, the counselor can specifically ask questions regarding the presence or absence of various symptoms and signs of Marfan syndrome and/or other connective tissue disorders. In this situation the following questions could be asked to identify if the patient has any ophthalmologic findings consistent with Marfan syndrome:

- Have you ever had an eye exam?
- Were you seen by an optometrist or an ophthalmologist?
- Were any vision abnormalities identified?
- Do you wear glasses?
- If you wear glasses, what do you specifically wear them for?
- Have you ever been diagnosed with an eye condition called *ectopia lentis*, which is a displacement of the lens of the eye from the center of the pupil?

It is often useful when collecting a patient's HPI to gather as much "specific" information as possible regarding a medical problem. "Specific (distinct, exact or precise)" is used intentionally to contrast with "nonspecific (general, wide-ranging, undetailed)." In the Marfan syndrome example, questions about "vision problems" or "the wearing of glasses" are very broad and have the potential to yield few useful details if not followed up with more probing inquiry. Although patients may not have the needed information, it is best practice to attempt to gather as much specific information as possible regarding a patient's medical problems, especially those relevant to the reason for referral.

While in many situations patients will have never seen a medical genetics professional in the past, there are increasing numbers of patients who have previously undergone some form of genetic testing. Prior testing may have been ordered by a PCP, another provider type, or even at the time of a previous evaluation by a medical genetics specialist. Alternatively, a patient may have results from direct-to-consumer testing that were not previously discussed with a genetics professional. Prior test results are often relevant to the evaluation and may contribute to establishing the differential diagnosis. If the patient in the above example had prior negative genetic testing for Marfan syndrome, this condition would be less concerning as a cause for the aortic abnormality. In all situations, it is ideal to have reviewed test results prior to the clinic visit, although invariably they may only be shared by the patient during the visit or when specifically asked about prior testing.

Past Medical History

After collecting the HPI, it is important to document additional medical problems affecting the patient; this is referred to as the past medical history (PMH). The PMH is not only important for understanding other medical problems affecting a patient, but may also reveal additional symptoms, signs, and conditions that may contribute to the differential diagnosis and the reason for referral. Components of the PMH vary depending on whether the patient is an adult, child, or adolescent and on the type of evaluation being performed; for example, comprehensive, targeted, reproductive/prenatal. These components of the PMH, some of which are discussed below, may include a reproductive, pregnancy and birth, developmental, medication and allergy, and surgical history.

Pregnancy/birth history There are many aspects of a patient's birth and prenatal history that can contribute to future medical problems. This includes teratogen exposures such as alcohol, illicit drugs, and certain medications. A maternal health history such as uncontrolled diabetes or phenylketonuria are known causes of congenital anomalies; this type of information is likely to significantly influence a clinician's concern for a genetic disorder in a child. The presence or absence of prenatal care, a history of pregnancy complications, and whether prenatal genetic testing has been performed are also relevant. While not diagnostic, if there is a noninvasive prenatal test result that is associated with a low or high risk for chromosomal disorders it is important to document this finding.

Developmental history Development is fundamental to the history gathered for a pediatric patient, and sometimes it also is vital to the assessment of an adult who may have been referred for intellectual disability or another neurodevelopmental disorder. It is helpful to ask about specific developmental milestones based on a patient's given age and to identify developmental services that are being provided as a result of noted developmental concerns. Focusing on developmental milestones (including both gains and losses) is most useful for children younger than 6 years of age, although obtaining early milestones in older children, albeit in less detail, is also helpful. In addition, asking about school progress and performance, whether extra support in school is being provided, such as physical, occupational, and/or speech therapy, and/or whether an individualized education program (IEP) is in place, will usually provide insight into overall developmental level and progress. Results of formalized school testing and/or other neurodevelopmental evaluations are valuable sources of information, if available. A general sense of development and cognitive ability can also be obtained by genetic counselors based on a patient's responses to questions in both pediatric and adult patients. This may be useful when planning how to discuss genetic testing and/or when providing genetic counseling to a patient and their family. There are numerous easily accessible resources available that describe age-specific developmental milestones (CDC Developmental Milestones, n.d.; Zubler et al., 2022).

Medication/Allergy/Surgical history   The final aspects of the PMH include documenting medications, medication allergies, and surgical history, depending on the clinical setting. The surgical history can be useful information as occasionally a previous surgery will reveal a history of a congenital anomaly forgotten by the patient or family. For example, the surgical correction of a heart malformation may reveal a PMH of a congenital heart malformation. If the malformation was corrected early, it may have been omitted as an actual medical diagnosis, especially if there was no need for ongoing cardiology follow-up.

The Social History

The social history assists with the counseling and management aspects of a patient's and family's medical care. The collection of information on housing, food security, transportation, child care, employment, education, personal safety, and finances may identify barriers to receiving medical care, potentially impacting the ability to follow through with medical management recommendations. The social history portion of the medical genetics evaluation may also provide pertinent details about the support systems in place, or lack thereof, for a patient and family. This information may suggest how well a genetic diagnosis involving complex health care needs might be managed or mismanaged. Additionally, this history may also help in understanding your patient's and family's coping mechanisms as they adjust to and begin to integrate a new diagnosis and its implications into their lives. Social determinants of health (SDOH), including the economic and social influences impacting a patient's health status and their access to care, are discussed in more detail in Chapter 10.

The Family History

The family health history is a critical component of the medical history, especially in genetics, given the relevance of symptoms and signs of a genetic diagnosis in family members to the diagnostic process and the potential implications of making a diagnosis in members of the patient's family. This component of the patient's history is covered in Chapter 3.

The Incomplete History

For a multitude of reasons, the components of a patient's history may be incomplete and/or inaccurate. With respect to adult patients, a pregnancy and or early developmental history may be impossible to obtain. Pediatric patients, depending on their age, are typically unable to provide their own history and depend on their parents or other caregivers to provide the majority of the history. While parents are often excellent sources of information, this is sometimes not the case. Examples include pediatric patients referred for developmental delay and/or intellectual disability who inherited the condition from an affected parent. In these situations, it may be difficult to obtain an accurate history from the parent secondary to their own intellectual disability. Additionally, adoptive or foster parents may be uncertain about various aspects of a child's history, such as the prenatal history and family history. In these circumstances there may be alternative sources of information, but often the evaluation must be done with incomplete information. Many clinical situations require medical genetics professionals to make decisions without all of the necessary information. Physicians may be forced to choose the best path forward in a patient's care while attempting to identify alternative sources of information that could possibly be obtained following the initial visit. Examples of this include obtaining medical records from an outside institution or collecting genetic test results from family members that may be available.

PHYSICAL EXAMINATION

The physical examination provides patient data, such as growth and observable characteristics, that may or may not support or further refine the differential diagnosis. In cases where genetic testing has been performed, the patient's physical findings may also impact the interpretation of the test results.

The physical examination is typically performed by the physician and consists of a general evaluation of the major organ systems, such as the lungs, heart, abdomen, and skin, usually in a systematic fashion (see Table 7-2). Each individual organ system could theoretically be extensively evaluated, but typically the focus is on the systems that may be affected by a genetic disorder and the identification of major abnormalities. Patients may be referred to other specialists if there is a

TABLE 7-2. **Basic components of a general physical examination**

* General health
* Vital signs
* Assessment of growth, body habitus, general proportions
* Examination by system or structure as appropriate
  * Head
  * Neck
  * Thorax
  * Cardiac
  * Pulmonary
  * Breast
  * Abdomen
  * Genitourinary
  * Pelvic
  * Rectal
  * Musculoskeletal
  * Neurological

concerning finding identified or if a need for a more specialized evaluation, such as a cardiology or neurology examination, is deemed necessary for the patient's diagnostic workup or management.

The following aspects of the examination, such as growth, development, and dysmorphology, and certain organ systems are highlighted given they are particularly relevant to a genetics evaluation and/or are more likely to be seen in various genetic conditions.

Growth

A growth assessment is a vitally important aspect of the exam. Since many genetic conditions adversely affect growth, obtaining growth parameters has important implications for the diagnostic process as well as for ensuring the patient, in particular the young patient, is at a healthy weight and height. In many clinical settings medical assistants will obtain a patient's height and weight, in addition to documenting a patient's vital signs which include temperature, blood pressure, pulse rate, and occasionally respiratory rate. The head circumference is of particular importance in the pediatric patient, but is also of value when certain adult conditions such as PTEN hamartoma tumor syndrome are within the differential. Growth parameters are plotted on age- and condition-appropriate growth charts. Any growth parameter that falls over 2 standard deviations above or below the 50th percentile for a patient's age should be considered abnormal. Many electronic medical record systems will automatically display a patient's growth percentiles and it may be possible to view a patient's growth trajectory over time, if they have had multiple evaluations in the same or a connected health care system.

Standard growth charts are based on a reference population and are available from various groups including the Center of Disease Control (based on a nationally representative sample) and the World Health Organization (which uses an internationally based sample, representing Brazil, Ghana, India, Norway, Oman and the US) (CDC, 2022; WHO, 2022). In the event a patient is being seen for a previously diagnosed condition, there may be condition-specific growth curves available and/or a chart based on the appropriate reference population. The use of condition-specific growth curves is important for both medical decision-making and genetic counseling. For example, patients with Russell-Silver syndrome (RSS) have short stature and failure to thrive (low weight) as cardinal features of the condition (Wollmann et al., 1995). If patients with RSS are plotted on a standard growth curve, they will appear to be greatly underweight and may even have been admitted to the hospital for an evaluation and management of their low weight. After an RSS diagnosis is made, plotting growth on an RSS-specific growth chart can provide a significant amount of reassurance to both the parents and members of the health care team as the patient may be at a healthy weight compared to other patients with RSS. In situations like this, parents will often express a significant amount of relief (and appreciation), as prior to the diagnosis they may have felt guilt or sensed blame from others for their child's growth delays.

Assessment of Dysmorphology

Dysmorphology is the study of the abnormal formation of body structures and, like many aspects of the physical examination, ranges from a general appreciation of abnormalities to a detailed examination that requires years of training to master. While this chapter will not detail the entirety of a comprehensive dysmorphology examination, it will provide an overview that will aid in the understanding of how the presence of specific findings can contribute to the evaluation of a patient in a genetics clinic.

Facial dysmorphology is considered the "hallmark" of a dysmorphology examination; however, there can be anomalies of essentially any body part. Major anomalies are malformations that significantly impact morbidity and mortality if not treated or surgically repaired. Examples of these include congenital heart malformations, cleft palate, and multicystic dysplastic kidneys. Minor anomalies are atypical morphologic features that do not significantly affect morbidity and mortality and occur in the general population. These most commonly involve the face, ears, hands, and feet and include findings such as epicanthal folds, single palmar creases, and a thin upper lip. While the presence of one or two minor anomalies can be seen in the general population, more than two in the same individual raises concern for an undiagnosed major anomaly and even the potential for an underlying disorder.

The dysmorphology examination is often performed along with portions of the general physical examination, especially the head, eyes, ears, nose, and throat (HEENT), as it is of particular importance due the presence or absence of dysmorphic features involving these structures. Dysmorphism and minor anomalies are most common in areas of complex and variable features such as the face. Patients and their family members may have questions about what is being seen, and depending on a parent's level of concern, certain findings may provoke anxiety. It is therefore often helpful to explain the purpose of the dysmorphology examination to patients and families. Statements such as:

All individuals have unique features which are identifiable and describing those features can occasionally assist with the medical genetics evaluation we are performing today. During this portion of the examination, you may hear us mention a number of findings; in most instances each finding by itself does not mean anything is wrong or abnormal. We will be sure to explain the significance of any finding if it raises concern, but you should also feel free to ask questions about what we are saying as well.

While most dysmorphic features are readily identifiable, there are findings such as palpebral fissure length and finger length which require accessing various resources to identify the significance of the finding. Resources that document age-specific norms of multiple physical examination findings are a vital tool for accurate assessment of their significance (Hall, 2007).

Perhaps the important consideration when performing a dysmorphology exam of the face, is whether the patient resembles other family members. For example, a 3-year-old girl may be undergoing an evaluation in the pediatric genetics clinic for a history of autism and seizures without a reported family history of the same conditions. If epicanthal folds are noted on examination, they may be a finding consistent with an underlying syndromic genetic diagnosis also associated with autism and seizures. However, if a parent also has epicanthal folds, it is possible that they are a familial trait and unrelated to the history of autism and seizures. Experienced dysmorphologists will compare a patient's features to those in the parents and siblings, occasionally looking at family photos if a family member is not present. Additionally, certain features may be more common in specific ancestral groups, making it important to consider whether a physical examination finding is actually atypical or not for each individual patient.

The *cardiac* examination typically includes auscultation of a patient's heart with a stethoscope to evaluate for murmurs (abnormal heart sounds) that may suggest an abnormally functioning or formed heart. Often heart abnormalities will have been diagnosed prior to a patient's genetic evaluation but occasionally, as is the case with any organ system, a genetics evaluation may be the first time a medical problem is suspected.

The *abdominal* examination is a very important aspect of pediatric genetic evaluations as various inborn errors of metabolism, such as lysosomal storage disorders and glycogen storage disorders, may present with organomegaly including hepatomegaly (liver enlargement) or splenomegaly (spleen enlargement).

The *dermatologic* examination provides important diagnostic information in both specialty-specific and comprehensive medical genetics clinics. Certain dermatologic abnormalities require a skin biopsy and microscopic analysis to provide a specific diagnosis, but findings such as café au lait macules (CAMs), hemangiomas, abnormal skin pigmentation, hypomelanotic macules, and shagreen patches are readily identifiable. A Wood's lamp, which is an ultraviolet light source, is a great aid when conducting a skin examination, specifically allowing for better detection of pigmented and hypopigmented skin lesions. Providers should also be aware of racial differences between lighter and darker skinned individuals.

Café au lait macules (CAMs) are features of many disorders such as neurofibromatosis type 1 (NF1), neurofibromatosis type 2 (NF2), McCune-Albright syndrome, and constitutional mismatch repair deficiency syndrome (CMMRD). CAMs are most commonly encountered in the evaluation of NF1, as their presence is a major criterion utilized when making a clinical diagnosis (Legius et al., 2021). The presence, size, appearance, and quantity of CAMs are important to document. Patients with NF1 often have CAMs with smooth borders ("coast of California"), while CAMs in patients with McCune-Albright syndrome classically have irregular borders ("coast of Maine"). Hypopigmented macules are identified in other conditions, such as tuberous sclerosis complex, but may also be present in unaffected individuals and are identified in 0.8% of normal newborns (Alper and Holmes, 1983).

The *neurological* exam typically includes a detailed assessment of a patient's cranial nerve function, reflexes, muscle tone and strength, although its components depend on the specific clinic as well as the reason for evaluation. For example, a 30-year-old woman being seen for presymptomatic *BRCA1* testing based on a positive family history likely requires a very limited physical and neurologic examination. In contrast, a 30-year-old woman being evaluated for a possible NF1 diagnosis will require detailed physical and neurologic exams given the various neurologic manifestations associated with NF1.

Many neurologic findings are nonspecific as they are seen in many conditions. These include findings such as hypotonia, hypertonia, speech and developmental delay, and attention-deficit/hyperactivity disorder. Observations about a patient's cognitive ability can be made while performing the physical examination as well as while collecting HPI and family history. This may be relevant to the evaluation of an adult patient as mild cognitive impairment may be undiagnosed or undocumented in this patient population and may have implications for diagnostic considerations, obtaining consent for testing, and for pre-test and post-test counseling.

TOOLS UTILIZED IN A MEDICAL GENETICS EVALUATION

Various tools and tests are regularly utilized by physicians to assist with the diagnosis and management of patients with confirmed or suspected genetic conditions. These tools can identify findings not apparent on the physical exam and may support a suspected genetic diagnosis or are a part of the medical management recommendations after a diagnosis is made. Often these tests, while not genetic testing *per se*, can indicate a specific condition. These include laboratory tests which measure levels of electrolytes, hormones, or other proteins and compounds present in the blood and urine. There are also condition-specific tests such as the measurement of enzyme activities for various lysosomal storage disorders or other metabolic disorders, and mitochondrial respiratory chain enzyme analysis for mitochondrial disorders. Other examples of testing include iron studies when evaluating a patient for hemochromatosis or urine organic acids when assessing for various inborn errors of metabolism. In general, these tests are very condition-specific and referring to published resources that include recommendations for medical management may be useful.

In addition to blood and urine testing, various imaging studies such as x-rays, ultrasounds, and MRIs may be utilized. Like blood and urine testing, these studies are used in both the workup and management of genetic disorders. Especially when evaluating very young children for a genetic disorder, physicians will recommend various studies to evaluate for the presence of undiagnosed congenital anomalies. In patients being evaluated for short stature, physicians may obtain a skeletal survey, which is an x-ray of the entirety of a patient's skeletal system. These x-rays may identify a pattern of skeletal abnormalities consistent with a specific condition or skeletal dysplasia, assisting with the initial workup. Subsequent genetic testing can then be ordered based on the x-ray findings. In patients evaluated for Marfan syndrome, physicians may recommend an echocardiogram to evaluate the aortic root, as the presence or absence of dilatation can aid in the workup of these patients. Abdominal ultrasounds may be utilized to evaluate for renal malformations or to evaluate the size and appearance of a patient's liver as hepatomegaly can be seen in various conditions including lysosomal storage disorders and Beckwith-Wiedemann syndrome.

Genetics Rounds and Case Conferencing

Collaboration with other professionals, case discussion with colleagues, and conferencing with multidisciplinary teams are often essential for the diagnostic evaluation of a patient. Given the rarity of most genetic disorders, it is a certainty that each individual genetic provider will never have seen every genetic disorder. For this reason, collaboration with other genetic providers is invaluable in the workup and management of many genetic conditions. Many clinics hold weekly or monthly case conferences to discuss puzzling or complicated cases. During these conferences, geneticists and genetic counselors may present a patient's history, family history, and physical examination (occasionally showing pictures or videos, if available) to gather the opinions and recommendations of other genetic specialists regarding a diagnosis, further diagnostic workup, and/or needed management. In the event photographs or videos are shared, it is important to document a patient or family's consent for their use. Often clinics will have specific consent forms for this purpose.

There are multiple additional venues where collaborative discussion of a patient's evaluation may occur. These include tumor boards where patients with cancer are discussed by various specialists and morbidity and mortality conferences which are held by various departments and specialties. Occasionally at these multidisciplinary conferences, genetic counselors are the only genetic experts present and may be asked to discuss either a patient's diagnosis or ongoing workup, as well as the implications for a patient's management.

FUTURE CARE CONSIDERATION FOLLOWING A GENETIC DIAGNOSIS

While certain conditions may require lifelong follow-up in a medical genetics clinic, many patients with genetic diagnoses are managed by their PCP. Given this, it is important to consider how a patient's diagnosis will be incorporated into their future medical care. While certain conditions such as trisomy 21 and achondroplasia have well established management guidelines, other rarer conditions do not (Hoover-Fong et al., 2020; Bull et al., 2022). In the case of a rare genetic diagnosis, it is important to equip the patient and their family, as well as their care team, with the information needed to support condition-specific medical care. This may be in the form of a clinical summary, recommendations for medical management, genetic counseling and risk assessment, test results, and relevant resources. For example, in males diagnosed with hereditary breast and ovarian cancer, recommended management and surveillance is often coordinated by the PCP who can perform clinical breast examinations, prostate-specific antigen monitoring, and digital rectal exams. In some situations, it may be necessary for a patient or family to be seen for a return visit in the genetics clinic. This may be the case if there is a new finding or medical problem requiring assessment. For example, pediatric patients may experience unexpected changes in growth and/or development requiring re-evaluation, especially if there are questions about how the new finding relates to a previously made diagnosis.

In certain genetic conditions it may be important to add other specialists to a patient's medical team. For example, in patients with Prader-Willi syndrome (PWS), an endocrinologist is a necessary member of the care team as patients with PWS experience significant benefit from growth hormone supplementation. For patients with a high risk of seizures, it may be appropriate to consider a referral to neurology for evaluation and management of a possible future epilepsy diagnosis.

A new diagnosis can be overwhelming for a patient and family. Ensuring all members of a patient's care team are comfortable with a new diagnosis may significantly reduce anxiety and positively impact care for the patient. Medical genetics clinics should expect and encourage clear lines of communication regarding a patient's diagnosis from both patients, families and the health care professionals who care for them.

PATIENT FOLLOW-UP WHEN A DIAGNOSIS IS NOT ESTABLISHED

While the goal of the medical genetics evaluation is to provide a patient with a genetic diagnosis, it is important to acknowledge that not all patients are given a confirmed diagnosis at the completion of the workup. In fact, the lack of an established diagnosis is not uncommon in the medical genetics clinic. This is especially true after the initial evaluation, even in cases in which there is a strong clinical suspicion for the presence of a genetic disorder (Findley et al., 2023; Lunke et al., 2023). In some instances, this may be related to an incomplete understanding of the genetic contribution to disease and the inability to identify, characterize, and interpret genomic variation in an individual. Other patients may have a medical problem caused by either a nongenetic etiology (such as an *in utero* teratogen exposure) or a multifactorial condition not amenable to current genetic testing paradigms. Additional evaluations and/or results of nongenetic based tests may also be needed to make a diagnosis.

The potential for the lack of a diagnosis is an important consideration when ensuring a patient's expectations align with those of the medical genetics team. Normal genetic test results may be surprising and confusing to the patient and family. Follow-up and additional testing in the genetics clinic may be recommended, and it is important to discuss their importance. The appropriate interval for follow-up may depend on the patient's symptoms and signs, the availability of additional testing—such as exome/genome testing if not previously performed, financial resources, and patient and family preferences for additional testing, as each genetic test may be accompanied by a significant emotional investment by the patient and family.

SUMMARY

A diagnosis is fundamental to the provision of care for patients and their families with genetic disorders. Although the evaluation of a patient has evolved over the past decade with advances in genetic testing capabilities and strategies, the medical genetics evaluation remains vital to the diagnostic process for the patient and family. Genetic counselors have a critical role in this process and therefore need to develop expertise in many of the elements of the evaluation.

REFERENCES

Alper JC & Holmes LB. (1983) The incidence and significance of birthmarks in a cohort of 4,641 newborns. *Pediatr Dermatol* 1:58–68.

Bull MJ, Trotter T, Santoro SL., et al. (2022) Health supervision for children and adolescents with Down syndrome. *Pediatrics* 149(5):e2022057010. doi:10.1542/PEDS. 2022-057010.

Centers for Disease Control and Prevention (CDC) (n.d) Developmental Milestones. https://www.cdc.gov/ncbddd/actearly/milestones/index.html Accessed May 30, 2022.

Centers for Disease Control and Prevention (CDC) (2022) Growth Charts - Clinical Growth Charts. https://www.cdc.gov/growthcharts/clinical_charts.htm Accessed May 28, 2024.

Devlin L & Morrison P. (2004) Accuracy of the clinical diagnosis of Down syndrome. *Ulster Med J* 73(1):4–12.

Findley T, Parchem J, Ramdaney A, & Morton, S. (2023) Challenges in the clinical understanding of genetic testing in birth defects and pediatric diseases. *Transl Pediatr* 12(5):1028–1040. doi: 10.21037/tp-23-54. Epub 2023 May 4.

Hall JG, Allenson KW, Gripp K, & Slavotinek A. (2007) *Handbook of Physical Measurements* Oxford: Oxford University Press.

Hoover-Fong J, Scott CI, & Jones MC. (2020) Health supervision for people with achondroplasia. *Pediatrics* 145(6):e20201010. doi:10.1542/PEDS.2020-1010/76908

Legius E, Messiaen L, Wolkenstein P, et al. (2021) Revised diagnostic criteria for neurofibromatosis type 1 and Legius syndrome: an international consensus recommendation. *Genet Med* 23:1506–1513.

Lionel AC, Costain G, Monfared N, *et al.* (2018) Improved diagnostic yield compared with targeted gene sequencing panels suggests a role for whole-genome sequencing as a first-tier genetic test. *Genet Med* 20(4):435–443. doi:10.1038/GIM.2017.119.

Lunke S, Bouffler S, Patel C, et al. (2023) Integrated multi-omics for rapid rare disease diagnosis on a national scale. *Nat Med* 29(7):1681–1691. doi: 10.1038/s41591-023-02401-9.

Nowaczyk MJM & Wassif AC. (2020) Smith-Lemli-Opitz syndrome. In: Adam MP, Feldman J, Mirzaa GM, et al. (eds.) GeneReviews [Internet]. Seattle, WA: University of Washington. https://www.ncbi.nlm.nih.gov/books/NBK1143/ Accessed May 28, 2024.

McDonald-McGinn S, Hain H, Emmanuel B, & Zackai E. (2020) 22q11.2 deletion syndrome. In: Adam MP, Feldman J, Mirzaa GM, et al. (eds) GeneReviews [Internet]. Seattle, WA: University of Washington. https://www.ncbi.nlm.nih.gov/books/NBK1523/ Accessed May 28, 2024.

Petty E. (2009) The Medical Genetics Evaluation. In: Uhlmann, Schuette, Yashar (eds.) *A Guide to Genetic Counseling*, Second Edition, New York: John Wiley & Sons, Inc.

World Health Organization (WHO). (2022) Child growth standards. https://www.who.int/tools/child-growth-standards/standards Accessed June 17, 2024.

Wollmann HA, Kirchner T, Enders H, et al. (1995) Growth and symptoms in Silver-Russell syndrome: review on the basis of 386 patients. *Eur J Pediatr* 154(12):958–68. doi: 10.1007/BF01958638

Zubler JM, Wiggins LD, Macias MM, et al. (2022) Evidence-informed milestones for developmental surveillance tools. *Pediatrics* 149(3):e2021052138. doi: 10.1542/peds.2021-052138.

8

Thinking it all Through: Case Preparation and Management

Lauren E. Hipp and Wendy R. Uhlmann

INTRODUCTION

Human genetics is an evolving landscape shaped by continuing discoveries, expanding technologies, and new applications to health and medical management. The training and expertise of a genetic counselor makes it possible to utilize these advances when providing genetic counseling, while appreciating the lived experience of patients and families. So, how does one navigate the horizon of information to provide counseling on conditions that can be difficult to spell, pronounce, or that have been rarely observed? Developing skills in case preparation and management are key to the practice of genetic counseling. Case preparation allows genetic counselors to anticipate a patient's needs and to build knowledge to confidently implement a plan for the visit. Building skills in case management will allow a genetic counselor to coordinate the components of a clinic visit, while being adaptable to the changing goals and needs of the patient and their medical team.

A Guide to Genetic Counseling, Third Edition. Edited by Vivian Y. Pan, Jane L. Schuette,
Karen E. Wain, and Beverly M. Yashar.
© 2025 John Wiley & Sons Ltd. Published 2025 by John Wiley & Sons Ltd.

It is important to note that genetic counselors have varied ways of conducting case preparation and management. This chapter aims to provide a general overview, while acknowledging that not all presented components will be applicable in all scenarios. Genetic counselors may also vary their approaches to case preparation as they develop their individualized counseling style. While specific approaches to case preparation and management may differ between clinic setting or even between clinic visits, these skills provide the foundation for a genetic counselor to provide genetic counseling and evolve with the changing nature of the field.

CASE PREPARATION

Case preparation for a genetic counseling visit is a process through which the genetic counselor uses baseline referral information about the indication to identify the key questions to address, gather relevant information, and formulate a plan for the appointment. Case preparation for individual cases can take anywhere from a few minutes to several hours depending on the clinical setting, the indication, and what the genetic counselor already knows about the genetic condition(s). Given the rapid advances being made in genetics, even indications that are more commonly seen may require preparation to ensure that information is current and that unique circumstances for your patient are identified and considered in your case plan. While preparation may be extensive, the goal is to establish a framework for comprehensive and quality patient care.

Case preparation is also a key component of professional development because it offers the opportunity for a genetic counselor to expand their knowledge base by researching new medical or genetic conditions, investigating new testing technologies, and considering new approaches to treatment and patient follow-up. Case preparation also provides the opportunity to hone skills in medical records review, critical assessment of the primary medical and genetics literature, and to experiment with different ways to organize information for use in a visit. While information gathering remains a primary component, case preparation provides the opportunity to reflect on the patient's perspective and to consider an approach that addresses both medical and psychosocial needs.

Formulating a Plan for the Clinic Visit

A primary goal of case preparation is to identify the key components for your genetic counseling case and to organize the components into a plan for the visit. The case plan may be guided by a number of factors, outlined below.

- **Consider the reason for referral and establish the goal(s) for the appointment.**

   When approaching case preparation, it is useful to first identify who the patient is and why the patient is being seen. Is the patient seeking a genetics evaluation for personal medical issues where the goal is to establish, confirm, or rule out a genetic condition? For an asymptomatic patient with a family history of a known condition, your goals may be focused on providing risk assessment and facilitating decision-making surrounding genetic testing. If your patient is being seen to discuss genetic test results, goals may include education and focus on medical management strategies. Of note, a visit may include more than one "patient" (e.g., patient and partner, parent and child, pregnant person and fetus) and, therefore, multiple individuals' goals may need to be considered. Additional information on working simultaneously with multiple family members is provided later in the chapter.

Knowing and anticipating the key questions to address will guide what information you gather as you prepare for the visit. The referral indication may assist in generating differential diagnoses; that is, a list of genetic conditions that warrant evaluation or testing. When reviewing a referral, the urgency of the evaluation should also be considered as time constraints may dictate scheduling, the availability of certain testing options, and/or timing of medical decisions. Common indications for urgent referrals include life-limiting conditions, pending surgical or treatment decisions, pregnancy or delivery management, and pending *in vitro* fertilization (IVF).

- **Anticipate your patient's expectations and needs**.

Think about why the patient is seeking genetic counseling at this time and what you anticipate are the patient's expectations and needs. As you gain experience as a genetic counselor, you will start to identify common questions asked by patients, both generally and in specific clinical contexts. This information can be useful in multiple ways. When planning the educational component of your genetic counseling session, it is helpful to consider the lived experience of your patients and how that may influence the information they are seeking, the decisions they may make during the visit, and their perception of the health care team. Acknowledging your patient's journey can assist in creating a counseling space where your patient feels comfortable, safe, and open to sharing.

- **Organize your session**.

Once the goals of your session are identified, you will need to determine what information to present and how it should be presented. A genetic counseling case may include components of history taking (i.e., medical and family history review), risk assessment, education, as well as discussion of genetic testing and/or medical management options. As part of case preparation, one should consider how each of these components can be used to meet the goals of the session, how to integrate and order components so the visit flows naturally, and which components may not be necessary. For example, medical history review could be a natural first step when evaluating a patient for signs or symptoms of a genetic condition. In contrast, a patient being seen to discuss a new genetic test result or newly established diagnosis may be eager to start with the education section of the visit and medical history review may be secondary. Perhaps the patient's medical history is well documented in the medical record and a brief summary rather than full review will suffice. Genetic counselors may choose to use organizational or counseling aids—such as outlines, sticky notes with key points, pictures, or slides—to guide both the patient and themselves during the visit. Additional discussion on the use of aids and the associated benefits and limitations is provided later in this chapter.

• **Consider your role as a member of the patient's health care team.**

Depending on your team and whether you live in a state with licensure, you may see patients as an independent provider or in conjunction with physicians or other advanced practice providers (e.g., physician's assistants, nurse practitioners). Of note, in some clinic settings, a genetic counselor may be the only team member trained in the field of genetics. It is important to determine each team members' roles within their individual scopes of practice and to establish who will be responsible for specific parts of the patient's visit and in what order. Planning for a session may be done as a team during a pre-clinic case conference or through email, phone, or video call; however, it may also occur simultaneously during the clinic visit, in a physical or virtual staff room. Genetic counselors working in teaching hospitals may also need to account for the role of trainees or other learners assigned to see a patient. Such preparation makes for smoother transitions in a session, less duplication of information for the patient, and ultimately a better patient experience and higher quality of care.

Review of medical and family records

Medical record review in preparation for a patient's visit provides the opportunity to learn more about a patient's journey, specifically the signs and symptoms that are of concern, the diagnostic evaluations completed to date, and the current medical management plan. A patient's medical record can also provide insight into psychosocial circumstances, including information on a patient's social support system, barriers that may impact their care, and personal wishes regarding their care. Such information can be useful in identifying needs or questions that may arise; however, critical thinking should be used given the possibility of documentation error and the potential for record entries to be reflective of provider implicit bias. Medical records to request and information to obtain for case preparation are presented in Table 8-1, organized by referral indication.

Medical records can be extensive to review. Many institutions will have electronic medical records that make it possible to easily access a large volume of documents from multiple health care institutions where a patient has received care. Relevant scanned documents (e.g., test reports, pedigrees) may be stored in

TABLE 8-1. Helpful medical records and other case preparation needs by referral indication

Diagnostic evaluation of a patient for a specified genetic condition

- Medical records on any prior genetic test results and genetics evaluations
- Medical records documenting symptoms relevant to the referral indication
- Medical records documenting diagnostic evaluations and tests completed (genetic and nongenetic) to date
- Family history information
- Information on the condition: diagnostic criteria, typical age of onset, and inheritance
- Testing options: test type, laboratory options, test sensitivity
- Need for other diagnostic studies: radiology or other imaging studies

Asymptomatic patient with family history of a specified genetic condition/ Asymptomatic patient requesting predictive genetic testing

- Medical records on any prior genetic testing completed in relative(s) (results from an affected relative are most informative; if unavailable, medical records documenting the genetic diagnosis in an affected relative)
- Family history information
- Information on the condition: diagnostic criteria, typical age of onset, inheritance, and relevant impacts to medical management if results return positive
- Testing options: test type, laboratory options, test sensitivity
- Assessment of the patient's personal risk to inherit the condition and/or to be a carrier
- Patient educational resources regarding the genetic condition
- Information about the Genetic Information Nondiscrimination Act (GINA), or country-specific protective legislation (for predictive testing cases)

Symptomatic patient with confirmed genetic diagnosis/ Symptomatic patient with positive genetic test results

- Medical records summarizing patient signs and symptoms relevant to the indication
- Medical records documenting genetic test results
- Family history information
- Information on the condition: diagnostic criteria, typical age of onset, and inheritance
- Assessment of risk to family members and discussion on communication with at-risk relatives (e.g., provision of family notification letter)
- Guidelines for surveillance, treatment, or other medical management/intervention
- Patient educational resources regarding the genetic condition
- Support group information

Symptomatic patient with unconfirmed genetic diagnosis/Symptomatic patient with negative genetic test results or variant of uncertain significance (VUS)

- Medical records summarizing patient signs and symptoms relevant to the indication
- Medical records documenting genetic test results
- Family history information
- Considerations for differential diagnosis
- Additional testing options: test type, laboratory options, test sensitivity
- For VUS results, information on the specific variant: consider laboratory report, clinical gene variant databases, primary literature review, contact with lab
- For VUS results, consider options for additional evidence: family segregation studies, RNA studies, enzyme testing (if relevant), diagnostic imaging studies (if relevant)

(continued)

TABLE 8-1. *(Continued)*

Patient presenting for preconception counseling (no specific genetic indioation)

- Medical records documenting pregnancy history, if relevant
- Family history information
- Assessment of age-related risk for chromosome abnormalities
- Baseline risk for congenital anomalies
- Testing options: carrier screening and information on test sensitivity/residual risks
- Information on available prenatal diagnostic testing options and assisted reproductive technologies (if indicated)
- Information about the Genetic Information Nondiscrimination Act (GINA), or country-specific protective legislation

Pregnant patient presenting to discuss fetal risk and prenatal testing options

- Medical (specifically obstetric) records
- Family history information
- Fetal ultrasound reports
- Genetic testing, carrier screening, or prenatal screening results, if previously completed
- If not previously completed, test options: test type, laboratory options, test sensitivity (not all laboratories accept prenatal samples)
- If personal/family history of known genetic condition, see relevant sections above

a separate "media" tab. Historical records may be stored off-site or in physical shadow charts and may require advance planning to obtain. When sorting records, it is helpful to first review the referral for genetic evaluation/genetic counseling and accompanying records to ascertain the key medical concerns and any questions posed by the referring health care team. Relevant specialist notes may be a good next step to learn more about a patient's clinical course and current management plan. The first visit note for each relevant specialist is likely to contain the most complete patient summary, while the most recent note from that specialist will likely provide the patient's current health status and ongoing care/follow-up plan.

Identifying the diagnostic tests and evaluations already done can reduce the likelihood of unnecessary or duplicate studies. Given the pace of advances in genetic testing, reports from testing previously completed will be useful in determining whether new or additional genetic testing should be considered, or whether reclassification of previously identified variants has new relevance to the patient's workup. Critical review and filtering of available records during case preparation can help determine whether additional medical records are needed prior to the appointment and can help you draft the list of questions to ask during the history review with your patient.

For patients being seen for a family history of a genetic condition, records from an affected relative (and potentially multiple relatives) are optimal to verify the genetic condition(s) in the family and to determine if the causative familial gene variant(s) is known. However, testing for the affected relative may not have been done or, if done, may not be available to the patient. Often these records are challenging to obtain, either because the patient is reluctant to make the request or relatives may not wish to share them. Additionally, patients may not complete family history forms in advance or may have limited or no knowledge about their family history. Considering these limitations, possible gaps in information, and potential alternatives to obtaining information are important steps in case preparation for your visit.

Identifying pertinent information during case preparation

Once the referral indication has been defined, information is then gathered to support the plan for the session. Key resources to use for case preparation are provided in Appendix A. While researching information, the goals are two-fold: to expand one's knowledge base and expertise on the clinical indication; and to identify information to communicate during the visit. Sample questions to guide information gathering and overall case preparation are provided in Table 8-2. Reviewing information on the signs, symptoms, and natural history of a condition will guide the questions to ask during history taking and will inform the education provided during the visit. Learning the inheritance pattern(s) for the genetic condition(s) will prepare you to provide genetic counseling regarding recurrence risk in relatives and/or whether testing in other relatives is indicated based on available family history. Investigating genetic conditions with similar or overlapping clinical features will assist in considering a differential diagnosis for the patient, which may also impact history taking and education. Knowing the genetic testing options available and the billing practices of commonly used genetic testing laboratories will be informative when determining genetic testing options, coordinating the logistics of testing, or when questions regarding out-of-pocket expenses arise. Lastly, investigating general screening options, therapies, treatments, or available research options for a condition will allow you to confidently participate in discussions surrounding the medical management plan with the medical team.

While the examples outlined above represent common questions addressed during a genetic counseling visit, a genetic counselor should also be prepared to handle new information or "surprises" that arise during the session. New signs and symptoms may be uncovered during the clinic visit that may change the original diagnosis being considered, or a patient may present to clinic with results of genetic testing that you were unaware were previously completed. Additional conditions may be noted in the family history that pose a genetic risk. For example, a patient seen for Neurofibromatosis type 1 may also have a family history of cancer that can either be addressed at the visit, deferred to a return visit, or referred to a cancer genetics clinic for dedicated counseling.

When gathering information during case preparation, a genetic counselor may also seek out printed or online resources to supplement their session and provide post-visit educational and/or psychosocial support to patients and families. A list of some established organizations that provide patient-directed resources is available

TABLE 8-2. Key questions to guide case preparation (not all questions will be relevant for each patient seen).

What is the referral indication? Why is the patient seeking genetics evaluation/counseling?

Is the patient being seen for diagnostic evaluation to rule in or out a genetic condition?
Is the patient being seen for genetic counseling for a previously established diagnosis or positive family history?

What information do you need to address the question posed in the referral?

What medical records will you need to review on the patient?
Are medical records from relative(s) needed?
Are there published diagnostic or testing criteria that are applicable to the evaluation?
What information do you need to obtain from genetics resources and primary literature to provide relevant information and to address anticipated questions?
What questions will you need to ask while taking the family and medical history?

What information can be conveyed about the suspected or confirmed genetic condition?

What are the known features of the condition? What is unknown?
What is the age of onset, natural history, and prognosis of the condition?
What is the penetrance of the condition? The expressivity?
Is the specific gene or variant identified in the family associated with specific features (i.e., genotype–phenotype correlations)?
Are there screening options, treatments options, or other interventions for the condition?
Additionally for chromosome rearrangements, what chromosome(s) are involved and what is the etiology/how does it occur?

What is your assessment of the patient's risk?

What is the incidence of the condition? The carrier frequency?
What is the inheritance pattern(s) for the suspected or confirmed genetic condition?
Does the inheritance pattern fit with what you are seeing in the family history?
Has *de novo* inheritance been reported for the condition? If so, at what frequency?
Are there unique aspects to the inheritance of the condition (e.g., anticipation, germline mosaicism, reduced penetrance)?
For multifactorial conditions, are there empiric risk figures that are relevant to provide?
What are the risks for infertility, pregnancy loss, or to have a liveborn child with the condition?
Is there another relative who is a better candidate for initial evaluation?

Will genetic testing or other diagnostic evaluations be indicated?

What type of testing should be offered (e.g., karyotype, chromosomal microarray analysis, gene panel, genomic sequencing, etc.)?
What are the benefits, risks, and limitations of available testing options?
What is the sensitivity of the proposed testing options? Will additional testing be needed if negative?
What laboratory will perform the test?
What are the patient's reproductive options, if relevant (e.g., prenatal diagnostic testing, assisted reproductive technologies, adoption)?
Will testing be covered by insurance or what are the out-of-pocket costs?

How do you plan to present information to your patient?

In what order will information be presented?
Does your patient have any specific needs that you should consider (e.g., vision or hearing impairment, color blindness)?
Would visual aids or other educational tools be helpful?
Are there written resources or educational videos that would be helpful for the patient?

How do you think the patient will respond to the information?

Can you anticipate your patient's questions and concerns?
Can you anticipate what decisions will need to be made?
What psychosocial concerns can you anticipate?
Are there support groups available for the suspected or confirmed genetic condition?
Could there be implications for insurance eligibility, military status, employment, etc.?

---

in the resource toolkit in Appendix A. Resources should be reviewed to confirm that the information provided is updated and accurate, written at a level appropriate for your patient's interests and needs, and that resources are free from bias, coercion, or commercial/financial interest. Resources may be selected to provide general background on a medical or genetic condition for the patient to reference later or to share with their family members. Identifying local, national, or even international registries and support groups may provide the opportunity for patients to connect with others living with the genetic condition, and to be kept abreast of new discoveries and research opportunities. Support groups can be a powerful outlet (virtually or in-person) for individuals living with rare conditions by providing a venue for psychosocial support, mentorship, and an opportunity to share their experience and learn from others who have navigated similar challenges and successes. It should be noted, however, that not all patients will be interested or accepting of such connections, or patients may seek alternative avenues for education and support at different times in their medical journey. While key resources can be identified during the case preparation process in anticipation of the patients' needs, the presentation of such materials may be guided by the desires and needs of the patient that unfold during the visit.

Conducting a literature search

With online access to the medical and scientific literature, genetic databases, and clinical resources, information needed for case preparation is often just a few keystrokes away. There may be practice guidelines for genetics evaluation and testing for specific clinical indications which you can ascertain through national genetics and specialists' professional organizations' websites and in the literature. Conducting literature searches of both the medical and scientific literature will assist in identifying relevant, accurate, and timely information to address the questions in Table 8-2. There are several factors that need to be considered during a literature review, including whether the journal is reputable, quality of the research/paper, type of study done, and limitations. If available, working with an informatician or library curator may provide insight into search tips and tools, appropriate key words for searches, and access to large databases to streamline your searches and to critically evaluate identified content.

Literature searches for some genetic conditions may yield numerous case reports and medical studies that require extensive time for review, critical analysis, and integration into the case plan. Literature review for rare genetic conditions can be equally challenging when searches are met with a paucity of data. In cases of rare genetic conditions or when the information the patient is requesting is not known, it can be helpful to inform the patient about the extent of your literature review and team discussions. This acknowledges the patient's inquiry, and assures the patient that you are prepared and have done the relevant investigations, but the information is simply not known.

Use of counseling aids and other organizational techniques

Genetic counselors may employ a variety of techniques for organizing information for use in a counseling session. Case outlines may be used to highlight pertinent information for quick reference and may ensure that relevant information is readily accessible. By organizing information in outline form, the order of session components can be previewed to check that the session flows in a comprehensible manner. Case outlines, however, should not be seen as a rigid framework for the genetic counseling session and flexibility should be maintained as patient questions and concerns unfold. While an outline can serve as a useful case preparation tool and a potential guide in sessions (especially for new learners), care should be taken to avoid dependence on the document during counseling. Familiarity with the content of the outline will allow the genetic counselor to maintain engagement and eye contact with the patient and be attuned to nonverbal cues that may otherwise be missed if frequently accessing the outlined text.

Counseling aids, created in advance or drawn out during the visit, can also help organize a session and promote patient understanding and engagement by presenting complex information in a visual manner. Similar to case outlines, counseling aids allow the genetic counselor to plan the content of their session, but also provide flexibility. Counseling aids can be drawn on, the presentation order can be changed in real time, and aids can be re-presented to address questions or misconceptions that may arise later in the session. Counseling aids can be shared with patients and, for the counselor, used in clinic visit documentation.

Images, if used for counseling aids, should be carefully selected and consideration given to diversity, inclusion, and patient representation. One should also consider whether such images are appropriate for a patient's particular presentation and risk and should be modified accordingly. Of note, visual aids will have limited utility if a patient has low vision but may still help the genetic counselor in determining the key content to convey when providing genetic counseling. When genetic counseling is provided by phone, consider sending counseling aids to the patient either pre- or post-visit.

Additional techniques for session organization include use of templates to organize information from patient chart reviews and use of sticky notes with key questions or bullet points. The techniques employed may vary depending on a genetic counselor's personal style, the counselor's familiarity with the given indication, the specific needs of the patient, or the goals of the session. Ultimately, the chosen organizational style should allow the genetic counselor to readily access the information they plan to present, feel confident in their knowledge base, and remain flexible as they tailor the information to the patient's specific needs and questions.

PERFORMING A RISK ASSESSMENT

Patients often seek information about the risk of a genetic condition for themselves, their children/future children, and other relatives. The steps and variables to consider in conducting a risk assessment are presented in Figure 8-1,

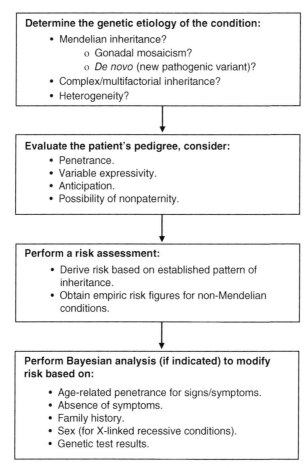

FIGURE 8-1. *Steps to consider in genetic counseling risk assessment*

and risk figures to provide are in Table 8-3. A key step is to determine the pattern(s) of inheritance for the genetic condition. Familiarity with the hallmark features and risk figures for each pattern of inheritance will allow you to readily assess pedigrees. Keep in mind that varied factors can affect pedigree interpretation, including variable expressivity, reduced penetrance, heterogeneity, mosaicism, and nonpaternity.

If the pattern of inheritance for a genetic condition is known, calculating the risks can be straightforward. However, if the genetic condition can be inherited in different ways (i.e., autosomal dominant, autosomal recessive, etc.), it is important to take this into account when evaluating the pedigree and to recognize that a range of risk figures may need to be provided. While it is important to be global in considering different patterns of inheritance, you also need to be practical and think about the most likely pattern(s) of inheritance and the fact that certain patterns of inheritance are less common (e.g., X-linked dominant, mitochondrial, Y-linked). If the mode of inheritance is not known for the genetic

TABLE 8-3. General risk figures to consider providing in a genetic counseling session

Incidence of ...

- The genetic condition in the population
- The carrier frequency in the general population
- The carrier frequency in the patient's ethnic/ancestral group (if indicated)

Percent of cases ...

- That arise due to inherited (genetic) factors
- That arise sporadically in the general population
- That arise *de novo*
- That are related to germline (gonadal) mosaicism

Patient's risk to be ...

- Affected with the condition
- Unaffected by the condition (noncarrier)
- An unaffected carrier of the condition (if indicated)

Risk for children/future children, siblings, and other relatives to be ...

- Affected with the condition
- Unaffected by the condition (noncarrier)
- An unaffected carrier of the condition (if indicated)

Risk for specific health issues ...

- Lifetime risks
- Relative risks
- Penetrance estimates

Modifications of risks based on information previously known ...

- From genetic test results
- From inheritance pattern/family history review
- Bayesian analysis

* Note: Not all of these risk figures will be provided to the patient. Consider which risk figures are relevant for decision-making and which make sense for the goals of the visit.

condition, or if multifactorial inheritance may be contributing, you will likely need to seek data from empiric studies. Some tips for evaluating pedigrees are listed in Figure 8-1.

Knowing the general population risks and carrier frequencies for a genetic condition(s) will allow you to present risk figures in a global context. It is helpful for patients to know whether their risk is the same, lower, or higher than the general population risk. If a carrier frequency is not specified, this generally can be derived by applying the Hardy–Weinberg equation to calculate allele frequencies ($p^2 + 2pq + q^2 = 1$; p and q are allele frequencies ($p + q = 1$) and for rare conditions, p, the most common allele, will be approximately equal to 1 and the carrier frequency ($2pq$) will be equal to $2q$). For example, for the autosomal recessive genetic condition, cystic fibrosis (CF), that has an incidence (q^2) of 1/2500,

$q = 1/50$, p can be approximated as 1 and the carrier frequency of $2pq$ would be calculated as $(2)(1)(1/50) = 1/25$. It is worth noting that prevalence data for most genetic conditions is ascertained from data on majority populations and may not represent diverse groups. Consequently, the accuracy of Hardy–Weinberg calculations may be limited. It can be helpful to show calculations of risk before testing and how risk figures would be modified depending on test results when counseling patients on testing options. For some genetic conditions, there may be specific risk models available to calculate the risk of inheriting a pathogenic gene variant (e.g., *BRCA1/2*-related hereditary breast and ovarian cancer syndrome; hypertrophic cardiomyopathy).

Bayesian Analysis

Bayesian analysis is a calculation that uses the patient's baseline (*a priori* or prior) risk and modifies it based on their age, clinical status, family history, or test results (conditional probability). Performing a Bayesian analysis can significantly impact the risk figures you provide and potentially result in a risk reduction that negates the need for further testing. Bayesian analysis is often used to derive the risk modification figures seen in genetic test reports. The case below illustrates how Bayesian analysis can be used to modify carrier risk based on family history (in this case, the number of unaffected male children for an X-linked recessive condition).

> *Ann, age 35, comes to see you for preconception genetic counseling. She is concerned about her risk for having a son with hemophilia, given her family history of this condition (two maternal uncles, maternal aunt's son, maternal grandmother's brother, all deceased). Hemophilia is an X-linked recessive condition. Given this family history, Ann's maternal grandmother and maternal aunt would be obligate carriers. Ann's mother would have a 50% risk of being a hemophilia carrier, and therefore Ann would have a 25% carrier risk (50% chance mother is a carrier, multiplied by 50% chance that Ann would inherit the X chromosome with the pathogenic variant for hemophilia if her mother was a carrier = 25%). However, Ann's mother's carrier risk for hemophilia is actually less than 50% because she has three unaffected sons. By performing a Bayesian analysis (Table 8-4), her carrier risk can be reduced from 50% to 11%. Ann's carrier risk would be half this risk, which is 5.5%. Ann's risk to have a child with hemophilia would be 1.4% (5.5% chance Ann is a carrier multiplied by ½, the chance of having a son, multiplied by ½, the chance a son would receive the X chromosome with the pathogenic variant = 1.4%).*

The above example shows that by simply using pen and paper to perform a Bayesian analysis, Ann's risk for having a son with hemophilia was significantly reduced without doing any genetic or other testing.

TABLE 8-4. Performing Bayesian analysis to modify carrier risk for hemophilia based on family history information

Probability	Ann's mother carrier	Ann's mother noncarrier
Prior probability[a]	1/2	1/2
Conditional probability[b] (3 unaffected sons)	1/8	1
Joint probability[c]	1/16	1/2 (= 8/16)
Posterior probability[d]	(1/16)/(1/16+8/16) = 1/9 = 11%	(8/16)/(8/16+1/16) = 8/9=89%

[a] Ann's mother's prior probability of being a carrier of hemophilia is ½ (the chance that she inherited the X chromosome with the hemophilia gene pathogenic variant from her mother, who is an obligate carrier). Probability that Ann's mother is not a hemophilia carrier is also ½ (the chance that she inherited the X chromosome without the hemophilia gene pathogenic variant from her mother).
[b] If Ann's mother is a carrier of hemophilia, each son would have a ½ chance of receiving the X chromosome with the hemophilia gene pathogenic variant and a ½ chance of not inheriting the pathogenic variant (i.e., unaffected). The probability that all three sons would be unaffected if Ann's mother is a carrier is 1/8 (½ × ½ × ½ = 1/8). If Ann's mother is not a carrier of hemophilia, she would have a 100% (=1) chance of having unaffected sons.
[c] Joint probability = prior probability multiplied by conditional probability.
[d] Posterior probability = joint probability divided by the sum of joint probabilities for both possible outcomes. Posterior probabilities always add up to 1 (or 100%).

Risk Presentation

Equally important as performing an accurate risk assessment is effective risk presentation and communication. If using empiric studies where risk figures differ from study to study, try to determine the reasons for the differences and consider whether the studies have limitations. If more than one risk figure or a range is applicable, this information should be provided to the patient. The risk figures provided could significantly impact the decisions of patients and their family members. In summary, make sure that risk figures are accurate, and clearly presented and documented.

CONTRACTING: TURNING CASE PREPARATION INTO REALITY

You've reviewed the patient's medical records, gathered relevant information, and are now ready to see the patient. Will your plan for the session fit with your patient's expectations? The opening of your genetic counseling session, referred to as contracting, provides the opportunity to confirm that goals are aligned and there is mutual agreement on how to move forward. Members of the clinical team involved in the appointment should introduce themselves and their roles, including any students or trainees involved in the patient's care. The team should acknowledge the referral indication and plan for the visit and patients should be invited to share their own understanding of why they are being seen, what they are hoping to learn, as well as their questions and concerns. It can be helpful to provide the patient an overview of what will happen during the clinic visit, especially if you will not be able to address your patient's questions or concerns until later in the session. In turn, patients should be prompted to introduce any family members or support persons accompanying them.

For patients with intellectual disabilities and/or patients who are minors, it is especially important to engage them early in the session and to inquire about their questions and interests- both medical and personal (e.g., hobbies, daily activities). This not only invites the patient into the conversation, but also helps build a relationship that can make the patient more comfortable during current and future medical encounters. These interactions can also allow you to identify anxieties or fears that may be present and to address them up front if possible. For example, a child who is upset or anxious about the prospect of a blood draw may be calmed by knowing that the visit will only involve talking, or that testing will be done on a saliva or buccal swab. In addition, these early conversations can also provide information as to the patient's level of interest and/or ability to participate in decision-making and may give you the opportunity to observe interactions between family members and the roles they play in the patient's care.

It may be determined in the opening moments of a session that the goals and expectations of the patient and the genetic counselor do not align. In such scenarios, it is important to acknowledge the discrepancies and to be transparent with your patient regarding how you plan to resolve the discordance. For example, if the patient expresses that they want genetic testing and you know it is unavailable or will not be done that day, it may be helpful to acknowledge this at the start of the appointment to minimize potential frustration and to reframe the session around alternative diagnostic approaches, if available. If the patient presents with concerns that are not in line with the referral indication and, thus, have not been prepped for, it may be appropriate to offer alternative ways to address the additional concerns, possibly through phone follow-up, a return visit, or a brief break in the session to consult with other team members. In some situations, discrepancies that arise during contracting may be mitigated simply by reorganizing the planned components for your visit. For example, if you sense the patient is very anxious about their risk for a genetic condition and you know the risk is low or lower than what the patient stated, you may consider sharing this information at the start of the session rather than waiting until your planned education component. Whether contracting is brief or extended, the goal should be to build a cooperative relationship with your patient and reciprocal agreement on how you will use the time together during the session.

LOGISTICAL COMPONENTS OF CASE MANAGEMENT

Case management in genetic counseling is the process through which a genetic counselor assesses the needs of their patients, formulates a plan to meet such needs, and coordinates the plan to completion. Case management requires skills in risk assessment, patient education, and psychosocial counseling—topics that will be covered in other chapters in this book. The following sections focuses on common planning and logistical aspects of case management in genetic counseling sessions.

Considering your Counseling Environment

Genetic counseling services have traditionally deployed an in-person model of clinician–patient interaction. Virtual platforms for outpatient genetics visit have also become mainstream, through use of both phone and audiovisual devices. Service delivery platforms present their own benefits, as well as limitations and unique barriers to care. Increasing demand for genetic counseling services have also prompted the need to consider alternative service delivery models, including the use of group counseling, videos or patient-directed learning modules for pre- and post-test counseling, as well as interactive platforms like chatbots that can help patients explore genetic information on their own time and at their own pace (Cohen et al., 2013; Nazareth et al., 2020; Lee et al., 2023).

The different platforms of service delivery may facilitate care for some patients and exclude it for others, raising issues of access, equity of care, and disparities (Uhlmann et al., 2021). An "in-person" model of care allows for many components of a genetics evaluation to be completed on the same day, including any required physical examinations, signatures on informed consent or testing documents, and immediate sample collection for genetic testing. In-person visits, however, may be inflexible for patients with scheduling restrictions and may present challenges for patients who do not have reliable transportation, who have childcare needs, who have a chronic illness that limits travel or that poses an infection risk, or who do not reside in physical proximity to a genetics clinic. The use of virtual platforms may provide the patient the comfort of remaining at home or at a local health care facility, the flexibility to complete their genetics visit in the middle of their workday, and the support of being joined remotely by family members, friends, or caregivers that may otherwise be unavailable to join in-person. Virtual visits, however, may pose logistical challenges for the coordination of genetic testing, including the need to obtain required signatures electronically or via mailed documents, as well as the need to facilitate alternative methods for patient sample collection (e.g., in-home saliva or buccal kit, mobile phlebotomy) (Uhlmann et al., 2021). Finally, a service delivery model that relies on group counseling may provide the benefit of seeing multiple patients simultaneously and allowing patients the chance to interact; however, this raises issues related to patient confidentiality and guidance may be institution specific.

In selecting a service delivery model for a particular patient, the following questions can be considered:

- What service delivery models are available to patients at your institution?
- What are the goals of the visit and is it feasible to achieve these goals via the selected platform? Is there a better platform to achieve those goals?
- Are there aspects of patient care that may be enhanced or compromised by use of a particular service delivery model?
- Can the patient and their desired support person(s) easily access the service (e.g., is there physical space? Is the required technology/device available to the patient?)?
- Does the specified location or delivery model allow for all health care providers contributing to the evaluation to be present?
- Is the chosen location free from distraction or other barriers that may impede patient participation?
- Does the specified location or mode of delivery provide protections for patient privacy and/or confidentiality?
- Does the patient have a stated preference for a particular model of care?

It is possible that a service delivery model may be utilized that subsequently is not optimal for the patient. For example, sometimes a virtual visit needs to be converted to a phone visit, or rescheduled as an in-person visit or another virtual visit when technological or other issues arise. Sometimes an in-person visit for physical exam is clearly indicated but a virtual visit is pursued due to timing considerations or transportation barriers. Therefore, it is important to consider the above questions from both the patient and provider perspectives: be flexible, adaptable, and able to pivot as indicated.

Defining your Medical Team

The clinical indications for which a patient may present for genetics evaluation continue to expand, driving the integration of genetics services into multiple specialty and subspecialty clinics. As such, the defining members of the medical team during a genetics evaluation will be dependent on the clinic setting, the patient population being served, and the care goals of the evaluation itself. In some settings, genetic counselors may provide services as independent health care providers. In other settings, genetic counselors may provide services alongside a physician or advanced practice provider. For example, in a pediatric or general medical genetics clinic, a genetic counselor may work in parallel with a medical geneticist, while in a cancer genetics or cardiac genetics setting, physician colleagues may include oncologists and cardiologists, respectively. In such scenarios, the genetics knowledge may be shared but components of the patient visit may be divided between team members based on their individualized levels of expertise.

In some settings, genetic counseling assistants (GCAs) have become integral in case management by handling several logistical and administrative tasks that arise during a patient's evaluation. GCAs can perform various supportive pre- and post-clinic responsibilities including requests for medical records and family history information, pedigree construction from family history forms or by phone, and assistance with the logistics of genetic testing (Pirzadeh-Miller et al., 2017; Hallquist et al., 2020). GCAs may act as an initial point of contact for a patient and may be an ongoing resource for a family navigating extended genetics evaluations or complexities in care coordination. GCAs working in research or laboratory settings may also be key resources and a point of connection for genetic counselors to address questions regarding available laboratory services, sample requirements, test status, or any issues that arise during the genetic testing process.

In defining your team, it is important to consider other available clinical and administrative resources. Genetic counselors participating in clinical care generally work closely with intake staff responsible for scheduling appointments and triaging patient referrals. Medical assistants, clinic nurses, and child-life specialists may also be available to assist in fulfilling a variety of patient needs, including obtaining required health data during medical intakes or by making a patient more comfortable during their visit or performing any required medical procedures. Genetic counselors may help their patients connect with social workers, psychologists, psychiatrists, and behavioral health specialists within their institution or assist in identifying psychosocial support resources in the patient's community. Lastly, a patient's referring provider(s) may be contacted to gain additional insight into a patient's clinical presentation, may assist in coordinating imaging or diagnostic testing locally, and may be an ongoing point of contact for a patient's long-term medical management. Through their interactions with patients, these health care team members may contribute valuable information regarding a patient's psychosocial status, family dynamics, and relevant barriers to care that may not be readily identified through chart review or during time-limited patient visits.

Case management also involves connecting with others who can assist you with logistical components of patient care and addressing issues that arise. Building relationships with relevant experts at commonly used laboratories may be used to stay up to date on laboratory test offerings and to help answer questions related to genetic test results and coordination of family studies. Billing representatives within a GC's home institution and at genetic testing laboratories can assist in navigating insurance coverage for genetic testing and addressing billing issues as they arise. Many institutions have departments devoted to patient relations and medical compliance that can assist when patient care does not go smoothly.

Working with Interpreters

Optimally, patients should receive genetic counseling in their preferred language, ideally from a qualified and/or certified medical interpreter. Certified interpreters are generally required to interpret everything said in a session. While some interpreters may provide simultaneous interpretation (i.e., the interpreter delivers the translated speech with minimum delay and interruption) or whispered interpretation (i.e., the interpreter whispers the translated speech to the client simultaneously), the more typical encounter will involve consecutive translation (i.e., the interpreter waits for a pause or break in speech then delivers the interpretation). Therefore, sessions involving consecutive translation can be expected to take longer and information critical to decision-making and patient care should be prioritized.

Some patients may request using a family member for interpretation or a certified interpreter in the patient's native language may not be available. If interpretation is being done by a family member, it is possible that information may be conveyed differently if the family member has a different perspective. As with any genetic counseling case, it is possible that the patient may be influenced by a family member during decision making. Hospitals often have listings of employees who can serve as interpreters, or access to a phone/video interpreter service, and it will take some advance planning to make sure an interpreter is available.

It may be helpful to brief the interpreter prior to the start of the session so they are aware of the session plan and visit content. An interpreter may also act as a cultural broker, providing the clinical team with insight into a patient/family's perspectives of a medical condition or approaches to medical decisions to ensure that care remains patient centered (Rosenbaum et al., 2020). Although clinic rooms can be small, the seating should be positioned in a way that facilitates eye contact between the GC and the patient, and to allow the GC to assess the patient's body language and response to presented information. For virtual visits, focusing simultaneously on both the patient and interpreter is easier to accomplish. Etiquette when using an interpreter includes: speaking directly to the patient instead of the interpreter; using summary statements and pauses; making sure that the interpreter has time to interpret and that the patient has time to respond; presenting information succinctly and clearly; minimizing use of technical terms and abstract concepts; and using pictures/diagrams. These are general guidelines for use with any patient, but are especially important when there are language and/or comprehension issues. As much as possible, focus on and engage the patient as you work with the interpreter.

Family Members as Team Members

Family members can play various roles during the evaluation of a patient. They may accompany the patient due to being a partner or parent/guardian. They may provide psychosocial support and/or may take on a more active role and assist in providing history information. They may also present separately for their own visit to discuss personal medical concerns or questions. In some situations, simultaneous evaluations of multiple affected family members can enrich the information available to the clinical team to guide their differential diagnoses and genetic testing plan for the family as a whole. Relatives may also be called upon to provide a DNA sample for segregation analysis during variant interpretation. This is common practice during genomic sequencing studies (e.g., trio exome or genome sequencing), and may also be useful to provide more information to reclassify variants of uncertain significance.

It is best practice to ask the patient to initiate contact with their relatives and to connect such relatives back to the clinic staff or to a local genetics clinic. Direct contact from the clinic staff to such relatives without the permission of the relative or authorization from the patient is not permissible in the United States given the Health Information Portability and Accountability Act (HIPAA) of 1996 (United States Congress, 1996). Any release of patient information to relatives requires signed release of information forms.

Lastly, other individuals may be involved in a patient's genetics evaluation as a court-appointed legal guardian or Durable Power of Attorney (DPOA), someone designated to act on an individual's behalf for medical, legal, and/or business matters. While such roles will commonly be filled by a family member, medical decisions may also be facilitated or influenced by court orders, foster parents, or case workers. Legal guardians will be required to provide informed consent for the patient's care, including any genetic testing ordered. The genetic counselor should clarify the plan for follow-up with both the patient and the guardian (when applicable), including preferences for communication of results and establishing a "point-person" for any required follow-up.

Time Management in Genetic Counseling Sessions

Even with thorough case preparation and a well-defined plan, a genetic counseling session may not unfold as anticipated. Multiple circumstances can require extended visit time including language barriers, technology issues, patient comprehension and needs, psychosocial circumstances, and delays in provider availability. Flexibility, adaptability, and time management are key aspects of case management. Tips for time management include the following.

- Giving prompts to focus your patient on information that is needed and directions to allow them to follow your line of questioning.
- Asking clear, focused questions using patient-friendly language (e.g., for a patient with a cardiovascular genetic condition, ask if anyone else has the same condition or a heart condition).
- Considering closed-ended questions if a short response is sufficient. Open-ended questions can be used if encouraging an extended patient response, specifically during psychosocial exploration or patient decision-making. The pace of your questions can model for the patient the rate of responses.

- Acknowledging and summarizing relevant information to encourage a focused patient response.
- Reminding patients of time limitations for the visit as indicated.

It is challenging to politely redirect talkative patients and to bring them back to the question at hand. It can also be challenging to determine when a response to a question is not going to yield the desired information and needs to be asked in a different way. Generally, the most pertinent information will be given within the first few minutes after a question is asked; however, it is not unusual for patients to remember important information and provide it later in the session.

When multiple family members are present, this can pose additional time management issues. While family members may serve as a support and may ask relevant questions, they may also ask multiple questions regarding their own circumstances. Unless the clinic visit was specifically scheduled as a family visit, it will be important to convey that focus needs to be on the patient given time constraints and that relatives can be seen separately in clinic as indicated. If more time with the patient is needed, you will need to determine if it is possible to extend the visit by delaying or having another team member (if an option) see your next patient; otherwise, a return visit may be scheduled.

CASE DOCUMENTATION

Documentation is the process of providing a written summary of your encounter with a patient in their formal medical record. Medical documentation, also referred to as a chart note, serves both clinical and nonclinical (e.g., billing, legal) purposes, with key examples outlined in Figure 8-2. If a patient is provided with documentation of their clinic visit, it can be the same as the document sent to the referring health care provider(s) or one specifically written to the patient using less technical wording (often called a patient letter). These documents serve as a written reminder of the counseling provided during a patient's visit, including the medical management plan, and may also be helpful when sharing information with other health care providers and at-risk relatives. Documentation may also address the limitations of the genetic counseling provided, such as lack of family records to comment on a specific recurrence risk, or limitations in knowledge based on old or limited studies.

Standards in Medical Documentation

A list of general components in clinical documentation is provided in Table 8-5. The National Society of Genetic Counselors also provides a practice resource outlining standards in clinical documentation (Hunt Brendish et al., 2021). A chart note should accurately summarize the medical evaluation and the genetic counseling, especially risk figures, that was provided. Language should be concise, factual, and supported with evidence from the medical literature or

For the health care team:	For health care administration:
• Provides a summary of the genetic evaluation, genetic counseling provided, prior workup, and proposed next steps in a patient's evaluation and care. • Provides education on the genetic condition(s) for referring providers or other medical staff. • Allows for continuity of care between providers.	• Supports insurance billing and reimbursement for medical services rendered. • May be audited as part of institutional or federal agency oversight.
For patients and families:	**For legal purposes:**
• Provides a summary of the genetic evaluation, genetic counseling provided, prior workup, and proposed next steps in a patient's evaluation and care. • Can be shared with patient's health care providers. • Can be shared with family members to facilitate communication about the genetic condition and potential health risk. • Can be used to advocate for work/school accommodations.	• Serves as a summary of medical interactions in the event of a medical malpractice claim. • May assist in determining patient eligibility for social security and/or disability payments.

FIGURE 8-2. *Multifaceted uses of clinical documentation*

TABLE 8-5. **Common components used in clinic documentation for a genetics visit (not all components will be required for all forms of documentation)**

Opening

- Patient demographics (e.g., name, age)
- Date of visit
- Referring provider
- Reason for referral/question to be addressed
- Participants in the clinic visit
- Duration of visit (can alternatively be listed in closing)

History of presenting concern

- Summary of the key medical findings and/or family history prompting request for genetics evaluation
- Signs and/or symptoms related to the referral indication (pertinent positives)
- Absence of signs and/or symptoms specific to the condition in question (pertinent negatives)
- Pregnancy/gynecologic history, if appropriate
- Developmental history, if appropriate
- Date, location, and source of relevant diagnostic studies (e.g., genetic test reports, imaging studies)

TABLE 8-5. *(Continued)*

Past medical history: List of medical diagnoses
Past surgical history: List of past surgeries or medical procedures (with dates)
Family history

- Any relevant features present in family members, guided by referral indication
- Absence of relevant features in family members, guided by referral indication
- "Red flags" or indicators of genetic conditions within a family
- Summary of relevant or available family records, including date, location, and source
- Pedigree (may be imaged separately)

Physical examination/Review of systems (if applicable)
Assessment

- Critical assessment and interpretation of personal and family history, physical examination (if indicated), and available genetic test results with respect to the condition(s) considered
- Summary and application of clinical diagnostic criteria, if appropriate
- Clinical impression on the likelihood of a genetic diagnosis or genetic risk
- Alternatives to the diagnosis questioned
- Discussion of available genetic testing options including benefits, risks, limitations, and possible results
- Discussion of medical necessity for proposed testing options to support insurance coverage
- Review of available lines of evidence for identified gene variants
- Patient's risk based on observed mode of inheritance
- Residual risk estimation following genetic testing

Education/Counseling

- Summary of the genetic condition, including key features and natural history
- Prevalence, penetrance, and expressivity of the condition
- Inheritance pattern and identification of at-risk relatives

Plan

- Testing details (e.g., test ordered, reference laboratory, relevant CPT codes, anticipated turnaround time)
- Plan for results disclosure or follow-up with patient
- List of medical recommendations for surveillance, treatment, or other intervention Referrals placed
- Follow-up visits, scheduled or indicated

Closing

- Noteworthy patient concerns and responses to provided education/counseling and proposed plan
- Resources provided to patient/family
- Names and titles of health care providers involved in the visit
- Clinic contact information for future follow-up

published guidelines when appropriate. Documentation should be free from personal bias or opinion and any value-laden terminology should be avoided (e.g., "mistake" to describe gene variants). For example, use of terms like "nice young man," "challenging patient," or "noncompliant patient" give the writer's personal impression of a patient and may suggest bias in the medical evaluation or recommendations given. Such language may also be detrimental to the patient–provider relationship or may sway the opinions of other health care providers who may read the documentation in preparation for seeing the patient in the future. When the visit note is being sent to both the health care provider and the patient, attempts should be made to use patient-friendly language whenever possible, and to provide definitions for any medical terminology used. Abbreviations should also be avoided unless previously defined. When documenting a review of medical records, it is helpful to provide the source and date of the original records (e.g., genetic test result, imaging report, pathology report) that your assessment was based on. If confirmatory records are not available, it should be noted that information was provided "per patient" or "by verbal report." Similarly, if there are insufficient records available to support an accurate risk assessment, such limitations should be noted in the clinic note. While it is important to note the individuals participating in the visit, full names should be avoided when possible unless required for medical decision making, guardianship documentation, or family follow-up.

Various additions to medical documentation may be required to support billing practices or reimbursement of the medical services provided, and may be institution specific. This may include a statement of who referred the patient, the duration of time spent with the patient during consultation, the mode of service delivery, and whether the visit was for a new or established patient.

Types of Medical Documentation

Additional scenarios requiring documentation include patient referral triage and/or scheduling calls, phone calls to patients to coordinate visit logistics or follow-up, and disclosures of genetic test results. Documentation should include the individual who was contacted, the purpose of the call, a summary of the interaction, and the outcome. If a new genetic diagnosis is made, a genetic counselor may assist a patient in communicating results to at-risk relatives by drafting a "family notification letter" that includes relevant information on the familial genetic condition and how relatives can access genetic counseling and testing. Similarly, a genetic counselor may be asked to draft a "letter of medical necessity" to an insurance company to assist in obtaining authorizations for genetic testing or other required services for the surveillance or treatment of the genetic condition.

Though one should strive for accuracy in all forms of chart documentation, changes and updates may be needed if information is not recorded correctly or new information becomes available after a consult. Chart notes are considered a permanent part of the patient's medical record and should never be deleted or removed except under the direction of your institution's medical records or health information department. If modifications are required, one can draft an "addendum" which includes a statement of the information to be corrected or modified, the date the modification was made or the new information became available, and the author updating the entry.

CASE FOLLOW-UP AND CARE COORDINATION

Planning for Test Result Disclosures and Future Patient Contact

Content outlined below focuses on key considerations for developing a plan for results communication with your patient. Creation of a mutually agreed upon plan ensures that realistic expectations are conveyed to the patient and helps to identify barriers to disclosure before they present.

- **Method of disclosure**. Most initial communication of results is done by phone or electronic patient portal, with return visits scheduled as indicated. Generally, email is not utilized since many commercial email servers are not secure and, thus, are not HIPAA compliant. Consideration for in-person result disclosures include, but are not limited to, patient preference, anticipated comprehension and/or psychosocial issues, and technological issues.

- **Team member assigned to facilitate disclosure.** Results may be disclosed by a genetic counselor, medical geneticist, other attending physician, or by another designated medical team member, including a genetic counselor assistant in some settings. When assigning a team member for results disclosure, it is important to consider the medical expertise of that individual, their ability to anticipate and address the patient's additional questions and follow-up needs, the established relationship of that team member with the patient or family, and the availability of that team member to obtain and disclose the result in a timely manner.

- **Timing.** Providing your patient with an estimated turn-around-time for testing will allow them to anticipate your follow-up. This will also help identify times where a patient may be unavailable due to work (and lack of privacy), childcare, travel, or other circumstances. Patients may request that results be disclosed on certain days or times when they know they will be free from distractions and/or have social support available. While patient preferences can be ascertained, final plans for disclosure should be realistic based on genetic counselor work hours and availability. Informing your patient about turnaround times for result disclosure is particularly important to discuss for indications and/or circumstances where information is time sensitive. Lab delays in result reporting should also be communicated to patients as they arise.

- **Individuals designated to receive results**. The point of contact for result disclosure will vary by clinic context and the indication for testing. In pediatrics, results are most often disclosed to parents or a child's legal guardian. For prenatal evaluations, the pregnant person is commonly the point of contact. For adults undergoing genetics evaluations, the patient is often contacted directly for results. Across all clinic settings, there may be emotional, cultural, or logistical factors that arise where a patient may prefer that their test result be disclosed to a partner or another designated family member. Alternative arrangements may be made for disclosure of results to parents, siblings, or other legal guardians for adult patients with intellectual disability, cognitive decline, or other severe or chronic health conditions that pose challenges for direct results disclosure. For patients of advanced age or in the setting of life-limiting disease, it is important to help your patient identify a relative for future contact and to document the follow-up plan within the patient's chart for reference by other team members. As discussed previously, any required records release or medical authorization forms should be signed by the appropriate party at the time the disclosure plan is discussed.

Immediate Release of Patient Results to the Electronic Medical Record

The 21st Century Cures Act, a congressional act passed in 2016 and made effective April 5, 2021, stipulates that patients have immediate access to certain categories of health care documentation and medical test results through the electronic health record (Majumder et al., 2017). Under such legislation, patients may receive immediate access to the results of their genetics evaluation, often simultaneous with the return of results to their ordering provider. This access may be welcomed by patients as it allows them to own their health information and to review information at their discretion. It may give the patient the opportunity to do their own research and be ready with questions when their health care provider contacts them with results and recommendations. It should be noted, however, that results may be released after traditional work hours, on weekends, or holidays when the patient's clinical team is not accessible for immediate consult. While concerns have been raised that patients may learn sensitive or distressing information about their health without the support of their health care provider, early studies indicate patient preference for such immediate access even in the event of abnormal results (Steitz et al., 2023). By discussing these circumstances up front, a genetic counselor can better understand a patient's preferences and can help them make an informed choice about when and how they access their health information.

A genetic counselor can prepare their patient for results access by foreshadowing the possible results, explaining how the patient would be alerted, and how they can follow-up with their health care team with questions. They can help their patient consider privacy when accessing results, timing and location (e.g., home versus at work), and whether they would want a support person available when results are viewed. Patients should also be informed that their medical team may need additional time to review a new result or to gather information and that this may delay immediate contact or response. By being transparent about options for results access and procedures for patient contact, patients can be empowered to make their own decisions while still feeling supported by their health care team.

Tracking genetic test results and other patient follow-up

Available genetic tests vary in test type, test technology, laboratory utilized, need for insurance pre-authorization, and turnaround time. This makes it vital for a genetic counselor to develop a system for tracking test orders and pending results and to ensure that the health care team is notified once results become available. Options include use of Excel spreadsheets, clinic databases, alerts through the electronic medical record, and laboratory online portals with secure email alerts. Similar systems may be leveraged to track other aspects of medical management for patient's undergoing follow-up in clinic, including reminders to schedule annual return visits, for annual surveillance imaging, bloodwork, other diagnostic studies, or reminders for variant reinterpretations or reanalysis of genomic sequencing data. Identifying and implementing a system that will allow for shared access by all providers and staff on the health care team can be particularly useful by allowing for shared communication on the status of a patient's evaluation, clarifying who is assigned to results disclosure or follow-up tasks, and enabling a patient's care to be covered by another team member in the event a provider is unavailable.

Patient follow-up and identification of a patient medical "home"

While some patients may be seen for annual follow-up in a genetics clinic, many patients may present for only a single consultation. Closing the visit or medical encounter with your patient often includes discussion of the long-term plan for medical management, treatment, and/or surveillance. A genetic counselor may assist their patient in identifying a health care provider who can be responsible for their long-term care plan, whether that be the patient's primary care physician or through coordinating a referral to a specialist.

Even after the evaluation or visit is complete, a genetic counselor may remain an important link between the patient, the genetics clinic, and a patient's other health care providers. A patient may reach out to the genetic counselor with additional questions, to identify additional support resources, or to assist in coordinating evaluations for family members. Other health care providers may contact the genetic counselor to clarify a patient's follow-up plan or to obtain advice on whether additional genetics evaluations are necessary. A family may return to clinic for additional discussion as new medical conditions arise in a family, new testing technologies become available, or as knowledge of the natural history of genetic conditions expands.

With the continued expansion of knowledge surrounding human genetic conditions and technologic advances in genetic testing, it is also anticipated that the information and interpretation of a patient's genetic test result may be updated with time. Patients with an inconclusive genetic test result (variant of uncertain significance) or a nondiagnostic evaluation should be encouraged to recontact the genetics clinic for periodic updates on the classification of their variant and any new testing options that may become available. Many academic and commercial genetic testing laboratories have procedures in place to issue an amended genetic test report or to recontact an ordering health care provider if there are updates to the classification of a particular variant. Clinics may choose to handle variant reclassifications in a number of different ways, including phone calls (typically preferred in the setting of a pathogenic reclassification), messages via the patient's electronic health portal, or letters mailed to the patient's home. Patient follow-up is also common in situations where reanalysis of previously nondiagnostic exome or genome sequencing is indicated. It can be useful to set expectations for patient follow-up at the time of results disclosure so there is mutual agreement as to who should initiate recontact (e.g., patient versus health care team), when follow-up is indicated (e.g., if new symptoms present or at set time intervals), and how follow-up will be completed (e.g., phone call, return visit to clinic).

SUMMARY

Genetic counselors play a pivotal role in the journey of a patient navigating and adapting to a genetic condition or genetic risk. Building from the basics of a patient's referral indication, genetic counselors use key skills in case preparation to anticipate questions, to research and prioritize relevant information, to assess risk, and ultimately develop a patient-centered care plan to meet the goals of the visit. Case management requires skills in organization and adaptability to carry out the logistical elements of a genetic counseling case, but also communication and active listening to ensure that patient needs are identified and addressed.

Building such skills takes time. Your knowledge base and expertise will grow as you prep more cases and, with experience, you will learn shortcuts and organizational techniques to become more efficient. While the content of this chapter has focused on genetic counseling practice in a clinical setting, many skills gained through case preparation and management can be applied in nonclinical settings, including industry, public health, and leadership roles. Your case preparation and management skills will continue to evolve as your clinical experiences grow and each case will provide a new opportunity to implement, refine, and master these skills.

APPENDIX A
Resource Toolkit for Preparation and Management of Genetic Counseling Cases

Information on genetic conditions	
MedGen	Gateway to a compilation of genetics resources including links to databases of genetic conditions, clinical information, practice guidelines, genetic testing, genes and clinical variants, curated reviews of medical literature, and support resources.
GeneReviews	Peer-reviewed summaries of genetic conditions authored by experts in the field. Content includes information on the natural history of the condition, diagnostic criteria, associated Mendelian genes, prevalence, penetrance, expressivity, inheritance, options for genetic testing, medical management guidelines, genetic counseling considerations and available support group resources.
Online Mendelian Inheritance in Man (OMIM)	Database citing seminal studies on established Mendelian disease genes and candidate genes for human disease. Content includes information on gene mapping, relevant animal models, gene structure and function, pathogenesis, genotype–phenotype correlations, population genetics, in addition to relevant clinical features and references. *Clinical Synopsis* function provides a review of systems with relevant clinical features (internal and external). Information useful for diagnosis and guiding physical examination. *PheneGene Graphics* provides a schematic of genes related to phenotype for the selected condition. *Search* function can be used to identify relevant genetic conditions by entering key features as search terms. This can be useful in developing a differential diagnosis.
MedlinePlus	Available from the National Institute of Health's National Library of Medicine. This searchable database provides general information on genetics, Mendelian genetic syndromes, and some multifactorial conditions. Helpful information is also available on general medical conditions and health risks.
Orphanet	Database of rare diseases and orphan drugs. Downloadable information is available on clinical features of genetic conditions, etiology, prevalence, management, and prognosis, with translation into other languages. Patient-directed resources are also available.
National Society of Genetic Counselors	*Practice guidelines* are available for some genetic conditions and for select topics relevant to clinical practice. *Policy statements* drafted and published by the society are available on topics specific to genetic testing, public health, and clinical practice.
American College of Medical Genetics and Genomics	*Practice guidelines* are available for a number of genetic conditions. *Action (ACT) sheets* are available for the diagnostic workup and management steps for certain metabolic conditions, including follow-up on positive newborn screens.
National Comprehensive Cancer Network	*Practice guidelines* are available for genetic testing, diagnostic workup, and management of hereditary cancer syndromes. Guidelines are also available for general cancer screening, oncology management, and options for cancer risk-reduction.

(continued)

(*Continued*)

Information on genetic testing and variant interpretation	
Genetic Testing Registry	National Institute of Health searchable registry for commercial, academic, domestic, and international genetic testing options.
ClinVar	A public archive of gene variant classifications with supporting evidence.
Clinical Genome Resource (ClinGen)	National Institute of Health-funded resource with curated entries regarding the clinical relevance of genes and variants, as well as actionability for medical management.
University of California Santa Cruz (UCSC) Genome Browser	Interactive schematic of the human genome reference sequence, useful for evaluating copy number variations, including breakpoints and involved Mendelian disease genes.
The Human Gene Mutation Database (HGMD)	Database of reported clinical gene variants with curated references from the medical literature.

Patient-friendly educational and support group resources	
Genetic and Rare Diseases Information Center (GARD)	Public resource for evidence-based information on rare disease and genetic conditions, including available patient support organizations.
MedlinePlus	See entry above "Information on Genetic Conditions." *Help Me Understand Genetics* section is devoted to patient-friendly content on genes, inheritance, genetic testing, gene therapy, and other precision medicine topics.
Chromosome Disorder Outreach, Inc.	Nonprofit patient registry and education, advocacy, and support organization for those with chromosome disorders.
UNIQUE (Understanding Rare Chromosome and Gene Disorders)	Research and support organization focused on recurrent chromosome anomalies, including translocations, inversions, deletions and duplications, chromosomal copy number variations, and certain single gene disorders. *Disorder guides,* translated in different languages, are available with patient-friendly information collated from the organization's patient registry, including clinical features, inheritance, and diagrams for relevant chromosome variants.
National Organization for Rare Disorders (NORD)	Database providing information on rare disease, as well as articles, videos, webinars, and fact sheets for patient education and support.
Genetic Alliance	Nonprofit organization aimed at creating connections between medical, research, and patient communities. Includes searchable directory of support groups and educational resources on basic genetic concepts.
National Human Genome Research Institute	Compendium of resources related to genetics education, genomics research, and genomic policy issues for health care providers, medical researchers, and patients.

(*Continued*)

Patient-friendly educational and support group resources	
Share Pregnancy & Infant Loss Support	Organization aimed at providing support, education, and connections among individuals who have experienced loss of a pregnancy or infant.
Resolve	Support organization founded by The National Infertility Association. Patient resources are available to identify and access community and professional support, as well as to answer key questions regarding reproductive options and financial planning for fertility care.
American Heart Association	Organization focused on promoting awareness on cardiovascular health. Online resources provide general information on select cardiovascular diseases, lifestyle interventions, and other measures to reduce disease risk.
Sudden Arrhythmia Death Syndromes (SADS) Foundation	Organization comprised of health care providers, researchers, patients, and their family members dedicated to providing education, support, and advocacy surrounding cardiac arrhythmias. The foundation's website provides information on sporadic and inherited cardiac arrhythmias, as well as opportunities to connect with other patients/families.
American Cancer Society	Research, advocacy, and support group focused on cancer screening, treatment, and survivorship. Online educational resources are available for specific cancer types, pediatric cancers, genetics of hereditary cancer, among others. Additional resources are available for identifying support, financial planning, and for transportation to medical appointments. Live chat, video chat, and helpline are available for patient assistance.
National Cancer Institute	Sector of the National Institute of Health focused on research, training, and education related to cancer. Educational resources available online on general cancer facts, screening, and treatment options, as well as information related to coping, decision-making during cancer treatments, and resources for caregivers.
Information on genetics legislation	
National Human Genome Research Institute	*Policy Issues in Genomics* section provides content on genetic discrimination and protective legislation, as well as information regarding the rights of patients during informed consent and human subjects research. Includes searchable database by state for genetics legislation.
GINAhelp.org	Patient-friendly online resource addressing questions related to the use of genetic information and the Genetic Information Non-Discrimination Act (GINA).

Additional resources on genetic discrimination and GINA are also available from the National Society of Genetic Counselors and the American Society of Human Genetics.

REFERENCES

Cohen S, Marvin M, Riley B, et al. (2013) Identification of genetic counseling service delivery models in practice: a report from the NSGC Service Delivery Model Task Force. *J Genet Couns* 22(4):411–421.

Hallquist M, Tricou E, Hallquist M, et al. (2020) Positive impact of genetic counseling assistants on genetic counseling efficiency, patient volume, and cost in a cancer genetics clinic. *Genet Med* 22(8):1348–1354.

Hunt Brendish K, Patel D, Yu K, et al. (2021) Genetic counseling clinical documentation: Practice resource of the National Society of Genetic Counselors. *J Genet Couns* 30(5):1336–1353.

Lee W, Shickh S, Assamad D, et al. (2023) Patient-facing digital tools for delivering genetic services: a systematic review. *J Genet Couns* 60(1):1–10.

Majumder M, Guerrini C, Bollinger J, et al. (2017) Sharing data under the 21st Century Cures Act. *Genet Med* 19(12):1289–1294.

Nazareth S, Nussbaum R, Siglen E, et al. (2020) Chatbots & artificial intelligence to scale genetic information delivery. *J Genet Couns* 30:7–10.

Pirzadeh-Miller S, Robinson L, Read P, et al. (2017) Genetic counseling assistants: an integral piece of the evolving genetic counseling service delivery model. *J Genet Couns* 26(4):716–727.

Rosenbaum M, Dineen R, Schmitz K, et al. (2020) Interpreters' perceptions of culture bumps in genetic counseling. *J Genet Couns* 29(3):352–364.

Steitz B, Turer R, Lin C, et al. (2023) Perspective of patients about immediate access to test results through an online patient portal. *JAMA* 6(3):e233572.

Uhlmann W, McKeon A, & Wang C. (2021) Genetic counseling, virtual visits, and equity in the era of COVID-19 and beyond. *J Genet Couns* 30(4):1038–1045.

United States Congress. (1996) Kennedy-Kaussbaum Act. Pub.L (104–191).

9

Inclusion, Inclusivity, and Inclusiveness in Genetic Counseling: On Being an Authentic and Collaborative Community of Providers

Annie K. Bao, Deanna R. Darnes, and Liann H. Jimmons

What has become clear is that education for critical consciousness coupled with anti-racist activism that works to change all our thinking so that we construct identity and community on the basis of openness, shared struggle, and inclusive working together offers us the continued possibility of eradicating racism.

Bell Hooks, Belonging: A Culture of Place

A Guide to Genetic Counseling, Third Edition. Edited by Vivian Y. Pan, Jane L. Schuette, Karen E. Wain, and Beverly M. Yashar.
© 2025 John Wiley & Sons Ltd. Published 2025 by John Wiley & Sons Ltd.

INTRODUCTION

Issues of diversity, equity, and inclusion (DEI) and the practice of attending to them are currently in an unprecedented phase of transformation. As awareness of DEI continues to advance into the mainstream of our societal systems (Saha et al., 2003; Nivet, 2011; Marrast et al., 2014; Purnell and Fenkl, 2019), the subject of inclusion is increasingly becoming more visible in the public discourse of education, training, and practice for various fields and professions (Clark et al., 1995; Allen 2000; Williams et al., 2005; Ainscow et al., 2006; Collins et al., 2019; Borkowski and Meese, 2020; Hogan and Viji, 2022). Deliberate efforts to promote meaningful change continue to manifest and unfold with the universal understanding that "at its highest point, inclusion is expressed as feeling 'safe' to speak up without fear of embarrassment or retaliation, *and* when people feel 'empowered' to grow and do one's best work" (Bourke, 2018). This coupled with research showing that "overall sentiment on diversity was 52% positive and 31% negative, sentiment on inclusion was markedly worse at only 29% positive and 61% negative" (Dixon-Fyle et al., 2020), influences thoughts, actions, and changes made with regards to inclusion in varied systems and communities. Even so, as DEI is gaining more attention and recognition in research, publications, scholarship, and practice, this work can likely be traced back centuries previous to what may be collectively recorded, recognized, and known.

In some corners of the genetic counseling community, conversations and people dedicated to advancing the work of DEI have existed since the 1980s (Wilkerson, 1985, 1987; personal communication; Baker et al., 1987; Ota Wang, 1994, 1998; personal communication; Ota Wang and Punales-Morejon, 1992). These individuals and narratives carry a largely untold history of inclusion that intersects with the published oral history of the origin story of the genetic counseling profession (Heimler, 1997). While only time will tell whether present dialogue and actions are more than just a fleeting trend in the genetic counseling community, the intention for this chapter is to contribute to the discourse of DEI by privileging (e.g., to attribute value and importance to some and not others) fundamental principles of inclusion, highlighting the hidden history of inclusion (and exclusion) in the genetic counseling community, and centering the de-colonized stories and narratives of those who are positioned best to speak on their own experiences to inform the clandestine context of genetic counseling.

Inclusion, inclusivity, and inclusiveness are referred to as the phases of inclusion (POI) throughout this chapter because, like phases of matter, they are of one substance, or in this case, the same concept. Yet, each phase describes a distinct state (of knowing, of doing, of being) and is unique in purpose to the roots of POI for the practice of genetic counseling. As you explore and examine your own understanding of POI as a genetic counselor (GC), you are encouraged to take your time, pause to identify your thoughts and emotions, and create space to practice reflexivity (e.g., assess the influence and impact of your positionality on your values, how you think, and what you do) in what is offered. You are invited to honor your beliefs, emotions, reactions, thoughts, and insights in your learning and development experience. In doing so, ponder also on the wisdom that "the quality of light by which we scrutinize our lives has direct bearing upon the product which we live, and upon the changes which we hope to bring about through those lives" (Lorde, 2012). You are mutually influencing and influenced by the systems you contribute to, participate in, and are involved with. As a product of your environment, the culture of POI that is (non)existent in the relationships and communities you're engaged in and systems you identify with (i.e., personal, professional, social, global, virtual, etc.) is reciprocally representative, to some extent, of your own positionality and values related to inclusion as well.

Some parts of this chapter may feel more relatable and applicable than others at various stages of your GC identity development. Here, you will not find a definitive (e.g., superior or directive) standard or guide to POI. Rather, you may choose with what and how you participate. Being rooted in truths of the profession and the realities of those who are influential during your training may aide you in navigating genetic counseling relationships and systems in the future. You will likely have more questions than answers throughout your experience that are reflective of your learning process. In critically thinking about your own perspective, being honest with (and about) your "self" will serve to ground and guide you towards a genuine and authentic knowing of your POI. Reflecting deeply on your "self" within the context of genetic counseling's POI, liberated from oppressive ideologies or values, including those of the authors, might also be informative and empowering. Ultimately, what you decide to include in your learning experiences reflects your POI within relationships and systems (i.e., genetic counseling community, medical, academic, training, clinical, research, laboratory, industry, etc.).

AUTHORS' POSITIONALITY

> *If I'm gonna tell a real story, I'm gonna start with my name.*
> Kendrick Lamar

As a reader, you will more effectively engage with (i.e., receive, question, challenge, process) the principles, stories, and narratives presented in this chapter if you are aware of the authors' positionality, which informs our perspective. Being that this chapter is written specifically for genetic counseling students in their training, it is essential first for the authorship team to be honest and transparent about where we stand in the discourse of DEI in genetic counseling and acknowledge the power and privileges that we hold so that we may preserve the integrity and genuineness in matters of POI. How you perceive and participate in this offering is merely reflective of the congruence or divergence of your positionality with ours. Knowing our position serves simply as a point of reference for you to better know where and how you stand in the discourse of DEI in genetic counseling. Similarly, knowing and understanding who you are (i.e., what resonates with you, your intentions for action, how you commit to practicing principles that you privilege, and with whom you choose to engage in relationship) may help also to clarify your own potential and contributions as a GC and a human being.

Truth, knowledge, insight, and perspective about POI are complex, nuanced, and evolving. They can be covert and overt; intellectual and heart-centered; manipulated and empowered; subverted and amplified; rejected and accepted; original and revised; weaponized and compassionate; internalized and externalized; individual and relational; oppressed and liberated in a broader DEI discourse. With mindfulness and humility exist opportunity and space for all that is true to be seen when you are grounded and principled. In doing this work, it is fundamental to critically attend to your positionality, practice reflection, and exercise reflexivity.

We present our reflexivity exercise below as an opportunity for you to identify your own proximity to and positionality in POI. Take what serves (you versus others) and leave the rest. Consider the power and privilege in your position to disengage with that which does not serve.

Who. In the interest of meaningful change in the genetic counseling community, we aspire to engage with matters of POI in genetic counseling by committing to truth, fostering belonging, practicing humility, and cultivating liberation. Together, we identify as Black, Asian, Mixed-Race, Female, LGBTQIA+, Cisgender-Heterosexual (cis-het), Disabled, Neurodivergent, Non-Disabled, GCs, marriage and family therapist (MFT), patients, providers, clinicians, colleagues, educators, students, supervisors, scholars, advocates, activists, trauma survivors, daughters, siblings, mothers, partners, companions, friends, women, American citizens, and human beings. We occupy space on land originally settled and occupied by the Caddo, Wichita, Comanche, Kānaka ʻōiwi, Ojibwe, Odawa, Potawatomi, Miami, Ho-Chunk, Menominee, Sac, and Fox and recognize the legacy of harm and colonization caused by the forced removal of Indigenous people from these lands. This is the collective land of traditional, ancestral, and contemporary Indigenous people and their civilization. We acknowledge their sovereignty as we continue to embrace and celebrate the oldest cultures in America.

Individually, our identities have been shaped by diverse and varied cultural positions, origins of societal power, and access to privilege within various systems, including the genetic counseling community. Collectively, our positionality represents both earned and unearned power and privilege in the socially constructed genetic counseling context to be authors of this inaugural chapter on inclusion, in a textbook for genetic counseling students. This perspective of POI was conceived from a position of marginalization and minoritization within the professional system of oppression by a majority caste of GCs (e.g., overrepresentation of white, middle-upper class, nondisabled, cis-het, women; their values, interests, and agendas). This positionality influences our perspectives, helps us to challenge our own assumptions and biases, and empowers us to change and evolve over time. Thich Nhat Hanh's lesson that "every thought you produce, anything you say, any action you do, it bears your signature" aligns with our positionality. Only with continuous reflexivity of our positionality, values, beliefs, behavior, and actions can we then be accountable for their impact as we strive to nurture POI in all (not just the genetic counseling community) of the systems in which we occupy and hold space.

What. During a time of growth for the genetic counseling community, universal social uncertainty, and shifts in global perspective, the authors, chapter contributors, and allies have all convened in solidarity to present one collective narrative for a legion of POI perspectives. People and communities have had to navigate the landscape of systemic oppression and white supremacy, while also advancing DEI in the interest of justice, for generations beyond what is written in the books of history. What is recorded is surely not representative of all that has been done or what is known. Knowledge and wisdom can also be transmitted through song, art, design, ritual, nature, etc. Thus, it is probable that lived experiences of challenges and successes in DEI exponentially outnumber what is included in the privileged pages of any publication.

Within the genetic counseling community, a landscape of competing priorities, varied benefits to stakeholders, and a homogeneous representation of those chosen as gatekeepers and leaders of the professional ecosystem to maintain or disrupt its status quo have existed (NSGC Professional Status Survey, 2022). The homogeneity of the profession is reflected in the fact that the manuscript for this chapter was submitted with reference to the Professional Status Survey (PSS) published in 2022 reflecting little change in the racial demographics of the field since its inception in 1980 (Professional Status Survey, 1980). During the final phase of edits for the textbook, the publication of the 2024 PSS further substantiates a continued preservation of status quo and lack of diversity in the field (Professional Status Survey, 2024). The inherent intricacies to constructing a cohesive offering about POI call on us to consistently practice with community-centered discipline, embody cultural humility, exercise complex discretion, and make decisions that are exclusionary of anything that may compromise inclusiveness. We avow, with resolve, that centering certain stories does not necessarily reflect excluding, or not being inclusive of, others. Instead, doing so is integral in the purpose of POI to privilege efforts that recognize and interrupt differentials of power and privilege that are inherent in systems of oppression and white supremacy.

Truth and reflexivity remain of the utmost importance in the construction of this chapter. The double bind that exists in "truth-telling" is that what we choose to include, in actuality, must also be to the exclusion of any notions in conflict with DEI principles that would be harmful, oppressive, or noninclusive to marginalized and minoritized individuals (MMIs). In examining the prisms of POI in genetic counseling, we invite and welcome the perspectives of those who are unseen, unheard, and unknown in service of equity in spaces typically dominated by those afforded preference in context of socially constructed notions of supremacy in whiteness. Even if issues do not impact us personally or directly, they matter and it is quintessential to embrace them as such. We include and celebrate what holds significance for one another as valuable to our relationships with each other and strengths within the genetic counseling community system.

By agreeing to author this chapter, we recognize the compromises and consequences that accompany whole-hearted commitment and contribution to the momentum for justice. We reflected frequently and deeply on the dangers and threats to our own safety and peace by engaging in the DEI discourse within genetic counseling, with its legacy of cultural hegemony and coddling of the majority. It is apropos to be mindful and forthcoming of our own limits in knowing, our instincts for safety and survival, and the reality that POI in genetic counseling supersedes all else here. What those in positions of power choose to privilege and assert as reality have the potential to impose and distort narratives for individual gain. As authors, we acknowledge that we too hold power and privilege to influence POI of the genetic counseling community and must refrain from any inclination to impose, project, or distort content to serve any personal interests.

Why. Ours is a perspective inextricably linked with the profoundly rich, valuable, and confronting background of all the people, places, and things that experience, contribute, and bear witness to how mechanisms of POI in the genetic counseling community system are built and preserved. This chapter is committed to first amplifying the untold, hidden, and erased lived experiences of those GCs who are not typically afforded the opportunity to be heard, seen, and known. The priority of the content included is intended to benefit the genetic counseling community as a whole (rather than any one individual or agenda) and lean firmly into the arc of the moral universe that bends towards justice for advancing POI in the genetic counseling culture. Together, this collective knowledge has the potential to influence patient care, community engagement, outcome measures, training standards, and future innovations. It is important, it matters, and we care.

We are dedicated to seeking and uplifting those who have been historically marginalized and minoritized within the genetic counseling community (e.g., chapter contributors) to join us in informing the dialogue of genetic counseling POI. In an effort to present a de-colonized, anti-racist, and heart-centered chapter about becoming inclusive in the genetic counseling community, we understand the risks, challenges, and rewards that may come in assuming this position (and mantle) to offer this experience during a consequential stage of identity formation for you in your training. These stories told and the narratives shared are important, they matter, and we care about them and those who dare to share.

How. Offering our position and process of seeking out stories, listening to unheard (oppressed, silenced, and erased) voices, recording their stories and narratives, and creating space for them to be known is our attempt to model the progression of POI. By examining how we contribute to non-inclusive behaviors and healing from the impact of systemic inequities, we aim to interrupt cycles of betrayal and harm. It is with intention that this chapter may disrupt the status quo of oppressive and exclusionary norms, demystify hidden historics that influence POI, and amplify stories that may better inform your perspective of DEI within the genetic counseling community. Our positionality in the discourse about DEI in genetic counseling reminds us to continue to normalize discussions and dialogue about POI, rather than ignore or avoid them.

You will not find a prescriptive guideline of "best practices" to be(come) inclusive as a GC. You will instead be invited to examine and explore your own sense of "self" as it relates to the relationships and systems that you are engaged with, to inform your own stance on POI as a GC. In presenting this de-colonized perspective on POI, you may notice our resistance to justifying humanity. The truth is sacred and does not need to be convincing or defended to be true. It is not in our interest (or yours) to appeal to any one person, identity, or group by rationalizing our (or our contributors') truths or presenting a "more digestible" (comfortable) version of the collective realities shared. We will accordingly abstain from expending energy or space explaining the imperative to humanize those who have been dehumanized within (and by) the genetic counseling community.

Furthermore, in refusing to claim supremacy of our own growing knowledge and understanding of POI, you may also notice an absence of absolute definitions of words and language. We are deliberate in our refusal to subscribe to any one approach or to impose a dominant perspective of how to be in relationship with others. At the forefront, it remains that we cannot effectively confront, deconstruct, and disrupt white supremacy and oppression *with* supremacy and oppression to co-construct another matrix of unjust power. Alas, it is incumbent on you and those you engage with to determine what you, individually and collectively, are capable and willing to do about POI in the genetic counseling community.

As authors, we identify as diverse MMIs who occupy space within the genetic counseling community. We are faithful to perpetual self-reflective practice (i.e., reflexivity, cultural humility, accountability, etc.). Reflexivity helps us recognize our individual and collective positionality that contributes to the homogeneous norms of genetic counseling and also informs opportunities to create meaningful change for POI in genetic counseling (Sikes, 2004; Bahari, 2010; Foote and Bartell, 2011; Scotland, 2012; Savin-Baden and Major, 2013; Ormston et al., 2014; Rowe, 2014; Marsh et al., 2018; Grix, 2019). A devotion to transparency, curiosity, and reflection serves to preserve the integrity, honesty, and humility of our position in the discourse on POI in genetic counseling. Being forthcoming of our own challenges and mistakes by taking accountability and steps towards atonement for repairing the harm we cause also advances collective efforts towards being authentic, genuine, and collaborative in a community. Practices in mindfulness, self-awareness, self-reflection, and reflexivity are essential to sustain accountability in the principled discipline of POI, remain heart-centered in our patient encounters, and be empathic colleagues within the genetic counseling system we persist in.

In the formation of this chapter, we remain grounded in the South African philosophy of Ubuntu that Desmond Tutu describes as "the very essence of being human" and to mean "I am because we are." We return (and encourage you to do so as you are able and see fruitful) to the Archbishop's description as a guiding principle: "a person with ubuntu is open and available to others, affirming of others, does not feel threatened that others are able and good, for he or she has a proper self-assurance that comes from knowing that he or she belongs in a greater whole and is diminished when others are humiliated or diminished, when others are tortured or oppressed, or treated as if they were less than who they are."

PAUSE.

What part of this mindfulness reflection and reflexivity practice resonates with your understanding of your "self?" Why do you feel the way you feel about who and what is being centered in this chapter? What does the (mis)alignment reflect about others? What does the dissonance or resonance reflect about you? What are you aware of and what do you acknowledge as the influence and impact of your own power, privilege, and positionality?

PHASES OF INCLUSION: PRINCIPLES FOR PRACTICE

We need to give each other the space to grow, to be ourselves, to exercise our diversity. We need to give each other space so that we may both give and receive such beautiful things as ideas, openness, dignity, joy, healing, and inclusion.

Max de Pree

A universally accepted definition and consensus of procedures or steps to becoming inclusive or practicing inclusion does not exist. While establishing a common language to communicate ideas is necessary, so too is resisting the inclination to colonize minds, subvert experiences, and establish supremacy of knowledge. POI takes many forms depending on context, though it is most prolific in the contexts of education for those with special needs, championed by disability rights and justice scholars and activists. For all intents and purposes, the definitions of inclusion, inclusivity, and inclusiveness depend mostly on you, those you dialogue with about POI, and the systems where you are navigating the discourse. Only once learned biases and behaviors of the genetic counseling community are named, owned, and interrupted (Bao et al., 2020) may those within this system of GCs reflect honestly on their impact and bridge the gaps of their own cognitive dissonance to aspire to become inclusive.

PAUSE.

As you consider your perspective on POI, please be mindful of what resonates for you and the reactions you have, and critically examine the epistemological origins (e.g., who, what, where, why, and how you know what you know) of your values, beliefs, thoughts, insights, perspectives, intentions, behaviors, and actions. Notice and ponder the areas of synergy and times of resistance in your learning. Creativity and wonder are welcome here too.

Phases of Inclusion (POI): Inclusion, Inclusivity, and Inclusiveness

Differentiating the phases of inclusion (POI) may serve to support your under-standing and clarify your position within the broader DEI discourse. The term *inclusion* conveys a collective understanding and knowing of what it is and looks like to maintain a system that includes all diverse people, places, and things. It is meant to refer to *what* a community system "aspires" to achieve. The absence of distinctly characterizing what inclusion objectively looks like, feels like, and acts like in a system constrains subsequent initiatives in practicing inclusivity or being inclusive.

Inclusivity refers to practices you implement to move towards being inclusive and achieving inclusion in a system. It denotes *how* inclusion is practiced and achieved in a system. Transparency and accountability in inclusion are reified by creating clear action items of inclusivity to fortify POI. Clear and explicit descrip-tions of inclusivity practices can pave the path towards objectively determining whether or not those actions are aligned with intentions.

Lastly, *inclusiveness* is a state of being that demonstrates your (and your sys-tems') *current state* of inclusion. Inclusiveness reflects the depth of inclusion and norms of inclusivity that are internalized within the collective genetic counseling community. While you examine how to become (more) inclusive, it may also be constructive to explore why you haven't already been inclusive and what keeps you from being (more) inclusive. Bear in mind that MMIs are the only ones with the power to determine who and what is genuinely inclusive, if practices employed reflect authentic inclusivity, and whether claims of a state of being inclusive have integrity and are trustworthy. Any attempts to incorporate POI are effectively exposed by whether patients, students, colleagues, and employees experience you or your actions as being inclusive (or not). As such, when MMIs do not actually have the experience of inclusivity with people, places, and things, those claims of inclusiveness fall short of truly being inclusive and may, in reality, be considered performative, manipulative, or harmful both in intent and impact.

PAUSE.

You are invited to distinguish, explore, and examine the following principles for the practice of POI that resonate (or don't) for you in your identity as a GC. Consider naming, examining, discussing, and clarifying how and why you feel, think, and react to the principles presented below. A deep understanding of your "self" may help to guide you in the evolution of your POI. A recognition of "self" may then further help you acknowledge others' POI.

Power and Privilege: Oppression, White supremacy, and Liberation

Scholars, educators and philosophers have been examining and writing about oppression, white supremacy, and liberation for decades (Collective, 1977; Lorde, 1977, 1981, 2003, 2021; Hooks, 1981, 2003, 2008; Frye, 1983; Morrison, 1984, 1993, 2017; Olson, 1986; Sniderman and Tetlock, 1986; Abberley, 1987; Wilkerson, 1987; McIntosh, 1989; Bell, 1991, 2018; Van Dijk, 1993; Brewer, 1999; Okun, 1999; Bartky, 2015; Bonilla-Silva and Forman, 2000; 2019; Jones, 2000; Ota Wang, 2001; Ota Wang and Sue, 2005; Wong, 2020). Centuries before that, the global majority and (US) domestic minority have been subjected to navigating colonized structures and systems that were rooted in the belief of a hierarchy in human value and supremacy that excluded them and was not built to resource their potential to thrive and succeed (Bell, 1975, 1988, 1995; McConahay et al., 1981; Kovel, 1984; Fredrickson, 1988; Morrison, 1993, 2000; Wellman, 1993; Berry, 1995; Feagin, 1995; Bonilla-Silva, 1997; Boeckmann, 2000; Harrell, 2000; Lorde, 2003, 2012; Christopher, 2021). In the spaces, places, and systems where worth is determined by labor, the resulting outcome has been generations of people being othered and exploited, with their cultures and essences coopted and appropriated, for the benefit of the few who hold power and privilege within colonized systems. As descendants of ancestral histories of oppression/castes/imperialism/colonization, these individuals represent a proportion of any community that carry with them an unaccounted weight of this reality and the intergenerational proclivity for survival and liberation from oppressors, imperialists, and colonists as an added (often ignored) burden in their experiences.

Within varied systems of oppression, white supremacy, and liberation (Bronfenbrenner, 1965, 1979, 1986, 1989; Bell, 1980, 2004; Baker et al., 1987; Wilkerson, 1987; Ota Wang, 1994; Van Ryn and Fu, 2003; Williams et al., 2005; Morrison, 2007, 2017; Roberts, 2011; Wong, 2018, 2000; Purnell and Fenkl, 2019; Borkowski and Meese, 2020; Lorde, 2020), one's identity formation is impacted by external systemic forces during whatever stage of development an individual is navigating (Erikson 1959, 1963, 1968). During this uniquely individual and personal kismet of interactions, various dimensions of experience and perspective come together to nurture growth within, towards finding and knowing a sense of "self." All things considered, you cannot underestimate the capacity of systems you engage with to impact who you are and influence how POI emerges for you in relationship with patients, students, and colleagues. Your "self" is thus grounded at the intersection of your environment and the all-encompassing complexities of your visible and hidden identity (Cross, Jr., 1971, 1991; Kim, 1981; Helms 1990, 1995; Poston, 1990; Phinney and Kohatsu, 1997; Ferdman and Gallegos, 2001; Horse, 2001, 2005; Wong, 2022).

PAUSE.

Within what systems do you occupy? How do you take up space? What positions of power and privilege do your patients hold within systems of oppression, white supremacy, and liberation? What positions of power and privilege have your role models, mentors, and representative leadership been afforded (earned and unearned) in the genetic counseling community? What power and privilege do you possess as a genetic counseling student at the intersection of your training experience and learning to facilitate encounters with others? Why and why not?

You are, in effect, the company that you keep. How those in positions of authority in the systems you exist within exercise their power and privilege is representative of the mechanisms of oppression, white supremacy, and liberation of those systems. They hold the most power to privilege and promote (or minimize and erase) POI in a community. These individuals are most endowed to either foster or destroy mechanisms of inclusion. In this way they either establish or reject practices of inclusivity, for the betterment or to the detriment of inclusiveness in microsystems (i.e., training programs, clinics, labs, teams, etc.) and the genetic counseling community macrosystem. Whoever holds power to establish and reinforce norms, standards, and rules of a system, is also permitted the privilege to set structures that have the ability to either be inclusive and collaborative or exclusive and ego-centered. "It is certain, in any case, that ignorance, allied with power, is the most ferocious enemy justice can have" (Baldwin, 1972). Those who seek to rule and dominate can only do so with followers. Therefore, it is incumbent that as members of any system (e.g., profession, organization, community, society, culture), you are diligent and fully informed of the mechanisms and structures you are representing and upholding (Tajfel, 1974; Tajfel et al., 1979; Tajfel and Turner, 2004). It is also essential for you to know the truth about those that influence and represent you and your values. Knowing who you are associated with, your positionality within certain contexts, and how you choose to engage (disengage, distance, or ignore) the reality of others' experiences, particularly those dissimilar to your own, will inexorably be linked to and influence your POI.

Ignorance is one thing. Willful ignorance and (pro)active avoidance or denial is another: a leverage of one's own position of power and privilege to "not know" the issues and avoid naming the people, places, and things that directly impact and constrain progress towards inclusion. A deliberate effort to maintain status quo, without directly assuming accountability for the impact of harm and choosing to "not know," "don't ask, don't tell," and so on, is upheld only by those with socially constructed power and privilege that is based on the hierarchy of human value. It is a position that many who do not hold majority identities in a system (i.e., the genetic counseling community) do not have the power and privilege to take. Therein lies an invitation for you to deeply examine the systems of oppression, white supremacy, and liberation that influence you, while also recognizing the (un)earned positions of power and privilege that you hold as a GC. The power and privilege you possess is dependent upon proximity to where they are concentrated, access to spaces for you to benefit, and those you are in relationship with (i.e., patients, educators, colleagues, employers, etc.) in any given system. To best understand your POI, it is indispensable to be aware of systems that indoctrinate you into knowing and belonging, as well as the systems of those in positions of power and privilege to include and represent you. Malcolm X suggested that "progress is healing the wound that the blow made. They haven't pulled the knife out; they won't even admit that it's there." With this in mind, only when those with the power and privilege in a system acknowledge and account for their own contributions to oppression and white supremacy can opportunity for liberation and progress in POI survive.

Pipelines of Inclusion (and Exclusion)

Just as the following pipelines are opportunities to impact and engage in meaningful change towards inclusion, they may also be coopted, exploited, appropriated, and coerced into becoming avenues for exclusion too. While you explore various pipelines, you may consider also identifying and reflecting upon the reciprocal, relational, and systemic nature that upholds or dismantles how these pipelines operate. As you work to advance POI, understanding reciprocity, relationships, and systems might also aid you in acknowledging the productive or harmful impact within the context of these varying pipelines.

Language   Language matters. Knowing and understanding language hold power. "Multiple studies reinforce the existence of racial bias and its negative implications for patient care" (Chapman et al., 2013). Words matter. The people (i.e., patients, mentees, colleagues, educators, mentors, etc.) that you engage with language and your words matter. A "minority tax" assumed by MMIs is a demand for code-switching to navigate and survive systems of codified (languages of) oppression, discrimination, misogynoir, and racism. In that, there is often an unaccounted for burden placed upon MMIs that along with tasks of invisible labor, serves to widen the gap of inequity. The impact of the language and words privileged within the genetic counseling community also matter. In fact, the use of coded language and words that validate oppression and white supremacy (e.g., to reify a hierarchy of human value) can also generate an impact that is divergent from what may be intended to be inclusive. The potential confusion, suffering, and harm (intended or not) that comes with using certain language and words may ultimately result in (deliberate or inadvertent) consequences for those with whom you choose to use them. Collectively, it is MMIs who are also most vulnerable to harm and damage with the lack of transparency, reframing, or manipulation of "well-intended" words and language.

Definitions of inclusion, inclusivity, and inclusiveness are varied and there is no "universal consensus" regarding these terms. This is reflected in the genetic counseling community's governing organizations with the spectrum by which POI are defined, acknowledged, and addressed. While organizations, including the National Society of Genetic Counselors (NSGC) and the National Academies of Sciences, Engineering, and Medicine (NASEM) have adopted the term "JEDI" (e.g., justice, equity, diversity, and inclusion) to brand social justice initiatives and committees, (amongst other problematic aspects of using this term) the broader association to *Star Wars* may distract from the seriousness of issues and "can inadvertently associate our justice work with stories and stereotypes that are a galaxy far, far away from the values of justice, equity, diversity, and inclusion" (Hammond et al., 2021).

DEI strategist and consultant Lily Zheng shared that they "cannot in good faith call myself a DEIJ consultant ... I worry that the more we take the deceptively small step of selling 'justice' in DEI work, the more we are giving the corporations and powerful organizations we work with the power to co-opt, dilute, and undermine it" (Zheng, 2022). Some asserted that "after a summer of uprisings for racial justice during a global pandemic ... we felt this era required us to lead with Justice and so renamed our office JEDI to reflect our paradigm shift in 2020" (Martinez and Truong, 2021). In 2021, the American Board of Genetic Counseling (ABGC) hired Nonprofit HR to conduct a DEIJ Certification Assessment (2021) to perform an "environmental scan of regulatory authorities and professional associations ... to learn what (they) are doing or recommending for DEIJ" (p. 11). The report by Nonprofit HR (2021), in comparison to the executive summary of that same report published by ABGC (2022), reveals how semantics can be just that or represent vastly varied positions. This is exemplary of how those in positions of power possess the ability to shape narratives by amplifying, oppressing, hiding, or erasing truths, findings, and meaning with strategic use of words and language.

For MMIs, DEIJ statements are meaningless, even unsafe, when actions and accountability are not congruent with the language and words used. A lack of clarity and ambiguity of the meaning of language and words used may also result in confusion and even harm. For example, the Association of Genetic Counseling Program Directors (AGCPD) does not appear to have a clearly defined position of justice (diversity, equity, or inclusiveness) in its stated mission "to build a diverse community of graduate-level educators to define best practices, facilitate resource-sharing, and foster collaborations to promote equitable, inclusive, and just education for genetic counselors." Merely having a general DEIJ statement leaves space for (mis)interpretation and exploitation such that those with the most power and privilege benefit most by evading accountability if diversity, equity, inclusivity, and justice are not upheld or when there is harm caused in these areas. Furthermore, DEIJ statements may also operate as distractions from the truth and reality of the state of the genetic counseling profession. Where language and words are oppressed, silenced, and erased, actions and behaviors of MMIs of any system often speak more to the truth than crafted public announcements. A composite review of the identities of individuals who dominate spaces of power and leadership (i.e., program directors, journal editors, board members, etc.) and the persistent lack of representation seem more reflective of POI in the genetic counseling that cannot be circumvented with a DEIJ statement.

Just as with inclusivity, inclusiveness, and inclusion, the meaning of justice is subjective and expansive in nature. While the DEI lens is just one approach to achieving justice, the term DEI is used in this chapter for the purpose of maintaining focus on POI within this context. Angela Davis famously noted that "'diversity' by itself may simply mean that previously marginalized individuals have been recruited to guarantee more efficient operation of oppressive systems." Diversity, without equity and inclusion, can therefore be coopted or appropriated to benefit those in power or maintain the status quo of oppression and perpetuation of harm to a group, community, system, and/or society's MMIs to preserve white supremacy. Within a broader discourse of DEI, the complexities of POI invite you to exercise patience, grace, and radical honesty with yourself and others as everyone continues to engage in the work.

PAUSE.

Who holds power and privilege in the genetic counseling community system with words and language? What is the intention behind the words that you choose with others? What is the impact of the words that you use with your patients, educators (students in the future), and colleagues who are marginalized and minoritized in a system? How is language utilized to include or exclude others, disrupt or protect the status quo? How is language used in promoting or interrupting oppression, white supremacy, and liberation?

Norms, Rules, Expectations, and Accountability Accreditation and regulatory boards have the power and privilege to build infrastructure and create policy, procedures, and processes of POI for a system. They can also be gatekeeping structures to reinforce or dismantle institutional and systemic mechanisms of oppression, white supremacy, or liberation. The individuals who occupy positions on these boards hold a certain level of power and privilege to be given titles and roles to make larger system decisions. They also hold the power and privilege to develop mechanisms that reinforce (or neglect) those policies, procedures, and processes by creating clear and transparent consequences and accountability measures. Those who are accustomed to exceptionalism and impunity being the same individuals who consider accountability as the injustice, add further complexity to this pipeline. The NSGC description explains that "Inclusion is the way we create environments in which an individual or group can feel accepted, respected, and valued. Inclusivity strives to create a sense of belonging for all individuals, regardless of different identities … true inclusion requires that we recognize and address our biases and actively work to decrease barriers within our profession and for the communities we serve." The Accreditation Council for Genetic Counseling (ACGC) does not seem to have any statements on DEI or definitions by which genetic counseling programs and faculty would uniformly operate or abide with matters of diversity, equity, and inclusion. And, the ABGC makes claims of being "committed to fostering diversity and inclusion, which embraces, but is not limited to" various listed identities, without a definition of inclusion by which accountability could be enforced. The collective composition of association, board, program, publication, and team leadership is reflective of AGCPD, ACGC, ABGC, and NSGC persistently preserving mechanisms and criteria that systematically maintain the status quo of white supremacy in who occupies or "qualifies" to be(come) program directors (save associate or assistant positions) or occupy leadership roles of any consequence.

The specific examples and models used to establish norms, rules, expectations, and accountability inevitably influence the manner in which a profession strives to pursue meaningful changes in problematic systems. It is also notable to acknowledge whether these are used to be models for aspirational growth or examples to validate the status quo. Nonprofit HR identified the Institute for Credentialing Excellence (ICE) and the National Commission for Certifying Agencies (NCCA) as comparable to NSGC and ACGC to conduct the ABGC environmental scan (2021). According to the report (Nonprofit HR, 2021), ICE "does not appear to have a DEIJ statement" or definition of inclusion while making an assertion as "a credible voice on DE&I practices and thought leadership." It also notes that the NCCA standards "appear to address DEIJ at least minimally" and is lacking in description of inclusion. In reviewing their own standards, it may be prudent to also ponder on why these were chosen as "comparable" and how ABGC, NSGC, and ACGC compare to the DEI efforts of other systems such as the National Human Genome Research Institute (NHGRI), the Department of Health and Human Services (HSS), or the American Society of Human Genetics (ASHG).

Mechanisms of accountability can either be created by and for those who preserve a privileged status quo and prosper in negative peace, as described in Dr Martin Luther King's *Letter from the Birmingham Jail,* or by and for all those who are impacted, including MMIs. By attending to the words, actions, and policies built by leaders, educators, and members of a system, their POI will be revealed to you. NSGC will be enacting disciplinary procedures that are effective January 1, 2024 "to ensure that the high standards of ethics, professionalism, and mutual respect outlined in all of NSGC's policies are upheld by NSGC members and staff" and "to establish NSGC as a safe and inclusive organization." It remains unclear how "true inclusion" (by its own definition "we recognize and address our biases and actively work to decrease barriers within our profession and for the communities we serve") has informed the development of this accountability mechanism. Negative peace, as we know it to be the absence of tension, thrives in environments where the harsh light of accountability can be too much to bear. Therefore, transparency in the details for how accountability will take place are necessary. Without this transparency in accountability, it is merely presumptive to associate it with POI.

PAUSE.

What is the positionality of "governing" systems for the genetic counseling community in establishing norms, rules, expectations, and accountability in POI? Who determines "regulations" of the entire genetic counseling community and how individuals engage (disengage, distance, or ignore) with patients, others, and each other? In what ways are power and privilege being used to empower others? How do those who influence and establish genetic counseling community standards utilize their power and privilege as it relates to POI?

Microsystems of the genetic counseling community macrosystem

While not an exhaustive list, the following are some microsystems that have the potential to foster inclusion (or exclusion) in their pipelines within the genetic counseling community macrosystem. Take note of what aligns with your sense of self and what may influence your viability as an arbiter of POI.

- Patient engagement: care, encounters, advocacy, oversight/accountability, and policy.
- Training programs: recruitment, admissions, standards, and educators.
- Supervisory and educational relationships: director, faculty, supervisor, advisor, and peer.
- Professional and social representation: mentorship, sponsorship, and belonging.
- Leadership, titles, and roles: recruiting/criteria, giving/granting, receiving/ accepting.
- Opportunity/proximity to power and privilege: paid versus volunteer work.
- History and narratives: research, publication, policy, and awards.

Authentic, Genuine, and Collaborative Community

As you reflect on claims made by individuals, institutions, and professional societies of "who we are (and are not) as GCs," "what we stand for as a genetic counseling community," "why we do what we do as GCs," "how we must proceed together," also examine these statements and if the actions that are informed by them are genuinely representative of you and include the realities of MMIs in the community. The cognitive dissonance between who you say you are, who you want to be, and who others see you as is just as meaningful for an individual as it is a community; the gap between the intentions and aspirations of a system is reflective of how others (outside of that system) experience the impact and actions of POI. Self-awareness and courage could be factors in sustaining honest, uncomfortable, and challenging dialogue to bridge that gap where harm to MMIs may occur.

An authentic community is socially constructed, relationally fostered, and collectively maintained (Taylor, 1992; Erickson, 1995; Trilling, 2009). Building and cultivating a community is often driven by subjective notions of POI. Upholding a community as one that is authentic, genuine, and collaborative is based on the personal perspectives that occupy space within a system. Furthermore, those who control levers of power and privilege in that system ultimately dictate if, when, and how a community presents itself based on their biased understanding of POI. The importance of transparency in the authors' positionality in the discourse of DEI in genetic counseling is relevant again here; independent of discipline, humility, and integrity (all three, driving accountability), each of us is merely degrees away from also becoming the oppressors, imperialists, and colonizers who have caused harm to MMI populations in systems we belong to (Mendelsohn, 1958; Walker, 1977, 1989; Roberts, 1983, 2000; Browne and Finkelhor, 1986; Widom and Ames, 1994).

A community is only as genuine as its leaders and members. Trust and safety to maintain DEI initiatives within a community are impossible to sustain in the absence of truth and authenticity. The depths to which each person is willing to be honest and transparent about their principles of POI and the extent to which they are humble and forthcoming about misdirection, missteps, and mistakes made are imperatives to repair and (re)build a more inclusive community. Within the community, the level of freedom to provide truthful reflection and feedback to each other about their principles and actions without fear of retaliation, shame, and blame can also be indicative of the capacity by which it can grow to become more inclusive.

PAUSE.

Is the genetic counseling profession reflective of who you want to be or who you know yourself to be, within? Is this Ubuntu? What matters as your POI emerge? How have you been misdirected in POI? What missteps have you taken in the evolution of POI? How have you accounted for mistakes in your POI? Have you identified models to help guide your POI?

As Toni Morrison aptly stated, "if you can only be tall because somebody is on their knees, then you have a serious problem." Is superiority (others being inferior) a requisite for advancement? Is belittling others reflective of confidence or prominence? Is dominance of knowledge indicative of status? To be collaborative is to embrace the needs of the community and resist sentiments of exceptionalism, oppression, and colonization that are based on any beliefs or values in a hierarchy of human value. Without clear goals, models, and examples of what a collaborative community looks like or leaders to drive those initiatives and efforts, it may seem evermore challenging to be collaborative. In individualistic, capitalistic, and hierarchical systems (i.e., medicine, academia, corporate, etc.), where conflicts of interest exist, it may be impossible to preserve a functional collaborative community. Those who privilege POI in genetic counseling as a practice (rather than as an item to be performed) towards improving DEI might also experience covert and overt resistance to meaningful change. How you perceive the rewards to cultivate a collaborative community will be directly proportionate to your level of dedication to POI in genetic counseling. Similarly, fear and perceived risk to that end will contribute to either expanding or limiting your willingness to be collaborative. The very nature of community requires individuals to serve the ultimate good of a collective system over all else (Hawley, 1950; Whittaker, 1970; Cody et al., 1975; Vellend, 2010). Leaders, mechanisms, and structures that uphold a collaborative community must then also be representative in serving the interests of all rather than a few or themselves.

Beyond defining community, authenticity, genuineness, and collaboration together, every member of a system uniquely contributes to the success and failure of "intentions" for progress in POI (Sue, 1978; Pheterson, 1986; Sonn and Fisher, 1998; Luchenski et al., 2018). You make the decision to be complicit, dismissive, complacent, or silent about discrepancies or distortions. You have the capacity to seize the opportunity to make meaningful change in maladaptive systems or assimilate in a community. The nature of leaders appointed are often reflective of the collaborative nature of an environment. Those who hold power and privilege to nurture a culture of inclusion that is collaborative are accountable to others in the community for both the celebration and the criticism of what may come. This does not absolve anyone of the responsibility (perhaps duty) to uphold principles of POI. Rather, it stresses that those with power and privilege have an added obligation to account for their position as agents of change or accessories to the status quo of oppression, white supremacy, or liberation.

PAUSE.

What are your definitions for community, authenticity, genuineness, and collaboration? What do these look like? How does it feel to be in an authentic, genuine, and collaborative community? Why does what you care about matter to you and your community?

What you perceive an authentic, genuine, and collaborative community to look like and feel like might be amplified or subverted, depending on the systems you are engaged with and how congruent your perspective is with those with the most power and privilege within them (Tajfel, 1974; Tajfel et al., 1979; Tajfel and Turner, 2004). Some of the lenses employed to understand POI may change and approaches to attending to mechanisms that constrain (or destroy) movement towards inclusion could evolve. As you continue to encounter, struggle, absorb, learn, err, advocate, grapple, rumble, and process the problems of DEI in the genetic counseling community, it is prudent to know and understand the (un)spoken principles of POI to ground your "self" and hold others accountable for upholding them for the purpose of bridging any "say–do" gaps. Absent of authenticity, genuineness, and collaboration, a system's potential to create meaningful change for POI in the genetic counseling community becomes null and void. Absence in community is ultimately reflective of absence in its members.

Just as all actions have equal and opposite reactions, all values, beliefs, thoughts, and insights will also have equal and opposite perspectives in any system that includes diverse individuals whose differences are genuinely respected (rather than coopted, exploited, appropriated, subverted, silenced, or erased). An authentic, genuine, and collaborative community that establishes guiding principles to promote POI in genetic counseling is able to give rise to the iterative process of repairing and (re)building those mechanisms and systems. With a "community agreement," all are welcome to discuss, disagree, and dissent in the DEI discourse. As such, being mindful of what in this chapter resonates with you, what does not; your thoughts, emotions, and insights; the origins of you that may or may not contribute to mechanisms of POI are of paramount worth in authentically, genuinely, and collaboratively being within the systems you are engaged in.

CONTEXT: GENETIC COUNSELING COMMUNITY STORIES AND NARRATIVES

One of the things that has always afflicted the American reality and the American vision is that aversion to history. History is not something you read about in a book; history is not even the past, it's the present, because everybody operates, whether or not we know it, out of assumptions which are produced only by our history.

James Baldwin

The History We've Told Ourselves

The practice of genetic counseling in the United States began through Hereditary Clinics in the early 1940s (Turner, 2012). Initial clinics, like the Dight Institute of Human Genetics, provided consultations for families as a basis for future studies and then progressed to providing risk assessments (Turner, 2012). The term genetic counselor itself was suggested and established in 1947, by Dr Sheldon C. Reed, a geneticist with a background in biology and human genetics (Reed, 1974). During his time consulting in London during World War II, his work was referred to as "genetic hygiene" (Turner, 2012). But given its strong association with the eugenics movement he developed the term genetic counseling instead. This term was chosen in part to avoid the association between hygiene and "tooth pastes and deodorants" as well as give an appropriate description to the process; which he likened to "genetic social work without eugenic connotations" (Reed, 1974). However, the beginning of our history that is viewed as canon is 1997's *An Oral History of the National Society of Genetic Counselors* by Audrey Heimler, which describes the profession's origins and how NSGC began (Heimler, 1997).

Here, genetic counseling history unfolds against the backdrop of several medical geneticists influencing the debate over the name of the "new" genetic counseling profession. One most notable was Charles Epstein, MD, who presented a paper in 1972 about who could identify as GCs in an effort to deter the usage of the term as it was presently "understood." From their positions of power (via gatekeeping and thereby upholding a system of oppression), some asserted that GCs should instead be named "genetic associates," further suggesting that the terms "assistant, aides, collaborators" would be acceptable, but not "counselor" (Heimler, 1997). This belief was predicated on the notion that "non-medically trained individuals" were not prepared to provide genetic counseling to patients, along with all that it would entail (Heimler, 1997). It was not only non-GC professionals who agreed with this sentiment. Some within the genetic counseling community, who felt their role was more so based in providing information and assisting the physician, agreed with Epstein by suggesting that "associate" was a "flexible title applicable to individuals who were not primarily counselors" (Heimler, 1997; Wilkerson, personal communication, 2022). But the belief that only a medically trained individual should be called a genetic counselor was an interesting stance to take given the history of both the term and individuals who first performed this service.

Notable shifts towards physicians providing genetic counseling began when the term "Human Genetics" was swapped out in favor of "Medical Genetics," when the ability to clinically order chromosome analysis became available, and when the demand for genetic counseling rose higher than the availability of Hereditary Clinics (Reed, 1974; Turner, 2012). But even with these changes and physicians taking over this role the belief that *only* physicians can do genetic counseling was never the endgame. As Reed put it, that idea was erroneous as "… not all genetic counseling is related to medical traits. There are several other reasons why genetic counseling should not necessarily be done only by physicians" (Reed, 1974). Nevertheless, with little challenge to Epstein's pronouncement, Heimler recognized that "genetic counselors would have to define, and possibly defend, their place in the medical genetics community" (Heimler, 1997). Though Epstein was later able to reflect on his viewpoint as "foolish" and come to value GCs, the history stands as an example of gatekeeping and the demand for outside (of the GC identity) stakeholders to be "proven wrong" in order to respectfully recognize the field (Heimler 1997; Baker et al., 1998, pp. xv–xvi).

Though time has moved forward, this mentality remains steadfast as the American College of Medical Genetics and Genomics (ACMG), the primary professional organization of MD clinical geneticists, who revoked their support for H.R. 3235 (e.g., a bill that would provide coverage under Medicare of genetic counseling services that are delivered by genetic counselors) due to their belief that ordering genetic testing constitutes practicing medicine (Raths, 2020). This known history shows us how mechanisms of exclusion can operate and the way in which it can manifest itself with nuance. Additionally, this and the further history to be discussed are also lessons in the importance of implementing inclusivity as an endeavor and not just a performance.

History of DEI

Saini (2020) noted in a world view publication of *Nature* that "when science is viewed in isolation from the past and politics, it's easier for those with bad intentions to revive dangerous and discredited ideas." Grounded in this belief, the intersection of genetic counseling community stories and narratives with POI are enmeshed with the history of diversity training, which was born out of the Civil Rights Movement by Black Americans to resist and interrupt the cycle of being disenfranchised and devalued (Vaughn, 2007, pp. 11–16). A major shift occurred with the passage of Title VII of The Civil Rights Act of 1964, making it "illegal to discriminate in hiring, termination, promotion, compensation, job training, or any other term, condition, or privilege of employment based on race, color, religion, sex, or national origin" (Anand et al., 2008, pp. 3563–74; EEOC). Consequently, training in anti-discrimination practices was developed in order to avoid costly litigation, which birthed DEI training in corporate systems.

The rising in-group (e.g., white and male) sentiment of "reverse racism" presented itself in accusations of historically marginalized and minoritized groups receiving preferential treatment, animosity towards difference, and claims that those with majority representation were being excluded (Anand et al,. 2008, pp. 356–74). Fervor for DEI training declined in 1982 when Clarence Thomas was appointed head of the Equal Employment Opportunity Commission (EEOC) and relaxed federal scrutiny and accountability (Anand et al., 2008, pp. 356–74). Left to their own devices to create policies and then afforded the power to self-govern, corporate institutions reimagined diversity training with a focus on assimilation for success, sensitivity awareness, "adjectives" attributed to different groups, tolerance for difference, and role plays of discrimination (Anand et al., 2008, pp. 356–74; Greenlining Institute, 2018).

During the resurgence of diversity training in the late 1990s, the term "inclusivity" became part of the discourse. Diversity and Inclusion (D&I) training focused on employees being cross-culturally competent by "building skills and competencies that enabled learners not only to value differences but also to be able to utilize them in making better business decisions" (Anand et al., 2008, pp. 356–74). In this new era, inclusion also encompassed identities such as ability differences, ancestries, religion, LGBTQIA+, and other worldviews (Vaughn, 2007, pp. 11–16). As demographics began to shift towards a "majority minority" culture, equity became more present in training and discussion (Greenlining Institute, 2018). As DEI work continues to evolve, devolve, and recalibrate, it is essential to be mindful of the precarious nature of its emergence, centered on those with intentions to avoid being considered discriminatory rather than disrupting the practices of discrimination themselves. Herein lies an imperative that the work of POI is to focus on those who have experienced the offense and not on their offenders and their primary desires to avoid discomfort, being identified in the harm they caused, and/or avoiding accountability that serves others.

History of DEI in Genetic Counseling

Meanwhile, during these historical national movements in DEI, Dr. Lorna Wilkerson (1987) offered the first diversity workshop focused on cultural issues (influencing patient care, inter-, and intra-professional relationships) at the 1985 NSGC Annual Education Conference (AEC). During a time that 3% of NSGC members were estimated to identify as minorities, the aim for Wilkerson's workshop (1987) was "to see the inclusion of relevant and up-to-date information on cultural diversity in genetic counseling stressed in all the training programs." Prior to the conference, the Minority Issues Sub-Committee of the Social Issues Committee was formed and those of all backgrounds, including white GCs, were encouraged to join (Wilkerson, 1987). Attendance for the workshop was close to none and white GCs "expressed concern over the idea of a 'collusion' of minority counselors" (Wilkerson, 1987), parallel to verbiage used by present-day white supremacists, separatists, and great replacement theorists (Berbrier, 2000; Cottrell and Neuberg, 2005; Brown, 2009; Consentino, 2020; Obaidi et al., 2022).

Until 1993, no systematic curriculum regarding GCs of diverse cultures existed, which motivated the development of *The Handbook of Cross-Cultural Genetic Counseling* by Dr. Vivian Ota Wang (1998). Dr Ota Wang (1998) assessed the implementation of the handbook curriculum by surveying genetic counseling students and then meeting with program leadership. Although the curriculum was shown to be effective at increasing multicultural counseling competence, programs and faculty were still hesitant with its incorporation. "While most genetic counselors, students, and program directors may intellectually acknowledge and respect the necessity of multicultural genetic counseling education, the emotionality (e.g., feelings of anxiety, uncertainty, anger, and guilt) created by multicultural issues may also leave them consciously or unconsciously reluctant to taking the necessary self-evaluative steps toward achieving greater multicultural counseling competency" (Ota Wang, 1998). Similarly, Dr. Wilkerson observed in 1987 that "even if it is meant with love and good will, suggestions of change can often fuel a very defensive reaction." Consensus among program leadership was that adequate knowledge of multicultural counseling could be achieved in 10 hours *or less* of curriculum over a two-year training program (Ota Wang, 1998). Despite efforts to quantify and fast-track DEI work, presently there is no recognized level of "competence" to achieve and these efforts fail to acknowledge how the "self" work required for POI emerges over a lifetime, not hours.

PAUSE.

What do you know of the history of genetic counseling? What positions of power and privilege do those who have shared genetic counseling history (known by you) hold in the system? What does this historical context and who is centered in it mean to you? How does history impact your POI and ways you relate to patients and others in the genetic counseling community? What else would you like to know about the history of the profession you are currently training to be a part of?

Significance of Context

All context matters as you explore your POI and the systems in which you are engaged. "In a society that sees casual racism among its most powerful leaders, white people can ignore the power of racism all around, or they can choose to acknowledge and confront it." (Romano, 2018, p. 262). Where you choose to devote your energy and what (and whom) you decide to deny is derived from your positionality in the discourse of DEI. And the oppression and white supremacy inherent in determining context is worthy of consideration throughout the experience, exploration, and examination of your "self" in this work.

Inclusivity affects academic performance, professional practice, and overall wellbeing in one's personal life outside of their training or professions (Miller and Orsillo, 2020). The genetic counseling profession has repeatedly made the mistake of applying the same standards of evidence and "significance" used in academia to define real world truths (Ota Wang, 2006). In other words, the (spoken and unspoken) norms, rules, expectations, and accountability of the "in-group" genetic counseling community (i.e., culture) have been manipulated to dismiss issues of inclusion as existing within one-off, interpersonal interactions that are subverted as "exceptions" to "who 'we' are as GCs" rather than representing complex problems that function (multi)systemically. From 1982 to 2024, when the first Black genetic counselor began training to the current, shifting landscape of diversity among trainees and professionals today, MMIs in the genetic counseling community have been and continue to be treated as less than the visible and representative majority (The Exeter Group, 2021, pp. 106–7; 217–22). This context matters insofar as it echoes the truth in how the genetic counseling community POI operates and the ways GCs practice POI with patients, clients, educators, students, colleagues, and each other.

While more attention and resources have begun to be directed to these topics in genetic counseling, research results and literature are only considered for review, acceptance, and publication at the discretion of historically noninclusive, problematic institutions, by predominately white, female editors of the *Journal of Genetic Counseling*. This context could impact the productivity necessary for meaningful change. If context is only defined by a few (with visibility, titles, power, and privilege) and the narrative controlled through this biased channel, then it is not representative or inclusive of the many others who are intrinsically woven into the fabric of the genetic counseling community. Should these same few members of the genetic counseling community refuse to account for the impact of their power and privilege to take actionable steps to either be a disruptor or gatekeeper of the status quo, then the legacy of exclusion will consequently remain.

PAUSE.

What matters to you? Who has power and privilege to tell the truth and the courage to confront the reality of the genetic counseling community system? How is power and privilege being used to seek hidden truths, add subverted context, and include oppressed histories? Where do you stand?

Importance of Stories and Narratives

A story is a description of people and events from one individual perspective. A narrative is a collective series of stories from multiple people that reveals systemic sequences of patterns and influences thoughts, meaning, and decision-making of a community system. Stories matter. The narrative that emerges from the common factors of these stories matters. And, actively seeking and listening to hidden, oppressed, and erased stories and narratives of the genetic counseling community matters in order to be conscious contributors to the dialogues of POI and the broader DEI discourse.

Parts of the genetic counseling origin story and the current state of the profession reflect a lack of inclusion, which is rooted in external and internal forces that have persistently plagued American systems and society as a whole. The "official" history of the genetic counseling profession, as we recognize it today, was only documented from the perspective of a white woman (Heimler, 1997), which reflects the ways in which (un)conscious bias, oppression, and white supremacy/exceptionalism was planted at the beginning of the genetic counseling profession's formation. It is impossible to provide an inclusive and accurate history when much of it was never considered, published, or even recorded. Notable "firsts" in the field still remain unknown (oppressed, silenced, or erased) and many of these "firsts" remain difficult to trace because those individuals left the field in pursuit of more inclusive spaces and systems. A lack of representation of MMIs in the genetic counseling community may be attributed to several reasons, which include but are not limited to a level of exclusion, lack of resources, and absence of interest amongst their more privileged colleagues to enact any meaningful change (Baker, 1987; Wilkerson, 1987; Wilkerson, contributors, personal interviews, 2022).

The stories and narratives of experiences we present reveal truth in the reality of how perpetual oppression and white supremacy, overt and covert, have impacted MMIs within the genetic counseling community (and those patients, colleagues, and others engaged with it) over time. Zora Neale Hurston explains that "if you are silent about your pain, they'll kill you and say you enjoyed it." Sharing the truth is an act of solidarity and resistance to the silence. As the genetic counseling community continues to grow, authentic engagement and genuine progress require deeper exploration, examination, and reflection in order to form a robust understanding of history and how it informs norms, rules, expectations, and accountability in this system. Gathering and centering oppressed, silenced, and erased stories and narratives helps to weave the missing patches in the tapestry of the genetic counseling profession. Only then may it be known how POI may be promoted and sustained in the genetic counseling profession today. Sharing stories and narratives of inclusion and exclusion in the genetic counseling community will offer an infrastructure to better understand where you are in your phase of POI. Your transformation in each phase of POI within the DEI discourse begins first in knowing your "self," understanding history and context, and recognizing opportunities for change.

With the consent of contributors, we share unedited and de-colonized stories and narratives from a diversity of MMIs, who are either no longer engaged with or still exist within the genetic counseling community. These narratives were collected from 2022–2023 by public invite through various genetic counseling professional and social networks that amplify the voices and experiences of MMIs. Each narrative includes multiple stories of those with the courage to share, so you may understand the nuances of inclusion (and exclusion) more deeply. Maintaining the positionality that the truth is sacred and does not need to be translated, defended or retold through the prism of anyone else's perspective lenses, the authors have preserved and verified all stories and narratives from the listed and anonymous contributors of this chapter. We invite you to name and acknowledge emotions, reactions, thoughts, and insights that arise for you as you learn of only some of the untold stories and narratives in the genetic counseling community.

In the Admissions Process "Don't reinvent the wheel" is a cliche heard being conveniently used by program leaders and institutions to justify their failure to effectively envision how their training programs could foster inclusive spaces (Contributors, personal interviews, 2022–2023). However, new training programs are actually being built on the foundations of DEI, while established institutions are struggling to incorporate the same principles. For example, some admissions committees are moving away from application review processes that evaluate individuals solely based on numbers and rigid rubrics that are oftentimes rooted in oppression and white supremacy values. In a more holistic approach that places more value on experiences, reviewers from diverse backgrounds (who have the capacity to understand the diversity experiences being written about) are invited to join this crucial point of access to influence POI. The GRE, once a universal program requirement, has been removed from over 50 genetic counseling programs after research revealed that the standardized exam was biased in favor of whites, males, and individuals with higher socioeconomic status (Miller and Stassun, 2014).

Getting to the interview process is inherently stressful. However, it is even more so when you feel as though you have to make parts of yourself smaller, to seem more palatable or digestible as the only or other in the space. *"During the interview I wore muted colors to blend in. I made these choices deliberately. Drawing attention to myself as anything other than a good student was not my goal"* (Contributor, personal interview, 2022). When asked why they made this deliberate choice, they shared *"I shadowed GCs. I didn't get the impression of what this culture actually is: [the] sorority girl, club, exclusive mean girl thing that exists, was not something I got a whiff of [then]. What made me make these [clothing] choices in the interview process was that I knew it was a predominantly white profession and predominantly white women. And, I knew that there was a risk of being tokenized because they were looking to increase diversity"* (Contributor, personal interview, 2022).

After presenting independent, original research as a prospective student at a NSGC AEC, one contributor was personally invited to interview with a genetic counseling training program. However, they had previously tried to apply for this same program but were not considered due to a GRE score below the minimum program requirement. They were offered guidance to retake the exam, attain a higher score, and come for an interview. Upon paying to retake the exam and receiving scores that *"did not meet criteria for consideration,"* the program leadership decided not to grant an interview solely on these scores from a biased exam. As a prospective student, they demonstrated their knowledge, skills, and potential for growth which appealed to program leaders, but were excluded due to a socially constructed prediction of supremacy and success. After finding success with another program, they struggled with the board exam which led to their diagnosis of attention deficit disorder. The genetic counseling training program's subsequent boastfulness of progress by eliminating the GRE is difficult for this contributor to see, because this program ultimately excluded this contributor and continues to fail to acknowledge the harm caused in the past, while presently sharing spaces with them. They feel they were engaged as *"a token racial and gender minority whose research and experience could be shown off, but were tossed aside when I didn't match other problematic standards of worthiness"* (Contributor, personal interview, 2023). They presently lead a successful genetic counseling career, with authorship of research publications, involvement in the development of a genetic counseling graduate training program, elected leadership roles on governing boards, and with NSGC award recognition, and they feel great pride in their work to allow the next generation to experience inclusion through various initiatives.

In Training and Education   The original study of Imposter Syndrome (IS) sought to make people feel less alone in their emotional struggles with an inability to internalize their own success within the workplace (Clance and Imes, 1978).

However, what the initial study did not do was evaluate the social constructs that impact the feelings of IS and what can be done to combat them. It is predicated on centering problematic issues on an individual rather than considering the systemic consideration of oppression and white supremacy, the intersectionality of one's lived experiences that can produce symptoms of IS. The following was expressed by a then first-year student contributor when discussing their experiences of IS (personal interview, 2022): *"We were creating a student video that would go on our university's website and our program director wanted everyone to be involved, but emphasized [that] certain people especially should [be involved] based on their particular/certain backgrounds. She wanted a person who was from the state that the program was located in, a person who was from out-of-state, a person who took time between undergrad and grad school, a person who matched right after undergraduate studies, etc. A while later at a classmate's house one of [my] peers said out of the blue, 'No offense but the only reason the director wanted you in the video was because you're Black; she's totally using you.' No one defended me or challenged the suggestion, not even me. It was my first taste of how this was going to go. It was only a video, but based on that comment it was clear that they [e.g., my fellow students in the program] have certain beliefs for why I'm here."* Though the student was fully qualified and deserving of a place in the program, the feelings of doubt were exacerbated by the commentary from her cohort and thus created feelings of IS.

When we consider the principles of POI, an important concept to understand is the importance of belonging. As defined in "The Many Questions of Belonging," belonging is the evaluation of cues that indicate to one if they fit in or are welcomed (or not) based on observations, interactions, values, and past events that define a particular culture and environment (Walton and Brady, 2017). Belonging, or the lack of that feeling, was illustrated by a student (Contributor, personal interview, 2022) as they discussed how a supervisor told them that they spoke very slowly and wondered aloud if it was because they were from the South. Along with being the only Black student in the program, they now received constant comments about their Southern heritage, and the stereotypes that go along with it, that perpetuated feelings that perfection (based on standards of white supremacy) was the only accepted pathway, as any actions to the contrary would be called into question. To overcome Stereotype Threat, a fear and anxiety of confirming a negative stereotype about one's social group which can cause underperformance in evaluative situations, individuals have to work harder to maintain performance, which can cause stress in other domains of their lives (Casad and Bryant, 2016). Exemplified by the student in this story, *"The last thing you want to do in grad school is feel isolated, alone, and double-othered"* (Contributor, personal interview, 2022).

An international student discussed the recurring patterns of being made to feel "othered" by their program and faculty (Contributor, personal interview, 2022). Their badge was labeled as "special volunteer" instead of genetic counseling student, they were not eligible for the stipend all their other classmates (with citizenship status) had access to, and offensive and inappropriate comments were made regarding immigrants. Instead of acknowledging the impact of the harm xenophobic comments caused, their program director advised them that this behavior towards international students was *"normal"* and (negative) peace amongst the cohort was privileged over attending to discriminatory rhetoric. These actions left them feeling as if they *"didn't belong"* (within the genetic counseling community) and led them towards a "nontraditional" genetic counseling role, rather than pursuing certification in genetic counseling. After years of reflection, they felt that *"there are people leaving this field because you [the genetic counseling community] haven't let them have a place here."* This sentiment was echoed by a graduate who was now able to not only reflect upon their time as a student, but view their former institution through the eyes of a now potential employer:

> The NSGC AEC was never a welcoming space to me. The days I spent there were just a reminder of all the microaggressions I endured from supervisors and classmates, and then the subsequent need to push those thoughts aside as I had to get through "polite" conversations during the conference. So, I stopped going. However, years later I started to connect more with my grad program and a few current students, so I decided to go back to the AEC to see if anything had changed. I ran into a former supervisor and the conversation drifted towards how a current student was doing. Though that supervisor was still very heavily involved with the program, they claimed to not know this particular GC student. Mind you, the 1st and 2nd year classes combined amounted to less than 15 students and this student was the only one of color. But they continued denying they knew the student until, magically they knew who I was talking about.
>
> What came next was a torrent of anecdotes, all depicting the student as "performing poorly," "having a hard time," and overall "not doing well." This supervisor wasn't aware of my mentorship with this student and how well I knew them. And, most importantly that I knew how this student was being treated by the program. What was so striking to me was though this supervisor may have just been speaking with a "former student" they were also speaking to a potential employer of this and other GC graduates, as my company was hiring.
>
> Or maybe that was the point, to impair the employability of this student. There's a lot of hushed talk of backdoor references and their rampant nature in our community. It was an eye-opening experience to see it done in real time, with little concern given to its future impact on the student on the part of the storyteller. There's much to be said about leaving the past in the past. However, what this community has taught me is even if you are able to move forward, there will still be those who wish to shape your future. (Contributor, personal interview, 2022).

In Patient Care   *"It was just, 'This is genetics.' This is what we can test for. It didn't really come with the historical or cultural context"* (Contributor, personal interview, 2022). This frank recount of training in the 1980s highlights the lack of education of our field's roots in eugenics and continuations of harmful practices due to this willful ignorance. *"I remember one patient. Her fetus was* *trisomy 18. She was hellbent on having that kid and they would go, 'Didn't you explain to her?' That was a life lesson that I learned when I had people who decided that they were going to have these children because the way it was, [the program] was, a lot of the counselors [were], 'Okay, you're gonna tell them they have trisomy ... they're gonna have whatever they're gonna have ... let's make sure we get the resources set up for their terminations,' because that was presumed what they would do."* The focus in training seemed to be based on the assumption that parents would choose to terminate affected fetuses and lacked sufficient training for GCs to attend to the needs of patients and their families in supporting a child with a disability (Contributor, personal interview, 2022) (Rapp, 1993; Asch, 1999).

With the lack of resources available in poor and racial and ethnic minority communities, abortion of fetuses likely to be severely disabled was posed as the more logical decision (Nsiah-Jefferson, 1989, p. 328). Success of some prenatal screening programs were measured by higher rates of termination that led to cost effectiveness, referring to costs saved by individual families and by government programs who would not have to support a disabled individual (Wilkerson 1985; Asch, 1999). These attitudes occurred at a time where parents who declined obstetrical interventions, such as prenatal screening and therapeutic abortion, could be court ordered to undergo such procedures. This was based on the assumption that fully informed patients would not have a "good" reason to disagree with the recommendation of their medical provider unless they were unfit to make such a decision in the first place (Nsiah-Jefferson, 1989, p. 329). In 1987, it was found that 81% of court ordered, compulsory obstetrical interventions were for Black, Hispanic, and Asian women (Nsiah-Jefferson, 1989, p. 329). While this may be distressing to you as a current GC student, it is necessary to note that the concept of "nondirective counseling" was once novel and radical, while ableism was acceptable.

Furthermore, "nondirective" does not mean "without bias" as both directive and non-directive methods can influence patients when providers do not check their personal biases (Kessler, 1992; Rapp, 1993). Despite apparent deficits in training about disability, this contributor was able to develop their own practice philosophy to be more inclusive, *"I gave everybody the full package ... I respected you, even if you had a sixth-grade education. I was going to explain it to you or let you see the options, that is if you wanted to see it, and then help you decide, as opposed to 'something's wrong, let's terminate'"* (Contributor, personal interview, 2022).

At another genetic training program, a contributor remarked that *"Healthcare disparities weren't talked about, but they were evident"* (Contributor, personal interview, 2023). They were revealed in the way supervisors spoke of certain neighborhoods and how they treated specific patients. This narrative exemplifies the very norms of a system (and members of the genetic counseling community) with the power and privilege to marginalize and minoritize individuals, based upon a hierarchy of human value. MMIs on the other hand, have little to no power and privilege to transform parts of their identities that are considered "marginal" or "minority" other than hide or assimilate to that which is not considered "on the margins" in a system.

This contributor continued by noting that disparaging comments (not just one or a few, but many that are indicative of a pattern of behavior) were made regarding *"safety"* of certain neighborhoods and people were reluctant to work in those areas. All the while, students lived in those same neighborhoods (Contributor, personal interview, 2023). Codified language of "safety," "professionalism," "aggressiveness," "niceness," and so on are oftentimes weaponized to reinforce the status quo of oppression and white supremacy. The contributor further described that hospitals within some areas lack comprehensive access to genetic testing and some patients can't be seen at all if they don't have the right insurance (Contributor, personal interview, 2023). Regardless of the hospital, it was clear to this contributor that supervisors treated non-white patients with impatience and intolerance, and discrimination worsened if an interpreter needed to be used. However, during this time they noted that even if an interpreter was not needed and the patient's culture differed from the supervisor, the patient was still met with the same dismissive behavior. Nonetheless, it was in these clinic situations where the student felt they learned how to be a better GC, as they *"learned what not to do."*

A key factor of implicit bias is that it's automatic and unintentional, which means that one cannot "clock in and clock out" of these biases in order to not affect the way we work. In *Killing the Black Body: Race, Reproduction, and the Meaning of Liberty*, Dorothy Roberts discusses racial steering where health care providers "import their social views into the clinical setting" and steer Black women towards certain reproductive decisions (Roberts, 2000). From this book, below is a confession of a GC to Rayna Rapp in 1987 on this very issue:

> It is often hard for a counselor to be value-free. Oh, I know I'm supposed to be value-free, but when I see a welfare mother having a third baby with a man who is not gonna support her, and the fetus has sickle cell anemia, it's hard not to steer her toward abortion. What does she need this added problem for, I'm thinking.
>
> (Roberts, 2000)

Though the above quote was from 1987, another contributor can attest to similar sentiments they observed from health care professionals. *"No doctor would go take care of the Black women. The white doctors wouldn't go to these people in [my state]. I always grew up knowing that there's certainty [that] white people would never take care of us because my grandmother basically died, 'cause nobody would come to the house when she was bleeding out"* (Contributor, personal interview, 2022). After growing up witnessing their family members' experiences of neglect in the health care system and early deaths due to racism in 1960/1970s, this GC was motivated to address these patient care gaps by *"working where no one else wanted to work."* *"I never quite fit in, and when I would explain where I worked (e.g., Harlem) and what I did (sickle cell counseling) they would start clutching their pearls."* During their time as a prenatal GC, they would take hours-long subway rides in the wee hours of the morning to attend deliveries of their patients who lacked a personal support system. Word spread around the community that they had someone *"they could trust on the inside,"* someone they could be honest with about their hopes and fears and feel safe with (Contributor, personal interview, 2022). It is currently known that Black maternal mortality is almost three times as high as white maternal mortality (Singh, 2021). Though we also know that marginalized and minoritized physicians provide care for the majority of MMIs and underserved patients (Marrast et al., 2014), the proportion of care in this manner for genetic counseling patients is unmeasured and likely undervalued.

Solicited advice from a contributor (Contributor, personal interview, 2022):

Don't downplay people's culture or practice. Different is not bad.
Different for different. Be adaptable.
Have a level of respect for how people think.
To [teach and promote] inclusion among staff and students: give case examples, room to discuss and process, encourage openness …
For example, coping in different cultures and allowing practices that may not be clinically impactful but are culturally significant.
Promote listening to community.

PAUSE.

How do your (and others') experiences in admissions, training, and education intersect with the stories and narratives of the genetic counseling history to influence your encounters with patients and colleagues? What is acceptable "then" and may not be "now?" What is acceptable "now" that may not be "in the future?" In a majority white profession, how can you motivate the majority to serve marginalized and minoritized communities where they may not have personal gain?

What is your positionality, power, and privilege in this context and how does it influence your genetic counseling practice? Where do you find motivation to engage with what is unfamiliar or uncomfortable for you? How do you build confidence and prepare to go where you will be most needed? In what ways do you practice at the intersection of POI and unconditional positive regard?

In Research   One contributor (personal interview, 2022) shared the difficulty in moving forward with research that would help advance DEI initiatives. The faculty advisors and principal investigators had their own agendas that biased student projects. Advisors were reluctant to allocate limited funds for translators and interpreters to expand the participant base to be more inclusive. With the rigidity and length of IRB processes, cuts were made in order to complete the study and reach high enough metrics to *"make it count."* This contributor's advising team prioritized and privileged statistical power when designing the study rather than considering the meaning and purpose. And, the student was not in a position of power to dissent.

Some students have had such harmful experiences (beyond that of inclusion) in their genetic counseling training programs that they have dissociated from the entire experience altogether, even if it means neglecting once meaningful initiatives and projects. One contributor revealed, "*I never published my thesis. The experience is so painful still. I couldn't bring myself to, so it took a lot away from me, but it's also taking a lot away from the community as well.*" They felt their optimism and motivation was slowly "*squashed*" and depleted by each racist or xenophobic incident. By the time it came to celebrate and amplify their work, they didn't have the energy or bandwidth left to engage. They feel guilt that they don't have the capacity to continue to engage in their genetic counseling community and in their research like they once hoped, but instead are taking time to focus on healing and finding their joy in it again (Contributor, personal interview, 2022).

PAUSE.

How relatable are these stories and narratives to you in your stage of genetic counseling training and POI? Where do opportunities to intervene for meaningful change present themselves? What power and privilege do you hold as a genetic counseling student and with your own identity to engage (disengage, distance, or ignore) with these stories and narratives? How do they provide context (or not)?

In Leadership Roles/Representation   Leadership roles hold an immense amount of power and privilege in any system. For the genetic counseling community, these roles also come with name recognition and, oftentimes, reputation and narratives that offer social capital to an individual within both micro- and macro-systems. Common tropes of MMIs can be manipulated and weaponized to justify excluding people from certain positions of power and are also used to create discord amongst the oppressed to create a scarcity mindset amongst those who are not represented by the genetic counseling majority (Contributors, personal interviews, 2022). As a thread in the narrative, if someone from a marginalized and minoritized identity "*causes too many issues*" or stands to disrupt the status quo "*too much,*" the reality of what little power and privilege they actually possess becomes more apparent. Access and proximity to whiteness and the power and privilege of leadership roles for those from marginalized and minoritized identities are often reduced as tokens to prove that a person or system is "*not racist.*"

One contributor (personal interview, 2022) noted that as a person of color, "*I have to work twice as hard as others in order to even be noticed by others. And even then, I know that if I make one misstep to disrupt the apple cart, there are a dozen others who are waiting to take my position to prove their worth (to themselves and others).*" None of us are liberated entirely from ego and desire to hold power and privilege in a system. You do not have to be white to be seduced and motivated by white supremacy and proximity to the power and privilege that it holds in our society. Thus, some MMIs may be made to feel exceptional to other MMIs, as though they were "chosen" by those in positions of power and privilege to make meaningful changes. Proximity to whiteness offers a false sense of power and privilege that may motivate MMIs to deceive, lie, and betray their sense of self and relation with others to achieve their positions. The concept of the model minority myth is predicated on the notion of being the better and a more acceptable minority from other MMIs in a torrid game of "oppression Olympics." Consequently, you might have certain leaders who seek "*goodness of fit*" or "*a good team player,*" which is codified language to mean those willing to maintain the status quo of oppression and white supremacy. Despite the truth and reality of these oppressive systems, common illusions emerge that can lead to thoughts of exceptionalism where "*I can truly make change,*" "*I'm better than others,*" and "*I can't pass up this opportunity*" become beliefs in an effort to move the needle forward.

While access to leadership roles matter, so do the actions of leaders, especially those who represent marginalized and minoritized identities. One contributor (personal interview, 2022) recounts a program director, who consistently called one student, a MMI, by the name of the only other student of the same marginalized and minoritized identity. As detailed by this contributor, "*Despite being told repeatedly of the harm this caused, [this program director] appeared to feign outrage of any insinuation that her behavior was problematic and made no attempt to account for her mistakes.*" This was not just limited to students, as this program director "*tended to mistake the names of faculty from overlapping marginalized and minoritized identities as well.*" In one particularly disturbing instance, in making this mistake during students' research presentations, "*she laughed it off as an innocent mistake and proceeded on.*" Another program director, apprised of this and many other instances of problematic behavior by leadership, "*dismissed the seriousness of the issue. Instead [the program director] justified the behavior and further placed blame on those who made the reports as 'the ones causing harm to the program and its directors.'*" This is an instance of program directors modelling for students and faculty that program directors are not to be questioned, challenged, or given critical feedback, because reputations and opportunities of those reporting would be affected "*in this small profession where everyone talks.*" Even more jarring for this contributor was that "*it was in a room full of bystanders (who claimed to be allies and took upstander and DEI trainings) and no one seemed to be affected by this behavior because we understand the negative consequences and how retaliatory program directors can be.*" This experience suggested that mistaking MMIs had become normalized, rather than an being an incident of exception. "*Program directors using their power to harm others and their privilege to ignore the impact of their actions seemingly had no boundaries or accountability.*"

Currently, the genetic counseling field is seeing new leaders and faculty disrupt the status quo and employ innovative teaching styles and learning environments.

In this (r)evolution, emerging leaders are modelling how to be inclusive providers by first demonstrating to their students how to be inclusive of each other. Genetic counseling educators who are open to honest and genuine feedback from their students model the benefits and necessity of practicing reciprocal humility and authenticity at all levels of seniority and expertise. One contributor recalled program leaders modeling POI and experiencing its impact during their training (personal interview, 2023):

> *For a white woman who had been a GC for three decades to open a class and intro-duce herself by acknowledging her deficits, her privilege, and her intentions to also learn from us [students] even as our educator... mind blowing. From that, I felt safe to be honest with my leadership and my classmates.*

This contributor went on to share about a time their white classmate made a harmful assumption about non-English speakers. When confronted by the contributor, the white classmate apologized. They were able to openly discuss how their backgrounds influenced their feelings and reactions, including the white classmate addressing their initial instinct to get defensive. The contributor was surprised because they had never experienced confronting a white person about a micro- or macro-aggression and had it end positively. They believe the positive outcome of this interaction was largely influenced by the examples set by program leadership. Their takeaway is this:

> *My expectations will stay high and I don't have to accept excuses from people who refuse to grow and neither do our patients. For the privileged people who feel "this is so hard," they need to look at themselves and figure out why.*

Leaders may consider modelling the same level of respect and compassion we expect to engage with our patients and other health care professionals in the way they address their students. Those leaders who respect their students' gender identities by using correct pronouns and advocating for them to be addressed respectfully and correctly by others are likely more inclined to do so for their patients. And, those who deny or refuse to (un)learn their biases of gender identity and sexual orientation are necessarily prone to engage in oppressive behaviors towards others with dissimilar identities to their own as well. One approach to mitigate this normalized harm might be to attend to the homogeneous representation of majority white women in positions of the genetic counseling community's leadership roles, seats on governing boards, regulatory organizations, and positions (and titles) on graduate program training programs. While the previous narrative was exemplary of white women leveraging their power and privilege to be allies and accomplices to MMIs, this is currently an exception.

Multiple contributors were brought to tears remembering the first time their identities were supported after being dismissed, minimized, or having faced backlash from their peers (personal interviews, 2022 and 2023). One contributor reflected, *"before this I was feeling so defeated, but now I know people and clinics like this exist. Like, I'm not asking too much.*" Some contributors (personal interviews, 2022 and 2023) are still struggling to name the harm they endured for fear of seeming ungrateful to their educators or disrespectful of their expertise. Teaching students that they are to accept abuse by their superiors in the name of respect and to exercise "unconditional positive regard" for their leadership (that they are not in positions of power or privilege to also expect in return), will predictably increase rates of burnout and attrition by the diverse voices and minds we are already lacking. Contributors' accounts related to genetic counseling community norms of complicity, authoritarianism, colonialism, oppression, and white supremacy influence future generations of GCs to uphold (or not) this system or risk being erased or worse even, villainized.

PAUSE.

What is your experience as a genetic counseling student of patients, peers, educators, supervisors, and directors? What do you know? What don't you know? What power and privilege do you hold that contributes to your ability to engage (disengage, distance, or ignore) with these GCs' stories and narratives?

Contributors (personal interviews, 2022 and 2023) felt that movement towards inclusivity cannot happen when a leader …

… encourages complacency and silence to keep the peace: "*Being tolerant of being intolerant is a long-winded way of upholding the status quo.*"

… is defensive and centers their own discomfort: "*I always try to say as clearly as I can, 'I don't think you're a racist. But what you did was racist.' I do all the stuff they tell you, call out the behavior not the person, call in instead of call out, and so on. But still they're just so in their own feelings they can't see how they've affected me or others. Or they double down and you realize they maybe are actually racist [laughs]. Sorry, we have to laugh to cope.*"

… closes themselves off to constructive feedback: "*This is why I love the term cultural humility. [Earlier trained] GCs were already told they're competent and they don't want to listen to young people or people earlier in their career because how could we possibly know more than them? But if they showed some humility and let go of some ego, we could actually get somewhere. We're not trying to attack anyone or say that we know more about genetic counseling than them. We don't. We know they're just using the tools they were given. But they need to accept that there are new tools now.*"

Simply put, when it comes to systemic and institutional change, "*it needs to come from the top*" (Contributor, personal interview, 2022).

Inter-professionally In the context of men as a statistical minority in genetic counseling, their minority status doesn't equate to an oppressed status as related to greater society. Because of this, men encountering exclusion who have tried to bring up their concerns have been dismissed *"because there are bigger problems"* (Contributors, personal interviews, 2022). However, this attitude is a part of the continuing pattern of ignoring exclusion. While just one symptom of a larger issue, multiple contributors pondered if it would be easier to start with addressing what some have deemed *"smaller"* problems (personal interviews, 2022). It is necessary to interrupt the identification of the entire genetic counseling profession as ladies, sisters, sister chromatids, gals, SIGsters, and other gendered terms and become more inclusive of all gender diversity. Additionally, continuing to create policies, procedures, norms, rules, regulations, and accountability as though the genetic counseling community is only composed of white, cis-het women reinforces early characterizations of genetic counseling as a woman's job.

To center those who have the most power and privilege in a system poses an issue as it relates to engagement with other systems and other professions' perceptions of the genetic counseling community. A problematic characterization of the genetic counseling profession as being a woman's job contributed to the narrative of male physicians who saw GCs as their assistants and supporters, not independently qualified professionals and providers in their own right (Contributors, personal interviews, 2022) (Heimler, 1997). Notably, contributors who were men identified and acknowledged the ways they had power and privilege because of their gender despite also experiencing some hardships for the same reason (Contributors, personal interviews, 2022).

Another contributor felt fortunate to have had what felt like the ideal working dynamics with the geneticists that oversaw the pediatric clinics they have worked in and said,

> We have unique training, unique titles, and unique expertise. If everyone on the team recognizes that from MD to GC to nurse to office staff, if everyone can respect and trust each other to fulfill their role instead of focusing on the hierarchy, we could get a lot more done.

The working relationship was collaborative and not authoritative. Everyone had established and agreed upon roles before, during, and after each consultation and, in that process, had the opportunity to exercise their own expertise. Their working philosophy was that, at the end of the day, *"if you want the patient to have the most comprehensive care, you need to utilize each member of your team's knowledge and strengths and put all egos aside."* At any level or title, providers have the opportunity to be humble to the moments their colleague may know something they don't. And those moments are exactly why each person on that team is there (Contributor, personal interview, 2022).

Intra-professionally Disabled GCs report feeling devalued and dehumanized when their needs are overlooked and requests for accommodations are ignored or outright denied (Contributors, personal interviews, 2022). Some contributors report that supervisors, managers, and colleagues fail "*to recognize the barriers to access of the physical clinic space for myself and patients in clinic, let alone utilize resources to accommodate individuals with (visible and invisible) disabilities.*" One contributor reported stigmatization of their mental health diagnosis by program directors and "*rather than offering support or taking the time to listen to my challenges, they shamed and disparaged my diagnosis by 'just joking' about it, creating additional stress during my training*" (Contributor, personal interview, 2023). Another contributor (personal interview, 2023) shared that while they were shadowing clinics as a prospective student, who was living with an invisible disability, "*observing how some GCs spoke about their disabled patients in clinic was discouraging.*"

Hosting professional or social events in spaces that are not accessible to disabled individuals excludes them from professional networking, forming social connections, and engaging in educational opportunities that their nondisabled peers have access to. For example, the lack of masking requirements in the midst of a pandemic at the 2022 NSGC and ACMG annual conferences excluded immunocompromised people and caregivers from attending in-person. With limited content available online, these individuals had utterly unequal access to the conference. Assuming all GCs are nondisabled propagates inequitable norms, rules, expectations, and accountability. It separates GCs from patients who identify as disabled while perpetuating ableism and othering, breeding an even greater power disparity in the patient-provider relationship. "*It feels hypocritical to encourage patients to be self-advocates while at the same time not respond to or be allies for our peers who have been trying to advocate for themselves*" (Contributor, personal interview, 2022).

PAUSE.

How will you encourage patients to be active and advocate for patients in your care when some GCs are excluded from participation in their training programs, clinics, industries, or professional activities?

"*Something that caught me off guard when I was preparing to apply to genetic counseling programs was the recommendation to read 'the green book' and how often white women in this majority white profession, that have ties to the perpetuation of white supremacy, would throw around the term 'the green book' without ever acknowledging the irony considering the historical meaning of a green book.*" While they were referring to the distinct, bright green cover of the earlier edition of this textbook and likely had no intentions of harm, assigning a new meaning to a term that represents anti-Black racism and violence is another example of erasure of relevant history and willful ignorance to its enduring effects. Jim Crow and the Civil Rights Movement are not that far back in history and we will continue to have patients, colleagues, and leaders who have had to use a real "green book" for their survival for many years to come (Contributor, personal interview, 2022).

After the greater publicization of anti-Black police brutality in 2020 and the new wave of privileged individuals responding to pressure to learn about and acknowledge that racism and discrimination still exist, DEI statements emerged at academic institutions everywhere (Esparza et al., 2022). Towards the final publication stages of this chapter, several states passed legislation attacking and politicizing DEIJ. In some cases, institutions and states initiated opposing actions that significantly impact DEIJ recognition, representation, and funding. Contributors who experienced discrimination at these institutions and saw these statements felt reassured or optimistic, yet were still left questioning if what they experienced was truly rooted in racism, homophobia, misogyny, ableism, etc. Self-appointed "allies" and those in leadership roles seemed to have been presented with the easiest pipeline to become abusers, consciously or unconsciously, of the communities and MMIs they claimed to support. These individuals, being products of systems of oppression and white supremacy themselves, were perceived as presenting themselves (and each other) as "*competent*" and "*humanitarian*" enough to be perfect and infallible in the work of justice. Afterall, how can someone who has read the "right" books, listened to the "right" podcasts, and quoted the "right" activists be harmful?

> "*The worst part is these are the same people who scream anti-racism, and all that bullshit while making your life miserable*" (Contributor, personal interview, 2022).

> "*I'm so embarrassed to be a GC. I've heard about white GCs behaving badly. I saw it for myself in the things that people had the audacity to say in 2020 because I appeared to be 'on their side.' They made assumptions about me and chose to freely speak in the most offensive ways. Hiding behind humor and willful ignorance of 'we don't know what we don't know' seems to [be] the norm ... they know*" (Contributor, personal interview, 2022).

> "*White liberals are even more spiteful when you speak up because they think, 'How dare you be so ungrateful for all we've done for you'*" (Contributor, personal interview, 2022).

> "*The people that hurt me don't think it applies to them ... because they know the [DEI] buzz words*" (Contributor, personal interview, 2022).

> "*History is repeating itself. When will white GCs realize that not everything is about them and that when we gather in our affinity spaces, it is one of the only places of peace for us in this profession? Not everything exists to serve you and you don't get to claim supremacy in all the places, especially in DEI*" (Contributor, personal interview, 2022).

> "*GCs in positions of power and privilege will do anything to defend and justify their positions of authority and leadership even, especially if it [is], at the expense of marginalized and minoritized people*" (Contributor, personal interview, 2023).

> "*I have come to know that the most visible and vocal GCs, leaders, and programs had the most to prove because they caused the most harm. I don't know what it is, but guilt, shame, and denial seem to be relevant here*" (Contributor, personal interview, 2023).

"We had our majority white leadership team (e.g., white program directors and 'other' faculty leaders) stand in front of us during orientation to 'confess' their power and privilege in a performative announcement of a revised 'anti-racist curriculum' led by two white faculty leaders. One program director actually altered her voice to a weepy tone as she shared that her family came from immense wealth but travelled to 'the bad parts of the city' to help others. She seemed to force emotions of pain and empathy, but there were no actual tears or authenticity in her act. In contrast, the MMI leaders who shared their experiences of racism in the genetic counseling community were doing all they could to steady their voices and contain their tears in the white gaze of power and privilege of their 'superiors.' The white program directors using scripts in their performances revealed more than I think they intended to or realized" (Contributor, personal interview, 2023).

PAUSE.

What meaning do you make of the stories and narratives shared? What emotions, reactions, thoughts, and insights do you have of POI after processing what you now know?

REFLECTIVE EXERCISES

We need to hold ourselves accountable. We need to have conversations about inclusion and diversity but back them with actions, policies, and practices.

Alice Wong

Discomfort is a part of facing the truth and reflecting on it, which is inherent in self-awareness and effective learning processes. Engaging in learning inevitably changes you. Resistance to learning likely results in contributing to status quo. As you continue to reflect upon your own role in systems of oppression, white supremacy, and liberation and the beliefs, emotions, thoughts, and actions that have upheld (mal)adaptive patterns within them, you can begin to internalize the impact of your behaviors. Only then will you recognize how you can grow and change your POI mindfully.

Your POI as a GC

In addition to the spaces to pause throughout the chapter, this is a list of prompts for you to reflect upon your own values, beliefs, and principles of POI in genetic counseling. At various stages of your training, you may find that your reflections are related to varying states of your identity development and the systems you are exposed to (and being indoctrinated in to). As you become liberated to allow yourself to change, grow, and know your own truth as a GC, please be mindful of who and what you allow to water the seeds of your core sense of "self." As POI and the work of DEI is evergreen, you are invited and encouraged to continue returning to these exercises in self-reflection (i.e., reflexivity, cultural humility, accountability, etc.) iteratively, reciprocally, relationally, and systemically (Bronfenbrenner 1965, 1979, 1986, 1989).

> **Exercise 1:** Identify your own positionality and perspective of POI as a budding GC. *Who* are you? *What* is the context of the system you are positioned in? Describe your "*why*" as a GC. *How* do you deliberately and unintentionally practice inclusivity??
>
> **Exercise 2:** Explore, examine, and identify principles of POI in genetic counseling that resonate for you (or don't). *How* do you experience power and privilege as a GC? In *what ways* do you exert your own power and privilege in the genetic counseling community system? *What* are the phases of inclusion that you embody in the systems you occupy space in? *When* do you maintain and promote exclusion? *Describe* how you are becoming authentic, genuine, and collaborative in the genetic counseling community. *Identify* pipelines of inclusion you envision yourself in as you evolve as a GC.
>
> **Exercise 3:** *Name* the emotions, reactions, thoughts, and insights that came up for you in reading the genetic counseling community stories and narratives. *Identify* moments of resonance with and the times of dissonance from other GCs' stories. *What* are you holding on to that may be holding you back from sharing your "self" with authenticity? *How* did you engage with (i.e., receive, question, challenge, process) the principles, history, and context presented? *Consider* the ways you related to other GCs and how it now informs your position and perspective about POI in genetic counseling.

CONCLUSION

Throughout this experiential learning of a de-colonized perspective on POI in the genetic counseling community, you have been called in as a future GC to consider your positionality about POI in the DEI discourse. A recognition of truth will inform how you create space, take space, and hold space for others as a GC. You have been invited to seek, know, and reflect deeply upon the truth of systems in which you enter. Additional context for the known history of genetic counseling at its intersections with DEI, and more specifically POI, was offered in the collective stories and narratives of current and former members of the genetic counseling community. The unknown, erased, and untold lived experiences of MMIs in the micro- and macro-systems of the genetic counseling profession have been offered for you to explore, examine, and reflect upon in relation to your own and others' positions, powers, and privileges in this context.

In acknowledging your emotions, reactions, thoughts, and insights, you will likely have more clarity and questions with where you stand and the opportunities you have to impact meaningful change in POI. Even though you have come to the conclusion of this chapter, the understanding of your own POI and the epistemological origins of your reality throughout the stages of your identity development as a GC have only just begun. That is the purpose of this work. The answers to the truth and transformation in your understanding of POI cannot be found in the pages of textbooks, the suggestions of your supervisors, or the instruction of your educators. This is an eternal process for those committed to the justice that inclusion promises for a community. For you, the reality and the opportunity to pursue and be part of the changes in POI as a genetic counselor and within the genetic counseling community lie within … you.

ACKNOWLEDGEMENTS: CONTRIBUTORS AND ALLIES

Inclusion is a right, not a privilege for a select few.
Judge Geary, Oberti v. Board of Education

We acknowledge those who wished to remain anonymous and the following named individuals whose energy, experiences, thoughts, ideas, insights, and support influenced and informed this chapter. It is with these contributors and allies that we conceived and wrote about inclusion, inclusivity, and inclusiveness in genetic counseling together in community. And, it is with our gratitude and their consent that we share this offering for future genetic counseling students together with our contributors and allies.

We are grateful to you all, who graciously and courageously shared your experiences to develop a perspective on the phases of inclusion in genetic counseling. We could not have imagined writing this chapter without including your voices and energy in these pages. Your stories and narratives watered the seeds of possibility for this chapter to grow and allowed us to preserve the heart-centered energy of this work. In community, we stand in solidarity with and for justice for you and us all. Ase/Ashe (from the Yoruba of Nigeria) and so it is.

Lila Aiyar, Janel Barbee, Austin Bland, Claudia Borodziuk, Jada Boyd, Eden Brush, Jason Carmichael, Amanda Chan, Gayun Chan-Smutko, Valerie Chu, Cheyla Clark, Jack Colleran, Jessica Giordano, Maylie Gonzales, Carlos Dominguez Gonzalez, Jennifer Eichmeyer, Grace-Ann Fasaye, Michelle Florido, Anna Gao, Shreshtha Garg, Damara Hamlin, Barbara Harrison, Sarah Jackson, Susheela Jayaraman, Shontiara Johnson, Sammy Jony, Kristen Kelly, Helen Kim, Neha Kumar, Zameena Lakhani, Priya Marathe, Carla McGruder, Mythili Merchant, Camille Miller, Vivian Ota Wang, Brenden Phung, Lex Powers, Nikhila Ramesh, Kyra Ramsey, Stephanie Smith-Jefferson, Cessalee Smith-Stovall, Anne Spencer, Tyler Stokes, Amy Swanson, Michelle Takemoto, Elise Travis, Janelle Villiers, Lorna Wilkerson, Carmen Williams, Alice Wong, Kim Zayhowski, Holly Zimmerman, and all of our past and present patients, students, mentors, advisors, and colleagues.

REFERENCES

Abberley P. (1987) The concept of oppression and the development of a social theory of disability. *Disability, Handicap & Society* 2(1):5–19.

Ainscow M, Booth T, & Dyson A. (2006) *Improving Schools, Developing Inclusion.* New York, NY: Routledge.

Allen KR. (2000) A conscious and inclusive family studies. *J Marriage Fam* 62(1):4–17.

American Board of Genetic Counseling (2022) ABGC executive summary: Diversity, equity, inclusion and justice (DEIJ) certification assessment report.

Anand R & Winters MF. (2008) A retrospective view of corporate diversity training from 1964 to the present. *Acad Manag Learn & Educ* 7(3):356–372. https://doi.org/10.5465/AMLE.2008.34251673

Asch A. (1999) Prenatal diagnosis and selective abortion: a challenge to practice and policy. *Am J Pub Health* 89(11):1649–1657. https://doi.org/10.2105/ajph.89.11.1649

Baker D, Schuette J, Uhlmann W, (eds.) (1998) *A Guide to Genetic Counseling.* New York: Wiley-Liss.

Baker TL, Diaz V, Sanchez GA, et al. (1987) Defining our cultures: bridging the gap. *Strategies in Genetic Counseling: Religious, Cultural and Ethnic Influences on the Counseling Process* 23(6):162–182.

Bahari, SF. (2010) Qualitative versus quantitative research strategies: contrasting epistemological and ontological assumptions. *Journal Teknologi* 52:17–28.

Baldwin JA. (1972) *No Name in the Street.* New York, NY: The Dial Press.

Bao AK, Bergner AL, Chan-Smutko G, & Villiers J. (2020) Reflections on diversity, equity, and inclusion in genetic counseling education. *J Genet Couns* 29:315–323. https://doi.org/10.1002/jgc4.1242

Bartky SL. (2015) *Femininity and Domination: Studies in the Phenomenology of Oppression.* New York, NY: Routledge.

Bell D. (1991) Racial realism. *Conn L Rev* 24:363.

Bell DA. (1975) Serving two masters: integration ideals and client interests in school desegregation litigation. *Yale LJ* 85:470.

Bell DA, Jr. (1980) Brown v. Board of Education and the interest-convergence dilemma. *Harvard Law Review* 93(3):518–533. https://harvardlawreview.org/print/no-volume/brown-v-board-of-education-and-the-interest-convergence-dilemma/ Accessed May 28, 2024.

Bell DA. (1988) White superiority in America: its legal legacy, its economic costs. *Vill L Rev* 33:767.

Bell DA. (1995) Who's afraid of critical race theory. *U Ill L Rev* 1995(4):893–910.

Bell DA. (2004) *Silent Covenants: Brown v. Board of Education and the Unfulfilled Hopes for Racial Reform.* Oxford: Oxford University Press.

Bell DA. (2018) *Faces at the Bottom of the Well: The Permanence of Racism.* London: Hachette.

Berbrier M. (2000) The victim ideology of white supremacists and white separatists in the United States, *Sociol Focus* 33(2):175–191. DOI: 10.1080/00380237.2000.10571164

Berry MF. (1995) *Black Resistance/White Law: A History of Constitutional Racism in America.* New York, NY: Penguin.

Boeckmann C. (2000) *A Question of Character: Scientific Racism and the Genres of American Fiction, 1892–1912.* Tuscaloosa, AL: University of Alabama Press.

Bonilla-Silva E & Forman TA. (2000) "I Am Not a Racist But...": Mapping white college students' racial ideology in the USA. *Discourse & Soc* 11(1):50–85.

Bonilla-Silva E. (1997) Rethinking racism: toward a structural interpretation. *Am Soc Rev* 62(3):465–480. https://doi.org/10.2307/2657316

Borkowski N & Meese KA. (2020) *Organizational Behavior in Health Care*. Burlington, MA: Jones & Bartlett Learning.

Bourke J. (2018) *Deloitte Review*, Issue 22. https://www2.deloitte.com/content/dam/insights/us/articles/4209_Diversity-and-inclusion-revolution/DI_Diversity-and-inclusion-revolution.pdf Accessed May 28, 2024.

Brewer MB. (1999) The psychology of prejudice: ingroup love and outgroup hate? *J Soc Issues* 55(3):429–444.

Bronfenbrenner U. (1965) *Two Worlds of Childhood*. London: Penguin.

Bronfenbrenner U. (1979) The *Ecology of Human Development: Experiments by Nature And Design*. Cambridge, MA: Harvard University Press.

Bronfenbrenner U. (1986) Ecology of the family as a context for human development: Research perspectives. *Dev Psychol* 22(6):723.

Bronfenbrenner U. (1989) Ecological systems theory. *Annals of Child Development* 6:187–249.

Brown C. (2009) WWW.HATE.COM: white supremacist discourse on the internet and the construction of whiteness ideology. *Howard Journal of Communications* 20(2):189–208, DOI: 10.1080/10646170902869544

Browne A & Finkelhor D. (1986) Impact of child sexual abuse: a review of the research. *Psychol Bull* 99(1):66.

Chapman EN, Kaatz A, & Carnes M. (2013) Physicians and implicit bias: how doctors may unwittingly perpetuate health care disparities. *J Gen Intern Med* 28(11):1504–1510

Christopher GC. (2021) Truth, racial healing, and transformation: creating public sentiment *Health Equity* 5(1):668–674. DOI: 10.1089/heq.2021.29008.ncl.

Clance PR & Imes SA. (1978) The imposter phenomenon in high achieving women: Dynamics and therapeutic intervention. *Psychol Psychother: Theor, Res & Pract* 15(3):241–247. https://doi.org/10.1037/h0086006

Clark C, Dyson A, & Millward A (eds.) (1995) *Towards Inclusive Schools?* London: Routledge.https://doi.org/10.4324/9780429469084

Cody ML, MacArthur RH, & Diamond JM. (1975) *Ecology and Evolution of Communities*. Cambridge, MA: Harvard University Press.

The Combahee River Collective. (1977) '*A Black Feminist Statement*.' pp. 210–218.

Collins A, Azmat F, & Rentschler R. (2019) 'Bringing everyone on the same journey': revisiting inclusion in higher education. *Studies in Higher Education* 44(8):1475–1487. https://doi.org/10.1080/03075079.2018.1450852

Cosentino G. (2020) From Pizzagate to the great replacement: the globalization of conspiracy theories. In: *Social Media and the Post-Truth World Order*, pp. 59–86. Cham: Palgrave Pivot.

Cottrell CA & Neuberg SL. (2005) Different emotional reactions to different groups: a sociofunctional threat-based approach to "prejudice." *J Personality Soc Psych* 8:770–789. https://doi.org/10.1037/0022-3514.88.5.770

Cross W. (1991) *Shades of Black: Diversity in African-American identity*. Philadelphia, PA: Temple University Press.

Cross WE, Jr. (1971) The Negro-to-Black conversion experience: Toward a psychology of Black liberation. *Black World* 20:13–27. DOI: 10.1177/00957984780050010

Dixon-Fyle S, Hunt V, Dolan K, & Prince S. (2020) *Diversity Wins: How inclusion matters*. McKinsey & Company. https://www.mckinsey.com/~/media/mckinsey/featured%20insights/diversity%20and%20inclusion/diversity%20wins%20how%20inclusion%20matters/diversity-wins-how-inclusion-matters-vf Accessed May 28, 2024.

Erikson EH. (1959) *Identity and the Life Cycle.* New York, NY: International University Press.

Erikson EH. (1963) *Childhood and Society.* New York, NY: Norton.

Erikson EH. (1968) *Identity, Youth, and Crisis.* New York, NY: Norton.

Erickson RJ. (1995) The importance of authenticity for self and society. *Symbolic interaction* 18(2):121–144.

Esparza CJ, Simon M, Bath E, & Ko M. (2022) Doing the Work-or Not: The Promise and Limitations of Diversity, Equity, and Inclusion in US Medical Schools and Academic Medical Centers. *Frontiers in Public Health* 10:900283. https://doi.org/10.3389/fpubh.2022.900283

Feagin JR. (1995) *Living with Racism: The Black Middle-Class Experience.* Boston, MA: Beacon Press.

Ferdman BM & Gallegos PI. (2001) Latinos and racial identity development. In: CL Wijeyesinghe & BW Jackson III (eds.) *New Perspectives on Racial Identity Development: A Theoretical and Practical Anthology*, pp. 32–66. New York, NY: New York University Press.

Foote MQ & Bartell TG. (2011) *Pathways to equity in mathematics education: how life experiences impact researcher positionality. Educ Stud in Math* 78:45–68.

Fredrickson GM. (1988) *The Arrogance of Race: Historical Perspectives on Slavery, Racism, and Social Inequality.* Middletown, CT: Wesleyan University Press.

Frye M. (1983) *The Politics of Reality: Essays in Feminist Theory.* New York, NY: Crossing Press.

Frye M. (2019) Oppression. In: T Ball, R Dagger, & D O'Neill (eds.) *Ideals and Ideologies*, pp. 411–419. New York, NY: Routledge.

Geary in Oberti v. Board of Education (1992): https://law.justia.com/cases/federal/district-courts/FSupp/801/1392/1945004/ Accessed June 17, 2024.

Greenlining Institute. (2018) Diversity, Equity and Inclusion Framework: Reclaiming Diversity, Equity and Inclusion for Racial Justice. https://greenlining.org/wp-content/uploads/2018/03/DEI-Framework.pdf Accessed May 28, 2024.

Grix, J. (2019) *The Foundations of Research.* London: Macmillan International.

Hammersley M. (1993) On the teacher as researcher. *Educ Act Res* 1(3):425–445.

Hammond JW, Brownwell SE, Kedharnath NA, et al. (2021). Why the term "JEDI" is problematic for describing programs that promote justice, equity, diversity and inclusion. *Scientific American.* https://www.scientificamerican.com/article/why-the-term-jedi-is-problematic-for-describing-programs-that-promote-justice-equity-diversity-and-inclusion/ Accessed May 28, 2024.

Harrell SP. (2000) A multidimensional conceptualization of racism-related stress: Implications for the well-being of people of color. *Am J Orthopsychiatry* 70(1):42–57.

Hawley AH. (1950) *Human Ecology; A Theory of Community Structure.* New York, NY: The Ronald Press

Heimler A. (1997) An oral history of the National Society of Genetic Counselors. *J Genet Couns* 6(3):315–336. DOI: 10.1023/A:1025680306348

Helms JE. (1990) *Black and White Racial Identity: Theory, Research and Practice.* Westport, CT: Greenwood Press.

Helms JE. (1995) An update of Helms's White and people of color racial identity models. In JG Ponterotto, JM Casas, LA Suzuki, & CM Alexander (eds.) *Handbook of Multicultural Counseling.* Thousand Oaks, CA: Sage.

Hogan KA & Viji S. (2022) *Inclusive Teaching: Strategies for Promoting Equity in the College Classroom.* Morgantown, VA: West Virginia University Press.

Hooks B. (1981) *Ain't I a Woman? Black Women and Feminism*. Boston: South End Press.

Hooks, B. (2003) *Teaching Community: A Pedagogy of Hope*. New York, NY: Routledge.

Hooks B. (2008) *Belonging: A Culture of Place*. New York, NY: Routledge.

Horse PG. (2005) Native American identity. *New Directions for Student Services* 109:61–68.

Jones CP. (2000) Levels of racism: a theoretic framework and a gardener's tale. *Am J Public Health* 90(8):1212.

Kim J. (1981) Processes of Asian American identity development: A study of Japanese American women's perceptions of their struggle to achieve positive identities as Americans of Asian ancestry. Doctoral Dissertation, University of Massachusetts Amherst. Available from Proquest. AAI8118010.

Kim J. (2001) Asian American racial identity theory. In: CL Wijeyesinghe & BW Jackson III (eds.) *New Perspectives on Racial Identity Development: A Theoretical and Practical Anthology* pp. 138 –161. New York, NY: New York University Press.

Kovel J. (1984) *White Racism: A Psychohistory*. New York, NY: Columbia University Press.

Lorde A. (1977) The transformation of silence into language and action. In: B Ryan (ed) *Identity Politics in the Women's Movement*, pp. 81–84. New York, NY: NYU Press.

Lorde A. (1981) The uses of anger. *WSQ* 25(1/2):278–285.

Lorde A. (2003) The master's tools will never dismantle the master's house. In: R Lewis and S Mills (eds) *Feminist Postcolonial Theory: A Reader*, p. 27. New York, NY: Routledge.

Lorde A. (2012) *Sister Outsider: Essays and Speeches*. Berkeley, CA: Crossing Press.

Lorde A. (2020) *The Cancer Journals*. London: Penguin.

Lorde A. (2021) Age, race, class, and sex: Women redefining difference. In: J Arthur, *Campus Wars: Multiculturalism And The Politics Of Difference* pp. 191–198, New York, NY: Routledge.

Luchenski S, Maguire N, Aldridge RW, et al. (2018) What works in inclusion health: overview of effective interventions for marginalised and excluded populations. *Lancet* 391(10117):266–280. https://doi.org/10.1016/S0140-6736(17)31959-1

Marrast LM, Zallman L, Woolhandler S, et al. (2014) Minority physicians' role in the care of underserved patients: diversifying the physician workforce may be key in addressing health disparities. *JAMA Internal Medicine* 174(2):289–291. https://doi.org/10.1001/jamainternmed.2013.12756

Martinez K & Truong KA. (2021) Opinion: From DEI to JEDI. *Diverse Issues in Higher Education*. https://www.diverseeducation.com/opinion/article/15109001/from-dei-to-jedi Accessed May 28, 2024.

Marsh D, Ercan S, Furlong P. (2017) A skin not a sweater: ontology and epistemology in political science. In: V Lowndes (ed.) *Theory and Methods in Political Science* London: Palgrave Macmillan Education.

McConahay JB, Hardee BB, & Batts V. (1981) Has racism declined in America? It depends on who is asking and what is asked. *Journal of Conflict Resolution* 25(4):563–579.

McIntosh P. (1989) White privilege: Unpacking the invisible knapsack. *Peace and Freedom Magazine* July/August:10–12.

Mendelsohn B. (1958) La victimologie. *Revue Française de Psychanalyse* 22(1) :95–119.

Miller AN & Orsillo SM. (2020). Values, acceptance, and belongingness in graduate school: perspectives from underrepresented minority students. *J Contextual Behav Sci* 15:197–206. https://doi.org/10.1016/j.jcbs.2020.01.002.

Miller C & Stassun K. (2014) A test that fails. *Nature* 510:303–304. https://doi.org/10.1038/nj7504-303a

Morrison T. (1984) Memory, creation, and writing. *Thought: Fordham University Quarterly* 59(4):385–390.

Morrison T. (1993) On the backs of blacks. *Time* 142(21):57.

Morrison T. (2007) *Playing in the Dark: Whiteness and the Literary Imagination.* New York, NY: Vintage.

Morrison T. (2000). Unspeakable things unspoken: the Afro-American presence in American literature (1990) In: FW Hayes (ed.) *A Turbulent Voyage: Readings in African American Studies* Third edition, p. 246. Lanham, MD: Rowman & Littlefield.

Morrison T. (2017) The origin of others. In: *The Origin of Others (The Charles Eliot Norton Lectures).* Cambridge, MA: Harvard University Press.

Nivet MA. (2011. Commentary: Diversity 3.0: a necessary systems upgrade. *Acad Med* 86 (12):1487–1489. https://doi.org/10.1097/ACM.0b013e3182351f79

Nonprofit HR. (2021) American Board of Genetic Counseling: DEIJ Certification Assessment Report. https://www.abgc.net/for-diplomates/diplomate-spotlight/diplomates/nonprofit-hr/

Nsiah-Jefferson L. (1989) Reproductive laws, women of color, and low-income women. In: S Cohen & N Taub (eds.) *Reproductive Laws for the 1990s. Contemporary Issues in Biomedicine, Ethics, and Society.* Totowa NJ: Humana Press.

Obaidi M, Kunst J, Ozer S & Kimel SY. (2022) The "Great Replacement" conspiracy: how the perceived ousting of Whites can evoke violent extremism and Islamophobia. *Group Processes & Intergroup Relations* 25(7):1675–1695. https://doi.org/10.1177/1368430 2211028293

Okun T. (1999) White Supremacy Culture. https://www.whitesupremacyculture.info/ Accessed May 29, 2024.

Olson J. (1986) Cultural Bridges to Justice: Training and Resources for Building Just Communities. www.culturalbridgestojustice.org Accessed May 29, 2024.

Ormston, R (2014) The foundations of qualitative research. In: J Ritchie, J Lewis, C MacNaughton-Nicholls, & R Ormston (eds.) *Qualitative Research Practice: A Guide for Social Science Students and Researchers* London: Sage.

Ota Wang V. (1994) Cultural competency in genetic counseling. *J Genet Couns* 3(4):267–277.

Ota Wang V. (1998) Curriculum evaluation and assessment of multicultural genetic counselor education. *J Genet Couns* 7(1):87–111.

Ota Wang V. (2001) Multicultural genetic counseling: then, now, and in the 21st century. *Am J Med Genet (Semin Med Genet)* 106:208–215.

Ota Wang V & Sue S. (2005) In the eye of the storm: race and genomics in research and practice. *Am Psychol* 60(1):37–45.

Pheterson, G. (1986) Alliances between women: overcoming internalized oppression and internalized domination. *Signs: Journal of Women in Culture and Society* 12(1):146–160.

Phinney JS & Kohatsu EL. (1997) Ethnic and racial identity development and mental health. In: J Schulenberg, JL Maggs and K Hurrelmann (eds.) *Health Risks and Developmental Transitions During Adolescence* pp. 420–443. Cambridge: Cambridge University Press.

Poston WSC. (1990) The biracial identity development model: a needed addition. *J Couns Dev* 69(2):152–155.

Purnell LD & Fenkl EA. (2019) Transcultural diversity and health care. In: LD Purnell & EA Fenkl (eds.) *Handbook for Culturally Competent Care.* Cham: Springer.

Rapp R. (1993) Amniocentesis in sociocultural perspective. *J Genet Counsel* 2:183–196. https://doi.org/10.1007/BF00962079

Raths D. (2020) ACMG Faces Backlash for Stance on Bill That Would Allow Genetic Counselors to Order Tests. Available at: https://www.hcinnovationgroup.com/clinical-it/genomics-precision-medicine/article/21121549/acmg-faces-backlash-for-stance-on-bill-that-would-allow-genetic-counselors-to-order-tests Accessed May 29, 2024.

Roberts DE. (2011) What's wrong with race-based medicine? genes, drugs, and health disparities. *Minnesota J Law, Sci & Tech* 12(1):1–21.

Roberts SJ. (1983) Oppressed group behavior: implications for nursing. *ANS Adv Nurs Sci* 5(4):21–30.

Roberts SJ. (2000) Development of a positive professional identity: liberating oneself from the oppressor within. *ANS Adv Nurs Sci* 22(4):71–82.

Romano MJ. (2018) White privilege in a white coat: how racism shaped my medical education. *Ann Fam Med* 16(3):261–263. doi:10.1370/afm.2231. PMID: 29760032; PMCID: PMC5951257.

Rowe, WE. (2014) Positionality. In: D Coghlan & M Brydon-Miller (eds.) *The Sage Encyclopedia of Action Research* London: Sage.

Saini A. (2020) Want to do better in science? Admit you're not objective. *Nature* 579:175. https://doi.org/10.1038/d41586-020-00669-2

Saha S, Arbelaez JJ, & Coope, LA. (2003) Patient-physician relationships and racial disparities in the quality of healthcare. *Am J Public Health* 93(10):1713–1719. https://doi.org/10.2105/ajph.93.10.1713

Reed SC. (1974) A short history of genetic counseling. *Soc Biol* 21:4:332–339. https://doi.org/10.1080/19485565.1974.9988131

Savin-Baden M & Howell Major C. (2013) *Qualitative Research: The Essential Guide to Theory and Practice*. London: Routledge

Scotland, J. (2012) Exploring the philosophical underpinnings of research: relating ontology and epistemology to the methodology and methods of the scientific, interpretive, and critical research paradigms. *Eng Lang Teaching* 5(9):9–16.

Sikes, P. (2004) Methodology, procedures and ethical concerns. In C Opie (ed.) *Doing Educational Research: A Guide for First Time Researchers*. London: Sage.

Singh GK. (2021) Trends and social inequalities in maternal mortality in the United States, 1969–2018. *Int J MCH AIDS* 10(1):29–42. https://doi.org/0.21106/ijma.444

Sniderman PM & Tetlock PE. (1986) Reflections on American racism. *J Soc Issues* 42(2):173–187.

Sonn CC & Fisher AT. (1998) Sense of community: community resilient responses to oppression and change. *J Community Psychol* 26(5)457–472.

Sue DW. (1978) Eliminating cultural oppression in counseling: toward a general theory. *J Couns Psychol* 25(5):419.

Tajfel H. (1974) Social identity and intergroup behavior. *Social Science Information (International Social Science Council)* 13(2):65–93. https://doi.org/10.1177/053901847401300204

Tajfel H, Turner JC, Austin WG, & Worchel S. (1979) An integrative theory of intergroup conflict. In: MJ Hatch and M Schultz (eds.) *Organizational Identity: A Reader*. Oxford: Oxford University Press.

Tajfel H & Turner JC. (2004) The social identity theory of intergroup behavior. In: JT Jost and J Sidanius (eds.) *Political Psychology*, pp. 276–293. New York, NY: Psychology Press.

Taylor C. (1992) *The Ethics of Authenticity*. Cambridge, MA: Harvard University Press.

The Exeter Group. (2021) National Society of Genetic Counselors Diversity, Equity, and Inclusion Assessment. https://www.nsgc.org/Portals/0/Docs/Policy/JEDI/NSGC%20

DEI%20Assessment%20Report%20of%20Findings%20and%20
Recommendations%20-%20Executive%20Summary.pdf?ver=7yIXuQLddI61mquIW
w2VVA%3D%3D#:~:text=Exeter%20administered%20the%20Diversity%2C%20
Equlty,%2C%20and%20inclusion%20(DEI) Accessed 17 June, 2024.

Trilling L. (2009) *Sincerity and Authenticity*. Cambridge, MA: Harvard University Press.

Turner AL. (2012) Will My Baby Be Normal? A History of Genetic Counseling in the United States, 1940-1970. MA Thesis, University of Oregon https://citeseerx.ist.psu.edu/document?repid=rep1&type=pdf&doi=3185183bcd412f7a2de8837e5dc496d7c6e248df Accessed May 29, 2024.

United States Equal Employment Opportunity Commission (EEOC). Washington, DC.

Vellend M. (2010) Conceptual synthesis in community ecology. *Q Rev Biol* 85(2):183–206.

Van Dijk TA. (1993) *Elite Discourse and Racism*. Thousand Oaks, CA: Sage Publications, Inc. https://doi.org/10.4135/9781483326184

Van Ryn M & Fu SS. (2003) Paved with good intentions: do public health and human service providers contribute to racial/ethnic disparities in health? *Am J Public Health* 93(2):248–255.

Vaughn BE. (2007) Strategic diversity and inclusion. Management Magazine 1(1):11– 16. DTUI.com Publications Division.

Walker LE. (1989) *Terrifying Love: Why Battered Women Kill and How Society Responds*. New York, NY: Harper & Row Publishers.

Walker LE. (1977) Who are the battered women? *Frontiers: A Journal of Women Studies*, 2(1):52–57. https://doi.org/10.2307/3346107

Walton GM & Brady ST. (2017) The many questions of belonging. In: AJ Elliot, CS Dweck, & DS Yeager (eds.) *Handbook of Competence and Motivation: Theory and Application*. New York, NY: The Guilford Press.

Wang V & Punales-Morejon D. (1992) Evaluating cultural awareness, knowledge, and skills: a prototype for the development of multiculturalism in genetic counseling. Paper presented at the 1992 Annual Education Conference of the National Society of Genetic Counseling, San Francisco, CA. *J Genet Counsel* 1(abst):340–341.

Wellman DT. (1993) *Portraits of White Racism*. Cambridge: Cambridge University Press.

Whittaker RH. (1970) *Communities and Ecosystems*. New York, NY: MacMillan.

Widom CS & Ames MA. (1994) Criminal consequences of childhood sexual victimization. *Child Abuse & Neglect* 18(4):303–318.

Wilkerson L. (1985) Defining our Cultures Workshop. 5th National Society of Genetic Counselors National Conference. Salt Lake City, UT.

Wilkerson L. (1987) Defining our cultures: bridging the gap (Introduction). *Strategies in Genetic Counseling: Religious, Cultural and Ethnic Influences on the Counseling Process* 23(6):162–163.

Williams DA, Berger JB, & McClendon SA. (2005) *Toward a Model of Inclusive Excellence and Change in Postsecondary Institutions* p. 39. Washington, DC: Association of American Colleges and Universities.

Wong A (ed). (2020) *Disability Visibility: First-Person Stories from the Twenty-First Century*. New York, NY: Vintage.

Wong A (ed). (2018) *Resistance and Hope: Essays by Disabled People*. Disability Visibility Project. https://disabilityvisibilityproject.com/ Accessed May 28, 2024.

Wong A. (2000) The work of disabled women seeking reproductive health care. *Sexuality and Disability* 18(4):301–306.

Wong A. (2022) *Year of the Tiger: An Activist's Life*. New York, NY: Vintage.

Zheng L. (2022) *LinkedIn* post.

10

Health Disparities and Opportunities for Equity in Genetic Counseling

Nadine Channaoui, Altovise T. Ewing-Crawford,
Barbara W. Harrison, and Vivian Y. Pan

INTRODUCTION

Genetic and genomic information is increasingly utilized in health care, heralding a precision medicine era in which prevention and treatment options are individually tailored to improve health outcomes. Yet, the reality is that our medical system in its current form does not adequately, equitably, or reliably serve all individuals. Just as medical providers and existing structures aid in getting patients to genetic counselors, genetic counselors have an opportunity and responsibility to impact the medical care people receive beyond their genetic counseling appointments. The actions we take as genetic counselors can impact the downstream care patients receive, the confidence and ability they have to navigate future appointments, and the ways in which they understand their

A Guide to Genetic Counseling, Third Edition. Edited by Vivian Y. Pan, Jane L. Schuette,
Karen E. Wain, and Beverly M. Yashar.
© 2025 John Wiley & Sons Ltd. Published 2025 by John Wiley & Sons Ltd.

health and medical management. If the goal of medical care is to enhance individuals' wellbeing, then the goal of genetic counseling must also include enhancing the functionality and effectiveness of the system in which we serve.

This chapter illustrates a multitude of factors that contribute to an individual's pursuit of health care related to genetic counseling and beyond, provides context and terminology to characterize disparities in genetic counseling services and healthcare, and invites you to reflect on a public health perspective to move towards equity and justice.

EQUALITY, EQUITY, AND JUSTICE

The development of a durable health care system that is designed to benefit and serve all must be grounded in the principles of equality, equity, and justice. *Equality* requires that each individual or group of people are provided with the same resources or opportunities, whereas *equity* recognizes the differing circumstances of each person and allocates tailored resources and opportunities needed to reach an equal outcome. To take it a step further, *justice* recognizes systemic biases and addresses the fundamental causes of inequity so that everyone has the opportunity and resources to reach the best outcome possible. Figure 10-1 illustrates these concepts.

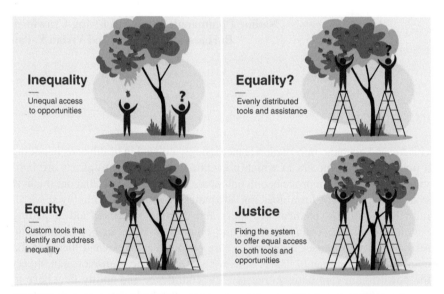

FIGURE 10-1. *Variations in fruit tree resources to illustrate principles of equity, equality, and justice Note. From "Is your data inclusive?: Optimizing results by eliminating the hidden costs of research participation," by A. Shipow and A. Singh, 2020, The Busara Blog (https://medium.com/busara-center-blog/is-your-data-inclusive-ddd59933f108). Copyright 2020 by The Busara Center. Reprinted with permission*

In Figure 10-1, the fruit tree can symbolize a medical system while the two individuals picking fruit can symbolize patients from different communities. The ladders, rods, and ropes can be considered actions of genetic counselors, health care providers, and others working toward justice in the medical system. It is important to note that although the shape of the tree seems naturally occurring, social and medical systems are historically constructed and reinforced over time to benefit certain populations. Our existing systems may seem natural or innate because they have been considered the norm for a long duration of time, but in fact, they are rooted in discriminatory practices and beliefs (Master of Public Health Program at George Washington University, 2020).

Health equity in genomics can be viewed as "the global applicability of genomic knowledge, fair and even access to genomic services such as testing and counseling, and unbiased implementation of genomic medicine" (Jooma et al., 2019). In this context, then, we must apply the health equity lens to all aspects of genomic medicine in our quest to provide quality services to all of our patients, including evaluating the sources of our genomic knowledge, the methods of genomics research, the development of clinically available genetic testing, and the process and delivery of genetic counseling. Table 10-1 offers examples of equality, equity, and justice in genomic medicine.

Health inequities and disparities

Observations of differences are expected in any population. Differences in health outcomes may be a result of differences in biological risk factors, environmental risk factors, and/or social risk factors. A difference becomes a disparity when certain populations have different access to resources to manage their differential risks, which then results in poorer outcomes in these populations. In other words, health *disparities* refer to the differences in outcomes or disease burden between disparate populations, health *inequities* are what caused those differences. Health disparities adversely affect groups of people who have systematically experienced greater social or economic obstacles to health based on their racial or ethnic group, religion, socioeconomic status, gender, mental health, cognitive, sensory, or physical disability, sexual orientation, geographic location, or other characteristics historically linked to discrimination or exclusion. Although these issues are not unique to the field of genetic and genomic medicine, existing health disparities may be exacerbated if we do not intentionally focus on health equity in the delivery of genetic services. For example, inequities in genomic databases lead to disparities in variant interpretation and thus decreased clinical utility for populations whose data are underrepresented in databases. The cascading effect of this may widen existing gaps in utilization of genetic services, reinforce biases and mistrust of the medical system, and result in worsening disparities in health outcomes between populations. Other known barriers to accessing genetic and genomic services include inconsistent and complex insurance coverage policies

TABLE 10-1. **Examples of equality, equity, and justice in genetics and genomic medicine**

Equality	Equity	Justice
Genetic testing lab lowers the cost of genetic testing for everyone so that testing is cheaper for everyone.	Genetic testing lab offers a sliding scale based on the patient's income and insurance status.	Genetic testing lab provides genetic testing to patients regardless of financial status. Additionally, everyone has reliable compensation from health insurance and/or subsidizing bodies to cover the cost of testing and any costs related to downstream care.
Everyone who attends a genetic counseling visit receives care in English, even though approximately 1 in 5 Americans do not speak English at home and approximately 1 in 12 Americans speak English less than "very well."	Genetic counseling clinics provide interpreters to individuals preferring to receive service in a language other than English.	Patients receive services in their preferred language from a genetic counselor who speaks their language and is able to complete medical forms in their own language.
All patients in a prenatal clinic are invited to participate in a research project, designed to elicit thoughts on prenatal genomic sequencing.	Because there is limited data on the perspectives of individuals from marginalized backgrounds, the researchers engage leaders from targeted communities in the development of the research project, with the intention of engaging them in all aspects of the project.	Understanding that participation in the project requires time and effort, the researchers secure adequate compensation for all participants. Additionally, researchers partner with payors and providers to integrate validated research findings and participant preferences into covered health care services and interventions.

for genetic testing and genetic services, uncertain availability of technology and genetic specialists in low-resourced areas, low genetic and genomic competency among primary care providers, and use of language in some educational materials that entails implicit biases and/or perpetuates myths related to genetic services (National Academies of Sciences, Engineering, and Medicine, 2018).

Potential Dangers of Genetic Determinism

Genetic determinism is a belief that our behaviors, diseases, attributes, and overall phenotypes are mostly due to our underlying genomic sequence, while simultaneously minimizing the role of epigenetics, environmental, and societal factors (Dar-Nimrod and Heine, 2011). On the other end of the spectrum, some may hold a belief system that emphasizes spiritual determinism, and more importantly, that we should not use genetics as a way to predict or prevent disease since health is determined by existential forces (e.g., divine power or purpose). There is evidence that one's belief in this regard has an impact on ascribing the importance of sharing family health history and the value of changing one's health behaviors for the goal of better health outcomes. Most people fall along the spectrum of these beliefs; a patient's belief pattern can impact their motivation to follow through on recommendations for care and dissemination of information in the family (Hong, 2019).

As genetic counselors, we have a responsibility to explore and help patients navigate scientific information in context of their beliefs. It can be tempting for genetic counselors to consider a patient's health only from the genetic/genomic perspective. A risk of focusing solely on a medical perspective is perpetuating biases and wrongfully placing blame on individuals rather than seeing the structural context in which they are living (e.g., blaming an individual's eating habits on self-control rather than noticing a lack of affordable, healthy food options accessible to them). Historically, "genetic data" has been used to exploit cultural beliefs or reinforce discrimination; for example, research on the genetic factors of violent behaviors have fostered racial and sex-based prejudices, the search for the "gay" gene has also been controversial in its role in pathologizing sexual orientation and perpetuating homophobic views (Stochholm et al., 2012; Smiley and Fakunle, 2016; HammackAviran et al., 2022). The concepts of race (a social construct) and genetic ancestry continue to be conflated in research and literature today (Roberts, 2008; Jones, 2018). Indeed, the veneer of objectivity and "pure" science often associated with genetic medicine can be weaponized. To guard against the dangers of genetic determinism, we must acknowledge the complex biological, social, environmental, and structural factors that impact each individual patient's health and behaviors. To provide equitable care, we must center our patient's experiences— all of their experiences, not just their genes.

A PATIENT'S LIVED JOURNEY: CENTERING THE EXPERIENCES OF PATIENTS FROM MARGINALIZED COMMUNITIES

The next section of this chapter centers on the story of Rachel, a fictional patient inspired by the lived experiences of numerous real patients from marginalized communities. Specifically, this scenario is drawn from experiences of this chapter's authors. We recognize that we do not, nor would it be possible to, represent all experiences from marginalized communities. Of note, we provide a detailed description of Rachel—more details than a genetic counselor would be expected to know—as a means to center the patient's point of view rather than the genetic counselor's. With guided prompts, we ask readers to reflect on their reactions, feelings, and strategies. We also provide descriptive analyses that incorporate history, present-day systemic factors, and other situational considerations that may affect a patient's journey in genetic counseling.

Background

Rachel Cohen (Rachel) uses pronouns of *she, her,* and *hers* and is a 35-year-old mixed ancestry (African and European) female (sex assigned at birth)/cis woman (gender identity) born in Washington, District of Columbia (DC) at a southeast community hospital in 1988. The hospital, the only one in this area of DC, has since closed its doors (in year 2005). Of note, southeast DC is one of the most racially and ethnically diverse and socioeconomically poor wards in the city.

Rachel was raised by a single mother, Elizabeth, of European descent. Elizabeth was born and raised in northwest Washington, DC, a region characterized by a highly educated and affluent population.

Rachel's late father, Joseph, a gentleman of African American descent, was born and raised in a rural area of Georgia (GA). He had a high school education and worked as a blue-collar employee in a factory outside of Atlanta, GA until he died at age 25. While growing up, Joseph's family depended on government insurance, and Joseph seldom saw a health care provider. Joseph would share stories from his childhood where he and his sister were often required to visit a White physician who would "stick" them with a needle. He mentioned that he and his sister, Christina, often experienced headaches and severe stomach pains after seeing the doctor. He never understood the purpose of medication the doctor administered to him and his sister, but the fact that his mother had finished schooling only through middle-school seemed to frustrate the physician. These experiences negatively impacted Joseph's willingness to interact with the medical system, even into adulthood. He always said, "there was no need for him to go looking for trouble at the doctor's office." Joseph also expressed his frustration with the fact that he had felt the doctors never took his questions or symptoms seriously, and that they always used words he did not understand. As a result, Joseph's suspicion of health care professionals and disinterest in seeking medical care persisted.

Rachel's parents met and fell in love in Washington, DC in 1987. Joseph was unable to find work in Washington, DC, and decided to move back to GA until he could get on his feet well enough to move the family to GA with him. During that time, Elizabeth and 3-month-old Rachel lived in a rented basement apartment in a quaint neighborhood in southeast Washington, DC. Within one year of returning to GA, Joseph died suddenly and unexpectedly. It was not until Rachel was in her mid-20s that she was informed by her mother that Joseph had had blood in his stool for two months leading up to his death. Neither a medical diagnosis nor cause of death were rendered because Joseph refused to visit a doctor or health care provider, and an autopsy was declined by surviving family members.

Rachel graduated from a Historically Black College and University (HBCU) in Washington, DC. Upon graduating, Rachel's deep roots and commitment to her community inspired her to stay in Washington, DC. Despite numerous socio-political challenges within the area, Rachel always knew southeast DC would be home for her. Rachel was also passionate about the endless opportunities to actively eliminate disparities and foster equity across health, economic, and educational boundaries.

REFLECTION PROMPTS

What are you noticing about Rachel's neighborhood, upbringing, education, and parents' experiences that might influence confidence in the medical system? For example, how might Joseph's experiences at the doctor during childhood impact his pursuit of medical diagnoses, and how might this then impact Rachel's ability to recount paternal family history?

Analysis of Relevant Topics

Several issues arise as we consider Rachel's background and how it affects her interaction with the medical system. We will delve into some below.

Systemic Racism in Health care The existence of multiple layers of systematic and institutionalized racism in our society from America's conception has led to substandard economic, educational, and financial circumstances for disproportionate numbers of individuals from marginalized backgrounds. According to the Center for Healthcare Quality and Payment Reform, over 130 rural hospitals have closed over the past decade, and 30% more are at risk of closing (Center for Healthcare Quality and Payment Reform, n.d.). This phenomenon also affects urban areas, where public hospitals are closing due to lack of appropriate government funding and a trend toward privatization of hospitals. Another consequence experienced by individuals in these under-resourced communities is inequitable access to jobs that typically provide commercial health insurance, and therefore depend on government-based health insurance (IOM, 2003; Artiga, et al., 2021; Lee et al., 2021; Yearby et al., 2022). Both of these factors have a negative effect on health care utilization, accessibility of prior health records, and maintenance of long-term relationships with health care providers.

Medical Mistrust The medical system, as an institution, is wrought with practices influenced by racism, sexism, xenophobia, classism, and homophobia (Casey et al., 2019; Jaiswal & Hailkitis, 2019). This leads to not only generalized suspicion of the health care system, but also active distrust toward and reluctance to engage with it. There is a collective consciousness built by a history of inconsistent health outcomes that continually maximize benefit for those of the majority culture, primarily those of middle- to upper-class, White, cis-gendered, able-bodied backgrounds, at the expense of those who do not fit that demographic. For example, there are numerous instances of using enslaved people for experimentation based on an argument that they were "subhuman," yet the information gained from these experiments was used to inform medical care for White patients (Washington, 2006). Further, the primary reason medical care was sought for enslaved people was to ensure they could continue to work for their masters. Medical distrust is an adaptive response to historical discrimination (Box 10-1). Thus, instead of asking how we might "cure" our patients of distrust, we must ask ourselves what we have done to demonstrate our worthiness of our patients' trust.

In our story, we can see that medical mistrust affected the medical care received and sought by Rachel's father, Joseph. His negative interactions with the medical system as a child, such as being "poked" by needles without explanation from the

---

BOX 10-1. NOTORIOUS EXAMPLE OF RACISM IN MEDICAL RESEARCH

Through Reconstruction Era in the US (1861–1900) to modern times, there have been many examples of medical research with negative impact on communities of color, those of lower social class, differently-abled communities, and other marginalized communities (Randall, 1996; Reilly, 2015; Strauss, et al., 2021; Arjunan, et al., 2022). One of the most infamous examples is the US Public Health Service Syphilis Study, officially named the Tuskegee Study of Untreated Syphilis in the Negro Male, which was conducted between 1932 and 1972. For this study of the natural progression of syphilis, African American men who were economically and socially disadvantaged were recruited, deceived, and kept from receiving penicillin treatment. Participants were promised medical care to treat "bad blood," which was a guise for collecting biospecimens without the men's knowledge of the actual intent for research, in addition to free meals and burial assistance. Not only were the human rights and health of these 600 men sacrificed in the name of research, but their spouses, sexual partners, and children also contracted the disease. The eventual revealing of the atrocities committed by this study led to the writing of the Belmont Report in 1979, which contributed to the establishment of institutional review boards to provide oversight for research. However, to many in the Black community, as well as those who are economically or socially disadvantaged, this study contributed (and continues to contribute) to mistrust for the medical system. Unfortunately, despite the existence of human protections measures, unjust and unethical medical research continues to take place, further eroding the fragile relationship between marginalized communities and the health care system.

physician, were reinforced when he felt unheard by doctors who were not vested in productive physician–patient relationships with him. This collection of experiences led him to completely disengage and refuse to see a doctor when he was very sick and likely had developed cancer.

It is critical to understand the legacy of medical mistrust and consider its impact on the genetic counseling encounter. In addition to potentially affecting the comfort a client with marginalized identities may have with health care providers (e.g., genetic counselors), medical mistrust can also impact the level of detail a patient has about family health history. For example, Rachel faced challenges collecting paternal family health history due to her father's experience of justified medical mistrust. Rachel had no way of knowing the medical cause of her father's early death nor what his medical history was prior to his passing. The absence of confirmed cause of death would then affect the genetic counselor's use of risk models and could even limit genetic testing options or insurance coverage available to Rachel.

Considerations of Personal and Organizational Health Literacy

Personal health literacy is "the degree to which individuals have the ability to find, understand, and use information and services to inform health-related decisions and actions for themselves and others" and organizational health literacy is "the degree to which organizations equitably enable individuals to find, understand, and use information and services to inform health-related decisions and actions for themselves and others" (Health Resources & Services Administration, 2019; CDC, 2023). Note that these definitions emphasize people's ability to *use* health information rather than simply reading it. Genetic literacy is more specific, defined as the "sufficient knowledge and understanding of genetic principles to make decisions that sustain personal well-being and effective participation in social decisions on genetic issues" (Kaye and Korf, 2013; Abrams et al., 2015). Individuals with low health literacy tend to have poorer health outcomes, partly due to challenges with sharing their medical and family health history, navigating the health care system to access appropriate services, and engaging in the decision-making process. According to the 2003 National Assessment of Health Literacy, White and Asian/Pacific Islander adults had higher average health literacy scores than those of Black, Hispanic, American Indian/Alaska Native, and multiracial adults (Kutner et al., 2006). Further, individuals without higher education or who never finished high school have lower levels of both health and genetic literacy (Krakow et al., 2017), and are therefore at a disadvantage in the genetic counseling setting unless the provider takes the time to ensure patient understanding. The Agency for Healthcare Research and Quality (2024) encourages practitioners to implement "health literacy universal precautions", which provide a supportive environment for all patients, including those with lower health literacy levels. This includes utilizing simple communication, confirming understanding at regular intervals, and making the practice environment easier to navigate. Indeed, these precautions align with principles of client-centered genetic counseling and their implementation should be considered in the genetic counseling setting.

PRE-APPOINTMENT

One Saturday morning in September at a public health community outreach event, Rachel learned about a medical service that had never been presented to her before: genetic counseling. She instantly recognized that genetic counseling could help her better manage her health and possibly prevent some of the diseases she knew ran in the family.

Rachel had heard that there were relatives on her dad's side of the family who died of cancer. However, a number of factors limited Rachel's ability to connect with her paternal relatives. Not only was her dad's side of the family limited in number, but her grandmother and only aunt died at early ages. Rachel saw the potential of a genetic counseling consultation to serve as the perfect impetus to reconnect with relatives and learn more about her family health history.

The day after the public health community outreach event, Rachel went to her mom and asked if she had contact information for her paternal relatives. After searching through a stack of papers for more than 30 minutes, Rachel's mother found a sheet of textured and stained paper with phone numbers and the names *Anna* and *Christina*. Those names did not ring a bell to Rachel at first, but Rachel's mom quickly told her that Anna was her cousin and the daughter of Aunt Christina. Rachel grabbed her cell phone and scaled the stairs as she dialed the phone numbers. To her surprise, someone picked up. Rachel was so surprised by this that it took her a little longer than usual to respond to the warm greeting on the other side of the phone. "Hello," the voice repeated. Rachel stuttered and responded, "Hi, this is Rachel. I know that this call is completely unexpected, but I am Joseph's daughter." Anna quickly asked Rachel to hold for a second; when she came back to the phone, she shared with Rachel that she was hard of hearing and needed to access her audio induction/hearing loop for the conversation.

Rachel shared that she had recently learned about genetic counseling and wanted to explore it as a service, since she was aware of their shared family history of cancer. Anna shared that she was quite familiar with genetic counseling and had actually undergone cancer genetic testing approximately two years prior. Anna also shared that she remembered the genetic counseling experience being slightly uncomfortable. Once she had informed the counselor that she was hard of hearing, the genetic counselor began speaking loudly and in short, basic words. Anna said she recalled the genetic counselor telling her that there was no gene mutation seen, but that her genetic testing revealed a change in a "braca" gene that had unknown meaning. Anna had figured that she would revisit cancer prevention and screening when she approached age 40. Anna left the genetic counseling consultation with the understanding that there was nothing she needed to share with her family members, so the visit was "out of sight, out of mind" for her.

Rachel took several notes about Anna's experience and proceeded to ask questions about their grandmother's cancer diagnosis as well as details about Aunt Christina's cancer experience. Rachel learned that her paternal grandmother was diagnosed with ovarian cancer at age 42 and that her Aunt Christina was diagnosed with breast cancer for the first time at age 45 and again in her opposite breast at age 49. Both women were now deceased.

Rachel recalled learning about a website that she could use to help identify genetic counselors in her area. She quickly determined that there were only five cancer genetic counselors within Washington, DC. She called two of the cancer genetic counselors on the generated list and was informed that the wait time for new appointments was over two months for each of them. The medical center where a third genetic counselor was located did not accept Rachel's health insurance. Luckily, Rachel was able to schedule an appointment with the fourth genetic counselor she called, who was based at a hospital over one hour away, to take place two months later. Rachel got a referral from her doctor's office, though they were initially reluctant to provide this as they had not believed Rachel to be at elevated risk of cancer.

REFLECTION PROMPTS

How might you prepare for individuals with differing abilities or who may need accommodation to optimize their experience? How might have the genetic counseling experience of Rachel's cousin, Anna, impacted the timeline of Rachel's pursuit of genetic counseling consultation? Rachel felt inspired to seek out genetic counseling after attending the public health fair; what do you think she experienced at that event that was inspiring to her? What might aid in the effectiveness of outreach for various communities? What factors might have impacted Rachel's ability to access a genetic counselor?

Analysis of Relevant Topics

A patient's experience with genetics begins before they reach a genetic counselor. Below we discuss some of the factors that may have impacted Rachel's experience and access to genetic counseling services.

Differences in Access to Family History   There are various challenges people may face to collect robust family history. For all families, healthcare has been different over the generations, including diagnosis, prognosis, and shame related to illness. Additionally, families can have incredibly variable communication with one another, whether that be regarding health or other life experiences. For family history to be shared and documented correctly, there has to be a trifecta of clear and accurate diagnosis shared first from provider to their patient, then from patient to their family member, and then from family member to their health care provider. As you might imagine, there can be holes in that pipeline of communication.

For people of color, there are additional considerations beyond those addressed above regarding medical mistrust. For example, systemic racism in American society has led to an unjust prison system, resulting in the rampant incarceration of tens of thousands of Black people, especially Black men, since the Reconstruction era in the US (approximate years 1861–1900). Indeed, according to the Federal Bureau of Prisons, in May 2022, Blacks accounted for over 38% of the prison population (Federal Bureau of Prisons, 2022), but only 13.4% of the US population in 2021 (United States Census Bureau, 2021). Historically (and presently), some people with African ancestry or Black race try to avoid discrimination by "passing" for White, at times dissociating from family to do so. Others traveled (and continue to travel) across the country to avoid racially motivated violence, Jim Crow segregation, or to find adequate work, as experienced by Rachel's father. All of these trends can affect amount and accuracy of family medical history shared.

For patients of immigrant families or immigrant lineage, there may be limitations to communication with family members in their home country or country of origin. Some families may go decades without seeing each other in person. Further, under-resourced medical systems in other countries may not be equipped to diagnose and/or manage rare diseases, and the limited services available may not be readily accessible to those who are affected. Influences of culture, belief systems, and faith can also reduce the openness between family members to discuss disease diagnoses, prognoses, and/or disabilities. This can limit the ability to collect family health history. Individual situations may also influence an individual's ability to gather family history information. For example, adoptees may not have access to health information from their biological relatives.

Inclusivity Gaps in Patient Communication and Resources   Given the substantial time, effort, and courage required to gather family health history—as demonstrated by Rachel's extensive efforts to connect with her paternal side—it becomes crucial for patients to fully grasp the significance of genetic counseling and of possible genetic testing. This awareness can serve as the driving force to surmount obstacles such as obtaining referrals, compiling family health data, or navigating the health care system to arrange a genetic counseling session. However, bias can exist in educational materials that discuss the advantages of genetic counseling and testing. For instance, these materials might lack clarity and accessibility in language (Early, 2020). Brochures may feature images that exclusively represent individuals who are White, able-bodied, cis-gender, and heterosexual, and these materials may only be available in English. While efforts to be more inclusive could involve altering images and providing translations, there may still be a lack of cultural context necessary for individuals to relate to and understand the materials. These deficiencies could have detrimental consequences, leading people from underrepresented backgrounds to feel excluded from the potential benefits of genetic medicine. As an illustration, information about genetic causes of breast cancer might disproportionately focus on Ashkenazi Jewish women due to the historical dominance of marketing tools highlighting the three founder *BRCA1/BRCA2* variants in this population. Although our understanding of breast cancer risks has expanded, the influence of these early efforts continues to shape themes of marketing campaigns. Notably, patient literature about breast cancer testing often neglects to include people with gender identity different from cis women, even though there are elevated cancer risks across sexes and genders who harbor certain pathogenic variants. For instance, if a Spanish-speaking patient with a *BRCA1* pathogenic variant conducts an internet search, they frequently encounter information in English centered around White, cis gender women. This exclusionary approach can further perpetuate disparities by discouraging these individuals from seeking engagement in genetic services.

Disparities in Referrals   Accessing specialty care in our current US health care system often requires a referral from a primary care provider. Despite professional guidelines from organizations such as the American College of Obstetrics and Gynecology (ACOG Committee Opinion, Number 691, 2017; ACOG Committee Opinion, Number 793, 2019; ACOG Practice Bulletin, 2020), the American Society of Clinical Oncologists (Hassett, et al., 2020; Konstantinopoulos et al., 2020), and the National Comprehensive Cancer Network (Daly et al., 2021), disparate referral of patients of underrepresented backgrounds to cancer genetic counseling have been documented (Williams et al., 2019; Lin et al., 2021). As advances in precision medicine lead to promising strategies of personalized care for individuals at risk for or diagnosed with certain conditions— including familial hypercholesterolemia, Lynch syndrome, or hereditary breast and ovarian cancer syndrome—these advances are not being optimally realized by individuals of minority racial and ethnic groups, people with gender and/or sex different from cis man, people living in rural communities, people who are uninsured or underinsured, and those with lower education and/or income (Khoury et al., 2022). This can have detrimental effects on the health management of these patients, as well as increasing feelings of mistrust of the health care system from the perspective of these communities. Further, a significant portion of these health care settings are underfunded, and providers are overworked, managing large numbers of patients who have not only medical needs, but are under significant social and economic stressors (Fiscella and Sanders, 2016; Essien et al., 2019). This can lead to gaps in medical management, and the possibility for both over- and underutilization of referrals to specialty care, including genetic counseling.

Limitations in Availability of Genetic Counseling Services   Traditional genetic service delivery models (i.e., in-person appointments in specialty care settings) have inherent barriers that disproportionately affect certain communities. Some challenges that affect the availability of services include the location of facilities where genetic counselors are employed, the limited number of genetics counselors, long wait times for appointments due in part to the labor-intensive nature of genetic counseling, and issues regarding reimbursement and licensure (Boothe et al., 2021; Raspa et al., 2021). According to the 2024 Professional Status Survey, approximately 68% of genetic counselors who provide direct patient care work in an academic medical center or private hospital (National Society of Genetic Counselors, 2024). However, 1 in 4 individuals who live in poverty receive services at federally qualified health centers (FQHC), which act as a safety net to provide health care services to rural and other underserved areas. Indeed, 10–13% of those identifying as Black, Hispanic, and Native American depend on FQHCs for care (Nath et al., 2016). Only 19% of genetic counselors involved in direct patient care are employed by public hospitals and FQHCs (National Society of Genetic Counselors, 2024). The lack of recognition and reimbursement for genetic counseling services by Medicare and some Medicaid plans has a detrimental effect on access for underserved communities in the US. If a hospital or health care system is not able to bill the majority, or even a portion, of their patients for services provided by a genetic counselor, this can discourage a decision to hire genetic counselors. For lower-income populations who depend on government-funded health insurance, their access to genetic counselors is therefore limited. Even amongst the population of individuals with private health insurance, the precedent set by the Centers for Medicare and Medicaid Services (CMS) has a strong influence on coverage decisions and may therefore have a similar effect.

In addition to the limited number of genetic counselors in the US, the time-measured workload of each genetic counselor is extensive (e.g., the majority of genetic counselors spend 30 to 60 minutes face-to-face with a new patient and another 30 to 45 minutes on follow-up for each case). Thus, patients often experience significant and frustrating wait times for appointments—both for booking appointments and for waiting room times—particularly in certain specialties such as pediatric or cancer genetics, and especially when a physician is required for evaluation (National Society of Genetic Counselors, 2024). Positive effects have been seen on health outcomes and on patient satisfaction when wait times are reduced for medical appointments (Kubendran et al., 2017; Lewis et al., 2018; Gorrie et al., 2021).

APPOINTMENT DAY

As Rachel set out for her 9:00 AM genetic counseling session, she gathered notes that she had collected during conversations with immediate and distant relatives. During Rachel's commute, she quickly found herself sitting in standstill traffic for over 30 minutes. She realized she was not going to make it to her genetic counseling session on time and could not run the additional risk of being late for work that day. Rachel was hesitant to reschedule the genetic counseling appointment for the next available opening because she would be starting a new job two weeks later as a patient health navigator/community health worker. That also prompted Rachel to remember that coverage by her new employer-based health insurance would not start until she had worked with them for four weeks. Despite the reluctance to reschedule and the obstacles in doing so, Rachel called the genetic counselor's office and requested to reschedule her session until mid-December (three months later than the originally booked appointment).

The morning of Rachel's rescheduled genetic counseling appointment had inclement weather—snow and ice—throughout the city. Though she recognized driving would be quicker than public transportation, Rachel decided it would be safer to take public transportation rather than driving her own vehicle on the potentially icy roads. Rachel was relieved to arrive safely, albeit approximately 15 minutes after the scheduled start time of the genetic counseling session. She was also glad to have saved money on parking fare when she noticed how expensive the hospital parking rates were.

As Rachel entered the hospital, she instantly felt unwelcome and out of place. Rachel observed that most of the people of color at the hospital were staff members responsible for maintaining the hospital grounds or cleaning the facility. Additionally, those were the only individuals who appeared to "see" Rachel and greet her with a warm smile and eye contact. There were limited to no clinicians of color who looked like Rachel cascading the hallways with badges hanging on lanyards, and this caused Rachel to question the quality of care, comfort, and satisfaction that she would experience at the hospital. Rachel approached the visitor's information desk to ask for directions to the genetics clinic and was told that she had arrived at the wrong entrance, and due to hospital construction, she would need to leave the building and walk around the hospital to get to the clinic.

When Rachel finally made it to the room of her genetic counseling session and before she could even take off her winter gear, the genetic counselor started telling her that they would have no more than 15 minutes together due to Rachel's tardiness.

During the appointment, the genetic counselor asked about Rachel's family history and recorded it in a pedigree. Early in the session, Rachel mentioned she had been raised by a single mother, a disclosure she soon recognized might have contributed to an abbreviated genetic counseling encounter. It seemed as though the genetic counselor had made the assumption that Rachel would have no information on paternal family history. Rachel was asked only about maternal family members before the genetic counselor said there was not elevated chance for a hereditary cancer syndrome.

As the genetic counselor prepared to wrap up the counseling session and exit the room, Rachel interjected and specifically asked if she could undergo genetic testing. The genetic counselor sat back down and explained that because she did not have a family history of cancer, Rachel was not an appropriate candidate for testing. Rachel pulled her notes out and explained that her father died of what was suspected to be cancer, her paternal grandmother died of ovarian cancer in her early 40s, and her paternal aunt died from breast cancer at age 50. Rachel also explained that one of her paternal cousins had undergone genetic testing a couple years prior and had learned of a variant of unknown significance (VUS). The cousin had been encouraged to recontact the genetic counselor or health care provider every couple of years to receive updates on the status of the variant.

While Rachel was interested in pursuing genetic testing, she was concerned about the out-of-pocket cost. Rachel had a new health insurance plan, which came with a new deductible. Although Rachel was worried about the cost, she did not raise her concern with the genetic counselor because she felt the genetic counselor was rushing to wrap up the visit. Rachel signed the consented forms for multigene cancer panel. A separate appointment was scheduled for Rachel at a nearby lab for a sample collection. Once the testing was ordered, the genetic counselor informed Rachel that they would notify her within 2 to 4 weeks when her results returned. Unfortunately, the lab was in the same neighborhood as the hospital (one hour from Rachel's home) and was open only from 8:00 AM until noon. These hours conflicted with Rachel's work schedule. Ultimately, because of the concern regarding the cost of testing, the pending deductible, and the scheduling barriers for the blood draw, Rachel decided to wait until January to undergo genetic testing so that she would have accumulated another vacation day at her new job and could take time off work for the blood draw.

REFLECTION PROMPTS

Often genetic counselors can view appointment cancellations, no-shows, and check-in times of a patient. On a busy day of clinic, when you see a patient has previously canceled and arrived late, what feelings might you have about the patient? How might that affect the way you provide genetic counseling to them? For Rachel, how do you think the genetic counseling session might have reinforced the lack of belonging Rachel had felt when she walked into the hospital? It is important to understand your own biases, as we all have them. What resources do you know about to explore biases you might have? What are ways you can demonstrate trustworthiness for your patients?

Analysis of Relevant Topics

Factors outside of the appointment can interact and shape the experience of the patient–genetic counselor relationship. Below we discuss some of the factors that may have impacted Rachel's genetic counseling experience.

Inequitable Distribution of Community Resources

In Rachel's case, recall the community hospital in her neighborhood had closed. This could have been due to inequitable distribution of resources rooted in biased political and economic systems, including racial biases and fragmentation of community health care. Further, the closing of urban hospitals can raise health care costs on individuals who must then go to other medical facilities that require additional travel time and potentially increased cost for out-of-network services (Andreyeva et al., 2022). For Rachel, even if the local hospital had still been open, it is possible a genetic counselor would not have been employed there. Regardless, she had to travel to a different part of the city to see a genetic counselor. The allocation of resources to infrastructure, including roads and public transportation, also created obstacles for Rachel to get from one end of the city to another, for her genetic counseling appointment, in a timely and safe manner. Rachel ultimately utilized public transportation, which is a common modality for individuals who may not have the financial means to have and maintain costs associated with a private automobile or, as in Rachel's case, for increased feeling of safety on unsafe roads. The time required to travel to a distant clinic can also be an issue for those who do not have a salaried job; time off from work may equate to no pay. Patients in rural areas may have to travel hours to access genetic counseling services.

After navigating numerous barriers to prepare for and schedule a genetic counseling appointment, there may be additional hurdles to an on-time arrival to an appointment. Balancing issues such as securing childcare, negotiating time off from work, and navigating public transportation can create additional stress as a client prepares to attend an appointment, and disruption of any of them can cause a client to be late for or miss their appointment. These issues disproportionately affect those from historically under-resourced communities; for example, missing work for appointments may not be an option for individuals who have been systematically siphoned into wage versus salaried positions. Inevitably, clients may be labeled as "noncompliant" or stigmatized for chronically missing appointments by providers, without adequate efforts to alleviate the cause. In the story, Rachel had to reschedule her appointment because of traffic and also wanting to avoid being late to work. Further, although Rachel was well-intentioned and motivated to attend the rescheduled genetic counseling appointment, the fact that she had to travel across the city on public transportation in inclement weather created an almost inevitable situation of tardiness for the appointment.

Clinician Implicit Bias   The role of implicit bias and the effect it can have when there is a lack of cultural congruence between the counselor and the client, particularly how it may affect the level of care provided, should also be considered. The nature of this incongruence can span broad areas of diversity: racial, ethnic, religious, gender identity, sexual orientation, ability/disability, etc., as well as less recognized factors such as weight. Although one may feel as if they are immune to or can control biases, we know implicit bias to be inherently involuntary, subconsciously influencing our thoughts and behaviors. There is a tremendous body of work on the impact of implicit bias in health care more broadly, and genetic counseling in particular (Schaa et al., 2015; FitzGerald and Hurst 2019; Lowe et al., 2020). Multiple studies reveal that implicit bias exists among health care professionals, including genetic counselors, at similar levels as the general population. These biases have significant consequences on medical care for patients who are the subject of biased behavior, including less tailored genetic counseling communication; questioning of symptoms, particularly pain, leading to delayed diagnosis (Hoffman et al., 2016); stigmatizing language in the medical record and transmission of bias among providers (Goddu et al., 2019); and condemning and inappropriate comments during the health care interaction (Sabin et al., 2015; Casanova-Perez et al., 2022). Due to these negative outcomes and experiences, many individuals from marginalized communities subsequently avoid interacting with the health care system, perpetuating health care disparities.

Clinician Trustworthiness

The genetic counselor–patient relationship is crucial to the success of the genetic counseling encounter. In describing the reciprocal engagement model of genetic counseling, McCarthy Veach et al. state that relationship is at the core of the genetic counseling process. Patient education, decision making, and psychological support can only occur if there is "trust, rapport and good communication" between the counselor and client (McCarthy Veach et al., 2007). As the authoritative figure in the session, the temperament of the genetic counselor can communicate a willingness to engage in a holistic interaction with the client—one that will meet both informational and counseling needs. Individuals from marginalized communities may not instantly bond with or assume confidence in the genetic counselor. This is particularly true if the patient is being seen in a physical space that is unfamiliar to them, or surrounded by people who do not look, speak, or share similar experiences as them. The value of racial concordance in health care broadly and genetic counseling specifically has been documented (Johnson Shen et al., 2018; Lowe et al., 2020; Palmer Kelly et al., 2021). Being in a strange environment and/or having an unfamiliar provider can be intimidating and cause patients to feel less empowered to participate in the session. Before Rachel met the genetic counselor, she observed the hospital environment and the lack of individuals who looked like her among health care professionals in the facility. Thankfully, this lack of representation, which was then compounded by a general lack of connectedness between Rachel and the genetic counselor, did not dissuade Rachel from speaking up before the session ended and advocating for a fuller view of her family history. However, for another patient, this narrative could have taken a different turn and the appropriate testing may not have been offered. One can also reflect on the experience of Rachel's cousin Anna, earlier in the story. Anna was hard of hearing and described the genetic counseling session as being "slightly uncomfortable." How the counselor responds to the needs of patients—including identifying and using an interpreter, accommodating family members in a session, taking time to acknowledge a recent loss, etcetera—is critical to how the patient reflects on the session and on the genetic counseling process more generally.

POST-APPOINTMENT

Three weeks after Rachel had gotten her blood drawn, she received a phone call from the genetic counselor confirming that a likely pathogenic variant in *BRCA1* had been detected, the same variant detected previously in Rachel's cousin, Anna. The genetic counselor informed Rachel that this variant had been recently reclassified and upgraded to likely pathogenic status. The genetic counselor also informed Rachel that while the laboratory that performed her testing classified the variant as likely pathogenic, a few of the other laboratories still classified the variant as a VUS. The genetic counselor explained that the presence of this gene variant in Rachel would be reason to follow high-risk screening and prevention recommendations for *BRCA1*-related cancers.

Because Rachel did not want to risk jeopardizing her reputation at or income from her new job, she decided to wait at least three months before scheduling her first breast cancer screening.

REFLECTION PROMPTS

How might it feel for a patient to learn that their genetic test result was being interpreted differently by seemingly knowledgeable laboratories and clinicians? What amount of responsibility do you think Rachel has to inform her cousin, Anna, about the variant classification? What might aid Rachel in having such a conversation?

Analysis of Relevant Topics

Each patient–provider interaction has the potential to ripple through to the patient's family, their communities, and ultimately to the society we all belong to. Below we discuss some of the factors that may have influenced Rachel's health beyond her interaction with genetic counseling.

Lack of Diversity in Genomic Studies The importance of including diverse genomes in research has been acknowledged (Wojcik et al., 2019), but to date, this goal has not been realized to a large extent (Sirugo et al., 2019; Jones et al., 2021). The historic lack of effort to include ancestrally diverse populations has led to inequitable analysis and utility of genetic testing. The prevalence of VUS findings is higher in individuals with non-European ancestries (Ricks-Santi et al., 2017; Kurian et al., 2018). Results that have uncertain significance and/or differing classifications can cause confusion regarding the meaning of the result, lack of clear guidance for follow up, and decreased benefit of genetic testing, which may then be communicated to others in the community and defeat efforts to engage others in genetic services.

Barriers to Receiving Necessary Downstream Care After Genetic Testing In addition to differences in practical barriers to medical screening, such as insurance coverage or transportation issues, differences in physician or other provider recommendations for screening also plague those of marginalized communities. For example, multiple studies have demonstrated disparate referral rates for colon cancer screening in racial/ethnic minority populations (Ahmed et al., 2013; May et al., 2015), as well as heart disease hospitalizations (Lo et al., 2018; Eberly et al., 2019). These disparities also impact referrals for cancer genetic services and management of genetic-related risks (Cragun et al. 2017; Chapman-Davis et al., 2020; Peterson et al., 2020; Garland et al., 2021).

Having the resources to follow through on medical recommendations is critical to maximize the benefits of the genetic counseling and testing process. However, a patient's ability to do so may be negatively impacted by a number of factors, including health insurance coverage, the ability to navigate the healthcare system, transportation issues, family communication, and general conviction regarding the benefit of the information in the context of one's medical care. Accessibility to care is influenced heavily by health insurance. The enactment of the Patient Protection and Affordable Care Act of 2010 made significant strides in decreasing inequalities regarding the number of those with access to health care in the United States, but tens of millions still lack health coverage, and others are underinsured (Renna et al., 2021; Artiga et al., 2022). Further, despite professional guidelines that dictate when certain screening and testing procedures are recommended, both government and private health insurance companies make decisions regarding coverage that may not be congruent with those guidelines and lead to gaps in care. Improvements in coverage mandates lead to higher rates of screening among patients (Sabik and Bradley, 2016; Preston et al., 2021; Sun et al., 2022).

The US health care system is extremely complex, with genetic testing being covered, to some extent, by many health insurance plans. However, policies range significantly regarding what testing can be ordered for whom and by whom, and which laboratory can complete the test. A genetic counselor may identify an optimal laboratory for testing, but it may fall outside of a patient's health care network. Although many counselors take on the responsibility of confirming or completing steps to ensure that testing is covered, this varies and is a particularly burdensome process to navigate for both patients and genetic counselors alike. Even if insurance covers testing, the level of coverage varies and may depend on copayments and deductibles, leading to out-of-pocket costs for patients. Although some individuals and families can reasonably absorb those costs, there is a disparate impact on individuals from lower income levels who may not have the disposable income available for this purpose. Families with the lowest income pay proportionately higher amounts in out-of-pocket health care costs (Galbraith et al., 2005), with a three-fold difference between the lowest and highest income brackets. This can lead to individuals declining or delaying genetic testing and medical screening.

EPILOGUE

A year after receiving her genetic test results, Rachel continued to follow recommended screening for breast cancer and had discussion about ovarian cancer prevention options with her primary care physician.

Rachel connected with the sole genetic counselor at the local safety net hospital through her work as a community health educator. Rachel felt an immediate connection to the genetic counselor. As a result, Rachel transferred her subsequent genetics care to the safety net hospital. She and the genetic counselor exchanged emails quarterly as Rachel gathered additional family health history information. Additionally, the genetic counselor kept Rachel abreast of changes in clinical guideline recommendations regarding screening, treatment options available for *BRCA1* gene previvors, and research opportunities. As a way of keeping the lines of communication open with relatives and getting to know her paternal relatives better, Rachel started a quarterly Zoom virtual chat with her family. This opportunity allowed her and other family members to bond and occasionally share and obtain family health history information. Because Anna turned 40 around the time that Rachel was scheduled for one of her upcoming mammograms, Rachel invited Anna to schedule her breast screening at the same time, so that they could navigate the experience together and support one another. Ultimately, Rachel was able to experience personalized health care based on her hereditary risk for cancer, and her lived experiences and navigation of various barriers present within the health care system enabled her to serve as a critical resource for others, including her family.

Rachel also shared her experience with her manager after learning more about the Genetic Information Nondiscrimination Act (GINA) and the protections that it offered against employer and health insurance discrimination. Rachel's advocacy efforts enabled her to facilitate a partnership between her employer, the new safety net hospital where she received care, and several community-based organizations as a way to actively combat inequities in dissemination of genetic information and to address misinformation gaps. The following year, Rachel was presented an opportunity to serve as a clinical advisor and member of multiple community advisory groups to several university hospitals in DC.

REFLECTION PROMPTS

How much do you relate to Rachel? What aspects of Rachel's experiences are similar or different from your own experience as a patient? When in the story did you have feelings of surprise or discomfort? Why do you think these feelings arose? How might Rachel's experiences be similar or different from the patients you encounter?

It is natural to feel overwhelmed by the layers of inequity and unjust circumstances that plague our patients, ourselves, and the health care system. To better understand where we, as genetic counselors, might be able to make small and large advances toward equity and justice, let us consider how a public health approach to genetic counseling can promote inclusivity, awareness, and systemic changes.

A PUBLIC HEALTH APPROACH TO GENETIC COUNSELING

While genetic counseling traditionally focuses on individualized patient care, a public health approach recognizes that health outcomes are deeply influenced by a complex interplay of genetic, social, economic, and environmental factors (BARHII, 2022). By combining these approaches, we can create a more inclusive and impactful framework to promote equitable access to genetic services. By shifting the focus from individual care to a broader population-level perspective and integrating public health principles into genetic counseling, professionals can work more effectively to address health disparities and promote equitable access to genetic services.

Public health emphasizes the importance of social determinants of health, such as income, education, and access to health care. Genetic counselors, adopting a public health perspective, can assess and address these determinants when providing genetic counseling services (Public Health Genetics and Genomics Week, 2024). This includes recognizing barriers to access and tailoring counseling to the specific needs and circumstances of each patient. Public health initiatives often involve community-based interventions to reach underserved populations. Genetic counselors can collaborate with community organizations, clinics, and public health agencies to teach about genetics and genetic counseling, share relevant resource materials, and/or provide genetic counseling services. Community-based research is another avenue of merging genetic counseling skills with public health initiatives.

Social Determinants of Health

Health outcomes are influenced by complex interactions between personal health practices, individual capacity and coping skills, human biology, health service availability, as well as social, economic, and physical environments. These determinants of health often reach beyond the boundaries of traditional health care. Sectors such as education, housing, transportation, agriculture, and environment can be important allies in influencing health status and improving population health (Healthy People, 2022). These non-medical factors that affect health are often referred to as social determinants of health (SDH). The World Health Organization (2022) defines SDH as the conditions in which people are born, grow, work, live, and age. Examples of SDH include income, education, food insecurity, housing, early childhood development, violence, and transportation. Studies suggest that SDH account for the majority of the modifiable contributors to health outcomes for a population (County Health Rankings and Roadmaps, 2022).

Consider the fact that zip codes are strongly associated with health outcomes. A zip code is a label for a community and the environment that exists there— whether there is wealth, strong community investment, or availability of hospitals and health centers. People with lower socioeconomic status (SES) are more likely to live and work in areas with sparse availability of affordable and healthy food options (e.g., fresh fruits and vegetables), have limited opportunities for physical activity (e.g., access to parks or gyms), and have higher exposure to environmental toxins (e.g., air/water/soil pollution). They may also have less access to high quality health care due to inadequate health insurance, lower health literacy, and/or financial obstacles. Additionally, fewer health care providers serve low-income neighborhoods, and dissemination of early detection and treatment advances are often slower in these neighborhoods. Consequently, residents of low-income neighborhoods, irrespective of their biological predispositions, have a heightened risk of developing specific health conditions. They are frequently diagnosed at later stages of illness, receive suboptimal standards of care, and encounter reduced survival rates and quality of life.

The Social Ecological Model of Health

The Social Ecological Model of Health (SEM) is a framework used in public health to understand and address health-related issues within the context of multiple interacting levels of influence (McLeroy et al., 1988; CDC, 2022). Developed to emphasize the complexity of health determinants, the SEM recognizes that individual health is shaped by multiple interconnected factors. This model is one framework we can use to understand how different factors interact and contribute to health behaviors and outcomes. The SEM consists of four levels, each representing a different sphere of influence:

- *Individual Level*: This innermost level focuses on personal characteristics, including genetics, knowledge, attitudes, beliefs, and behaviors. It recognizes that individual health decisions are influenced by psychological factors, perceptions, and lifestyle choices.
- *Interpersonal Level*: This level considers the influence of relationships and interactions with family members, friends, peers, and health care providers. Social support, communication, and social norms play a crucial role in shaping behaviors and health outcomes.
- *Community Level*: This level refers to communities, which encompass the physical, social, and cultural environments in which individuals live. These environments influence health through factors like access to healthcare, availability of healthy food, safety, social networks, and community norms.
- *Societal (Structural) Level*: The outermost level encompasses the broader societal factors that shape health, such as policies, laws, economic systems, cultural norms, and media influences. These factors can impact health equity by creating opportunities or barriers for different groups.

The spheres of influence are illustrated below in Figure 10-2.

These four layers, or "levels," do not exist independently from one another, but rather interact and shape each other (Peterson et al., 2021). For example, an individual's knowledge is shaped by the interactions they have with their family members and peers, and the societal provision and accessibility of this information.

INDIVIDUAL	INTERPERSONAL RELATIONSHIPS
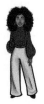 An **individual** has their own beliefs, behaviors, knowledge, skills, and (social and medical) identities and experiences.	Through contact, communication, and/or biology, an individual has **relationships** with other people, including their family, friends, partners, and social networks.
COMMUNITIES	**SOCIETY**
Communities are the physical and social settings, including institutions, where interactions between people take place. 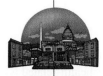	Communities are microcosms of a larger **society**, which is shaped by history, policy, and norms.

Note: Digital illustrations by Isaiah Johnson (2022)

FIGURE 10-2. *Levels of the social ecological model of health*

Rachel's story illustrated how her experience with genetic counseling was influenced by her individual qualities, values, and skills (e.g., ability to navigate health care system enough to schedule and attend genetic counseling session); relationships with her family members (e.g., conversation with her paternal cousin about family history); attendance at community events (e.g., public health community outreach event introducing service of genetic counseling); and surrounding societal history, policy, and norms (e.g., influence of inequitable distribution of municipal resources leading Rachel to get genetic counseling at a predominantly White medical center far from her home). Table 10-2 provides some examples of health disparities at the different levels of the SEM framework.

The SEM emphasizes that health outcomes are not solely determined by individual choices, but rather by the dynamic interactions among these multiple levels of influence. By understanding and addressing factors at each level, public health interventions can be more comprehensive and effective in promoting health and preventing disease. The model also highlights the need for multidisciplinary collaboration and policy changes to create supportive environments that foster health equity and overall wellbeing.

Rachel's story is just one illustration of a patient's experience within the medical system. As genetic counselors, we encounter countless stories, each with their own array of obstacles and propellants that influence the services we provide to our patients. Although this chapter is dedicated to centering the patient experience, importantly, our own journey to genetic counseling as a career and our own experiences in the medical system can be viewed and analyzed from the SEM lens.

TABLE 10-2. Examples of health disparities in genetic counseling through the lens of the Social Ecological Model of Health

Individual	• Differences in health literacy, socioeconomic status, education level, health insurance coverage may be barriers to accessing genetic services
	• Lack of awareness or misconceptions about genetic conditions may lead to delayed or missed opportunities in preventive care
Interpersonal	• Lack of open communication about health matters within family and social networks
	• Lack of experiences with genetic services among family members or friends
	• Reduced contact with biological family members
	• Negative medical experiences (medical mistrust) among family members or friends
	• Belonging to social networks that do not support/condone genetic services
	• Lack of family medical history knowledge can lead to disparities in genetic services
Community	• Lack of referral to genetic services
	• Unwelcoming environment within medical facility
	• Negative experience with genetic service provider
	• Unhelpful or absent patient education
	• Incorrect or incomplete rendering of genetic services
	• Services financially out of reach to patient
	• Challenges in infrastructure and transportation
	• Lack of medical facilities with genetic services
	• Geographical distance from medical care
Societal	• Health care service(s) provided only to individuals with (certain) health insurance plans, thus individuals with limited financial resources may face additional barriers
	• Past and present systemic racism, ableism, sexism (and other systems of oppression)
	• Genetic services perceived/treated as elite services (i.e., genetic determinism)
	• History of eugenics and its impact on cultural norms and policies exacerbating disparities

The intersections between genetic counseling and public health are significant. Both fields share the ultimate goals of improving health, facilitating increased patient option and navigation, and preventing or better understanding disease. Genetic counselors possess expertise in knowing about and communicating genetic information, while public health professionals excel in studying and implementing large-scale interventions. There are numerous health equity and public health frameworks that are outside the scope of this chapter. We encourage readers to engage in continuous learning and to consider collaborating with public health professionals. A partnership between the fields can enhance health equity by bridging gaps in knowledge and resources, leading to more informed decision making at both the individual and community levels.

Actions Toward Equity and Justice

Genetic counselors, adopting a public health lens, can prioritize culturally sensitive care, engage with diverse communities, and address social determinants of health that impact access to genetic services (Association of State and Territorial Health Officials, 2001). By focusing on community-based interventions, genetic counselors can take their services directly to underserved populations, reducing barriers and ensuring that traditionally marginalized groups justly receive benefits others experience. Integrating genetic counseling and public health can come with challenges. Overcoming differing philosophies and fostering collaboration between professionals from these two fields may require dedicated education and training efforts. Resource constraints, such as limited funding, can impede the implementation of integrated initiatives. Data sharing and privacy concerns must be managed thoughtfully to protect patient information while still enabling effective public health interventions. Cultural competence and sensitivity are crucial to ensure that integrated efforts resonate with diverse populations and do not (inadvertently) perpetuate disparities. To successfully integrate genetic counseling and public health for health equity, strategies such as interdisciplinary collaboration, advocacy for policy changes, and community engagement are vital. Establishing guidelines for data sharing, funding initiatives, and ongoing education can help bridge the gap between these fields. By navigating these challenges and implementing innovative solutions, the genetic counseling and public health fields can work in harmony to create a more equitable health care landscape, where every individual has access to the benefits of genetic services and improved health outcomes.

It is impossible for a single genetic counselor or the entire body of genetic counselors to repair all disparities in the medical system and society at large. We can, however, take actions that move toward equity and justice. Table 10-3 gives a few example strategies that could be taken to address factors currently obstructing the potential benefits of genetic counseling services.

SUMMARY

The integration of genetic and genomic information in health care ushers in a precision medicine era, but the existing medical system falls short in serving all individuals equitably. Just as genetic counselors guide patients to specialized care, they also have a responsibility to impact the broader medical care individuals receive beyond genetic counseling. In this chapter, health disparities and inequities were explored within the framework of genetics and genomics. Concepts of equality, equity, and justice were introduced. Equality, ensuring equal access to resources,

TABLE 10-3. **Examples of integrating a public health perspective to promote health equity**

Individual	• Empathy and Patient-Centered Care: Genetic counselors can practice patient-centered care by actively listening to patients' concerns, showing empathy, and tailoring counseling to individual needs.
	• Cultural Competency/Humility/Responsiveness: Genetic counselors should undergo cultural competence training to better understand the diverse backgrounds of their patients and of themselves. This helps in providing respectful and authentic care that reduces biases.
	• Accessible Communication: Genetic counselors can ensure that information is presented in a clear and understandable manner, tailored to the patient's literacy level and language preferences. This enhances patient understanding and decision making.
Interpersonal	• Cultivate Trustworthiness: Genetic counselors should be mindful of implicit biases provide empathetic, transparent, and culturally sensitive communication and create a safe and respectful environment for open dialogue and shared decision making.
	• Empowerment Through Education: Genetic counselors can identify moments in their life when an interaction with someone else (e.g., taxi cab, café, grocery store, barber shop, gym) naturally veers toward conversation about how and when to seek genetic services.
	• Collaboration: Genetic counselors can collaborate with healthcare providers from diverse disciplines, including social workers, physicians, and public health professionals, to develop holistic care plans that address patients' medical, psychological, and social needs.
Community	• Addressing Health Disparities: Genetic counselors can engage in quality improvement measures within their clinic or work setting that aim to address disparities.
	• Advocacy: Genetic counselors can advocate for policies that promote equitable access to genetic counseling services and genetic testing. They can also contribute their expertise to policy discussions related to genetic discrimination, insurance coverage, and privacy.
	• Community Engagement: Organizing workshops, support groups, and community events can raise awareness about genetics, promote preventive measures, and provide support for individuals and families affected by genetic conditions.
Societal	• Policy and Legislative Change: Genetic counselors can engage in advocacy efforts to influence policy changes that promote health equity, prevent genetic discrimination, and ensure equitable access to genetic testing and counseling services.
	• Research and Data Collection: Engaging in research on health disparities and outcomes in genetics can help identify gaps and areas for improvement. These results can inform interventions that aim to reduce disparities.

is distinct from equity, which considers individual circumstances to allocate tailored resources, and justice, addressing systemic biases for equitable outcomes. Health disparities stem from unequal access to resources that lead to poorer outcomes in certain populations.

By centering the experiences of patients from marginalized communities, various factors influencing an individual's health care journey through genetic counseling were explored. The presence of systemic racism in society has resulted in unequal economic, educational, and financial conditions for marginalized communities, leading to disparities in health care. Factors such as hospital closures, inadequate funding, and privatization affect access to health care in under-resourced urban and rural areas. Medical distrust, stemming from a history of discriminatory practices, has led to hesitancy in engaging with the health care system. Personal and organizational health literacy, along with biases in patient materials and lack of inclusivity, contribute to disparities in understanding and utilizing health care services. Challenges in accessing family history information arise from historical and current factors, including systemic racism, unjust incarceration rates, and limited resources in other countries. Disparities in referrals to genetic counseling result from biased practices and underfunding of health care settings, affecting care quality and patient engagement. Traditional genetic service models have inherent barriers for marginalized communities due to location, limited availability, and reimbursement issues. Implicit biases among clinicians, compounded by a lack of diversity in genomic studies, further perpetuate disparities in care provision. Lack of diversity in research studies leads to inequitable genetic testing outcomes and increased prevalence of variants of unknown significance. Barriers to downstream care after genetic testing, including insurance coverage, navigating the health care system, and disparities in coverage mandates, impact the overall benefits of genetic counseling and testing for marginalized populations. Addressing these systemic issues is crucial to achieving equitable health care access and outcomes for all individuals.

We acknowledge that this chapter does not provide an exhaustive review of all barriers and obstacles to health equity. The highlighted journey of "Rachel" does not capture all elements of marginalization. As the field of genetic counseling continues to center health equity and justice, we encourage critical analysis beyond the words of this chapter.

Genetic counselors, while traditionally focused on personalized care, have an opportunity and responsibility to impact broader health care. Integrating a public health approach with genetic counseling practice acknowledges the influence of genetic, social, economic, and environmental factors on health outcomes. By shifting the focus from individual care to a population-level perspective, genetic counselors can work more effectively to address health disparities and promote equitable access to genetic services. We underscored the significance of SDH in influencing health outcomes beyond traditional health care domains and introduced the SEM of Health as a framework to understand how various factors interact at different levels, from individual to societal, influencing health behaviors and outcomes. Genetic counselors can take proactive steps, guided by a public health lens, to prioritize equity, justice, and patient-centered care, ultimately contributing to a more equitable health care landscape.

KEY DEFINITIONS

Ableism: system of power, including beliefs and practices, that devalues and discriminates against people with physical, intellectual, or psychiatric disabilities (Center for Disability Rights).

Ancestry: lineage of an individual or group of individuals defined by geographical origins.

Anti-racism: work of actively opposing racism by advocating for changes in political, economic, and social life (Race Forward, 2015).

Community-based research and intervention: An approach to studying and addressing various issues within communities that involve active participation from community members, organizations, and researchers to collaboratively identify problems, develop research questions, and implement strategies for positive change (Wallerstein et al., 2018).

Cultural competency/humility/responsiveness: The term *cultural* refers to beliefs, values, and/or communities that make up a component of an individual's lived experience.
* *competency* denotes mastery of understanding
* *humility* denotes lessening of power or reducing one's own importance
* *responsiveness* denotes attentiveness and adaptive action or thought.

Determinants of health: range of personal, social, economic, and environmental factors that influence health status.

Health disparity: component of health status, access, or service that does not optimize health for all people and instead cultivates or maintains differences that harm those who have been historically disadvantaged.

Health equity: 1) the idea that everyone should have a fair opportunity to attain their full health potential and that no one should be disadvantaged from achieving this potential (Whitehead, 1992); 2) the process assuring the conditions for optimal health for all people (Jones et al., 2019).

Health inequity: health status, access, or service that is more beneficial to some individuals than others and simultaneously more harmful to some individuals than others.

Intersectionality: theory that a person's experience is shaped by multiple facets of their individual and perceived identity.

Public health: the science and art of society collectively preventing disease, prolonging life, promoting health, protecting the health of and improving the health of people and the communities where they live, learn, work and play (American Public Health Association, 2021; CDC Foundation, 2022).

Public health genomics: genome-based knowledge and technologies for the benefit of preventing disease, prolonging life, promoting health, protecting and improving the health of people and populations, responsibly, effectively and equitably (Burke et al., 2006).

Race: politically and socially charged construct/concept used to caste people into a hierarchical human-grouping system that leads to the marginalization of some groups across nations, regions and the world.

Racism: when one racially categorized group has the power to carry out systematic discrimination against other racially categorized groups through the institutional policies and practices of the society, while shaping the cultural beliefs and values that support those racist policies and practices.

Social determinants of health: conditions in which people are born, grow, live, work and age, including non-medical factors such as socioeconomic status, education, neighborhood and physical environment, employment, social support networks, access to health care, and the wider set of forces and systems that shape these conditions (Office of Disease Prevention and Health Promotion, 2022; World Health Organization, 2022)

Systemic (Systematic, Structural, Institutional) Racism: 1) policies and practices entrenched in established institutions, which result in the exclusion or promotion of designated racial groups; 2) inequalities rooted in the system-wide operation of a society that excludes substantial numbers of members of particular groups from significant participation in major social institutions (Banaji et al., 2021; Braveman et al., 2022).

REFERENCES

Abrams, LR, McBride CM, Hooker GW, et al. (2015) The many facets of genetic literacy: assessing the scalability of multiple measures for broad use in survey research. *PloS One* 10(10):e0141532. https://doi.org/10.1371/journal.pone.0141532

Ahmed NU, Pelletier V, Winter K, & Albatineh AN. (2013) Factors explaining racial/ethnic disparities in rates of physician recommendation for colorectal cancer screening. *Am J Public Health* 103(7):e91–e99. https://doi.org/10.2105/AJPH.2012.301034

Agency for Healthcare Research and Quality. (2022) AHRQ Health Literacy Universal Precautions Toolkit. https://www.ahrq.gov/health-literacy/improve/precautions/index.html Accessed May 23, 2022.

American College of Obstetricians and Gynecologists. (2017) Carrier screening for genetic conditions. Committee Opinion No. 691. *Obstet Gynecol* 129:e41–55.

American College of Obstetricians and Gynecologists. (2019) Hereditary Cancer Syndromes and Risk Assessment: Committee Opinion No. 793. (2019). *Obstet Gynecol,* 134(6):e143–e149. https://doi.org/10.1097/AOG.0000000000003562

American College of Obstetricians and Gynecologists' Committee on Practice Bulletins—Obstetrics; Committee on Genetics; Society for Maternal-Fetal Medicine. Screening for Fetal Chromosomal Abnormalities (2020) ACOG Practice Bulletin, Number 226. *Obstet Gynecol* 136(4):e48–e69. doi: 10.1097/AOG.00000000

American Public Health Association. (2021) *What is Public Health?* https://www.apha.org/what-is-public-health Accessed June 3, 2022.

Andreyeva E, Kash B, Averhart Preston V, et al. (2022) Rural hospital closures: effects on utilization and medical spending among commercially insured individuals. *Med Care* 60(6):437–443. https://doi.org/10.1097/MLR.0000000000001711

Arjunan A, Darnes DR, Sagaser KG, & Svenson AB. (2022) Addressing reproductive healthcare disparities through equitable carrier screening: medical racism and genetic discrimination in United States' history highlights the needs for change in obstetrical genetics care. *Societies* 12(2):33. https://doi.org/10.3390/soc12020033

Artiga S, Hill L, Orgera K, & Damico A. (2022) Health Coverage by Race and Ethnicity, 2010-2019; Published: Jul 16, 2021; https://www.kff.org/racial-equity-and-health-policy/issue-brief/health-coverage-by-race-and-ethnicity/ Accessed May 23, 2022.

Association of State and Territorial Health Officials, (2001) Framework for public health genetics policies and practices in state and local public health agencies. https://portal.ct.gov/-/media/Departments-and-Agencies/DPH/dph/Genomics/asthopdf.pdf Accessed May 23, 2022.

Banaji, M.R., Fiske, S.T. & Massey, D.S. Systemic racism: individuals and interactions, institutions and society. *Cogn. Research* 6, 82 (2021). https://doi.org/10.1186/s41235-021-00349-3

Bay Area Regional Health Inequities Initiative. (2020). A public health framework for reducing health inequities. https://www.phi.org/thought-leadership/a-public-health-framework-for-reducing-health-inequities/ Accessed 26 May 2022.

Boothe E, Greenberg S, Delaney C, & Cohen S. (2021) Genetic counseling service delivery models: a study of genetic counselors' interests, needs, and barriers to implementation. *J Genet Couns* 30(1):283–292.

Braveman PA, Arkin E, Proctor D, et al. (2022) Systemic and structural racism: definitions, examples, health damages, and approaches to dismantling. *Health Aff* (Millwood) 41(2):171–178. doi: 10.1377/hlthaff.2021.01394.

Burke W, Khoury MJ, Stewart A, & Zimmern RL. (2006) The path from genome-based research to population health: development of an international public health genomics network. *Genet Med* 8:451–458.

Casanova-Perez R, Apodaca C, Bascom E, et al. (2022) Broken down by bias: healthcare biases experienced by BIPOC and LGBTQ+ patients. *AMIA Annual Symposium proceedings*. AMIA Symposium, 2021 pp. 275–284.

Casey LS, Reisner SL, Findling MG, et al. (2019) Discrimination in the United States: experiences of lesbian, gay, bisexual, transgender, and queer Americans. *Health Serv Res* 54(Suppl 2):1454–1466. https://doi.org/10.1111/1475-6773.13229

CDC Foundation. (2022) *What is Public Health?* https://www.cdcfoundation.org/what-public-health Accessed June 3, 2022.

Center for Disease Control and Prevention. (2022) The Social-Ecological Model: A Framework for Prevention. https://www.cdc.gov/violenceprevention/about/social-ecologicalmodel.html Accessed October 7, 2023.

Center for Disease Control and Prevention. (2023) Health Literacy. https://www.cdc.gov/healthliteracy/learn/index.html Accessed October 7, 2023.

Center for Healthcare Quality and Payment Reform (n.d) Saving Rural Hospitals: Overview of Problems and Solutions. https://ruralhospitals.chqpr.org/Overview.html Accessed May 22, 2022.

Chapman-Davis E, Zhou ZN, Fields JC, et al. (2021) Racial and ethnic disparities in genetic testing at a hereditary breast and ovarian cancer center. *J Gen Intern Med* 36(1):35–42. https://doi.org/10.1007/s11606-020-06064-x

County Health Rankings and Roadmaps. (2022) County Health Rankings Model. https://www.countyhealthrankings.org/explore-health-rankings/measures-data-sources/county-health-rankings-model Accessed May 26, 2022.

Cragun D, Weidner A, Lewis C, et al. (2017) Racial disparities in BRCA testing and cancer risk management across a population-based sample of young breast cancer survivors. *Cancer* 123(13):2497–2505. https://doi.org/10.1002/cncr.30621

Daly, MB, Pal T, Berry MP, et al. (2021). Genetic/familial high-risk assessment: breast, ovarian, and pancreatic, Version 2.2021. NCCN clinical practice guidelines in oncology. *J Natl Compr Canc Netw* 19(1):77–102. https://doi.org/10.6004/jnccn.2021.0001

Dar-Nimrod I & Heine SJ. (2011) Genetic essentialism: on the deceptive determinism of DNA. *Psychol Bull.* 137(5):800–818. https://doi.org/10.1037/a0021860

Early ML, Kumar P, Marcell AV, et al. (2020) Literacy assessment of preimplantation genetic patient education materials exceed national reading levels. *J Assist Reprod Genet* 37(8):1913–1922. https://doi.org/10.1007/s10815-020-01837-z

Eberly LA, Richterman A, Beckett AG, et al. (2019) Identification of racial inequities in access to specialized inpatient heart failure care at an academic medical center. *Circ HeartFail* 12(11):e006214. https://doi.org/10.1161/CIRCHEARTFAILURE.119.006214

Essien UR, He W, Ray A, et al. (2019) Disparities in quality of primary care by resident and staff physicians: is there a conflict between training and equity? *J Gen Intern Med* 34(7):1184–1191. https://doi.org/10.1007/s11606-019-04960-5

Federal Bureau of Prisons. (2022) *Inmate Race.* https://www.bop.gov/about/statistics/statistics_inmate_race.jsp Accessed May 29, 2024.

Fiscella K & Sanders MR. (2016) Racial and ethnic disparities in the quality of health care. *Annu Rev Public Health* 37:375–394. https://doi.org/10.1146/annurev-publhealth-032315-021439

FitzGerald C & Hurst S. (2017) Implicit bias in healthcare professionals: a systematic review. *BMC Med Ethics* 18(1):19. https://doi.org/10.1186/s12910-017-0179-8

Galbraith AA, Wong ST, Kim SE, & Newacheck PW. (2005) Out-of-pocket financial burden for low-income families with children: socioeconomic disparities and effects of insurance. *Health Serv Res* 40(6 Part 1):1722–1736. https://doi.org/10.1111/j.1475-6773.2005.00421.x

Garland V, Cioffi J, Kirelik D, et al. (2021) African-Americans Are less frequently assessed for hereditary colon cancer. *J Nat Med Assoc* 113(3):336–341. https://doi.org/10.1016/j.jnma.2020.09.146

Goddu A, O'Conor KJ, Lanzkron S, et al. (2018) Do Words matter? Stigmatizing language and the transmission of bias in the medical record. *J Gen Intern Med* 33(5):685–691. https://doi.org/10.1007/s11606-017-4289-2

Gorrie A, Gold J, Cameron C, et al. (2021) Benefits and limitations of telegenetics: a literature review. *J Genet Couns* 30(4):924–937. https://doi.org/10.1002/jgc4.1418

Hammack-Aviran C, Eilmus A, Diehl C, et al. (2022) LGBTQ+ perspectives on conducting genomic research on sexual orientation and gender identity. *Behav Genet* 52:246–267. https://doi.org/10.1007/s10519-022-10105-y

Hassett MJ, Somerfield MR, Baker ER, et al. (2020) Management of male breast cancer: ASCO guideline. *J Clin Oncol* 38(16):1849–1863. https://doi.org/10.1200/JCO.19.03120

Health Resources & Services Administration. (2019) Health Literacy. https://www.hrsa.gov/about/organization/bureaus/ohe/health-literacy/ Accessed May 26, 2022.

Healthy People. (2022) https://wayback.archive-it.org/5774/20220415230635/ https://www.healthypeople.gov/2020/about/foundation-health-measures/Determinants-of-Health Accessed May 26, 2022.

Hoffman KM, Trawalter S, Axt JR, & Oliver MN. (2016) Racial bias in pain assessment and treatment recommendations, and false beliefs about biological differences between blacks and whites. *Proc Natl Acad Sci USA* 113(16):4296–4301. https://doi.org/10.1073/pnas.1516047113

Hong SJ. (2019) Cross-cultural differences in the influences of spiritual and religious tendencies on beliefs in genetic determinism and family health history communication: a teleological approach. *J Relig Health* 58(5):1516–1536. https://doi.org/10.1007/s10943-018-0729-5

Institute of Medicine (US) Committee on Understanding and Eliminating Racial and Ethnic Disparities in Health Care, Smedley, BD., Stith AY & Nelson AR (Eds.). (2003) *Unequal Treatment: Confronting Racial and Ethnic Disparities in Health Care.* Washington, DC: National Academies Press.

Jaiswal J & Halkitis PN. (2019) Towards a more inclusive and dynamic understanding of medical mistrust informed by science. *Behav Med* 45(2):79–85. https://doi.org/10.1080/08964289.2019.1619511

Jones CP. (2018) Toward the science and practice of anti-racism: launching a national campaign against racism. *Ethnicity & Disease* 28:231–234

Jones CP, Holden KB, & Belton A. (2019) Strategies for achieving health equity: concern about the whole plus concern about the hole. *Ethn Dis* 29(Suppl 2):345–348. https://doi.org/10.18865/ed.29.S2.345

Jones KM, Cook-Deegan R, Rotimi CN, et al. (2021) Complicated legacies: the human genome at 20. *Science* 371(6529):564–569. https://doi.org/10.1126/science.abg5266

Jooma S, Hahn MJ, Hindorff LA, & Bonham VL. (2019) Defining and achieving health equity in genomic medicine. *Ethn Dis* 29(Suppl 1):173–178. https://doi.org/10.18865/ed.29.S1.173

Kaye C & Korf B. (2013) Genetic literacy and competency. *Pediatrics* 132(Suppl 3):S224–S230. https://doi.org/10.1542/peds.2013-1032G

Khoury MJ, Bowen S, Dotson WD, et al. (2022) Health equity in the implementation of genomics and precision medicine: a public health imperative. *Genet Med* 24(8):1630–1639. https://doi.org/10.1016/j.gim.2022.04.009

Konstantinopoulos PA, Norquist B, Lacchetti C, et al. (2020) Germline and somatic tumor testing in epithelial ovarian cancer: ASCO guideline. *J Clin Oncology* 38(11):1222–1245. https://doi.org/10.1200/JCO.19.02960

Krakow M, Ratcliff CL, Hesse BW, & Greenberg-Worisek AJ. (2017) Assessing genetic literacy awareness and knowledge gaps in the US population: results from the Health Information National Trends Survey. *Public Health Genom* 20(6):343–348. https://doi.org/10.1159/000489117

Kubendran S, Sivamurthy S, & Schaefer GB. (2017) A novel approach in pediatric telegenetic services: geneticist, pediatrician and genetic counselor team. *Genet Med* 19(11):1260–1267. https://doi.org/10.1038/gim.2017.45

Kurian AW, Ward KC, Hamilton AS, et al. (2018). Uptake, results, and outcomes of germline multiple-gene sequencing after diagnosis of breast cancer. *JAMA Oncol* 4(8):1066–1072. https://doi.org/10.1001/jamaoncol.2018.0644

Kutner M, Greenberg E, Jin Y, & Paulsen C. (2006) The Health Literacy of America's Adults: Results from the 2003 National Assessment of Adult Literacy (NCES 2006–483). Washington, DC: U.S. Department of Education – National Center for Education Statistics. https://nces.ed.gov/pubsearch/pubsinfo.asp?pubid=2006483 Accessed May 30, 2024.

Lee DC, Liang H, & Shi L. (2021) The convergence of racial and income disparities in health insurance coverage in the United States. *Int J Equity Health* 20(1):96. https://doi.org/10.1186/s12939-021-01436-z

Lewis AK, Harding KE, Snowdon DA, & Taylor NF. (2018) Reducing wait time from referral to first visit for community outpatient services may contribute to better health outcomes: a systematic review. *BMC Health Serv Res* 18(1):869. https://doi.org/10.1186/s12913-018-3669-6

Lin J, Sharaf RN, Saganty R, et al. (2021). Achieving universal genetic assessment for women with ovarian cancer: are we there yet? A systematic review and meta-analysis. *Gynecol Oncol* 162(2):506–516. https://doi.org/10.1016/j.ygyno.2021.05.011

Lo AX, Donnelly JP, Durant RW, et al. (2018) A national study of U.S. emergency departments: racial disparities in hospitalizations for heart failure. *Am J Prev Med* 55(5 Suppl 1):S31–S39. https://doi.org/10.1016/j.amepre.2018.05.020

Lowe C, Beach MC, & Roter DL. (2020) Individuation and implicit racial bias in genetic counseling communication. *Patient Educ Couns* 103(4):804–810. https://doi.org/10.1016/j.pec.2019.10.016

Master of Public Health Program at George Washington University. (2020) *Equity vs. Equality: What's the Difference?* https://onlinepublichealth.gwu.edu/resources/equity-vs-equality/ Accessed May 26, 2022.

May FP, Almario CV, Ponce N, & Spiegel BM. (2015) Racial minorities are more likely than whites to report lack of provider recommendation for colon cancer screening. *Am J Gastroenterol* 110(10): 1388–1394. https://doi.org/10.1038/ajg.2015.138

McLeroy KR, Bibeau D, Steckler A, & Glanz K. (1988) An ecological perspective on health promotion programs. *Health Educ Q* 15(4)351–377. https://doi.org/10.1177/109019818801500401

Nath JB, Costigan S, & Hsia RY. (2016) Changes in demographics of patients seen at federally qualified health centers, 2005-2014. *JAMA Intern Med* 176(5):712–714. https://doi.org/10.1001/jamainternmed.2016.0705

National Academies of Sciences, Engineering, and Medicine. (2018) *Understanding Disparities in Access to Genomic Medicine: Proceedings of a Workshop*, Washington, DC: The National Academies Press.

National Society of Genetic Counselors. (2024). *2024 Professional Status Survey*, Chicago, IL: National Society of Genetic Counselors.

Office of Disease Prevention and Health Promotion. (2022) *Determinants of Health.* https://health.gov/healthypeople/priority-areas/social-determinants-health Accessed June 17, 2024.

Palmer Kelly E, McGee J, Obeng-Gyasi S, et al. (2021) Marginalized patient identities and the patient-physician relationship in the cancer care context: a systematic scoping review. *Support Care Cancer* 29(12):7195–7207. https://doi.org/10.1007/s00520-021-06382-8

Peterson A, Charles V, Yeung D, & Coyle K. (2021) The Health Equity Framework: A Science- and Justice-Based Model for Public Health Researchers and Practitioners. *Health Promot Prac* 22(6):741–746. https://doi.org/10.1177/1524839920950730

Peterson JM, Pepin A, Thomas R, et al. (2020) Racial disparities in breast cancer hereditary risk assessment referrals. *J Genet Couns* 29(4):587–593. https://doi.org/10.1002/jgc4.1250

Preston, MA, Ross, L, Chukmaitov, A, et al. (2021) Health insurance coverage mandates: colorectal cancer screening in the post-ACA era. *Cancer Prevent Res* 14(1):123–130.

Public Health Genetics and Genomics Week. (2024) About Public Health Genetics and Genomics. https://phgw.org/ Accessed June 12, 2024.

Race Forward. (2015) *Race Reporting Guide*. New York, NY: Race Forward. https://www. raceforward.org/reporting-guide#:~:text=Race%20Forward's%20Race%20 Reporting%20Guide,of%20people%20of%20all%20races Accessed May 30, 2024

Randall VR. (1996) Slavery, segregation and racism: trusting the health care system ain't always easy! An African American perspective on bioethics. *St Louis U Pub L Rev* 15(2):191–235.

Raspa M, Moultrie R, Toth D, & Haque SN. (2021) Barriers and facilitators to genetic service delivery models: scoping review. *Interact J* 10(1): e23523. https://doi.org/ 10.2196/23523

Renna F, Kosteas VD, & Dinkar K. (2021) Inequality in health insurance coverage before and after the Affordable Care Act. *Health Econ* 30(2), 384–402. https://doi.org/10.1002/ hec.4195

Reilly PR. (2015) Eugenics and Involuntary Sterilization: 1907–2015. *Annu Rev Genomics Hum Genet* 16:351–368. https://doi.org/10.1146/annurev-genom-090314-024930

Ricks-Santi L, McDonald JT, Gold B, et al. (2017). Next generation sequencing reveals high prevalence of BRCA1 and BRCA2 variants of unknown significance in early-onset breast cancer in African American women. *Ethn Dis* 27(2):169–178. https://doi. org/10.18865/ed.27.2.169

Roberts D. (2008) Is race-based medicine good for us?: African American approaches to race, biomedicine, and equality. *J Law Med Ethics* 36(3):537–545. doi: 10.1111/j.1748-720X.2008.302.x. PMID: 18840247.

Sabik LM & Bradley CJ. (2016) The impact of near-universal insurance coverage on breast and cervical cancer screening: evidence from Massachusetts. *Health Econ* 25(4):391–407. https://doi.org/10.1002/hec.3159

Sabin JA, Riskind RG, & Nosek BA. (2015) Health care providers' implicit and explicit attitudes toward lesbian women and gay men. *Am J Public Health* 105(9):1831–1841. https://doi.org/10.2105/AJPH.2015.302631

Schaa KL, Roter DL, Biesecker BB et al. (2015) Genetic counselors' implicit racial attitudes and their relationship to communication. *Health Psychol* 34(2):111–119. https://doi.org/10.1037/hea0000155

Shen MJ, Peterson, EB, Costas-Muñiz R, et al. (2018) The effects of race and racial concordance on patient-physician communication: a systematic review of the literature. *J Racial Ethn Health Disparities* 5(1):117–140. https://doi.org/10.1007/s40615-017-0350-4

Shipow A & Singh A. (2020, 26 June) Is Your Data Inclusive? https://medium.com/busara-center-blog/is-your-data-inclusive-ddd59933f108 Accessed May 26, 2022.

Sirugo G, Williams SM, & Tishkoff SA. (2019) The missing diversity in human genetic studies. *Cell* 177(1):26–31. https://doi.org/10.1016/j.cell.2019.02.048

Smiley C & Fakunle D. (2016) From "brute" to "thug:" the demonization and criminalization of unarmed Black male victims in America. *J Hum Behav Soc Environ* 26(3-4):350–366. doi: 10.1080/10911359.2015.1129256. PMID: 27594778; PMCID: PMC5004736.

Stochholm K, Bojesen A, Jensen A, et al. (2012) Criminality in men with Klinefelter's syndrome and XYY syndrome: a cohort study. *Brit Med J Open* 2(1):e000650. doi: 10.1136/bmjopen-2011-000650. PMID: 22357573; PMCID: PMC3289987.

Strauss D, de la Salle S, Sloshower J, & Williams MT. (2021) Research abuses against people of colour and other vulnerable groups in early psychedelic research. *J Med Ethics* Advance online publication. https://doi.org/10.1136/medethics-2021-107262

Sun J, Perraillon MC, & Myerson R. (2022) The impact of Medicare health insurance coverage on lung cancer screening. *Med Care* 60(1):29–36. https://doi.org/10.1097/MLR.0000000000001655

United States Census Bureau (2021) Quick Facts: United States. https://www.census.gov/quickfacts/fact/table/US/PST045221 Accessed May 26, 2022.

Veach PM, Bartels DM, & Leroy BS. (2007) Coming full circle: a reciprocal-engagement model of genetic counseling practice. *J Genet Couns* 16(6):713–728. https://doi.org/10.1007/s10897-007-9113-4

Wallerstein N, Duran B, Oetzel J, & Minkler M. (2018) *Community Based Participatory Research for Health: Advancing Social and Health Equity.* San Francisco, CA: Jossey-Bass.

Washington HA. (2006) *Medical Apartheid: The Dark History of Medical Experimentation on Black Americans From Colonial Times to the Present.* New York, NY: Doubleday.

Whitehead, M. (1992) The concepts and principles of equity in health. *Int J Health Service* 22(3):429–445. https://doi.org/10.2190/986L-LHQ6-2VTE-YRRN

Williams CD, Bullard AJ, O'Leary M, et al. (2019) Racial/ethnic disparities in BRCA counseling and testing: a narrative review. *J Racial Ethn Health Disparities* 6(3): 570–583. https://doi.org/10.1007/s40615-018-00556-7

Wojcik GL, Graff M, Nishimura KK, et al. (2019) Genetic analyses of diverse populations improves discovery for complex traits. *Nature* 570(7762):514–518. https://doi.org/10.1038/s41586-019-1310-4

World Health Organization. (2022) Social Determinants of Health. https://www.who.int/health-topics/social-determinants-of-health Accessed May 26, 2022.

Yearby R, Clark B, & Figueroa JF. (2022) Structural racism in historical and modern US health care policy. *Health Aff* 41(2):187–194. https://doi.org/10.1377/hlthaff.2021.01466

11

Genetic Counselors in the Healthcare Ecosystem: Navigating Policies, Payment and Professional Advocacy

Gillian W. Hooker and Katie Lang

INTRODUCTION

Genetic counselors work within the large and rapidly evolving ecosystem of health care, where there are widely variable practices and financial structures. In this chapter, we explore the economics of the health care systems that support the provision of genetic counseling services. We will touch on different models of health care delivery around the world and highlight particular challenges and opportunities when working within government and third-party payer systems, like health insurance companies. The chapter takes a deeper dive into the US health care system, not to imply supremacy of a system known to have significant dysfunction and

A Guide to Genetic Counseling, Third Edition. Edited by Vivian Y. Pan, Jane L. Schuette, Karen E. Wain, and Beverly M. Yashar.
© 2025 John Wiley & Sons Ltd. Published 2025 by John Wiley & Sons Ltd.

numerous disparities, but rather because it is the system best known to the authors who work within it and in recognition of the complex influence US health care has on the global population. Understanding the motivations and financial incentives of the health care systems in which most genetic counselors work is critical to the advancement of the profession. As we grow, we must deliver services that provide value to the patients and other stakeholders we serve, and we must be able to articulate that value across all of these groups. In doing so, we lay a path for a sustainable, thriving future for the profession of genetic counseling.

HEALTH CARE ECOSYSTEMS AROUND THE WORLD

Across the global health care ecosystem, there are different "biospheres" of health care that function according to different sets of rules, with different power structures and varying levels of hierarchy and government involvement. A major distinction between different countries' health care systems is whether or not they have Universal Healthcare Coverage (UHC) (Council on Foreign Relations, 2023). In many countries in the developing world, there is no national infrastructure for health care and health care is paid for by those who can afford it or who are supported by aid organizations. In a country with UHC, all people can go to the doctor when they are sick or for preventive care and governments ensure that they have the ability to pay for that care. Countries with UHC vary as to how payments for care are subsidized. In some cases, like Cuba and the United Kingdom, countries have a single, government-run and funded payer system. In these countries, health care is commonly delivered through hospitals and clinics run by the government and health care providers are often government employees. There may be a private insurance option that exists in parallel that people may buy into. Canada is also a country with universal, publicly funded care, with the additional complexity of health care being funded and administered at the provincial level across Canada's 13 provinces. Other countries, like Germany, France, and Japan, set up their UHC programs such that people are required to have health insurance and may purchase that insurance from competing insurers. Government funding is typically provided to cover a baseline level of insurance and individuals may opt to pay more for private insurance which may cover additional services or needs. Hospitals are either public, not-for-profit private, or for-profit privately-owned. Most health care providers work in private practices or are employed by hospitals (The Commonwealth Fund, 2020). Models of genetic counseling employment vary around the world and many new models are in development (Abacan et al., 2019).

THE US HEALTH CARE ECOSYSTEM

The United States is unique in being a multipayer system without universal coverage, since there is currently no mandate that requires everyone to have insurance. Multiple private companies sell insurance through employers and to a lesser extent directly to individuals or families. An estimated 65% of US residents have private insurance, also called commercial insurance. Public insurance is provided to those who are 65 or older via Medicare, to those who have a disability and or are below a specific income threshold via Medicaid, to those who are in the armed services via TriCare, or those who have served in the military via the Veterans Health Administration. As of 2020, an estimated 8.6% of US residents did not have health insurance (Table 11-1; Cohen et al., 2021; Rosso, 2022).

Hospitals in the US are a mix of public, private for-profit, and private non-profit, with the majority being private nonprofit hospitals owned by religious organizations, fraternal societies (like Shriners) or academic institutions (Rice et al., 2013). For those in the armed services or who have served in the military, individuals may receive services through a specific military or veteran's hospital within which all services are covered. Similarly, some private insurance companies are under an umbrella system, sometimes called an Accountable Care Organization (ACO) or Integrated Health System, that also owns hospitals and a care delivery system (e.g., Kaiser Permanente). In these models, the same overall entity acts as both an insurer and provides care so the system as a whole is incentivized to control costs while also providing quality care. Since the insurance company and the hospital are one and the same, financially speaking, providing efficient care both benefits patients and saves the system money.

Health care providers in the US may work in private practice or be employed by hospital systems, with a general trend toward more providers employed in larger systems (The Commonwealth Fund, 2020). Specialty care (inclusive of clinical genetics) is even more likely to be found in larger health systems, and in particular, academic medical centers. Academic medical centers are institutions that typically

TABLE 11-1. Insurance status across the US population

Type of Insurance	Covered Lives	Percent of US Residents Covered—2020 Enrollment*
Private Health Insurance	Individuals insured through their employer (group) and who purchase insurance for themselves (non-group)	64.9%
Medicare	Individuals over 65 years of age	18.4%
Medicaid	Individuals below a specific income threshold including children, pregnant women, adults and individuals with disabilities, and people aged 65 and older	17.8%
Armed Services/ TriCare	Military service members and their dependents	2.8%
Veterans Health Administration	Veterans of the military	0.9%
Indian Health Service	American Indians and Alaska Natives	0.008%
Uninsured	Individuals living without health insurance	8.6%

* Note: categories are not mutually exclusive.
Source: Rosso (2022)

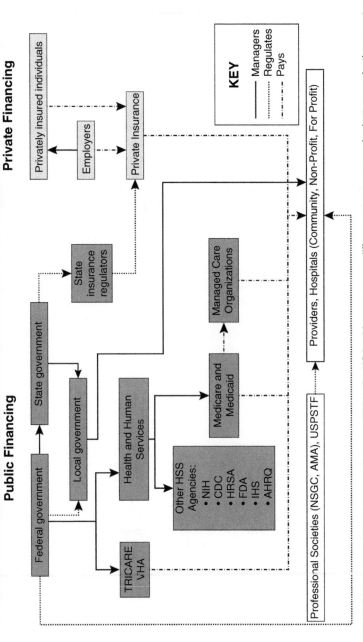

FIGURE 11-1. *The US health care biosphere. Within the US health care system, different government and private organizations must work together to deliver health care to the population via a complex network of payments and regulations. Adapted from Rice et al. by KF Mittendorf and GW Hooker*

have three goals: 1) to provide patient care; 2) to conduct research; and 3) to train the health care workforce (American Academy of Medical Colleges, 2022). They comprise about 5% of all US hospitals but provide a much higher percentage of care, often as a referral site for patients who need more specialized services (Burke et al., 2017; American Academy of Medical Colleges, 2022). Of those genetic counselors who work in a clinical role, historically a higher percentage work in academic medical centers than in private or public hospital settings (NSGC, 2024). Federally Qualified Health Centers (FQHCs) are centers designated to receive funds from the Health Services and Resource Administration under the US Department of Health and Human Services to provide community-based (largely primary care) services in underserved areas. FQHCs may exist under the umbrella of a larger health care system (Federally Qualified Health Centers, 2017).

A small number of genetic counselors report maintaining a private practice, and an increasing number of genetic counselors are providing remote care for patients via telehealth genetic counseling companies (NSGC, 2024). These companies may serve a number of different health care systems, insurers, or laboratories seeking to provide access to genetic counselors. A major barrier to expansion of access to genetic counselors, be it in person or by telehealth, remains reimbursement for genetic counseling services, discussed in more detail below.

Absent direct reimbursement for services, genetic counselors' salaries must be supported with other indirect value calculations. Many genetic counselors work in research settings (academic medical centers) where their salaries are subsidized with research dollars (often funded via the National Institutes of Health). Some are supported by state or federal public health programs, such as those for newborn screening. Other genetic counselors may provide services in conjunction with laboratories and the sale of genetic tests, such that the cost of the test subsidizes the clinical services provided ancillary to testing. Finally, downstream care provided by a hospital may be used to justify salary support for genetic counselors. This will be discussed later in the chapter as well. Sources of funding are critical to understand, as they shed light on the ways those dependent on that funding are financially incentivized within a system. In a system where genetic counselors salaries can only be partially supported by revenues for the clinical services they provide, there is a risk that conflicts can be created between the different interests that are also supporting them (i.e., research, laboratory, downstream service providers). In order to move toward autonomous practice free from incentives introduced by the various salary subsidies, policies to support direct payment of genetic counselors are critical.

FEDERAL POLICIES

Federal policies can have a significant impact on access to services and the way those services are provided. A review of all federal policies impacting the business of genetic counseling is beyond the scope of this chapter, but a few major legislative efforts that impact the business and practice of genetic counseling are summarized below.

Genetic Information Nondiscrimination Act (GINA)

The Genetic Information Nondiscrimination Act was enacted in 2008, to prevent Americans from being discriminated against based on genetic information (either from genetic tests or family history) by health insurers or employers (Hudson et al., 2008). Health insurers may not use genetic information to determine who is eligible for coverage or to set premiums for coverage. Employers may not use genetic information in hiring, firing, or in making decisions about promotions or job placements. Under the law, neither employers nor health insurance companies can request or require the provision of this information to make hiring or premium decisions. Carve outs to the law include: 1) the US Military *is* permitted to use genetic information in making employment decisions; 2) it does not apply to employers with fewer than 15 employees; and 3) it does not apply to benefits provided to veterans, federal employees, or through the Indian Health Service. Genetic counselors are frequently called upon to address patient concerns about genetic testing and discrimination and asked about the provisions of GINA. Advocates cite the legislation as a major step forward in building public trust in genetic testing. One key distinction to note is that GINA is intended to protect against discrimination based upon *predisposition* to disease, but not manifest disease, in which case the Americans with Disabilities Act provides protection in the employment setting and the Affordable Care Act has provisions in the health insurance setting (Baird and Rosenbaum, 2008; Blumenthal et al., 2015).

The Affordable Care Act

The Affordable Care Act (ACA) was signed into law in 2010, and represented the most significant health care legislative package signed into law since the introduction of Medicare and Medicaid in 1965 (Blumenthal et al., 2015). The law had the goal of making health insurance available and affordable for more people via subsidies or tax credits provided to individuals or families below a specific income threshold and by giving states the option of expanding state Medicaid programs. The law also includes provisions requiring insurers to provide coverage for those with pre-existing health conditions (including pregnancy) and preventing them from canceling coverage after health conditions are identified. Another key part of the law relevant to the practice of genetic counseling is mandatory coverage of a defined set of preventive health measures. The preventive health measures are covered when supported by strong recommendations from the US Preventive Services Task Force, the Advisory Committee on Immunization Practices (ACIP), the Health Resources and Services Administration's (HRSA's) Bright Futures Project, or the Institute of Medicine (IOM) committee on women's clinical preventive services. The preventive measures recommended for coverage include a broad swath of disease prevention measures, and among them are recommenda-tions for genetic testing and counseling for a select number of conditions. For example, because of this mandate, *BRCA1* and *BRCA2* germline testing is required to be covered for patients meeting certain high risk criteria (Blumenthal et al., 2015; US Preventive Services Task Force et al., 2019).

The 21st Century Cures Act

The 21st Century Cures Act was passed in 2016, and was a law designed to acceler-ate the development of new treatments for disease (and in particular rare diseases) and to bring these new treatments and innovations more quickly to patients who stand to benefit (21st Century Cures Act, 2016). The 21st Century Cures Act included many different provisions impacting the FDA, NIH funding (primarily for large initiatives like the All of Us / Precision Medicine Initiative and the Cancer Moonshot), funding for mental health care and addiction treatment, and a number of practices in health information technology. One piece of this legislation that gar-nered a lot of attention from hospitals systems and providers was that it proposed measures for the federal government to promote better communication between electronic health records belonging to different systems and included "information blocking" penalties for not providing patients timely access to medical records. Genetic counselors nationally and within their local systems were involved in con-versations about how and when genetic test results could be made available to patients via their health portals. On the long-term horizon, the 21st Century Cures Act has provided additional incentives and lower barriers to drug development for rare disease, expanding the footprint of the life science industry in addressing rare, genetic diseases and increasingly pulling genetic counselors into roles related to clinical trial recruitment and in the biopharma industry.

Access to Genetic Counselor Services Act

In order to be recognized as a provider of services to Medicare beneficiaries, and therefore reimbursed for their services to these patients, providers must be defined and added via an amendment to the Social Security Act. The Social Security Act was enacted as a part of President Franklin Roosevelt's New Deal program in 1935 and was amended in 1965 to establish the Medicare and Medicaid programs with the addition of Title XVIII (Klees et al., 2009). Within the law, definitions of the services and providers permitted by the law are articulated. Medicare benefi-ciaries may constitute a significant portion of some genetic counselors' patient populations, particularly in settings like oncology and cardiology. The Access to Genetic Counselor Services Act (introduced for legislative consideration at the time of publication of this book) would add genetic counselors as providers under the Social Security Act (The Access to Genetic Counselor Services Act, 2021). Enactment of a law requires passage through both the US House of Representatives and Senate and signature by the President. Significant work by many genetic counselors and patient and physician advocates has gone to promote passage of this legislation with the goal of positioning genetic counselors to serve more patients in settings where it has been challenging to provide the financial support for genetic counselors. Further, the ramifications of bill passage will likely extend beyond Medicare, as many Medicaid and commercial payers use Medicare as a guide in developing credentialing and payment processes.

This is far from an exhaustive analysis of policies impacting genetic counselor reimbursement and practice, but it is intended to provide a sense of the dramatic impact policies can have on the genetic counseling landscape. Many decisions within the health care system are driven by the financial and personal incentives of decision-makers or by policies compelling compliance with a standard established by law. To effect change in a system, it is critical to understand both incentives and policy structures, as well as the mechanisms through which policy is developed and enacted.

HEALTH AND HUMAN SERVICES

Many countries have a central Health Ministry or office tasked with overseeing implementation of health care policy. Within the US, the Department of Health and Human Services (HHS) is a cabinet-level department of the US Executive Branch. HHS is tasked with implementing health care and biomedical research laws passed by the Legislative Branch (Department of Health and Human Services, n.d.). Major operating agencies under the purview of HHS include:

- National Institutes of Health (NIH): tasked with overseeing biomedical and public health research.
- Centers for Disease Control and Prevention (CDC): tasked with the protection of public health and safety through the control and prevention of disease.
- Health Resources and Services Administration (HRSA): focused on improving access to health care for people who are uninsured, isolated or medically vulnerable.
- Food and Drug Administration (FDA): tasked with protecting and promoting public health through regulation of food safety, tobacco products, dietary supplements, prescription and over-the-counter pharmaceutical medications, vaccines, biopharmaceuticals, blood transfusions, medical devices, some diagnostics, electromagnetic radiation emitting devices (ERED), cosmetics, animal foods and feed, and veterinary products.
- Indian Health Service (IHS): tasked with providing direct medical care and public health services to federally recognized Native American Tribes and Alaska Native people.

- Agency for Healthcare Research and Quality (AHRQ): tasked with enhancing the quality, appropriateness, and effectiveness of health care services through research, guidelines and disseminating best-practices.
- Centers for Medicare and Medicaid Services (CMS): administers the Medicare program and works with states to administer the national Medicaid program.

Genetic counselors interact with the agencies of HHS in a number of ways. Genetic counselors have been employed within the NIH, CDC, and HRSA working both on the policy and research sides of these organizations. Funding from the NIH supports many research initiatives across the country, a number of which provide support for salaries of genetic counselors, an increasing number of whom are writing grants and serving as Principal Investigators (PIs) on NIH-funded studies. The CDC funds public health implementation programs and has funded specific programs intended to increase the identification of patients for whom genetic testing would be clinically impactful—and genetic counselors have led and been involved with a number of these efforts. Regulation of genetic tests and other diagnostics falls under the purview of the FDA, and discussions of how involved the FDA should be in the regulation of these tests are ongoing. Historically, the FDA has been most focused on tests provided direct-to-consumer, tests sold as kits that are performed across many different labs, and on tests that are "companion diagnostics" or intended to be used in conjunction with prescribing FDA-approved therapies. They have been less stringent with regard to most other Laboratory Developed Tests (LDTs)—historically defined as tests developed within a single lab for use within that lab, which are the tests most often utilized in clinic by genetic counselors. As policies have shifted and changed, genetic counselors have often been called upon to present the clinical perspective on test quality and regulation.

CMS establishes national policies for coverage and payment of services by Medicare for individuals over the age of 65. This includes setting national payment standards, or fee schedules, for how much Medicare will pay for specific services. There is a physician fee schedule that outlines payments to health care providers and also a laboratory fee schedule that CMS uses to set payments for tests. Rates on the laboratory fee schedule are informed by a committee of representatives from across the laboratory industry. A select set of medical policies, called National Coverage Determinations (NCDs), are issued by CMS and are intended to apply as a minimum standard for what should be covered for all Medicare beneficiaries. Most Medicare policies, however, are governed regionally by Medicare Administrative Contractors (MACs), which are private companies delegated by Medicare to process claims and establish policies. These policies are called Local Coverage Determinations (LCDs). LCDs apply to services provided within the region covered by a MAC and, importantly for genetic testing, will apply based on the location of the laboratory, not the location of the patient. Patients who have traditional Medicare will have coverage dictated by

MACs. Many Medicare beneficiaries have Medicare Advantage plans, administered by health insurance companies paid by Medicare usually per covered life, who must follow at a minimum the rules established by Medicare and the MACs, but who can choose to cover services above and beyond Medicare minimums. Medicaid and commercial payers will often look to Medicare policy as a guide for payments and policies.

Medicaid programs that cover individuals living with disabilities or below a specific income level are typically implemented at the state level, but with significant funding from the federal government. Many states have fee schedules defining by procedure code which services they will pay for and which are not coverable. Most often, states will delegate management of their Medicaid plans out to Managed Care Organizations (MCOs) who are paid per covered life to manage care while meeting specific standards for quality. MCOs will often have their own policies for coverage that provide specificity beyond state fee schedules and may also choose to cover services beyond those mandated by the state if they believe they will significantly improve quality and/or reduce overall costs. Anecdotally, genetic counselors in a number of states have reported success in being paid for services rendered to Medicaid beneficiaries, though expanding federal policies will likely be influential in making this standard practice in the future.

PRIVATE PAYERS

Private health insurance is an option in many of the countries in the world with Universal Health Coverage and in the US it is the means by which nearly two-thirds of Americans get coverage for their health care (Rosso, 2022). Most of the time in the US, health insurance is offered as a benefit paid by employers. The basic idea of insurance is that a group of individuals all contribute to a pool of money, which is then dispersed to cover their health care as needed, such that any one person won't face financial failure when their medical costs rise dramatically. Insurance plans vary in the extent to which the insurance plan or the employer customer of the insurance plan is at risk for the cost of an individual's health care. In some cases, those insured are "fully insured," meaning that the health insurance company is financially responsible for the costs of care for those insured under that plan, also known as the "risk pool" of members covered by that plan. In other cases, the risk pool is that of an employer or group of employees, and the insurance company is just paid to do the administrative work of managing payment for services but isn't actually at risk for the costs of care. Increasingly, employers are choosing to maintain their own risk pools or "self-fund," such that the insurance companies are not at risk for the cost of health care, but rather the employers are covering all of the costs of care for the pool of people. With employer-funded models, the insurance companies are motivated to control costs such that they can compete against other insurers for the employer's business by offering low premiums to be paid by employers seeking to manage their human resource costs (Claxton et al., 2021). In situations where genetic counselors are lobbying for changes in policies or procedures of a health insurance company, it is important to recognize these distinctions as sometimes those efforts may be better targeted toward employer groups, rather than the insurance company.

Included in the services offered by private payers are typically medical coverage policies for managing utilization of health care services, network contracts negotiated with different provider networks, labs and hospitals, and the management of claims submission and payment. Benefit packages outline the scope of the services to be managed and specific rules pertaining to services that a group may opt into coverage for (e.g., fertility services are often an "opt in" benefit for employers) and also the rules around co-pays and deductibles which may or may not differ depending upon whether a provider is "in network" or "out of network." A co-pay is a portion of a service that is paid by the member at the time of service, with the intention of creating a disincentive for individuals to seek services that they do not need or wouldn't want to pay for at all on their own. Balance billing is when a provider (e.g., a lab or a hospital) bills for the difference between the provider's charge and the allowed amount determined by the insurer. A deductible sets an amount, up to which the insured person pays for their own care, and after which the insurance company will pay for care. For instance, an individual with a $2,000 deductible in their benefit plan will pay $2,000 out of pocket for health care until they meet that deductible, after which point, their insurance will pay for their care, usually minus any co-pays. Often, individuals with a high-deductible benefit plan will use a health savings account (HSA), or portion of their paycheck that is set aside and not taxed, to pay for health care expenses.

Coverage policies are different from benefit packages in that a benefit package may lay out coverage for all medically necessary services within a particular area, and a coverage policy will articulate how a plan will define medical necessity across that range of services. State and federal laws governing insurance usually require health insurers to maintain accreditations that oversee how they develop, review, and implement medical policy and utilization management programs. For accreditation, they are required to review evidence and guidelines on a regular basis and maintain up-to-date policies and practices. Some health plans have specific coverage policies for genetic counseling and indications under which services are covered, and when policies do not exist coverage of services is typically determined by a general policy which lays out how the plan's clinical staff reviews for medical necessity. Far more commonly, plans have policies for coverage or noncoverage of genetic tests and often, as a part of coverage for genetic testing, they will also require that genetic counseling be performed. All plans have processes for appeals of claims that are denied, and most plans also have separate processes for providers to reach out with concerns or evidence to indicate a policy should be updated (Box 11-1).

BOX 11-1. APPROACHING HEALTH INSURANCE COMPANIES ON A PATIENT'S BEHALF

Clinical Scenario: A patient's insurance company denied a claim for payment of a genetic test that is recommended for the patient based on highly reputable national guidelines.

Questions to Ask of the Insurance Company:

1. What was the reason for the denial?
2. Was the test not covered under the medical policy?
3. Was there additional documentation that was needed?
4. Was the claim denied because of an administrative problem with the claim that was submitted by the hospital or lab?

Possible Approaches to Working with the Insurance Company

1. Consider writing a letter of medical necessity and/or appeal based on your patient, asking for an exception to the coverage decision articulating the national guidelines as well as the reasons this test will be important for care of your patient and how it will impact their medical management.
2. Make sure if documentation of genetic counseling is required, that that was provided along with any relevant family or medical history that may help.
3. If a test requires additional administrative steps be taken (e.g., prior authorization by the insurer, registration with the insurer's system), ask if those can be done retroactively.
4. Independently of your particular case, request a meeting with the health insurer's medical directors to talk about the policy and suggest edits to the policy based on national guidelines, emphasizing the benefits of this testing across all patients. If there are administrative challenges to payment, seek to understand why the insurer feels those systems are necessary.

Claims systems that process health insurance claims speak the language of CPT® (Current Procedural Terminology)[1] and ICD (International Classification of Diseases). CPT® is legislated into the federal HIPAA law as the official standard for communication about which medical procedure was performed between providers and health insurers (Health Insurance Portability and Accountability Act, 1996). CPT® codes are created by the American Medical Association (AMA) and those who use them must have a license from the AMA. They are created via a process

---

[1] CPT® is a registered trademark of the American Medical Association.

governed by the CPT® editorial panel who meets three times a year to review proposals from the clinical community, medical device manufactures, and diagnostic laboratories for new codes and code changes. The editorial panel can approve these updates to the code set which then allows those services to be billed. In 2007, the CPT® editorial panel approved the first code developed specifically for genetic counseling services provided by nonphysician providers which is used by many genetic counselors today. Given the evolving nature of CPT® codes, this chapter will not dive into specifics of their use by genetic counselors. However, any genetic counselor in a patient-facing role should work with their billing department about how the codes that cover our services are utilized at their institution.

When inquiring as to whether a service is covered by a health plan or not, it is useful to know which CPT® code might be used to bill for that service, as health insurer decision-making is frequently tied to the codes that are used. ICD codes lay out the diagnosis of the patient and the current standard in most places is to use the ICD-10, or 10th edition of ICD. These codes are used to communicate why a service is being provided and can, in some cases, be used to determine whether a service is covered or not. For instance, if a plan covers *BRCA1/2* testing for all individuals with ovarian cancer, and a claim is submitted with a procedure code for *BRCA1/2* testing and an ICD code for ovarian cancer, no further records would need to be reviewed to determine that the claim is payable. In practice, there are limitations in the specificity of both ICD and CPT® code sets since many genetic conditions and tests are not well represented by these codes, and it remains difficult for many patients to get clear cut answers about coverage for genetic counseling and testing services. In theory, prior authorization is a tool to provide feedback in advance about whether a service will be covered for a member of a health plan. Unfortunately, provider workflows, particularly related to genetic testing, do not fit well with prior authorization processes and commonly it is seen as an administrative burden to be overcome. There is wide variability across the practice of genetic counseling as to how counselors engage with prior authorization processes; in some clinics it is routine and may be requested before a patient is even seen in clinic and in some cases, it is managed largely by the laboratories who perform and bill for the tests.

As genetic counselors continue to grow into broader and more established roles within the health care biospheres in which they work, it is critical that we work with stakeholders across the health care system to build sustainable practices that bring value to all of the people who stand to benefit. In order to effectively work with payers to ensure our patients get the services they need, we need to understand their mandates and incentives and work within those structures to achieve shared goals. Life within an academic bubble can run the risk of insulating students and researchers from the realities of real-world health care and may minimize the importance of understanding payment and reimbursement systems. If we are truly going to move the needle on addressing the health disparities that are a reality of today's genomic medicine, we must be able to speak to the very systems that may exacerbate these disparities and be prepared to advocate for change within them.

THE INTEGRATION OF GENETIC COUNSELORS INTO THE HEALTH CARE ECOSYSTEM

As outlined so far in this chapter, the health care ecosystem is an interconnected web involving patients, providers, hospitals, private practices, laboratories, research programs, government agencies, insurance companies, and many other players. Genetic counselors that work outside of medical institutions are vital parts of this ecosystem by using their expertise in many ways, including helping to develop innovative new tests, advising on policies within government and the private sector, building new technology to enhance genetic counselor workflow, educating providers and patients around the country, and providing genetic counseling through more accessible means like telegenetics. These roles bring a huge amount of value to the larger system. In recognition of the fact the majority of genetic counselors work within hospital systems, and the fact that many of the current challenges related to billing, wait times, and staffing currently lie within hospital systems, the remainder of this chapter focuses heavily on this type of patient-facing clinical practice. Additionally, as with earlier parts of this chapter, the focus of this portion will be on health care structures within the US.

GENETIC COUNSELOR CERTIFICATION, LICENSURE, AND CREDENTIALING

For genetic counselors who opt to pursue a clinical role, integration into the complex medical system does not happen automatically. After completion of a graduate program, genetic counselors who want to provide direct patient care embark on a path that likely includes certification, possibly a license issued by the state government (depending on where they provide services), and for a small but increasing number, credentialing with third-party payers and/or their medical institution. With each of these steps, a genetic counselor becomes more integrated into this ecosystem, increasing both the visibility and viability of the profession.

The processes of certification, licensure, and credentialing are not undertaken by all genetic counselors. Depending on their role and work environment, they may not even be necessary. However, for those patient-facing genetic counselors who provide clinical care, especially if they bill payers for their services, these are interdependent steps that help genetic counselors become recognized and legitimized within the health care system. At their core, each of these processes is designed to ensure anyone receiving care from a genetic counselor can know that their provider is qualified. Each step is overseen by a different organization: certification is managed by a genetic counselor-led certifying body, licensure is governmental, and credentialing is taken on by an institution and/or private payer.

Certification

After completion of a training program, most graduates will sit for the board exam. Students may be surprised to learn that no one is required to take boards. It is technically voluntary. However, board certification is how the genetic counseling community, in alignment with most other health care providers, has collectively decided we measure competency to practice as a genetic counselor. This standardized demonstration of competency is also required for further integration into the larger health care system as a prerequisite for licensure, which will be discussed later in this chapter. Becoming board certified essentially shows that one has the adequate level of knowledge to practice independently. But just because one passes boards, does not guarantee the ability to practice on our own. In the real world, the ability of genetic counselors to practice independently, meaning without the supervision of a physician, is usually determined by scope of practice definitions, billing structures, and licensure laws within their state of practice.

The process of board certification is common across a wide array of professions, not just health care providers. There is a growing recognition that modalities other than standardized testing may have less bias and be more reflective of true competency. For example, some genetic counseling programs have already removed the GRE as a requirement for applications due to evidence that they reinforce or increase existing racial disparities in higher education (Knoester et al., 2017; Langin, 2019). In the future, the way in which genetic counselors demonstrate their knowledge and skills could look different; but whatever its shape, this step will always remain a vital bridge from student to practitioner.

Within the current structure, once someone completes their education, they opt to take a standardized test. If they pass that test, they receive the appropriate credential. For genetic counselors, the official "credential" is CGC® which stands for Certified Genetic Counselor (of note, this term credential is different from institutional and payer credentialing which we will discuss later in this chapter). The CGC credential allows genetic counselors to professionally display their training and expertise alongside their name.

Certifications are usually time-limited, meaning that they must be maintained and renewed after some period. For genetic counselors that means receiving continuing education to show ongoing competence as the field evolves and then recertifying after a certain period of time. If a genetic counselor does not renew and lets their certification lapse, they must retake the board exam again. Letting certification lapse would have downstream ramifications for their ability to practice if they are also licensed and/or credentialed by institutions or payers. because both of those typically depend first on active certification.

In the US, the board exam is administered by the American Board of Genetic Counseling (ABGC). As Box 11-2 explains, ABGC is a separate organization from the National Society of Genetic Counselors (NSGC) and is also separate from the body that accredits genetic counselor training programs, the Accreditation Council for Genetic Counseling (ACGC).

BOX 11-2. ALPHABET SOUP: WHAT ARE THESE DIFFERENT GROUPS?

NSGC: The National Society of Genetic Counselors (NSGC) promotes the professional interests of genetic counselors and provides a network for professional communications. Access to continuing education opportunities, professional resources, advocacy, and the discussion of all issues relevant to human genetics and the genetic counseling profession are an integral part of belonging to the NSGC. https://www.nsgc.org/About/About-NSGC

ABGC: ABGC is a not-for-profit organization incorporated in 1993 to establish standards of competence for Certified Genetic Counselors and advance their value as leaders in precision health to safeguard and serve the public. https://www.abgc.net/about-abgc/

ACGC: The stated purpose of ACGC is to advance "quality in genetic counseling education by developing and maintaining standards for educational and clinical training of genetic counseling students and implementing a peer-review process to evaluate programs". Essentially, they ensure GC programs provide adequate training for students to become genetic counselors. https://www.gceducation.org/about-acgc/

In the past, in order to be certified by ABGC, an individual needed to graduate from an accredited training program in the US or Canada. Starting in 2018, a pathway was developed for genetic counselors who trained in programs outside of these two countries to also take the ABGC exam. International accrediting bodies can apply to become a "Recognized Accrediting Body" and if they meet the quality standards put forth by ABGC, then students who graduate from programs accredited by these bodies will be considered eligible to sit for the US board examination (ABGC, n.d.).

While not every international accrediting body has been officially recognized by ABGC, throughout the world there are independent accrediting bodies who ensure patients in those countries are also receiving the highest quality care from qualified genetics providers. One area seeing increasing growth is Latin America. Genetic counseling is not yet a widely recognized profession in this region (Abacan et al., 2019). As of 2022, there are two genetic counseling training programs, one in Cuba and one in Brazil. To increase awareness of the profession of genetic counseling and support genetics providers and families in Latin America, the Latin American Professional Society of Genetic Counseling (SPLAgen) was created in 2020. This organization has compiled an extensive and evolving list of genetics professionals throughout Mexico, Central America, and South America to highlight the services and enable connections between providers (Simone, 2022). Table 11-2 provides a snapshot of genetic counselor training and oversight around the world.

TABLE 11-2. Summary of various genetic counselor certification and regulations around the world

Country	Year first training program started	Oversight Body	Requirements	Recertification Schedule
Australia/New Zealand	1995 (GradDip); 2011 (MS)	Certification (HGSA)	Min. 2 years of practice w/supervision, case logbook, case studies, reflective essay, lit review or 1st author publication	Under review
Canada	1985	Certification (CAGC)	Graduation from approved MS program; case logbook, letters of recommendation	Every 10 years by: work experience and continuing ed or exam
India	2007 (Cert.) 2014 (MS)	Certification (BGC)	2 levels w/ different requirements based on experience, including logged cases, essays, and case studies	Every 2–3 years; requires continuing ed or professional activities
Israel	1997	Licensure (Israeli Ministry of Health)	2 years postgrad work; 85 case logbook; certification one year after exam if criteria met	Every 5 years
Japan	2000s	Certification (JBGC)	Graduation from approved program; active membership in JSHG or JSGC for 2 years	Every 5 years by continuing ed
Saudi Arabia	2005 (GradDip); 2015 (MS)	Licensure (SCFHS)	Panel interview, testing, or exam by medical board	Under review
South Africa	1989	Registration (HPCSA)	Graduation from approved Master's degree program plus 2 years of internship after which portfolio is submitted; Logbook w/ min of 200 cases; case reports, reflective essay; research experience; supervisor reports; training assessment.	Every 2 years by continuing ed. A percentage of ed must pertain to ethics, human rights, or health law
Taiwan	2003	Certification (TAGC)	Based on a combination of education and work experience; 50 case log and other records review	Every 6 years by continuing ed
UK	1992	Registration (GCRB)	Approved 2-year MS and 2 years postgrad work experience. 50 cases, reference, essay, case studies, supervision, recorded consults, and professional development reflection	Every 5 years
US	1969	Certification (ABGC)	Graduation from ABGC approved accredited program; case logbook	Every 5 years by continuing ed or exam

GradDip: Graduate Diploma which in some countries is considered an advanced degree; HGSA: Human Genetics Society of Australasia; BGC: Board of Genetic Counseling; JBGC: Japanese Board of Genetic Counseling, JSHG: Japan Society of Human Genetics; JSGC: Japanese Society for Genetic Counseling; SCFHS: Saudi Commission for Health Specialties; HPCSA: Health Professions Council of South Africa; TAGC: Taiwan Association of Genetic Counseling; GCRB: Genetic Counsellor Registration Board Adapted with permission from Abacan et al. (2019)

Licensure

As previously discussed, certification is a voluntary process developed from within a profession to show competency. Licensure, on the other hand, is where the practice of genetic counseling becomes regulated by the government. A license conveys a legal authority to work in an occupation and is determined by state law. Essentially, at its core, licensure is about protecting the public from unqualified practitioners in any field, not just health care. As of 2020, the Bureau of Labor Statistics estimated that about 22% of the civilian workforce had a license including many nonmedical professions (Bureau of Labor Statistics, 2022).

Licenses are important for several reasons. First, and by far most importantly, they protect the public. If a profession is licensed, then there is an element of harm that can come if the duties of that profession are not carried out appropriately. If a state offers genetic counselor licensure, that means that at some point in the past, genetic counselors (and others) in that state took on the arduous task of getting a law passed. The process of getting these laws passed can be long and involve many stakeholders including physician's groups, hospital systems, elected officials, patient advocates, and lobbyists. There can be many steps and the process can last years (see Box 11-3) but achieving licensure in all 50 states has been a long-held priority for the profession (NSGC, n.d.a).

To build support for a profession to be licensed, it is helpful to illustrate the consequences of unqualified individuals working in that profession. These are referred to as "cases of harm." Genetic counselors across the country have compiled these cases which often include stories as heartbreaking as preventable deaths, unnecessary surgeries, or intense emotional stress, and range all the way to improper billing that cost the state government or state residents money.

Additional reasons licensure is important are the dual benefits of a defined scope of practice and title protection. Scope of practice essentially means an

---

BOX 11-3. HOW IS A BILL PASSED BY A STATE?

The process is different in every state but generally involves the following steps:

- draft bill
- identify sponsor and co-sponsors
- introduce bill
- gain additional co-sponsors
- committee hearings
- bill passage in both houses
- governor signs bill

outline of what genetic counselors are qualified to do in their roles. NSGC maintains a standard for how genetic counselors' scope of practice is defined (see Box 11-4), though each state may add or subtract to this standard within their own state laws. Title protection defines who is allowed to call themselves a genetic counselor in that state. In states without licensure, there is no limitation on who is allowed to practice using the title of genetic counselor. It is easy to imagine the harm that could come from unqualified individuals with inadequate training calling themselves a genetic counselor, setting up their own practice, and charging patients to interpret genetic test results, for example. When licensure does not exist, it is much harder for the state to protect residents from such activity because there's no legal definition of the profession. It should be clarified, however, that title protection relates to which professionals can *call* themselves a genetic counselor but does not restrict who can *provide* genetic counseling. For example, in a state that licenses genetic counselors, a physician can still provide genetic counseling to their patients since that would usually be considered part of their scope of practice based on their own license. This is an important distinction because

---

BOX 11-4. GENETIC COUNSELOR SCOPE OF PRACTICE

(a) obtain and evaluate individual, family, and medical histories to determine genetic risk for genetic/medical conditions and diseases in a patient, his/her offspring, and other family members;

(b) discuss the features, natural history, means of diagnosis, genetic and environmental factors, and management of risk for genetic/medical conditions and diseases;

(c) identify and coordinate genetic laboratory tests and other diagnostic studies as appropriate for the genetic assessment;

(d) integrate genetic laboratory test results and other diagnostic studies with personal and family medical history to assess and communicate risk factors for genetic/medical conditions and diseases;

(e) explain the clinical implications of genetic laboratory tests and other diagnostic studies and their results;

(f) evaluate the client's or family's responses to the condition or risk of recurrence and provide client-centered counseling and anticipatory guidance;

(g) identify and utilize community resources that provide medical, educational, financial, and psychosocial support and advocacy;

(h) provide written documentation of medical, genetic, and counseling information for families and health care professionals.

NSGC (n.d.b)

while one of the goals of genetic counseling licensure is to protect the public from unqualified providers, it is not meant to limit the responsible provision of genetic counseling by other health care providers, when appropriate.

Obtaining a License

If a genetic counselor is in a state with licensure, typically they will need to apply for a license with the state before they can see patients independently. Additional documentation is required which can be extensive and include things like a background check, copies of licenses in other states, and professional references. Licensure applications also cost money, which can also vary from state to state. Once an application is submitted, it is reviewed by a designated state board, often within the state's Department of Health. If all documentation is completed and the fee is paid, it would be unusual for an application to be denied. However, state boards can also receive complaints or concerns about providers applying for licensure, so each application is reviewed thoroughly by the designated board. If approved, a license will be issued. States have differing requirements for ongoing licensing but typically they require continuing education along the same lines as that needed to maintain certification. However, it is important for licensed genetic counselors to know their specific state's requirements because the timing, due dates, and documentation for submission of continuing education documentation can be different than that for recertification. Once licensure exists in a state, there is greater protection for residents because individuals without appropriate training will not meet the standards to obtain a license, and if a licensed provider is found to be doing harm by the designated state board, their license can be taken away and they can no longer lawfully practice in that state.

While licensure is a major goal for the profession, it should be noted that there can be some challenges when a state decides to pursue this aim. There may be individuals with a wealth of experience who began practicing before the current board examination structure or ACGC existed. There could be individuals practicing competently as genetic counselors who trained abroad. Depending on how a licensure law is written, the title protection language may exclude these individuals from calling themselves genetic counselors if, for example, the law requires someone to be board certified through ABGC. Some states may opt to include language that enables these individuals to obtain a license. However, it can be a delicate balance to ensure the standards that are set are not biased towards a particular group, but also are written so that unqualified individuals cannot become licensed because the language was broader than it was meant to be.

The emergence of multistate licensure (MSL) is another illustration of the challenges that can come with licensure. A growing number of genetic counselors are obtaining licenses in more than one, and sometimes all, licensing states, due to the evolving roles of genetic counselors. Many genetic counselors pursuing MSL are employed by national telegenetics companies or in private practice and want to provide care for patients in a broader region than just their state. This is necessary because the genetic counselor must be licensed where the patient is physically located at the time of the visit, not where the provider is or where the patient's home is located. So, if a genetic counselor wants to provide services to patients in multiple states, they have to hold a license in all of those states even if the services are virtual and the genetic counselor will always be in the same location. It is a major challenge for these genetic counselors to maintain so many licenses. There is significant time in tracking the various documentation requirements, since they are not the same in each state, in addition to paying each state's fees. Studies have shown that if a genetic counselor wanted to provide services nationally, the upfront cost of MSL would approach $5,000—not including recurring annual fees in the thousands for renewals (Tschirgi et al., 2022). This will undoubtedly increase as more states pass licensure laws.

Given this challenge, many understandably ask: why is there not just one license for the whole country? The answer is that there are some aspects of regulation that are traditionally handled state by state, and licensure is one of them, across all professions. This gives states the power to develop and oversee the process how they see fit. There is, however, a concept called a compact, which occurs when multiple states join together and pass the same bill. Under a compact, participating states grant one another reciprocity, meaning that a license in one state grants a license in all member states. This is already in existence for physicians and is called the Interstate Medical Licensure Compact. It covers more than 30 states and additional states are introducing legislation (Interstate Medical Licensure Compact, 2020). Passing an interstate compact is a complex process that requires states and stakeholders working together and each participating state would need to amend their existing genetic counselor licensing law (or pass one in the first place) to create a compact. Creating momentum for huge efforts like exploring a compact highlights why integration into the health care ecosystem better positions genetic counselors to tackle major initiatives.

Credentialing

The third component of integration into the health care ecosystem is credentialing. Because credentialing is dependent on both board certification and (usually) licensure, it is also the one that clinical genetic counselors report they are least likely to have (NSGC, 2024). As a reminder, passing the certification exam boards and using the CGC credential is not the same as being credentialed by a hospital or payer. Credentialing in this context is a process that institutions and third-party payers undertake to confirm that a person has the qualifications to perform their duties. Like licensure, at its core, credentialing is about patient protection. Health care institutions and payers have a huge incentive to ensure that services they are providing and services they are paying for, respectively, are being carried out by individuals with the appropriate training. So why aren't more genetic counselors credentialed? It likely is due to the relative size of the profession related to other health professionals employed by the institution. Credentialing is time intensive and usually is not a one-time event, but must be renewed. Therefore, if there is only a given amount of administrative bandwidth, coupled with the billing and reimbursement challenges genetic counselors face, some institutions may decide not to credential their genetic counselors and not attempt to get them credentialed with payers. A genetic counselor who is not credentialed can still bill for their services, but there may be more roadblocks to reimbursement.

Another barrier to credentialing is likely the lack of knowledge amongst genetic counselors about its importance (Williamson, 2021). While there is a long-term benefit, genetic counselors themselves may not be pushing for it at their own institutions. Genetic counselors have also reported that even when they ask to be credentialed, their institution did not move forward (NSGC, 2024). There will continue to be discussion throughout the genetic counselor community towards credentialing as it can contribute to better reimbursement and better integration into the health care system.

CODING AND BILLING FOR GENETICS SERVICES IN THE US

For genetic counselors who see patients in a hospital setting, more than half of them bill for their services (NSGC, 2024). The most common way genetic counselors bill is with CPT® codes. Codes and code descriptors can change over time. There has not always been a specific code for genetic counselors to use. It wasn't until 2006 that a CPT® code was developed and approved through work by NSGC in conjunction with the American Medical Association (AMA), who, as previously discussed, oversees the creation of CPT® codes. On January 1, 2007, a code became active and available for genetic counselors to bill (Harrison et al., 2010). Since then, usage of a genetic counseling-specific code for GC billing has steadily increased. A 2009 study found that 24% of genetic counselors who billed for their services used the code for at least some portion of visits (Harrison et al., 2010), and 2023 the reported usage was up to 75% (NSGC, 2024). In late 2023, additional changes to coding for genetic counseling were announced. It is vital as a practicing genetic counselor who bills, or wants to bill, for services to work closely with your institution's billing department and coding experts within NSGC to ensure up-to-date and appropriate coding for your services.

Evaluation and Management (E&M) Codes

Another common way genetic counselors bill is using different CPT® codes that fall into a category called "Evaluation and Management" or E&M codes. Whether or not genetic counselors are reimbursed for E&M codes depends on many factors including the policy of the individual payer being billed, and who was involved in the visit. Some clinics opt for "incident-to" billing. This type of billing has to meet specific criteria but essentially enables the genetic counselor's time to be reimbursed at the same rate as a physician (which is going to be higher than a genetic counselor alone). The challenge with "incident-to" billing is that both providers have to be involved with the same patient encounter which can present challenges to busy clinics who are attempting to improve efficiency. E&M codes vary based on the length and complexity of the visit. There are other "incident-to" codes that enable billing to Medicare when a genetic counselor and physician are both involved with a patient visit. As described earlier in this chapter, at the time of publication, Medicare does not recognize genetic counselors as independent providers (regardless of certification, licensure, or credentialing). Without this recognition, genetic counselors cannot bill Medicare directly unless a physician is also involved in that encounter.

It is important for billing genetic counselors to understand that just because a certain amount is billed for a particular encounter does not mean the full amount, or even any of the amount, will be paid by the health insurance company, regardless of credentialing or licensure. This is the same across the health care system. Payment can depend on many complex factors. One study documented that about 34.5% of genetic counselor visit costs billed with the genetic counseling CPT® code were reimbursed (Leonhard et al., 2017). This means that if $100 was billed, the institution was paid on average $34.50. This was just one study, and reimbursement may vary by region, institution, and other factors, but it highlights the importance of understanding reimbursement patterns in a specific genetics clinic which can help ensure the clinic is maximizing its financial contribution.

Billing using CPT® and/or E&M codes are examples of professional fees. This type of billing is designed to reimburse for a professional service. Facility fees are a different type of billing where the amount billed to the patient is related to the overhead cost of utilizing a physical space, like rent, air conditioning, and lighting. There are parameters under which these can be billed, and they usually require a space to be an outpatient hospital clinic. These are usually reimbursed at lower rates than professional fees but can also be simpler to bill, so some institutions opt for this over professional fees.

Because of the complexities of billing and reimbursement, it is extremely beneficial for a genetic counselor who bills or who is interested in billing to make connections with their billing team. Hospitals employ billing experts who can help a clinic access their claim and reimbursement data. The NSGC Professional Status Survey asks questions about billing in its annual survey. As of 2022, a very large percentage of genetic counselors who bill for their services answer "Do Not Know" when asked if there had been changes to their reimbursement the prior year. As genetics clinics are under increasing pressure to see more patients and feel pressure to hire more genetic counselors, understanding reimbursement and revenue generation for services is a huge component of building a strong business case which can help get positions approved. This will be discussed later in the Business Case section of this chapter.

CLINICAL PRACTICE CHALLENGES

Even as the roles and career paths available to genetic counselors become more diverse, all genetic counselors, either directly or indirectly, interact with the larger health care ecosystem. Understanding the fundamental components that go into clinical practice, beyond just seeing patients, can position genetic counselors to be in a better position to advocate for the profession.

Patient-Related Activities

Much of genetic counselor training is appropriately dedicated to the fundamentals of providing quality genetic counseling across a variety of specialties. For genetic counselors that enter clinical practice, they often find quickly that most of their time is not actually spent with patients. This is not unique to genetic counselors since many providers will be involved in clinic operations, administrative meetings, training program commitments, professional development and volunteer roles, and so on, in addition to their time seeing patients.

On top of those commitments, genetic counselors handle many activities related to the patients they see outside of the face-to-face appointment. These activities are called Patient-Related Activities, or PRAs and include note and letter writing, case preparation/medical record review, literature reviews, paperwork, coordination of care, among others. See Table 11-3 for more detail on what genetic counselors report as their most common PRAs, across specialties. Research on genetic counselor workload has found that for every 45-minute session with a patient, genetic counselors spent about 3 hours on PRAs for that same patient (Attard et al., 2019).

TABLE 11-3. **Average percentage of time spent on PRAs: average across specialties**

Patient-Related Activity	% of time per week (40-hr work week)
Letter writing/dictation	15.75%
Medical record review	9.75%
Patient-related paperwork	5.75%
Coordinating patient care	5.75%
Pre- or post-clinic meeting	3.75%
Other medical record documentation	3.25%
Case reporting to physician	3%
Literature search or review	3%

Adapted from Attard et al. (2019)

GENETIC COUNSELING SERVICE DELIVERY MODELS

The "traditional" model of genetic counseling typically encompasses a referral to a clinic, a pre-test consult including the common components of a visit (contracting, pedigree, education, risk assessment, decision making, plans for results/follow-up), then the coordination of testing, and lastly patients receiving results and follow-up as needed. Historically, these visits have been provided in-person and involve a genetic counselor, or genetic counselor and doctor, and one patient is seen at a time.

Given the evolving landscape of genetics, new ways to meet the needs of patients needing genetics services have been emerging (Cohen et al., 2019; Bednar et al., 2022). These are often referred to as service delivery models (SDMs). Service delivery is a very broad term that can refer to the mode in which patient visits are held: in-person, via telegenetics, by telephone, or in a group setting (Trepanier, 2020). SDMs can also include a new way to provide genetic counseling where some components of the "traditional" session are delivered in a new way, by someone other than a genetic counselor, or in some cases removed altogether. For an SDM to work well, it should enable the genetic counselor to work at the top of their scope, while also ensuring effective and high-quality patient care (Box 11-5).

IMPROVING ACCESS TO SERVICES

One of the major motivating factors for innovating the delivery of genetic counseling is improving patient access to genetics services. There is a broad perception that there is a "shortage" of genetic counselors. This can be difficult to untangle. On the one hand, many referring providers may perceive that there is a difficulty

---

BOX 11-5. WHAT IS "WORKING AT THE TOP OF YOUR SCOPE"?

You may hear people refer to the importance of genetic counselors "working at the top of their scope." But, what does this mean? The Genetic Counselors Scope of Practice, as defined by NSGC is shown in Box 11-4 of this chapter. This is the core set of skills that we have extensive training in. "Working at the top of your scope" means that as much of your workload as possible is dedicated to performing tasks you are uniquely trained to do. It also therefore means reducing administrative tasks like scheduling, answering phones, completing paperwork, and so on. It makes economic sense for an institution to have their providers working at the top of their scope because their compensation is based on a specialized set of skills and it is inefficient for them to spend their time on tasks unrelated to their training. Utilizing our skills also creates job satisfaction and enables us to help far more patients and their families while bringing the most possible value to our institutions.

getting their patients into a genetics clinic, but this can vary greatly by specialty and geography (Wallace et al., n.d.; Fogleman et al., 2019). Surveys of genetic counselors found that urgent patients can often be seen within an appropriate time period (Knapke et al., 2016). Additionally, NSGC's own workforce study suggested that the rapid growth of training programs is closing the supply/demand gap sooner than anticipated (Hoskovec et al., 2018; NSGC, 2022). On top of that, the rise of third-party telegenetics companies indicates that access should continue to improve. However, if the larger referral base for a genetics clinic is not aware of these changes, then they can't be utilized to improve access.

Telegenetics

While great strides have been made in the number of genetic counselors in practice, there is evidence that genetic counselor "deserts" remain. Demographic data shows that genetic counselors tend to be highly concentrated in more populated states, and within those states, are usually working within large metropolitan areas (NSGC, 2024). If patients do not have in-person genetics services within a reasonable distance of their home then these services are inaccessible (Wallace et al., no date). One solution to this geographic barrier is telegenetics which includes both virtual visits utilizing video, as well as telephone consults (Cohen et al., 2019). The use of telegenetics saw a rapid rise around 2021, almost certainly caused by the COVID19 pandemic which started in early 2020. The 2022 Professional Status Survey indicated that for the first time, video-based telemedicine was the most common mode of providing genetic counseling, with 82% of respondents reporting using this mode for at least some of their visits. In two years, the use of video-based telemedicine for at least some clinic visits jumped from 28% to 82% (NSGC, 2022). In addition, surveys of genetic counselors show that in many states, there have been more licenses issued than there are providers in that state, indicating a growth in the availability of telemedicine-based genetic counseling across the country (NSGC, 2022). That same time period also saw a dramatic, durable shift in the number of different modes utilized by genetic counselors, with almost half of genetic counselor respondents saying they use three different modes (in-person, video-based telemedicine, and phone-based telemedicine) compared to only 14% of respondents answering that way in 2019 (NSGC, 2022). Subsequent surveys did not find a significant drop over time, indicating this was not only a response to the pandemic, but likely will remain a primary way genetic counseling is delivered (NSGC, 2024).

While this data may represent a snapshot in time, they do show that clinics were able to rapidly pivot to alternative modes of delivery when necessary. The sustainability of these modes in the long run will likely largely depend on payer reimbursement, patient satisfaction, and accessibility. While health literacy, access to quality internet connection, patient preference, and other challenges may mean that telegenetics is not the solution for all patients facing geographic barriers to genetics services, it could go a long way in breaching this gap for many.

Group counseling

A lesser utilized mode of delivering genetic counseling is the group counseling model. Generally, this model is most beneficial when a group of patients have the same indication, and the major components of the visit, like providing education and discussion of testing options, can be provided all at once. An example of this model in action is the Veterans Health Administration (VA). To meet the needs of the influx of referrals, a process was designed so patients having similar indications participate in virtual group counseling sessions. For example, patients referred due to a family history of cancer but who have not had cancer themselves would be scheduled in the same group appointment. Genetic counselors at the VA report that this cut down on wait times and enabled more patients to be seen. Since the visits were virtual, the model also gave patients across the country access to genetic counselors, even though all the participating genetic counselors were based in a single city (Venne et al., 2019). Challenges to the group counseling model include a high level of coordination to triage patients into particular groups, late arrivals impacting the start time for the group, and reimbursement issues. Surveys of genetic counselors do not show a rapid growth of this model compared to other modes of service delivery, but the VA example illustrates this may work well for larger institutions with a broad geographic footprint (NSGC, 2024).

NEW SERVICE DELIVERY MODELS

While telegenetics and virtual group counseling are examples of new modes of conducting a genetic counselor visit, there are emerging changes to clinical workflow that can also fall under the category of SDMs. These attempt to address inefficiencies or barriers to care in multiple different areas. Some may tackle decreasing wait times, some attempt to increase testing volumes, and some may increase clinical efficiency by providing some components of genetic counseling outside of the visit itself, like pre-visit educational videos. Some clinics are utilizing different provider types like genetic counseling assistants (GCAs) to deliver some components of a traditional genetic counseling visit.

Surveys have shown a great interest in new SDMs among clinical genetic counselors, likely because most of them reported that their current model was inadequate to serve their patients' needs (Boothe et al., 2021). A variety of reasons were cited, but over three-quarters of genetic counselors desired "to increase the number of patients we can serve" (Khan et al., 2021).

Genetic Counseling Assistants

The adoption of GCAs has been one way that genetic counselors have tackled increasing demands for services. Typically, they are deployed to handle tasks that do not require a genetic counselor, like pedigree-drawing, records requests, and patient intakes. The GCA model has been shown to reduce genetic counselor time on PRAs, increase new patient volume, and decrease costs to patients in a sustainable way (Pirzadeh-Miller et al., 2017; Hallquist et al., 2020, Krutish et al., 2022). The major challenge with GCAs is whether or not their time will become billable like assistants in other areas of medicine (physical therapy assistants, physician assistants, etc.). It can be difficult to convince administrators to hire for positions that do not bring in revenue. Therefore, it is helpful for genetic counselors to understand how to build a business case and advocate for themselves.

Genetics Extenders and Point of Care Testing

Genetic counselors continue to innovate and think outside the traditional box in order to meet the needs of patients. Surveys of clinical genetic counselors have uncovered a wide array of changes to clinical workflows and alternative SDMs. Some of these new SDMs result in someone other than a genetic counselor actually seeing the patient. For example, the genetics "extender" model may involve training a non-genetics provider, like a medical assistant or a nurse, to provide some genetics education, facilitate testing, and ensure patients get results. In this model, the genetic counselor may never see the patient, but supervises and trains a group of extenders and performs periodic chart reviews for quality assurance. Another model involves "point of care" testing, sometimes also called "mainstreaming." In these models, providers who usually refer a patient to a genetics clinic for testing, instead order the testing themselves for a designated group of patients. This model has been shown to work in cancer centers where a single group of patients with the same diagnosis, like ovarian or pancreatic cancer, may need germline test results near the time of diagnosis for treatment planning, or to "update" cancer testing for previously negative patients (Symecko et al., 2019; Ranallo et al., 2021). In both of these examples, the patients don't necessarily have a visit with the genetic counselor. Instead, the genetic counselor can focus their time facilitating this workflow by providing oversight of the larger process, periodic chart review, and/or reserving their patient-facing visits for the cases that are more complex.

A body of literature around SDMs continues to grow which will be necessary to ensure we are not sacrificing patient outcomes for efficiency (Greenberg, 2020). Many of the challenges to delivery of care have some proposed solutions, but the solutions aren't without their own barriers. For example, telephone or video-based counseling may not be covered by insurance, could require licenses in multiple states and data suggest lower uptake of testing for underserved populations when patients aren't seen in-person (Butrick et al., 2015). Extender and point-of-care models may leave some patients who would greatly benefit from the one-on-one nature of traditional genetic counseling feeling confused or worried about their results. Studies of new models need to include diverse populations to ensure attempts to overcome some barriers don't introduce new disparities for certain populations.

Considerations for New Service Delivery Models

Before implementing a new model or workflow change, it is important to consider all the impacts on clinical staff. Who is going to be the point person for this new process? Do they have the bandwidth to take on extra duties? If it will fall to the genetic counselor, will it actually increase efficiency or just add a new list of tasks? Does it solve the main problem the clinic is facing, or could it unintentionally exacerbate other pain points? For example, an administrator may propose implementing a waiting room questionnaire to identify more patients for a genetics clinic and increase downstream revenue. Identifying patients who may be falling through the cracks for genetics services is undeniably a good thing. However, there are other considerations, too:

- Can the clinic handle this influx of patients?
- Could it increase wait times significantly?
- Who will be in charge of reviewing the patient answers to the questionnaire?
- Who will contact the high-risk patients?
- Will this be documented in their medical record? If so, how and by whom?
- Who will track whether those patients are ever seen and/or tested?
- Are there resources in place for uninsured or underinsured patients who may be identified as high risk to access the necessary follow-up services?
- Is the questionnaire accessible to patients who may speak a different language or have other accessibility challenges?
- If patients have questions, who will they contact?

Many of these challenges can likely be addressed, but it is important to examine these changes from all angles to ensure the net impact is positive for the system and the clinic, and not increased workload for staff who are already overwhelmed or create anxiety and confusion for patients in the process.

While overcoming clinical challenges is vital, genetic counselors still work within an economic system too. Considerations like the inability to bill for GCA services, concerns about reimbursement for telegenetics services, and the cost of hiring support staff to take on new roles within a genetics clinic means that these processes are not easy to develop, nor are they easy to convince institutional leadership to adopt, even if they result in more patients being seen. Next in this chapter we will discuss the creation of a "Business Case" to empower genetic counselors to advocate using data, relationship-building, and many of the other skills genetic counselors already have in their toolkit.

ARGUING THE BUSINESS CASE FOR GENETIC COUNSELING

In 2021, for the first time, NSGC convened a group of genetic counselors from a variety of patient care settings for the Business Case Summit (Babu et al., 2021). Despite the growth of the genetic counselor profession, genetic counseling remains a very small segment of the overall health care ecosystem. In addition, there are major billing and reimbursement challenges, as previously outlined. Therefore, it can be a huge challenge for genetic counselors employed by hospitals to measure and report the financial impact of genetic counseling services within their institution. However, as the Business Case workgroup determined, genetic counselors already have many of the skills and expertise needed to overcome these challenges.

A business case is a tool developed to show a target audience that a given proposal both solves a relevant problem and is a good investment (Babu et al., 2021). Most often, this will involve financial impact either through cost savings or increased revenue. This chapter has already touched on many of the issues that have hindered genetic counselors from developing business cases in the past: challenges in billing, lack of recognition by CMS, inconsistent reimbursement, low rates of credentialing, and lack of time due to increasing referrals and inefficiencies in clinic (Babu et al., 2021). There is never going to be a one-size-fits-all approach to a business case since clinics can vary. However, the work group did put forth some common themes from genetic counselors with experience in developing them including:

- collect data early to tell a compelling story;
- engage a variety of partners for success;
- clearly articulate and ask for your value;
- align on goals, priorities, and timing.

Practice Metrics

The starting point for any business case is metrics. Most commonly this would include number of visits, no-show rates, wait times, appointment type (initial/results/other), and mode of visit (video-based telemedicine, phone-based telemedicine, in-person, group, other). More advanced metrics could include:

- capturing the time between a referral and when the patient is scheduled and/or seen;
- last-minute cancellation rate (patients that cancel within 24 hours of appointment);
- unique referring providers (how many individual providers are sending patients);
- referrals by provider type (where and what type of providers are referrals coming from);
- completion rate for pre-appointment documentation, if requested;
- geographic footprint (where do your patients live and how far do they travel);

- what percentage of eligible patients from your institution are being referred;
- capturing race/ethnicity, language spoken, and other demographic information to explore disparities in access.

These metrics allow a clinic to better understand the state of their practice. While financial impact is one metric that can help grow a service line, metrics can also help improve workflow, for example:

- changes in referral patterns leads to physician outreach and education;
- expansion of clinics into high referral areas to increase patient access;
- sending reminders regarding appointments to reduce no-show rates and increase volume.

Revenue and Cost Savings

There are several ways health care providers can show they bring financial value to an institution. First is reimbursement, which is the payment received for the services billed. This is usually the most straightforward impact to track. Genetic counselors may not regularly be a part of financial meetings at their institution, so it's not uncommon for this data to be something that seems inaccessible. Any institution is going to have teams of people who are handling patient billing, which includes tracking charges, reviewing, and appealing denials, providing documentation (from clinical notes) to support the charges. It benefits all clinics to know how this is being handled and by whom. If possible, some reporting process could be set up so this could be tracked over time. It is possible that charges are going unreimbursed due to issues with documentation that could easily be resolved. Given that most institutions have far fewer genetic counselors than other types of providers, it may be that the billing providers are unaware of reimbursement problems because it is a small amount of revenue compared to the overall revenue for a center. However, if genetic counselors want to increase our presence, we should inquire and be involved in how billing is being handled so we can not only address any issues but also contribute to the overall financial case in support of our positions.

Another way to show value is to investigate downstream revenue. This is the revenue generated from other consults, imaging, surgeries, screenings, lab work, and so on that a patient may receive as the result of their genetics consult and/or test result. This revenue may be complicated to track depending on the structure of the institution, or whether a clinic is based on a community model where various types of follow-up may happen within private practices and not under the same financial umbrella or documented in the same EHR. It can be extremely helpful for genetic counselors in clinical practice to understand who has access to this type of data and how reporting could work. It could be something that is revisited over time and not continuously tracked (Mauer et al., 2021).

A third value added of genetic counselors is not based on revenue but instead on cost savings to an institution. Some institutions have laboratories that process both in-house tests and send-out genetic tests. Many studies have shown that by having genetic counselors review genetic testing orders they can save potentially millions of dollars by correcting improperly ordered tests that would not have been reimbursed by payers (Mathias et al., 2016; McWalter et al., 2018). This same cost savings has also been demonstrated when genetic counselors are employed directly by reference laboratories as well, illustrating that genetic counselors do not have to be directly seeing patients to make a positive impact on the overall health care ecosystem (Miller et al., 2014; Mathias et al., 2016; Larsen Haidle et al., 2017).

CONCLUSIONS

Regardless of where they are employed, genetic counselors contribute to the overall health care ecosystem. Historically, the business aspects of genetic counseling were not a major focus of genetics programs given the vast amount of information that needs to be covered in a genetic counselor training program. However, as the total number of genetic counselors continues to grow rapidly, and our profession becomes more in demand, it is vital that we understand how we are contributing value and, most importantly, are able to make that case with data. We are accustomed to using data in our practice and it is no different here. Understanding how business decisions are made within a hospital setting can mean the difference between a program that has long-term sustainability and one that is at risk of being eradicated as focus on health care costs and efficiency continue.

REFERENCES

21st Century Cures Act. (2016) *H.R.34.*

Abacan M-A, Alsubaie L, Barlow-Stewart K, et al. (2019) The Global State of the Genetic Counseling Profession. *Eur J Hum Genet* 27(2):183–197.

American Academy of Medical Colleges (n.d.) Who We Are. https://www.aamc.org/who-we-are Accessed May 30, 2022.

American Board of Genetic Counseling (ABGC). (n.d.) Eligibility Requirements https://www.abgc.net/Certify/Eligibility-Requirements Accessed June 7, 2024.

Attard CA, Carmany EP, & Trepanier AM. (2019) Genetic counselor workflow study: the times are they a-changin'? *J Genet Couns*,28(1):130–140.

Babu D, Miller EM, Roscow B, et al. (2021) An Introduction to the Genetic Counseling Business Case Experience: Learnings from NSGC's First Business Case Summit. National Society of Genetic Counselors. https://www.nsgc.org/Portals/0/ASD%20Cmtc%20Resources/An%20Introduction%20to%20the%20Genetic%20Counseling%20Business%20Case%20Experience_FINAL.pdf?ver=7Y34fExVWdAjGnbEdJ245w%3D%3D%C3%97tamp=1632411925369 Accessed May 30, 2024.

Baird RM & Rosenbaum SE. (2008) *Disability: The Social, Political, and Ethical Debate.* Buffalo, NY: Prometheus Books.

Bednar E, Nitecki R, Krause K, & Rauh-Hain J. (2022) Interventions to improve delivery of cancer genetics services in the United States: a scoping review. *Genet Med* 24(6): 1176–1186.

Blumenthal D, Abrams M, & Nuzum R. (2015) The Affordable Care Act at 5 years. *N Engl J Med* 372:2451–2458.

Boothe E, Greenberg S, Delaney CL, & Cohen, SA. (2021) Genetic counseling service delivery models: a study of genetic counselors' interests, needs, and barriers to implementation. *J Genet Couns* 30(1):283–292.

Bureau of Labor Statistics. (2022) Data on certifications and licenses. https://www.bls.gov/cps/certifications-and-licenses.htm Accessed May 30, 2022.

Burke LG, Frakt AB, Khullar D, et al. (2017) Association between teaching status and mortality in US hospitals. *JAMA* 317(20):2105–2113. https://jamanetwork.com/journals/jama/fullarticle/2627971 Accessed May 30, 2024.

Butrick M, Kelly S, Peshkin BN, et al. (2015) Disparities in uptake of BRCA1/2 genetic testing in a randomized trial of telephone counseling. *Genet Med* 17(6):467–475.

Claxton G, Rae M, Damico A, et al. (2021) Health benefits in 2021: employer programs evolving in response to the COVID-19 pandemic. *Health Aff* 40(12):1961–1971.

Cohen RA. (2021) Health insurance coverage: early release of estimates from the nmnmn -National Health Interview Survey, January–June 2020. https://stacks.cdc.gov/view/cdc/100469/cdc_100469_DS1.pdf . Accessed May 30, 2024.

Cohen, SA, Bradbury A, Henderson V, et al (2019) Genetic counseling and testing in a community setting: quality, access, and efficiency. *Am Soc Clin Oncol Educ Book* 39:e34–e44

Council on Foreign Relations. (2023) How Health Care Works Around the World (no date) World101 from the Council on Foreign Relations. https://world101.cfr.org/global-era-issues/global-health/how-health-care-works-around-world Accessed May 30, 2022.

Department of Health and Human Services. (n.d.) HHS.gov. https://www.hhs.gov/ Accessed May 30, 2022.

Federally Qualified Health Centers. (2017) Official web site of the U.S. Health Resources & Services Administration. https://www.hrsa.gov/opa/eligibility-and-registration/health-centers/fqhc/index.html Accessed May 30, 2022.

Fogleman AJ, Zahnd WE, Lipka AE, et al. (2019) Knowledge, attitudes, and perceived barriers towards genetic testing across three rural Illinois communities. *J Community Genet* 10(3):417–423.

Greenberg S, Boothe E, Delaney C, et al. (2020) Genetic Counseling Service Delivery Models in the United States: Assessment of Changes in Use from 2010 to 2017. *J Genet Couns* 29(6):1126–1141.

Hallquist MLG, Tricou EP, Hallquist MN, et al. (2020) Positive impact of genetic counseling assistants on genetic counseling efficiency, patient volume, and cost in a cancer genetics clinic *Genet Med* 22(8):1348–1354.

Harrison TA, Doyle DL, McGowan C, *et al.* (2010) Billing for medical genetics and genetic counseling services: a national survey. *J Genet Couns* 19(1):38–43.

Health Insurance Portability and Accountability Act. (1996) *100 Stat.* 2548.

Hoskovec JM, Bennett RL, Carey ME, et al. (2018) Projecting the supply and demand for certified genetic counselors: a workforce study. *J Genet Couns* 27(1):16–20.

Hudson KL, Holohan MK, & Collins FS. (2008) Keeping pace with the times–the Genetic Information Nondiscrimination Act of 2008. *N Engl J Med* 358(25):2661–2663.

Interstate Medical Licensure Compact. (2020) Physician Licensure. https://www.imlcc.org/a-faster-pathway-to-physician-licensure/ Accessed June 1, 2022.

Khan A. Cohen S, Weir C, & Greenberg S. (2021) Implementing innovative service delivery models in genetic counseling: a qualitative analysis of facilitators and barriers. *J Genet Counseling* 30(1):319–328.

Klees BS, Wolfe CJ, & Curtis CA. (2009) Brief summaries of Medicare & Medicaid. Title XVIII and Title XIX of The Social Security Act. Baltimore, MD: Centers for Medicare & Medicaid Services. https://www.cms.gov/research-statistics-data-and-systems/statistics-trends-and-reports/medicareprogramratesstats/downloads/medicaremedicaidsummaries2009.pdf Accessed May 30, 2024.

Knapke S, Larsen Haidle J, Nagy R, & Pirzadeh-Miller S. (2016) The current state of cancer genetic counseling access and availability. *Genet Med*http://paperpile.com/b/E4wpsW/kyxor 18(4):410–412.

Knoester M & Au W. (2017) Standardized testing and school segregation: like tinder for fire? *Race Ethn Educ* 20(1):1–14.

Krutish A, Balshaw RF, Jiang X, & Hartley JN. (2022) Integrating genetic assistants into the workforce: An 18-year productivity analysis and development of a staff mix planning tool. *J Genet Couns* 31(5):1183–1192. doi:10.1002/jgc4.1589.

Langin K. (2019) A wave of graduate programs drops the GRE application requirement. *Science*. 29 May 2019. doi: 10.5555/article.2427138

Larsen Haidle J, Sternen D, Dickerson J, et al. (2017) Genetic Counselors Save Costs Across the Genetic Testing Spectrum. *Am J Manag Care* 23(10 Spec No.):SP428–SP43:0.

Leonhard J, Munson, PJ, Flanagan JD, et al. (2017) Analysis of reimbursement of genetic counseling services at a single institution in a state requiring licensure. *J Genet Couns* 26(4):852–858.

Mathias PC Conta JH, Konnick EQ, et al. (2016) Preventing genetic testing order errors with a laboratory utilization management program. *Am J Clin Path* 146(2):221–226.

Mauer CB, Reys BD, Hall RE, et al. (2021) Downstream revenue generated by a cancer genetic counselor. *JCO Oncol Pract* 17(9)e1394–e1402.

McWalter K, Cho MT, Hart T, et al. (2018) Genetic counseling in industry settings: opportunities in the era of precision health. *Am J Med Genet* 178(1):46–53.

Miller CE, Krautscheid P, Baldwin EE, et al. (2014) Genetic counselor review of genetic test orders in a reference laboratory reduces unnecessary testing. *Am J Med Genet A* 164A(5):1094–1101. doi:10.1002/ajmg.a.36453.

NSGC. (2022) 2022 Professional Status Survey: Service Delivery and Access. Chicago, IL: National Society of Genetic Counselors.

NSGC. (2024) 2024 Professional Status Survey. Chicago, IL: National Society of Genetic Counselors.

NSGC. (n.d.a) States issuing licences. https://www.nsgc.org/Policy-Research-and-Publications/State-Licensure-for-Genetic-Counselors/States-Issuing-Licenses Accessed May 31, 2022.

NSGC.(n.d.b) Scope of Practice. Chicago, IL: National Society of Genetic Counselors.

Pirzadeh-Miller S, Robinson LS, Read P, & Ross TS. (2017) Genetic counseling assistants: An integral piece of the evolving genetic counseling service delivery model. *J Genet Couns* 26(4):716–727.

Ranallo L, Nye LE, Williams M, et al. (2021) Point of care genetic testing in a breast cancer survivorship clinic *J Clin Oncology* 39(15_suppl).10580–10580.

Rice T, Rosenau P, Unruh LY, et al. (2013) United States of America: health system review. *Health Syst Trans* 15(3):1–431.

Rosso R. (2022) *U.S. Health Care Coverage and Spending. IF10830.* Washington DC: Congressional Research Service.

Simone L, de Leon A, Diaz Caro D, & Margarit S. (2022) Creating a genetic counseling professional society in Latin America. NSGC Perspectives. March 3, 2022. https://perspectives.nsgc.org/Article/creating-a-genetic-counseling-professional-society-in-latin-america Accessed May 30, 2024.

Symecko H, Mueller R, Spielman K, et al. (2019) Ten-fold increase in genetic testing in pancreatic and metastatic prostate cancer with implementation of point of care (POC) testing. *J Clin Oncol* 37(15_suppl):1506–1506.

The Access to Genetic Counselor Services Act of 2021 (n. d.) *H.R. 2144 / S. 1450.* https://www.congress.gov/bill/117th-congress/house-bill/2144 Accessed May 30, 2024.

The Commonwealth Fund. (2020) Health System Features. https://www.commonwealthfund.org/international-health-policy-center/system-features . Accessed May 30, 2022.

Trepanier A & Allain DC. (2020) Adapting genetic counseling practice to different models of service delivery. In: Bonnie S LeRoy, Patricia M Veach, & Nancy P Callanan (eds.) *Genetic Counseling Practice: Advanced Concepts and Skills* Second Edition, pp. 317–39. Hoboken, NJ: Wiley.

Tschirgi, ML, Owens KM, Mackall MS, et al. (2022) Easing the burden of multi-state genetic counseling licensure in the United States: process, pitfalls, and possible solutions. *J Genet Couns* 31(1):41–48.

US Preventive Services Task Force *et al.* (2019) Risk assessment, genetic counseling, and genetic testing for BRCA-related cancer: US Preventive Services Task Force Recommendation Statement. *JAMA* 322(7):652–665.

Venne V, Arfons L, De Castro Maj. M, et al. (2019) Genomic medicine and genetic counseling in the department of veterans affairs and department of defense. Frontline Medical Communications. https://www.frontlinemedcom.com/genomic-medicine-genetic-counseling-in-the-va-and-dod/ Accessed May 30, 2022.

Wallace SE, Neben CL, Stedden W, et al. (no date) Geographical Barriers to Genetic Counseling for Hereditary Cancer and Cardiovascular Disease. https://www.color.com/wp-content/uploads/2019/11/2019-NSGC-SWallace_website.pdf Accessed May 30, 2024.

Williamson R, Lee DL, & Laprise J. (2021) Why you should care about genetic counselor credentialing, NSGC Perspectives (June 16, 2021). https://perspectives.nsgc.org/Article/why-you-should-care-about-genetic-counselor-credentialing Accessed May 30, 2022.

12

Ethical Genetic Counseling Practice

Curtis R. Coughlin II
and Kelly E. Ormond

INTRODUCTION

Importance of ethical practice in genetic counseling

Historically, the field of genetics has been synonymous with cutting edge medical advancements. The human genome project brought unprecedented promise to understand humanity, although it also raised philosophical questions about what it meant to be "human" (Venter et al., 2001; Nurk et al., 2022). Diagnostic advances have broadened potential testing from single genes to exome and genome sequencing, raising questions of what information should be returned in research studies and in clinical settings. Changes in diagnostic testing mean that now prenatal diagnosis, and possibly newborn screening in the near future, may include exome or genome sequencing, with predictive information available for a range of conditions (Bodian et al., 2016; Best et al., 2018). Recognition that these new technologies could raise important and unique ethical issues led to the National Human Genome Research Institute to establish an Ethical Legal and Social Issues (ELSI) research branch in 1989, when the human genome project was first beginning (Dolan et al., 2022).

A Guide to Genetic Counseling, Third Edition. Edited by Vivian Y. Pan, Jane L. Schuette,
Karen E. Wain, and Beverly M. Yashar.
© 2025 John Wiley & Sons Ltd. Published 2025 by John Wiley & Sons Ltd.

Advances in treatments such as gene therapy, including gene transfer, gene editing strategies, and functional interference strategies, have dramatically changed the natural history of some genetic diseases, although we have also suffered the tragic loss of research subjects (Kochenderfer et al., 2012; Finkel et al., 2017). While exciting from both a scientific and medical perspective, these technologies raise questions about whether we *should* be using these medical and scientific advancements (Ormond et al., 2019), as well as the broader social implications of gene therapies on the persons with various genetic conditions they are meant to treat. In particular, the promise (and worry) of human germline gene editing (Wrigley et al., 2015) has especially captured the interest of both scientific and regulatory organizations (Nuffield Council of Bioethics, 2016; Ormond et al., 2017; Howard et al., 2018; Allyse et al., 2019; Eriksson et al., 2020; Medicine, Sciences and Society, 2020) and popular media stories.

Although not as sensational as topics like gene therapies, the practice of genetic counseling often involves extremely difficult conversations and value-laden medical decisions. For example, genetic counselors may play a role in discussions about infertility, abortion, pursuing experimental treatment, whether and when to know about one's future risks for inherited illness, or withdrawing life sustaining measures. Although there are ethical frameworks to support these types of decisions (some of which will be discussed throughout this chapter), these conversations and clinical decisions are complex. Therefore, it is likely that any practicing genetic counselor will be faced with value-laden conflicts or ethical uncertainties.

Throughout this chapter, we will focus on the ethical practice of genetic counseling. Ethical practice is fundamental to all aspects of health care; bioethics and clinical medical ethics have been a part of medical practice for decades. Our work in clinical and research genetics may appear to have a special emphasis on ethics. In part, this is a response to the history of eugenics, which we will discuss below. In this chapter, we will also outline some common theoretical and methodological approaches to ethical issues. Often, we will use case-based examples to emphasize the utility of these approaches. The intent of this chapter is not to train bioethics professionals, but rather to aid the genetics provider in *identifying* ethical concerns or questions that arise in their practice, *being aware* of general ethical principles and resources that are available, and *formulating* potential responses.

Historical context: Our eugenic legacy

Eugenics is a term that was coined by Francis Galton in the late 1800s—it means "well born" and was focused on the concept of bettering the human race through "better breeding" (Galton, 1909). While eugenics is often most associated with the atrocities in Nazi Germany, it started primarily in the United Kingdom (UK) and United States (US) and by the 1920s eugenics programs were occurring globally. It took various forms. Positive eugenics was concerned with selecting for desirable traits, while negative eugenics was concerned with minimizing the number of people with what were seen as undesirable diseases or traits. Positive eugenics was the primary focus of eugenicists in the UK (for example, Galton) and included things like the "better baby" and "fittest family" competitions. Negative eugenics was a form of Social Darwinism and was an increasing focus of the US eugenicists (for example, Davenport, who started the Cold Spring Harbor Laboratory and the Eugenics Records Office), as well as those in Germany. Approaches to negative eugenics included abortion, involuntary sterilization, immigration restrictions and marriage restrictions, institutionalization, and ultimately infanticide and euthanasia (Garver and Garver, 1991).

Early eugenics succeeded because it appeared to simplify complex ideas regarding inheritance, and the scientific basis lent credence to the theory. However, it conflated science and politics, addressing issues that caused social or emotional turmoil by "blaming genes" and removing social responsibility for issues like poverty. While many of the early eugenicists appeared to have good intentions to improve the health of populations, their actions led to bad outcomes, most well-known being the Nazi Germany focus on racial supremacy through the Holocaust. The Holocaust began by targeting persons with disabilities, persons who were LGBTQ, and the elderly, and went on to target people of different ancestral backgrounds (with a heavy focus on people of Jewish background, but also people of Scinti and Roma backgrounds). Most obviously it went far beyond other eugenic programs by killing people. But it is equally important to realize that eugenic actions such as involuntary sterilization and other actions were occurring until the 1970s across the world, and that these were disproportionately focused on persons from historically marginalized groups across the world.

In 1979, federal sterilization regulations in the US were enacted in order to prevent sterilization of individuals who did not voluntarily consent to sterilization. While these regulations essentially ended eugenic-focused sterilization programs, many states have yet to repeal their laws. Unfortunately, forced or coerced sterilization has continued as a result of discrimination or racist ideology, with ongoing examples reported as recently as in the 2020s. For example, coerced sterilizations were reported in California prisons between 1997–2010 (Kouros, 2013), an increased number of tubal ligations were reported in aboriginal women in the Saskatoon Region of Canada (Collier, 2017), and in 2020 there were concerns about coerced sterilizations in many immigration and customs enforcement centers in the US (Ghandakly and Fabi, 2021). For those interested in a more detailed historical view of eugenics, we recommend eugenicsarchive. ca/discover/world (for a global view) and eugenicsarchive.org (for a deep view into American eugenics).

The field of human genetics has attempted to distance itself from the eugenics movements. But it is important to understand the impact of these events on the field of genetic counseling today, how it influences the way that the public or patients may view genetics, and to work within the profession to ensure that genetics is not misused in future eugenic ways. Our eugenic history has informed many of the approaches of genetics and genetic counseling, including nondirectiveness and a focus on autonomy when it comes to genetic decision-making, especially around reproductive decisions. It is also critical because we are often asked to consider whether a new technology is leading to eugenic behaviors. For example, does the ease of noninvasive prenatal screening (NIPS) and higher likelihood of pregnancy termination when Down syndrome is detected, including in the absence of confirmatory diagnostic testing, mean that the availability or offer of NIPS, particularly in the broad context to all pregnant persons, is eugenic (Gilbert, 2017)? Does the availability of ancestry testing or specific genome wide testing continue to promote the "scientific racism" and white supremacy that was the foundation of the Holocaust (Harmon, 2018)? Additionally, core principles of informed consent and voluntariness in scientific research ethics were only articulated after the inhumane acts that occurred before and during the Holocaust (Shuster, 1997). There are few areas of modern medical ethics that were not greatly impacted by the Holocaust. This is, in part, why there has been an effort to commemorate International Holocaust Remembrance Day in all health professions (Silvers et al., 2021; Wynia and Silvers, 2021).

MORALITY, ETHICS, AND THE LAW: SOME DEFINITIONS

The terms morality, ethics, and ethical issues are often used interchangeably, which can lead to confusion; we have defined them here and in Table 12-1. **Morality** refers to *personal* moral choices and is concerned with how one "should" behave. It considers actions to be morally right or wrong, and therefore permissible, required, or disallowed. One's personal view of morality can be based upon faith traditions, experiences, or a reflection of one's general beliefs. In contrast, **ethics** can be defined as a *formal process* to analyze the basis for moral choices, which aids in clarity and consistency, and **ethical issues** involve core values of a given practice (Glover, 2006). Ethical issues occur within many fields, including business, government, health care, and the sciences, including both medical practice and research.

TABLE 12-1. **Definitions**

Term	Definition	Example
Morality/moral values	Moral choices. How one "should" behave. These can be personal or professional	These are often based on faith traditions, culture, and/or personal experience
Ethics	A formal process to analyze the basis for moral choices	Provides a framework for clinical decision-making
Ethical issues	Core values in a given practice (e.g., health care, genetic counseling)	Privacy, respect for patients, truth telling, transparency
Bioethics	Ethical issues with health care and life sciences	Ethical implication of basic or translational science to the practice of health care

Ethical issues within health care settings and clinical research are somewhat unique. The term **bioethics** is often used to differentiate ethical issues within the health care and life sciences from other professional ethical issues. Others have argued that clinical ethics or even health care ethics is more appropriate terminology (Tarzian et al., 2015). Bioethics has its roots firmly planted in philosophy and theology, although it is a clinical discipline of ethics and emerged in response to mistreatment of human research subjects and questions arising from medical advancements (Jonsen, 1993). Ethical issues in health care involve the core values of health care (Table 12-1): respect for patients, truth telling (veracity), ensuring we are benefiting and not harming patients (beneficence and nonmaleficence), and professional integrity; these will be discussed in detail later in the chapter.

Professional ethics and personal morality

In health care settings, there is the potential for tension between personal values (morality) and professional values. Ethics provides a formal mechanism to evaluate this tension, to support a given health care choice, and aims to apply similar reasoning in future situations. As a genetic counselor, you are responsible for not only your personal actions, but also for your professional actions. Patients, colleagues, and the public do not know your personal moral values, but they do have expectations about your professional conduct. These professional expectations extend beyond you as the individual and reflect your training (Senter et al., 2018). For those genetic professionals not in private practice, patients may also have expectations about their care based on your institution or employer. For example, patients who seek care at a religiously affiliated center may assume a genetic counselor will not discuss certain options, such as pregnancy termination. But since many patients do not consider an institution's religious affiliation when choosing options for health care (Freedman et al., 2018; Guiahi et al., 2019), providers should be transparent about any institutional policies that restrict health care options and not assume that patients understand the impact of said policies.

Because of this tension between morality and professional ethics, it is possible that a health care decision could be ethical but inconsistent with a genetic counselor's personal values. For a moment consider the genetic counselor who does not personally support abortion, either in general or in the specific circumstances that are present, but who is caring for a patient who desires a pregnancy termination after prenatal diagnosis. Or a genetic counselor who highly values health in all situations and is caring for a patient who desires pre-implantation genetic diagnosis (PGD), wishes to implant *affected* embryos (or avoid implanting unaffected, carrier embryos), and is faced with decisions about what to do with remaining embryos later. Or a patient who has a severe genetic condition, is near the end of life, and wishes to consider physician-assisted death or to limit medically provided hydration or nutrition; the medical provider may be from a faith tradition that considers any method of hastening death to be immoral (Quill et al.,1997; Diekema et al., 2009).

Many institutions have a **conscientious objection** policy that outlines when a provider can decline to be part of medical care based on their own (deeply held and longstanding) religious beliefs or moral convictions. Common examples of medically indicated procedures where conscientious objection may apply include abortion, contraception, sterilization, procedures or treatments related to human embryos or stem cells, genital cutting procedures, gender affirming surgeries, and physician-assisted dying. For example, 10% of physicians in the UK refused to provide abortions and based on a report from the Italian Ministry of Health, nearly 70% of gynecologist in Italy refuse to perform abortions on moral grounds (Green, 1995; Zampas and Andión-Ibañez, 2012; Chavkin et al., 2013). In some situations, concerns have been raised that conscientious objection policies are used as a way to deny legal and ethically appropriate medical care (Curlin et al., 2007; Frader and Bosk, 2009). One could imagine that when a procedure is considered legal, but a high percentage of providers decline to perform it (such as the example above where 70% of doctors declined to perform abortions in a given location), there could be a significant impact on persons' ability to obtain access to medical information and medically indicated procedures. This may be particularly relevant in rural or underserved areas where alternative providers are scarce, whether by legal restrictions or by conscientious objection policies. This has downstream implications on providing just care and equal access, as well as impacts on patient autonomy, if these conscientious objections lead to limiting patient knowledge about choices and the ability to enact a choice consistent with their own values. As such, many governments (e.g., the US, EU), have rulings consistent with the obligation that if a provider chooses to utilize conscientious objection, they must "not prevent patients from obtaining access to services to which they are entitled." (*R.R. v. Poland* (2011), Application No. 27617/04, para. 206 (European Court of Human Rights).

Recent data suggests many genetic counselors are either unaware of—or unclear how— such conscientious objector policies pertain to the practice of genetic counseling (Bonine et al., 2021). Importantly, the NSGC Code of Ethics (National Society of Genetic Counselors, 2018) and its explication (Senter et al., 2018) specifically addresses this in section II.6 "Refer clients to an alternate genetic counselor or other qualified professional when situations arise in which a genetic counselor's personal values, attitudes and beliefs may impede his or her ability to counsel a client." Similar recommendations for referral are found in the relevant code of ethics or professional practice in (for example) Canada (CAGC—Canadian Association of Genetic Counsellors, 2006), Europe (European Board of Medical Genetics, 2013), and Australia (Human Genetics Society of Australasia, 2022). We also suggest that this is one of many examples where the individual genetic professional should investigate institutional policies, discuss their concerns with a local ethics committee, and seek advice from colleagues and mentors.

Ethics and the law

There are fundamental differences between ethics and the law. An ethical decision is focused on what *rules* (or ethical principles) someone should follow as well as the *character* (emphasized in virtue ethic approaches) of the provider. Although these frameworks are applied uniformly, an ethical decision is often based on the context of the case. For example, consider two cases where parents are requesting hysterectomy for an adolescent with intellectual disability. In one case, the family is concerned about their daughter's new romantic relationship and her ability to raise a child. In a second case, the daughter has a history of severe pelvic and perineal pain with significant bleeding and her medical team suggests either endometrial ablation or hysterectomy. It is possible that these two cases may result in different ethical decisions despite applying the same ethical framework. In contrast, the law demands a *minimum standard* that must be applied; a legal obligation, so to speak. In some US states it is not permissible to perform a procedure that results in sterilization of an individual with intellectual disability without a direct court order. In these states, this uniform standard is applied regardless of the situation. Of note, existing laws may hold standards that are quite different (and often lower) than what an ethical assessment might suggest should be considered, and such laws can differ quite significantly depending on the location. It may be obvious to the reader that the legal standard is different from country to country (i.e., between the US and the UK, or even within European countries of the EU) but the legal standard may also be different within a country (i.e., between different states in the US).

Another area where legal and ethical standards may differ is when determining who the proper medical decision-maker is in a given clinical situation. By the nature of the genetic counseling profession, the legal principle of competence and the ethical principle of decision-making capacity are most relevant when obtaining informed consent for genetic testing (or for treatment decisions). If a patient does not have competence, that patient cannot provide informed consent for any medical decision, including genetic testing. The more difficult cases involve patients who legally have competence but may not have medical decision-making capacity for a specific decision. As just discussed, medical decision-making capacity is a clinical decision and is usually determined by an attending physician or mental health professional. Legally, a surrogate or proxy decision-maker could consent to genetic testing. Although there are times when medical decisions may be time sensitive, it is also ethically justified to wait for a patient to regain medical decision-making when possible. This is true for medical interventions, decisions about advance directives, as well as genetic testing.

Of course, there are situations where an established law conflicts with ethical principles of a given profession or the moral values of an individual. As noted at the beginning of this chapter, at one time many places around the world had laws that supported sterilization programs; now we identify those laws as being unethical. A recent example in the United States is the Dobbs ruling in 2022, after which many states restricted abortion provision, impacting US-based genetic counselors and their prenatal patients (Hercher, 2022). Recently there have been calls for "professional civil disobedience" with the goal of changing government policies (Flynn et al., 2021; Howard, 2021; Wynia, 2022). An individual's obligation to enact social change is beyond the scope of this chapter, although it is worth pointing out that the NSGC Code of Ethics states that genetic counselors should "Adhere to applicable laws and regulations. However, when such laws are in conflict with the principles of the profession, genetic counselors work toward change that will benefit the public interest" (National Society of Genetic Counselors, 2018).

ETHICAL FOUNDATIONS

There are several theoretical and methodological approaches to health care ethics, and we will briefly highlight just a few. Some are based on rules that tell us how to act (deontological approaches, such as principlism), and others focus on the consequences of such actions (for example, consequentialism and utilitarianism). One common criticism of ethical theories is the suggestion that one could simply pick and choose a theory to suit a pre-decided clinical decision. While it is true that each ethical theory emphasizes a different value or principle, these ethical approaches often lead us to a similar recommendation. It would also be unusual for a clinical ethicist to only consider one principle or a single value when considering the ethical justification for a clinical decision. Finally, it is also important to state that these are just some common examples of approaches to ethical issues; other approaches exist. Table 12-2 summarizes key principles and values.

Principlism

Many readers will be familiar with the four principles of biomedical ethics, colloquially referred to as principlism (Beauchamp and Childress, 1979). Beauchamp and Childress attempted to identify fundamental obligations that underlie clinical ethics and described them by the following four concepts. The respect for **autonomy** is grounded in the dignity of each individual (respect for persons) and is often actualized as the obligation to respect a competent person's choices. **Beneficence** is the obligation to maximize benefits ("do good"), while **nonmaleficence** is the obligation to minimize harm ("do no harm"). And the principle of **justice** is concerned with distributing both those benefits and harms in an equitable manner.

Autonomy may be the most often discussed ethical principle within the field of genetic counseling, as the profession aims to guide and support individuals through complex medical decisions. In fact, the principle of autonomy is so often discussed that it is in danger of being oversimplified. Autonomy emphasizes that patients be appropriately informed to make the best possible decisions for themselves, and we often refer to the informed consent process as it relates

TABLE 12-2. **Definitions and examples of principles and concepts**

Term	Definition	Example
Ethical principles		
Beneficence	"Do good." May include clinical and personal utility, among other things.	Having a genetic test result may allow a patient to make an informed decision to undergo early screening, therefore detecting a cancer at an earlier stage.
Non-maleficence	Avoid/minimize harm (physical, emotional, social, financial).	Risks should be minimized and balanced against the potential for benefit.
Autonomy	Respect for persons, and for self-determination.	Informed consent allows a patient to make a decision that fits their values and preferences.
Justice	Treat a patient fairly, equitably, and appropriately.	Genetic research includes people from a wide range of ancestries, improving variant interpretation across populations.
Veracity	Honesty and truthfulness.	Genetics providers should tell the truth to patients; for example, about a diagnosis or prognosis.
Fidelity	Do as one says they will do; trustworthiness.	Genetics researchers should not use research data in ways that were not previously determined unless the consent process allows it.
Privacy	Desire to keep information to oneself.	A patient may not wish to share their diagnosis with others.
Confidentiality	The requirement for a medical provider to not disclose information without patient permission.	A medical provider should not disclose genetic test results or a diagnosis unless authorized by the patient or compelled by law.
Concepts		
Patient Preferences	Stated patient preferences and/or prioritized values.	A patient may have an advance directive, POLST, or may have told providers or family/friends what their wishes are. One might also examine past decisions for patterns.
Quality of Life	A subjective measure of happiness that may be based on factors such as health, relationships, economics, and both internal and external environments.	A patient may feel they have a high quality of life.

to supporting patient autonomy. We will discuss informed consent in more detail shortly. This entails more than providing facts, but rather that an individual be able to consider how a decision would align with their personal goals and values. It is also critical that autonomous decisions are voluntary. Decisions about issues such as pregnancy termination and end of life care are morally complex, and it is important that the patient can consider these medical options without being coerced into a decision.

Principlism is arguably the most widely recognized normative ethical framework and can be found in guidance documents such as the US-based Belmont Report (National Commission for the Protection of Human Subjects of Biomedical and Behavioral Research, 1979), which is one of the earlier documents to establish ethical principles for biomedical and behavioral research involving human subjects (Beauchamp, 2005). The principlist paradigm is quite popular among clinicians and educational programs due, in part, to the simplification of ethics into four principles, although this framework is often criticized for limiting the number of moral obligations identified by a clinical or researcher (Fiester, 2007). Additionally, there is no guidance within principlism about how one balances the principles when they are in conflict. For example, autonomy is not the only ethical principle and is balanced by the principles of beneficence and nonmaleficence. That is, an individual's medical decisions are limited to those choices that would promote an individual's wellbeing and limiting those decisions that may create harm.

One example of limitation of autonomy in health care is when a patient requests a treatment that is not expected to have a physiological benefit (sometimes referred to as medically or physiologically futile). Consider a patient with a viral infection who requests treatment with an antibiotic. In this situation, there would be no benefit to the patient to be treated with an antibiotic and a risk of harm. In these situations, a provider can essentially override a patient's autonomous decision about treatment (Consensus statement of the Society of Critical Care Medicine's Ethics Committee, 1997). In practice, requests for medically futile interventions are rare. There is growing consensus that providers have a limited obligation to provide potentially nonbeneficial or potentially inappropriate interventions (Kon et al., 2016). In short, these are interventions where there may be some physiological benefit although the intervention does not help achieve the goal(s) of care. In these complicated situations it is unclear how to balance autonomy with beneficence and justice, and other ethical principles or frameworks are often relied upon.

Virtue ethics

Virtue ethics may be the oldest known ethical theory and is often attributed to historical philosophers such as Plato, Aristotle, and Confucius. Virtue ethics focuses on the professional character or conduct of the clinician and emphasizes concepts such as honesty and truthfulness (veracity), trustworthiness (fidelity), and the protection of privacy (Oakley, 2010; Holland, 2011).

Veracity emphasizes one's obligation to be truthful or honest; in medical ethics this implies that health care providers will be truthful to patients about their diagnosis, prognosis, and options. It is based on the premise of respect for the patient, and that truthful information is a requirement for making informed and autonomous health care decisions. While one might assume that health care providers will always be truthful, and that no one enter a health care profession with the intent to be dishonest, there are many examples where a health care provider might soften or hide the full truth from a patient (minimizing severity, e.g. use a euphemism, such as saying "a growth" rather than "tumor" or "cancer"), usually with the intent to minimize harm.

For example, consider a genetic test result that identifies misattributed paternity or non-parentage. Should the genetic provider truthfully disclose this result; and, if so, to whom? The concept of veracity suggests that the clinician remain honest throughout the testing process, and, in the case of misattributed paternity, disclose the result to all parties (Ross, 1996; Hercher and Jamal, 2016). Some genetic professionals have elected to hide the truth or even lie rather than disclose the result (Wertz et al., 1990; Pencarinha et al., 1992). In these situations, there is a tension between the perceived duty to protect the biological mother's privacy and the duty to be truthful (Wertz et al., 1990), as well as a concern that such an approach would have limited medical benefit and potential harm (Botkin et al., 2015). This is another example of where a principles-based approach doesn't clarify which principle should take precedence (e.g., veracity versus nonmaleficence and confidentiality). One additional place where veracity comes up in both clinical and research practice is with the concept of transparency, particularly around potential conflicts of interest.

In a related concept, **fidelity** emphasizes the obligation to do as one says or the concept of trustworthiness. One clear application of this virtue is the duty to protect a patient's confidentiality. Again, this seems straightforward, and no genetic professional intends to not follow through on such a simple promise. For example, if patient samples or genomic data are routinely shared with a biotechnology company, the genetic counselor should be *honest and transparent* about that relationship. And if a patient is promised their data will not be aggregated into such a data set, the genetic counselor has an obligation to ensure that promise is fulfilled.

Finally, **privacy and confidentiality** are core ethical issues in all specialties of medicine. Privacy is about the desire of a patient to keep certain things to themselves so that they are "not known by others." The notion of privacy is a longstanding ethical concept and goes back to the time of Hippocrates, even if what is desired to be kept private may change based on culture or era. For example, it is worth noting that several cultures value family decision-making as opposed to individual decision making, which is not limited to a given geographical area (Clark, 2007; Deem and Stokes, 2018), but it is important to remember there may be nuances to such preferences, and clinicians should not make assumptions when sharing medical information or obtaining informed consent. Confidentiality is a related concept, based on a medical provider not purposefully disclosing private information without authorization. Medical confidentiality is the foundation of a trusting relationship between a medical provider and a patient; without it, patients will not feel comfortable truthfully disclosing things, particularly those that may be stigmatizing or embarrassing. On a very practical level, medical confidentiality does not mean that no person other than the provider will know the specific medical information; rather, in the course of conducting medical care, disclosures must occur. These may be to colleagues, to medical payors, or to administrative support personnel within a medical setting. However, any such disclosures should occur on a "need to know" basis and require discretion. This includes being sensitive to inadvertent disclosures in public locations (including social media discussions), and to the information that is shared in professional conferences and publications. Any additional disclosures, including to family members, should generally be authorized specifically by the patient. Many countries have specific laws and regulations about privacy; for example, in the US the Health Insurance Portability and Accountability Act (HIPAA) (United States, 1996), or in the EU, the General Data Protection Regulation (GDPR).

Ethics of care

The ethics of care approach focuses on the patient (and the health care professional) in the context of their relationships. Values such as **sympathy, compassion,** and **love** are emphasized over duties or ethical principles. These values are also predominant in feminist writing (or feminist ethics) and sometimes these terms are used interchangeably (Larrabee, 1992). One benefit of this approach is the move away from vagueness associated with principlism, although a common criticism is that the ethics of care approach lacks a well-defined basis for ethical justification. As a result, the ethics of care is often used to analyze how you *should* approach an ethical issue while keeping the context of the relationship central. This ethical framework has been applied to social programs such as universal health care and social issues such as LGBTQ and disability rights (Hamington and Miller, 2006). The NSGC code of ethics is also strongly influenced by the ethics of care model.

Consider, for example, an adolescent patient who was recently diagnosed with a genetic cause of cardiac disease. Their parents request that health care providers do not disclose this diagnosis, as they have told their child that everyone sees a cardiologist at that age. Several values are in tension in this case, including our respect of parental authority and our duty of veracity towards the adolescent. The ethics of care approach also emphasizes the impact that disclosing this diagnosis would have on the patient, and on the patient–parent relationship. It is equally important to consider the impact of disclosing the result on the therapeutic relationship between the health care provider and the patient/parents.

ETHICAL ANALYSIS

Bioethics is often referred to as a form of applied ethics, although that is controversial as it suggests the idea that ethical issues are simply moral dilemmas that can be solved by the well-trained philosopher (Agich, 2001; Magelssen et al., 2016). Of course, ethical theory alone is limited and perhaps even confusing when different ethical theories emphasize alternative approaches. For example, v irtue ethics may appear antithetical to principlism due to the emphasis on moral character over rules or obligations. In a recent edition of their seminal work, Beauchamp and Childress have stated that ethical theory is more complete with the addition of virtues, and that virtue-based and principle-based ethics are complementary approaches to most ethical or moral issues (Beauchamp and Childress, 2013). Clinical ethics, or ethics consultation, is a relatively new field that grew out of the unique ethical challenges present in health care (Singer et al., 2001; Siegler, 2019).

Ethical decision-making

There are several approaches to a clinical ethics consultation, and while we do not expect this chapter will create ethics consultants, there is a value in understanding how to think through an ethical conflict. These common ethical decision-making approaches aim to help facilitate the process of determining what to do when faced with an ethical conflict. Just as a pedigree software or interview techniques support the process of genetic counseling, none of these ethical frameworks should be conflated to be an actual ethics consult. Instead, these tools provide some structure to the thought process, and ensure that a standardized approach to ethics consultation occurs, with an emphasis on medical information, the social context, and the values of all stakeholders involved (Table 12-3).

One of the earlier approaches to ethics consultation is called the **"Four box method"** (Jonsen et al., 2010). In this process, the professional considers the medical indication, patient preferences, quality of life issues, and social/contextual issues with a focus on the bioethical principles that underlie them (autonomy, beneficence, nonmaleficence, and justice). Questions that one might ask include: How clear or uncertain is the diagnosis and prognosis, and what does it entail? What treatments or medical approaches are possible and what is their likelihood of impact? Who is the correct decision-maker? Has the patient expressed a view or preference? What are the impacts on quality of life if treatment is or is not pursued? Are there social issues that may impact access (e.g., financial considerations or allocation issues), conflicts of interest, or areas of religious or legal consideration?

Two additional common approaches to ethical issues were developed by the National Center for Ethics in Health Care (ethics.va.gov) and are described in Table 12-3. The **CASES** approach consists of five steps, which are also primarily focused on responding to a specific ethical or clinical question in an individual

TABLE 12-3. Ethical decision-making tools

CASES	ISSUES	Eight-steps	Four-box model
Clarify the consultant request	Identify an issue	1. What is the question?	• Medical indications
Assemble relevant information	Study the issue	2. What is my "gut reaction"	• Beneficence and nonmaleficence
Synthesize the information	Select a strategy	3. What are the facts?	• Patient and family preferences
Explain the synthesis	Undertake a plan	4. What are the values?	• Respect for autonomy
Support the consultation process	Evaluate and adjust	5. What are my options?	• Quality of life
	Sustain and spread	6. What should I do?	• Beneficence, non-maleficence, respect for autonomy
		7. What justifies my choice?	• Contextual features
		8. How can I prevent this problem?	• Justice

patient (Geppert and Chanko, 2016). This approach was intended to be reminiscent of taking a patient's history, performing a physical exam, and writing a clinic note. Similarly, the **ISSUES** approach consists of seven steps to identify and address ethical gaps in health care. With a focus on systems level issues, the ISSUES approach is commonly used in preventive ethics programs with the aim to avoid patient level ethical concerns.

Finally, there is the **Eight Steps** ethical decision-making matrix, which is a tool that organizes complex ethical problems (Glover, 2006) by combining the steps of an ethics consult (steps 1–7; CASES) and a focus on preventive ethics (step 8; ISSUES framework). What is unique in the eight-step method is the reminder to determine the primary values at stake. As mentioned above, the clinical or medical decisions are often value-laden, which is one reason that simple application of ethical theory is not practical. This is not the only ethical tool that highlights the values and perspectives of the patient.

In general, the methods or tools for an ethics consult all have the same goal: to progress from the medical facts of the case to a morally sound decision (Anderson-Shaw, 2015). Often there is more than one morally sound decision (or ethically justified decision) possible. The goal of ethics consultation is not to arise at a single decision, but rather create a deliberative process that promotes respect for values and interests of all participants. Although these tools were intended to assist the health care ethics consultant (or bioethicist), these same tools can be applied to a possible ethical issue and can assist the genetics professional when evaluating a possible ethical question.

INFORMED CONSENT AS A FOUNDATIONAL CONCEPT IN GENETIC COUNSELING

Informed consent

Building strongly on the principle of autonomy, the goal of **informed consent** (in either a research or clinical setting) is to gather *autonomous authorization* for a medical intervention or research participation. Informed consent is based on the premise of there being a competent person (the patient or their surrogate decision-maker), who receives and comprehends relevant information and makes a voluntary authorization (Faden and Beauchamp, 1986; Appelbaum, 2007), or an informed refusal. Informed consent is both an ethical and legal concept and is governed by laws that vary depending on your country and state of residence (see, for example, Spector-Bagdady et al., 2018). Importantly, informed consent is not the completion of a form, but rather a process.

Informed consent has always been a cornerstone of genetic counseling practice, in part due to the history of eugenics and our desire to ensure that decisions regarding genetic testing are not coerced. The NSGC Code of Ethics, for example, says in section II.4 that genetic counselors will work to "enable their clients to make informed decisions, free of coercion, by providing or illuminating the necessary facts, clarifying the alternatives and anticipated consequences."

The Nuremberg Code lays out requirements that the patient or research participant must receive enough information to make an informed decision, but there are few legal or ethical standards that help us operationalize this in practice (Trials of War Criminals Before the Nuremberg Military Tribunals Under Control Council Law No. 10. Nuremberg, October 1946-April 1949: Case 11: *U.S. v. von Weizsäecker (Ministries case)*, 1949). What information is required to be adequate for decision-making? Various standards have existed over time. First, the **professional standard**, which allows professionals to determine what the "reasonable" information for consent entails—this may be through professional guidelines, or through a local or national standard that is established. Next, the **reasonable person standard** for informed consent suggests that a provider should inform people to the degree in which most other typical persons would expect to be informed. In recent years, informed consent has evolved towards the **subjective standard**, which acknowledges that patients have different informational needs at the time of providing informed consent, and that the process should be tailored.

When providing informed consent for a genetic test, for example, a genetic counselor should identify the specific decision and options available, as well as who the correct decision-maker may be. Then, they should consider what information the patient or decision-maker will likely desire to determine their course of action, and plan to present the information at an appropriate educational level (including in the consent form, which is often written at too high a reading level) (Henderson et al., 2014). The amount of time needed may increase with the level of complexity in the informed consent process. It is also important to consider the difference between providing information and ensuring they comprehend the options and implications (Hammami et al., 2014); many research studies show that people do not understand relevant information even after an informed consent process (for further reading: Beardsley et al., 2007, Ormond et al., 2007; Albala ct al., 2010; Kass et al., 2011; Klima et al., 2014).

Finally, it is important to remember that standards for informed consent should vary depending on the potential implications and risks of the procedure or action being considered. For example, if a patient is considering a low-risk test where there is high certainty about its results and future outcomes, then simple consent may be appropriate. An example might be a diagnostic blood test where there was an effective treatment for the most likely diagnosis. Whereas, if a patient were considering something where there was high risk and low certainty, a higher bar for what was discussed in the informed consent process, including both more information as well as a discussion of patient values and preferences, would be appropriate (Whitney et al., 2004).

Shared decision-making

One approach to clinical ethical consultations (and in recent years, genetic counseling as well) is a shared decision-making model of care. This approach recognizes that the goals of care are often value-laden decisions and necessitate input from the patient. As in the principle of informed consent, for a patient to make a decision about goals of care they need to understand therapeutic options as well as the potential benefits and possible harm that may arise. However, shared decision-making goes beyond informed consent, in that the goal is to respect both the values of the patient and the expertise of the medical team. While the patient may decide on the ultimate goal of care, the health care provider is the expert on how to achieve the agreed upon goals of care.

Surrogate decision-makers

As we previously discussed, adult patients do not always have competency or decision-making capacity. In these situations, the health care team relies on a surrogate decision-maker to establish the goals of care. Ideally, the patient identifies a surrogate decision-maker through an advanced directive such as a living will or a medical durable power of attorney (MDPOA) document. Unfortunately, most patients have not identified a surrogate decision-maker, which means that the medical team must help identify appropriate decision maker(s). In the US, some states have specific statutes which specify a priority order for surrogate decision-makers, such as a spouse or domestic partner, followed by an adult child.

The role of a surrogate decision-maker is to make decisions on behalf of the patient using the **substituted judgment standard**. In brief, a surrogate decision-maker does not make the choice that they simply think is "best." But rather they should use their knowledge of the patient's preferences and values to determine what the patient would have decided for themselves. In an ideal case, the surrogate decision-maker can use previous discussions with the patient to make a choice that is consistent with the patient's own preferences.

Consider a 17-year-old with a life-limiting genetic condition who has consistently stated her preference to limit medical interventions such as cardiopulmonary resuscitation (CPR). While still a minor, the patient is brought to the emergency department and her parents request CPR. Who makes the decision about what medical care is provided?

This example highlights a common discussion between clinicians, ethicists, and lawyers: the concepts of competency and medical decision-making capacity. **Competency** is a legal term and is often discussed in health care when a patient reaches a legal age of maturity. Occasionally clinicians question whether a patient has general competency, and a court must determine the competency of an individual. If an individual is determined not to be competent, they cannot make any of their own decisions (including health care related decisions). In contrast, **medical decision-making capacity** is a clinical decision and limited to a specific medical decision. Although there may be varying legal standards for medical decision-making capacity, in general a patient should understand relevant information, appreciate medical consequences of the situation, be able to communicate a choice, and provide a rationale for the treatment choice (Appelbaum, 2007). Since it is based on a specific decision, it is possible for a patient to lose medical decision-making capacity for one decision (i.e., decision to leave a hospital) but to retain decision-making capacity for another at the same time (i.e., decline a recommended treatment). If an adult patient loses medical decision-making capacity, which can happen on a temporary (e.g., head trauma, active psychological illness) or permanent (dementia) basis, it is paramount to identify a surrogate or proxy decision-maker . Of note, the process for identifying a surrogate or proxy decision maker is often regional. As of 2020, 11 US states had no surrogate consent statute, although hospitals within these states generally follow local best practice guidelines.

If we return the above case example, it may be ethically appropriate to use the substituted judgment standard for this 17-year-old, which is used when an adult does not have capacity to make their decisions. Surrogate decision-makers have an obligation to use their knowledge of a patient's values and preferences to determine what a patient would have decided for themselves (Chaet, 2019). In this example, the patient has consistently stated her desire to limit medical interventions, including CPR. An appointed surrogate decision-maker could use these conversations to make a decision in line with the patient's stated values and goals of care. As a result, it is reasonable to assume that a surrogate decision maker would disagree with the parental request and support the patient's previous decision to limit CPR. Although this approach may be ethically justified, state law may limit a health care provider's ability to override a parental decision in a minor. This is one example where a decision may be ethically justified, in this case to support a minor's decision, but not legally appropriate. In situations when the ethical and legal decisions are in tension and cannot be resolved, clinicians usually have two options: to defer to the legal standard or to petition the court for guidance.

Parental authority and best interest standard

Of course, the substituted judgment standard would be difficult to apply in pediatric cases where a child may not have voiced their own preferences or values. In general, it is assumed that parents are better suited to understand the unique needs of their children and to make decisions that are beneficial to their children (Diekema, 2011). The parents' responsibility is to support the **best interest** of their child and to preserve family relationships, rather than to express their (the parents') own autonomous choice. **Parental authority** is not absolute. There may be disagreements between parents and medical providers about proposed treatments. One approach in such disagreements is to ask whether the requested treatment is harmful (Diekema, 2019). Hopefully the pediatrics case example provided below provides context for parental decision making and the limitation of parental authority.

CASE EXAMPLE: PEDIATRICS AND PARENTAL AUTHORITY

Blake is a 2-week-old infant who presented to care at 3 days of life with neonatal epilepsy and was diagnosed with a severe neurologic disorder. Although there is phenotypic variability, the genetic disorder is characterized by central nervous system involvement resulting in limited capacity to feed orally, and most patients die in early childhood. The genetic team joined a care conference to discuss the diagnosis with the family and were optimistic that Blake had an attenuated phenotype of the disease. During the care conference, Blake's parents stated they were worried about Blake's quality of life and decided to withdraw respiratory support. The genetic counselor on the team is concerned about this decision as some patients can live well into childhood and treatments for genetic diseases continue to improve.

It is possible that readers would have different reactions to this example based on the genetic diagnosis. The intent is not to focus on a specific genetic disorder, but rather how to make difficult medical decisions for pediatric patients who have not had an opportunity to voice their own values and decisions. In this case, the respect for parental decision-making and professional integrity is in tension. We will briefly discuss one possible approach to this ethics consult.

In general, the basis for making medical decisions in pediatrics is that of **best interest,** which can be defined as the best estimate of what a reasonable person would consider to be beneficial, given the probable harms or burdens. In general, it is assumed that parents are the persons best suited and most inclined to act in the best interest of their children (Katz et al., 2016). It is appropriate for parents to use predictions about survival or **quality of life** and evaluate which treatment options are consistent with the patient's interests (Beauchamp and Childress, 2013). Decisions about quality of life are complicated and rooted in a patient's (or family's) values, spirituality, and culture. Again, it is important to emphasize that parents are typically provided wide latitude to determine the quality of life for their child, assuming that such decisions do not create harm, although even the definition of harm is value laden (Diekema, 2019; Ross, 2019).

There is much published about the limitation of the best interest standard. One concern is the suggestion that there is one "best" or "right" choice, and that any other decision made by a parent or guardian is unethical. It is important to remind ourselves that parents and guardians have the right to make less than perfect decisions. And that as long as a decision is in the range of ethically appropriate options, those decisions should be respected (McDougall et al., 2018). As we have frequently mentioned, medical decisions about goals of care are often value laden. Patients (or in this case, parents of a patient) may make a different decision than you would have made in the same situation. Often, there is not one right decision but a range of ethically justified or acceptable decisions.

At times, it can be difficult to understand the decisions made by parents for their children, which can result in significant moral distress for health care providers. This may be due to a decision that is morally difficult for the health care provider, as in the examples of withdrawing or withholding life sustaining therapies. At times, a health care provider may be concerned that a parent is not acting in the best interest of their child. There are limits to parental authority, and the medical team has an independent obligation to the best interest of their patient. Typically, a court decision or involvement of a state agency (in the US often referred to as the Department of Human Services or DHS) is required to override a parental decision. The ethical framework for state involvement is based on the potential harm of the parental decision (Diekema, 2011). Just because a health care provider requests court or state agency involvement does not mean there will be agreement by the agency to remove parental decision-making rights. While the genetic professional has an independent obligation to the patient, it is reasonable to involve other institutional resources such as social worker service or a child protection team who have extensive experience involving DHS or other similar agencies.

CLINICAL EXAMPLES OF ETHICAL ISSUES IN GENETIC COUNSELING

Case example: Reproductive ethics: embryos, abortion, and the disability lens

You are seeing a couple, Chris and Susanne, in your reproductive genetics clinic. They are not yet pregnant, and are contemplating their reproductive choices, given that Susanne is a carrier of an X-linked condition. Susanne has a brother affected with this condition, so she is very familiar with the prognosis and reproductive risks. The couple has several questions that come up in your genetic counseling discussion, including around their reproductive options from pre-implantation genetic diagnosis (PGD) to prenatal testing and potential termination. The couple expressed they are unsure what is the morally right thing to do if they consider PGD and then have embryos that they will not use, and that they struggle in thinking about whether pregnancy termination feels like a morally acceptable choice. Susanne is also struggling to consider her options given her relationship with her affected sibling.

When thinking about embryos, one of the ways that bioethicists consider the issues is by thinking about their **moral status**. This foundational concept can ethically inform thinking about a range of reproductive issues including discarding unused embryos after IVF/PGD, germline gene editing, and pregnancy termination. To say that something or someone has moral status implies moral protections, rights, and obligations based on the interests of that entity. How do we decide what gets moral status? Philosophers have proposed several different theories that consider different features. For example, one could consider that human properties (e.g., that all biologic humans, meaning someone who has human DNA) entitle one to moral status. If one uses this criterion, all humans, no matter what characteristics, would be entitled to equal moral status; this approach to moral status protects vulnerable persons in a way that other approaches might not. However, it also means that no other species has any moral status and is therefore not entitled to rights or protections, and it doesn't clarify whether genetically modified humans would still be entitled to moral status. Other approaches to moral status might focus on cognitive properties, perhaps through demonstrating self-consciousness; intentional action; ability to give and appreciate reasons for acting; intelligence: capacity for beliefs, desires, thoughts; communication with language; rationality and higher order volition. These various models would enable both humans and some animals to have moral status but might exclude infants and individuals with dementia and/or cognitive impairments. Other approaches might require that in order to have moral status, you must first have moral agency (be capable of judging right and wrong), sentience (consciousness is required to have moral status, capacity to feel pain and pleasure), or that moral status is based on relationships (e.g., if there is an established social relationship, then there are moral obligations).

Regardless of which philosophical approach to moral status one uses, we assume that "people" (broadly) have moral status and therefore rights. But at what point does an embryo or a fetus become "a person" and how do we define that? Does a fetus have rights, and if so at what point? If, for example, we assume a zygote, embryo, or fetus is a full human being with moral status, including a right to life and protection, then would this mean that abortion or discarding embryos is morally wrong? On the other hand, if we assume they are simply biologic tissue, then there would be no moral problem with abortion or destroying embryonic tissue. Most people fall somewhere in the middle, believing that a fetus doesn't have the same rights as a living child or adult, but is somehow "special" and deserving of our respect (and therefore some measure of protection), and that moral status develops throughout the pregnancy. This raises new questions: at what point do we consider that moral status arises, and is it a developing concept, or a binary one? Is it with gametes when there is the *potential* of a new being? At conception, when there is a novel genetic code, or after twinning can no longer occur and there is a single human potential? Do we focus on location, such as at implantation or birth? Is an unborn 39-week fetus substantially different from a 1-week-old that was delivered at 38 weeks (Kuhse and Singer, 1990)? Do we rely upon objective biologic measures such as when the primitive streak has formed, or when the brain or heart begins to function? Do we rely on other features such as when fetal movement can be observed or felt, or when a fetus is viable or could survive independently from the mother? Principles such as viability (and even ability for fetal tissue to grow independently) remain a "moving target," with neo-natal technologies changing at what stage infants can live with support. Ensoulment, or other religious concepts, are equally challenging to define.

As a society we generally accept that it is wrong to kill or purposefully cause harm to a moral agent. Therefore, when considering the morality of abortion, this means we have to consider whether the fetus (at a particular gestational stage) has moral status, and therefore a right to life. And if we assume yes, how do we resolve conflict between mother's *autonomy* and *nonmaleficence* towards the fetus? Importantly, when does fetal moral agency equal/trump the woman's moral agency? In a thought-provoking paper, Judith Jarvis Thomson posits that the general argument against abortion is that a fetus is a person, who has a right to life, and that this very right to life trumps the rights to bodily integrity and autonomy of the mother (Thomson, 1971). She proposes an analogy that emphasizes the various roles of choice, self-defense, the extended time frame of pregnancy, and the medical and psychological impact of carrying a pregnancy as key issues that play a role in assessing where rights (in this case, the right of the fetus to use the mother's body) and duties (in this case the woman's duty to carry a pregnancy to term) may have limits.

> In the most ordinary sort of case, to deprive someone of what he has a right to is to treat him unjustly … You are surely not being unjust to him for you gave him no right to use your kidneys, and no one else can have given him any such right … The right to life consists not in the right not to be killed, but in the right not to be killed unjustly.
>
> (Thomson, 1971)

The legal aspects of abortion will vary significantly based on the country in which one is practicing, and in some cases the more local state or provincial laws. These laws may vary significantly in terms of the gestational ages when abortion is legal, and under what circumstances (e.g., there may be exceptions or require-ments for rape, incest, situations where the mother's life is endangered by the pregnancy, or when the fetus is diagnosed with a life threatening or other medical condition). Since these laws are in flux in many locations (Harris, 2022), we will encourage all readers to review the current state of these laws in their own jurisdictions.

If we go back to the case example, perhaps in part due to the worries about eugenics and coercion, autonomy seems paramount to genetic counselors when discussing reproductive genetic testing. For example, the NSGC Reproductive Freedom position statement (adopted 2010) says "NSGC firmly believes that reproductive decisions should be made in the context of unbiased and comprehensive information, free from discrimination or coercion" (NSGC, 2022). Autonomy in this sense is enacted through informed consent and the use of a nonjudgmental approach. The ethical obligations of a reproductive genetic counselor might include familiarity with the local laws (and knowledge of referral options when necessary), personal reflection regarding one's own stance towards the moral status of embryos and fetuses, and some thought about how they might discuss these issues with patients. In specific cases, a reproductive genetic counselor might also actively encourage the patient to reflect on the values that they and their partner hold and help them apply the values towards a choice that matches them.

One last important ethical topic that arises in regard to reproductive genetic counseling is the interface with disability studies. It is important to briefly discuss here the expressionist argument, most clearly put forward by Adrienne Asch and colleagues in various forms (e.g., Parens and Asch, 2000). Dr Asch posits that the mere availability of selective abortion of fetuses with disabling traits is morally problematic, because it expresses discriminatory views against the trait and the people who carry it. As Marsha Saxton said "The message at the heart of widespread selective abortion on the basis of prenatal diagnosis is the greatest insult; some of us are 'too flawed' in our very DNA to even exist; we are unworthy of being born" (Saxton, 1998). Additionally, prenatal diagnosis and selective abortion reinforces the medical model of disability and continues the social discrimination that our patients with genetic disease already face. On a more individual level, the expressionist argument also points out that selective termination of a fetus with a disability focuses on the "part" versus "whole" of an individual, suggests intolerance and may often be based on incorrect perceptions about quality of life with disabling conditions.

Genetic counselors may find themselves in an ethically challenging situation, balancing the autonomy of a pregnant patient and couple with their respect for persons with disabilities. It is important to remember that supporting parental autonomy in individual decisions is not incompatible with supporting people who have disabling conditions, and that genetic counselors can and should advocate for a more socially just environment for people with genetic conditions. Genetic counselors previously spoke of nondirectiveness as a way to help prospective parents make decisions when faced with a prenatal genetic diagnosis, and of course the principle of noncoercion and supporting patients' autonomy is critical here. But genetic counselors must also recognize that they come with their own personal biases and views about disability, just as our patients do; in each case they are based on our personal experiences and exposures. In order to support patients' autonomy, it is the responsibility of the genetic counselor to support informed decision-making by presenting descriptions of genetic conditions in as balanced a way as possible, ensuring that patients are offered resources that include other families who have lived experience with the condition, and letting patients know all the options that may be available to them without making assumptions about their preferences. While there is limited empiric data to say what genetic counselors do or do not say in prenatal genetic counseling sessions, the limited data available suggests that there is much work to do in this area (Farrelly et al., 2012).

Case example: Predictive genetic and genomic testing: Genetic testing of adolescents, duty to warn

Alex, age 21, has a family history of colon cancer. Alex's father, paternal aunt, and paternal grandparent all developed cancer in their early 50s. Alex's father died when Alex was 6, and the family has not stayed in contact with any relatives on that side of the family. But because of the cancer, Alex is worried, and wants genetic testing.

Predictive genetic testing has been available since the late 1990s in various settings, including various cancer predisposition syndromes (e.g., breast cancer, colon cancer, and others) and neurodegenerative conditions starting with Huntington disease. Because predictive testing may not always be associated with medical actionability, and because historically there was variable uptake for genetic testing (particularly for conditions like Huntington disease where there was limited clinical utility to the results), informed consent and patient autonomy has always been a key concept before genetic testing is performed.

Alex undergoes genetic testing and learns that they carry a pathogenic muta-tion in one of the Lynch syndrome genes. Alex has a 16-year-old sibling, Sam; their mother and step-father are very anxious after learning Alex's results, and want to test Sam.

Predictive testing for adolescents is a special case for genetics providers, and there are several relevant practice guidelines on the topic (Committee on Bioethics et al., 2013; Ross et al., 2013; Botkin et al., 2015). Adolescents do not yet have competence, though they have growing decision-making capacity. The major value claim in delaying predictive genetic testing until adulthood is to preserve the future autonomy of the child, particularly for conditions where there is variable or low uptake of genetic testing in adults (e.g., Huntington disease) or where there is limited medical actionability at young ages. There are also hypothetical concerns of harm, such as psychological impact on the child (increased anxiety or depres-sion), or differential parental treatment. While there is not much data that exist on these empirical risks, the limited data that exists does not support them as a significant risk (McConkie-Rosell et al., 2008; Wakefield et al., 2016).

In this case, there are a number of things that we could consider when making an ethical assessment. First, Sam is 16 years old. While age is not always directly correlated to decision-making capacity, one could assume that at 16, Sam has developed some autonomy and sense of values and personal desires. Sam's desires should be considered within this process—for example, if Sam's mother desires testing but Sam does not, this should certainly be taken strongly into account. On the other hand, if both Sam and Sam's parents want testing, this would support consideration of the process. Second, Sam's biologic father died of colon cancer when Sam was a baby. Sam may not know much about the family history or about cancer. At 16, not much would change medically for Sam, and screening would not likely start for several years.

Alex is not in touch with any paternal relatives, but knows that their father had, before they were born, two other children (Alex's half-siblings) who are now in their early 40s. You suggest that it would be useful to pass this genetic information along, but Alex's mother insists that they are not in touch with that side of the family, and that it is not possible.

Genetics is inherently a family event. When an individual is diagnosed with a genetic condition or pathogenic variant, it has implications for other at-risk family members. While in most cases, relatives are happy (at least in principle, if not in action) to share genetic risk information and enable cascade testing, there are some cases where family members are estranged, or simply do not wish to share information with relevant relatives. This discomfort with sharing genetic information can often be addressed with time and with support to address potential concerns about sharing (both informational and psychological). The main issue now, as the case evolves, is around what is called the **duty to warn**. Here, the duty of confidentiality towards ones' patient (in this case Alex) is weighed against any potential duties that one might have towards the at-risk half-siblings.

Medical confidentiality is foundational in establishing a trusting relationship between patient and medical care provider. It is both beneficent and respectful of autonomy to ask for a patient's authorization for disclosure rather than disclosing medical information without their permission. Despite this, in most countries there are some limits to medical confidentiality where there would be a public health or medical reason why disclosure of risks/exposure was important. These usually include infectious diseases (sexually transmitted diseases, highly infectious viruses that required contact tracing) or situations that involve harm (e.g., abuse, suspicious deaths, gunshots or knife wounds).

If one were to consider breaching confidentiality of a patient's private medical information (in this case, genetic testing results), a medical professional must ask themselves if it is *permissible* to breach confidentiality and disclose the medical information, and if so, is disclosure *obligatory*? Many of our decisions about duty to warn stem from a US legal case *Tarasoff v. Regents*, 1974. While this case dealt with a psychiatrist who became aware that his patient was threatening to murder another individual, it highlights that

> [w]hen a therapist determines, or pursuant to the standards of his profession should determine, that his patient presents a serious danger of violence to another, he incurs an obligation to use reasonable care to protect the intended victim against such danger. The discharge of this duty may require the therapist to take one or more of various steps, depending on the nature of the case. Thus, it may call for him to warn the intended victim or others likely to appraise the victim of the danger, to notify the police, or to take whatever other steps are reasonably necessary under the circumstances.
>
> *Tarasoff v. Board of Regents of the Universities of California*
> ($_{551}$ P.2d $_{334}$ [Cal. 1976])

The logic that derives from Tarasoff requires medical providers to ask themselves several questions when faced with the potential for nondisclosure of relevant genetic information. First, where does the providers' primary duty lie? Is it with the patient, the family, or another person, and can the potential others be identified and located? Second, what would the potential benefits (beneficence) and harms (nonmaleficence) be in disclosing this information? Specifically, what is the potential for harm and its magnitude if the risk is not disclosed? And what is the potential that harm can be averted if disclosed? Here it would be important to consider the specifics of the genetic condition within the family—what is the penetrance and severity, and what options are there for medical actions that would change the course of illness if disclosed? Is there a likelihood that the genetic risk or condition would have been otherwise identified without the disclosure? And finally, can you identify the person(s) at risk? These questions can help a genetic counselor think about what ethical obligations they may have, and to whom.

In practice, one would certainly not go immediately to breaching confidentiality. A reasonable first step would be to explore with the patient the reasons why they are concerned about disclosing the information themselves. A genetic counselor could help patients brainstorm ways to comfortably share hard information, including through offering assistance in sharing the information (letters, practice language) or even offering to provide the disclosure with the patient's permission. Sometimes all it takes is time for a patient to realize that they can and should disclose genetic information to others. As a last resort, if they still do not want the information disclosed, go back to the process and determine if it meets the criteria for breaking confidentiality (an identifiable person at high risk of serious harm). And of course, if one is ever considering disclosing genetic information without authorization, it would be prudent to discuss in advance with your hospital ethics committee or legal/risk management department.

In the event that a genetic counselor or another healthcare provider is considering disclosing genetic information, case law from around the world can also help

TABLE 12-4. Case law focused on disclosing genetic information

§ Australia: Privacy Amendment (Enhancing Privacy Protection) Act 2012; No. 197,2012

- Comment: legislation that permitted health care providers to breach patient confidentiality to inform family members

§ France: Code de la santé publique. Article - L1131-1. JORF

- Comment: Legal duty for patients to inform relatives, either directly or indirectly through the health care provider, about genetic risks relevant for their health

§ United Kingdom: *ABC v. St George's Healthcare NHS Trust & Ors* [2020] EWHC 455 (QB)

- Comment: Health care providers have a duty to balance the interests of the patients and their relatives

§ United States: *Pate v. Threlkel – 661 So. 2d 278* (Fla. 1995)

- Comment: A physician has a duty to warn all at risk parties when the physician knows of those third parties. Although warning the patient of a genetically transferable disease fulfills the physician obligation to warn third parties.

§ United States: *Safer v. Estate of Pack – 291 N.J. Super. 619,677 A.2d 118* (Super. Ct. App. Div. 1996)

- Comment: A physician has a duty to warn those at risk of avoidable harm from a genetic disease. No difference between genetic threat and that of an infection, contagion, or threat of physical harm.

us think through these situations. For the most part, cases where there has been an autosomal dominant, highly penetrant condition that has medical actionability have been the cases most likely to be seen as meeting duty to warn criteria. In Table 12-4 we provide a few legal cases from various countries with legal decisions about disclosing genetic information. These are just examples and are not intended to provide legal precedence for a specific case. This is another reminder to seek out local expertise, such as your institution's legal team, when difficult cases arise.

RESOURCES FOR ETHICAL DILEMMAS

Code of ethics

A code of ethics is a set of principles and standards, often endorsed by a specific professional group. These differ from medical oaths (e.g., the Hippocratic Oath, the Declaration of Geneva Physician's pledge), which are often inspirational and without any enforcement processes. Many genetics professional organizations have their own code of ethics. For example, the NSGC Code of Ethics, first approved in 1992, is a relational code of ethics and discusses behaviors and actions that a genetic counselor would have with themselves, their clients, their colleagues, and society (Benkendorf et al., 1992; National Society of Genetic

Counselors, 2018). While not an exhaustive list, the Canadian Association of Genetic Counselors (CAGC—Canadian Association of Genetic Counsellors, 2006), the British Association of Genetic Counselors and Nurses (Association of Genetic Nurses and Counsellors, 2021), and the Human Society of Genetics in Australasia (Human Genetics Society of Australasia, 2022) have similarly structured codes of ethics. Others, for example the European Board of Medical Genetics (European Board of Medical Genetics, 2013), present a code of professional practice standards.

A key point about codes of ethics: they are generally developed as a way to define specific values or ethical principles that the organization sees as important, and in some cases to apply specific ethical principles to the work that a professional does by describing specific behaviors; in this way they can serve as a guide to conduct. All new genetic counselors are encouraged to be familiar with the relevant codes of ethics or practice standards that are available in their respective locations. Some professional societies will ask new members to affirm that they will adhere to the code of ethics or professional standards that they have adopted. Importantly, these guidelines can be considered professional standards or the values (i.e., morals) of a given profession. Understanding professional and personal values are critical when confronted with an ethical challenge and can often help identify those ethical challenges that could benefit from a formal ethics consult.

Institutional ethics consultants and committees

One goal of this chapter is to familiarize the reader with common theoretical and methodological approaches to health care ethics, but we understand that few genetic providers will formally work in bioethics. Rather, it is important for the genetic professional to recognize when an ethical question arises, to have some fundamental ways to think through the ethical challenge and try to mediate it, and to be aware of local resources that can provide additional assistance in the event that an ethical challenge is especially complex or unresolved.

Many hospitals, including the majority in the United States, will have interdisciplinary ethics committees. These ethics committees are responsible for developing institutional policy, educating clinicians about ethical issues, and being available for consultation when a health care provider encounters an ethically difficult case. These ethics review committees were first formed in the US in the 1960s and 1970s around questions of abortion or scarce resources (e.g., dialysis machines). Since the 1970s, health care ethics committees have increased around the world (Hajibabaee et al., 2016).

Ethics consultants are individuals with specific clinical ethics training and/or expertise. They are often members of the aforementioned hospital ethics committees. In a 2007 survey of US hospitals, individuals performing ethics consultations were primarily physicians or nurses followed by social workers, chaplains, and administrations (Fox et al., 2007), although some genetic counselors and clinical geneticists have additional training and work as bioethicists. In the US, the

American Society for Bioethics and Humanities (ASBH) has offered a certification examination for health care ethics consultants (HEC) establishing expectations for training programs and evaluating competency of ethics consultants (Sawyer et al., 2021). The HEC-C program is still fairly new (established in 2018) and it is unclear whether this certification program, or other similar initiatives, will improve the quality of health care ethics consultation (Antommaria et al., 2020).

If a genetic counselor or other clinician has specific clinical ethics concerns (i.e., an ethical question related to a specific patient) or local institutional ethics issues, these should be reviewed by an institutional-based bioethicist or local ethics committee. Of note, some professional organizations (e.g., NSGC) will also have an ethics committee that accepts consultations on specific cases. For example, the NSGC Ethics Advisory Group serves as a resource to both the board of directors and the members at large on ethical issues in general. Individual members can also request an ethics inquiry review focused on the application of the NSGC code of ethics. Professional organizations can be useful adjuncts to the local ethics committees as they may be more familiar with specific issues that arise in genetics and genetic counseling, and with professional guidelines (e.g., regarding genetic testing in children).

RESEARCH ETHICS

The focus of this chapter is the ethical practice of genetic counseling, and, thus, we have focused on clinical ethics thus far. A detailed discussion of research ethics within the field of genetics is beyond the scope of this single chapter, but it is important to recognize basic research ethics principles. Importantly, the main difference between clinical practice and research is that clinical medicine offers the hope of individual treatment or management that has potential benefit for that individual. In research, the emphasis is generalizable knowledge, and therefore the potential risk–benefit ratio is quite different. Additionally, given the well-documented history of research harms internationally, specific research ethics guidelines have been developed, starting with the Nuremberg Code (1947) and Declaration of Helsinki (1964).

In the US, the National Commission for the Protection of Human Subjects of Biomedical and Behavioral Research was charged with establishing the ethical principles for biomedical and behavioral research involving human subjects in the 1970s. The Commission's final recommendations were detailed in The Belmont Report and included three basic principles. **Respect for Persons** is based on the idea that subjects are autonomous agents and also recognizes that individuals with diminished autonomy are entitled to protection. This may be due to physiological limitations, such as an individual without capacity, or circumstances that may limit one's liberty. The principle of **Beneficence** is often summarized as maximizing potential benefits to research participants and minimizing possible harms. And **Justice** is focused on ensuring that there is equitable distribution of both the benefits and burdens of participating in research. Hopefully these research ethical principles are familiar as they closely resemble the four ethical principles described by Beauchamp and Childress, discussed earlier in the text. That is probably due to the fact that the two texts were published less than one year apart and were heavily influenced by the other (Beauchamp, 2005).

Research ethics will be a part of most genetic counselor's practice in different ways. First, the majority of Master level genetic counseling programs will involve performing some sort of research as part of the graduation requirements. Trainees may design a project and obtain ethics committee approval, recruit participants, collect and analyze data, and publish their research work. Practicing genetic counselors may interact with clinical trials for treatment for genetic disease or may be a part of a team that writes up case reports, performs chart review studies, studies the impact of their genetic counseling practice, or many other types of research.

CONCLUSIONS

It is important for all health care providers to understand that ethics is an inherent part of clinical medicine. Our aim in this chapter was to do more than discuss the meaning of ethics and rather provide the genetic counselor with the tools to identify ethical issues or questions and formulate appropriate responses. In addition, it is important for the genetic counselor to be familiar with the various genetic counseling codes of ethics, institutional policies, and ethics consultants or committees. These resources are intended to aid the provider through complex ethical and moral difficulties in their genetic counseling practice.

REFERENCES

Agich GJ. (2001) The question of method in ethics consultation. *Am J Bioeth* 1(4):31–41. https://doi.org/10.1162/152651601317139360.

Albala I, Doyle M, & Appelbaum PS. (2010) The evolution of consent forms for research: a quarter century of changes. *IRB* 32(3):7–11.

Allyse M Bombard Y, Isasi R, et al. (2019) What do we do now? Responding to claims of germline gene editing in humans. *Genet Med* 21(10):2181–2183. https://doi.org/10.1038/s41436-019-0492-3.

Antommaria AHM, Feudtner C, Benner MB, & Cohn, F. (2020) The healthcare ethics consultant-certified program: fair, feasible, and defensible, but neither definitive nor finished. *Am J Bioeth* 20(3):1–5. https://doi.org/10.1080/15265161.2020.1718421.

Appelbaum PS. (2007) Clinical practice. Assessment of patients' competence to consent to treatment, *N Engl J Med* 357(18):1834–1840. https://doi.org/10.1056/NEJMcp074045.

Anderson-Shaw L. (2015) *Improving Competencies in Clinical Ethics Consultation: An Education Guide* Second edition. Chicago, IL: American Society for Bioethics and Humanities.

Association of Genetic Nurses and Counsellors. (2021) https://www.agnc.org.uk/info-education/documents-websites/ Accessed July 1, 2022.

Beardsley E, Jefford M & Mileshkin L. (2007) Longer consent forms for clinical trials compromise patient understanding: so why are they lengthening? *J Clin Oncol* 25(9):e13–14. https://doi.org/10.1200/JCO.2006.10.3341.

Beauchamp T & Childress J. (1979) *Principles of Biomedical Ethics.* New York, NY: Oxford University Press.

Beauchamp TL. (2005) The Origins and Evolution of the Belmont Report. In: James F Childress, Eric M Meslin and Harold T. Shapiro *Belmont Revisted: Ethical Principles for Research with Human Subjects.* Washington, DC: Georgetown University Press, pp. 12–25.

Beauchamp TL & Childress JF. (2013) *Principles of Biomedical Ethics.* New York, NY: Oxford University Press.

Benkendorf JL, Callanan NP, Grobstein R, et al. (1992) An explication of the National Society of Genetic Counselors (NSGC) code of ethics. *J Genetic Couns* 1(1):31–39.

Best S, Wou K, Vora N, et al. (2018) Promises, pitfalls and practicalities of prenatal whole exome sequencing. *Prenatl Diagn* 38(1):10–19. https://doi.org/10.1002/pd.5102.

Bodian DL, Klein E, Iyer RK, et al. (2016) Utility of whole-genome sequencing for detection of newborn screening disorders in a population cohort of 1,696 neonates. *Genet Med* 18(3):221–230. https://doi.org/10.1038/gim.2015.111.

Bonine S, Bell M, Fishler K, et al. (2021) Conscience clauses in genetic counseling: awareness and attitudes. *J Genet Couns* 30(5):1468–1479. https://doi.org/10.1002/jgc4.1414.

Botkin JR, Belmont JW, Berg JS, et al. (2015) points to consider: ethical, legal, and psychosocial implications of genetic testing in children and adolescents. *Am J Hum Genet* 97(1):6–21. https://doi.org/10.1016/j.ajhg.2015.05.022.

Canadian Association of Genetic Counsellors (CAGC). (2006) Code of Ethics. https://www.cagc-accg.ca/?page=354 Accessed July 1, 2022.

Chaet DH. (2019) AMA Code of Medical Ethics' opinions related to unrepresented patients. *AMA J Ethics* 21(7):E600–602. https://doi.org/10.1001/amajethics.2019.600.

Chavkin W, Leitman L, & Polin K, *et al.* (2013) Conscientious objection and refusal to provide reproductive healthcare: a White Paper examining prevalence, health consequences, and policy responses. *Int J Gynaecol Obstet* 123Suppl 3:S41–56. https://doi.org/10.1016/S0020-7292(13)60002-8.

Clark PA. (2007) Intensive care patients' evaluations of the informed consent process. *Dimens Crit Care Nurs* 26(5):207–226. https://doi.org/10.1097/01.DCC.0000286826.57603.6a.

Collier R. (2017) Reports of coerced sterilization of Indigenous women in Canada mirrors shameful past. *CMAJ* 189(33):E1080–E1081. https://doi.org/10.1503/cmaj.1095471.

Committee on Bioethics, Committee on Genetics, American College of Medical Genetics, & Genomics Social; Ethical; Legal Issues Committee. (2013) Ethical and policy issues in genetic testing and screening of children. *Pediatrics* 131(3):620–622. https://doi.org/10.1542/peds.2012-3680.

Consensus statement of the Society of Critical Care Medicines Ethics Committee regarding futile and other possibly inadvisable treatments (1997) *Crit Care Med* 25(5):887–891. https://doi.org/10.1097/00003246-199705000-00028.

Curlin FA, Lawrence RE, Chin MH & Lantos JD. (2007) Religion, conscience, and controversial clinical practices. *N Engl J Med* 356(6):593–600. https://doi.org/10.1056/NEJMsa065316.

Dee, MJ & Stokes F. (2018) Culture and consent in clinical care: a critical review of nursing and nursing ethics literature. *Annu Rev Nurs Res* 37(1):223–259. https://doi.org/10.1891/0739-6686.37.1.223.

Diekema DS. (2011) Revisiting the best interest standard: uses and misuses. *J Clin Ethics* 22(2):128–133.

Diekema DS. (2019) Decision making on behalf of children: understanding the role of the harm principle. *J Clin Ethics* 30(3):207–212.

Diekema DS, Botkin JR & Committee on Bioethics. (2009) Clinical report–Forgoing medically provided nutrition and hydration in children. *Pediatrics* 124(2):813–822. https://doi.org/10.1542/peds.2009-1299.

Dolan DD, Lee SS-J, & Cho MK. (2022) Three decades of ethical, legal, and social implications research: Looking back to chart a path forward. *Cell Genom* p. 100150. https://doi.org/10.1016/j.xgen.2022.100150.

Eriksson D, Custers R, Edvardsson Björnberg K, et al. (2020) Options to reform the European Union Legislation on GMOs: risk governance. *Trends Biotechnol* 38(4):349–351. https://doi.org/10.1016/j.tibtech.2019.12.016.

European Board of Medical Genetics. (2013) Code of Professional Practice for Genetic Counsellors in Europe. https://www.ebmg.eu/fileadmin/GCGN_Downloads/EBMG CodeofprofessionalpracticeforgeneticcounsellorsinEurope.pdf https://www.ebmg.eu/413.0.html Accessed June 4, 2024.

Faden RR & Beauchamp TL. (1986) *A History and Theory of Informed Consent.* Oxford: Oxford University Press.

Farrelly E, Cho MK, Erby L, et al. (2012) Genetic counseling for prenatal testing: where is the discussion about disability? *J GenetCouns* 21(6):814–824. https://doi.org/10.1007/s10897-012-9484-z.

Fiester A. (2007) Viewpoint: why the clinical ethics we teach fails patients. *Acad Med* 82(7):684–689. https://doi.org/10.1097/ACM.0b013e318067456d.

Finkel RS, Mercuri E, Darras BT, et al. (2017) Nusinersen versus sham control in infantile-onset spinal muscular atrophy. *N Engl J Med* 377(18):1723–1732. https://doi.org/10.1056/NEJMoa1702752.

Flynn AWP, Domínguez S, Jordan R, et al. (2021) When the political is professional: civil disobedience in psychology *Am Psychol* 76(8):1217–1231. https://doi.org/10.1037/amp0000867.

Fox E, Myers S, & Pearlman RA. (2007) Ethics consultation in United States hospitals: a national survey. *American J Bioeth* 7(2):13–25. https://doi.org/10.1080/15265160601109085.

Frader J & Bosk CL. (2009) The personal is political, the professional is not: conscientious objection to obtaining/providing/acting on genetic information, *Am J Med Genet C.* 151C(1):62–67. https://doi.org/10.1002/ajmg.c.30200.

Freedman LR, Hebert LE, Battistelli MF, & Stulberg DB. (2018) Religious hospital policies on reproductive care: what do patients want to know? *Am J Obstet Gynecol* 218(2):251.e1–251.e9. https://doi.org/10.1016/j.ajog.2017.11.595.

Galton F. (1909) Eugenic qualities of primary importance. *The Eugenics Review* 1(2):74–76.

Garver KL & Garver B. (1991) Eugenics: past, present, and the future. *Am J Hum Genet* 49(5):1109–1118.

Nuffield Council on Bioethics. (2016) Genome Editing: An Ethical Review. London. file:///C:/Users/user/Downloads/Genome-editing-an-ethical-review%20(1).pdf Accessed June 4, 2024

Geppert C & Chanko BL. (2016) The CASES approach to ethics consultation: the centrality of the ethics question. *Am J Bioeth* 16(2):80–82. https://doi.org/10.1080/15265161.
2015.1132054.

Ghandakly EC & Fabi R. (2021) Sterilization in US immigration and customs enforcement's (ICE's) detention: ethical failures and systemic injustice. *Am J Public Health*
111(5):832–834. https://doi.org/10.2105/AJPH.2021.306186.

Gilbert, S. (2017, December 13) Is Noninvasive Prenatal Genetic Testing Eugenic? The
HastingsCenter.https://www.thehastingscenter.org/noninvasive-prenatal-genetic-testing-
eugenic/ Accessed June 30, 2022).

Glover JJ. (2006) Ethical decision-making guidelines and tools. In: L Beebe Harman (ed)
Ethical Challenges in the Management of Health Information Second Edition. Sudbury,
MA: Jones and Bartlett, p. 24.

Green JM. (1995) Obstetricians views on prenatal diagnosis and termination of pregnancy:
1980 compared with 1993. *Br J Obstet Gynaecol* 102(3):228–232. https://doi.
org/10.1111/j.1471-0528.1995.tb09099.x.

Guiahi M, Helbin PE, Teal SB, et al. (2019) Patient views on religious institutional
health care, *JAMA Netw Open* 2(12), p. e1917008. https://doi.org/10.1001/
jamanetworkopen.2019.17008.

Hajibabaee F, Soodabeh Joolaee S, Cheraghi MA, et al. (2016) Hospital/clinical ethics
committees' notion: an overview, *J Med Ethics Hist Med* 9:17.

Hamington M & Miller DC. (2006) *Socializing Care: Feminist Ethics and Public Issues.*
Lanham, MD: Rowman & Littlefield.

Hammami MM, Al-Jawarneh Y, Hammami MB & Al Qadire M. (2014) Information disclosure in clinical informed consent: "reasonable" patient's perception of norm in high-
context communication culture, *BMC Med Ethics* 15:3. https://doi.org/10.1186/
1472-6939-15-3.

Harmon A. (2018, October 19) Geneticists Criticize Use of Science by White Nationalists
to Justify "Racial Purity".*The New York Times.* https://www.nytimes.com/2018/10/19/
us/white-supremacists-science-genetics.html Accessed July 1, 2022.

Harris LH. (2022) Navigating loss of abortion services - a large academic medical center
prepares for the overturn of Roe v. Wade, *N Engl J Med* 386(22):2061–2064. https://doi.
org/10.1056/NEJMp2206246.

Henderson GE, Wolf SM, Kuczynski KJ, et al. (2014) The challenge of informed consent
and return of results in translational genomics: empirical analysis and recommendations, *J Law Med Ethics* 42(3):344–355. https://doi.org/10.1111/jlme.12151.

Hercher L. (2022, August 3) Genetic Counselors Scramble Post- Roe to Provide
Routine Pregnancy Services without Being Accused of a Crime *Scientific American.*
https://www.scientificamerican.com/article/genetic-counselors-scramble-post-
roe-to-provide-routine-pregnancy-services-without-being-accused-of-a-crime/
Accessed September 23, 2022.

Hercher L & Jamal L. (2016) An old problem in a new age: revisiting the clinical dilemma
of misattributed paternity. *Appl Transl Genom* 8:36–39. https://doi.org/10.1016/
j.atg.2016.01.004.

Holland S. (2011) The virtue ethics approach to bioethics. *Bioethics* 25(4):192–201.
https://doi.org/10.1111/j.1467-8519.2009.01758.x.

Howard D. (2021) Civil disobedience, not merely conscientious objection, in medicine,
HEC Forum 33(3):215–232. https://doi.org/10.1007/s10730-020-09417-5.

Howard HC, van El CG, Forzano F, et al. (2018) One small edit for humans, one giant edit for humankind? Points and questions to consider for a responsible way forward for gene editing in humans. *Eur J Hum Genet* 26(1):1–11. https://doi.org/10.1038/s41431-017-0024-z.

Human Genetics Society of Australasia. (2022). https://www.hgsa.org.au/common/Uploaded%20files/pdfs/policies,%20position%20statements%20and%20guidelines/genetic%20counselling/Code%20of%20Ethics%20for%20GC.pdf Accessed 1 July 2022.

Jonsen A, Siegler M. & Winslade, W. (2010) *Clinical Ethics: A Practical Approach to Ethical Decisions in Clinical Medicine* Seventh Edition. New York,NY: McGraw Hill Professional.

Jonsen AR. (1993) The birth of bioethics. *Hastings Cent Rep.* 23(6):S1–4.

Kass NE, Chaisson L, Taylor HA & Lohse J. (2011) Length and complexity of US and international HIV consent forms from federal HIV network trials *J Gen Intern Med* 26(11):1324–1328. https://doi.org/10.1007/s11606-011-1778-6.

Katz AL, Webb SA & Committee on Bioethics (2016) Informed consent in decision-making in pediatric practice. *Pediatrics* 138(2):e20161485. https://doi.org/10.1542/peds.2016-1485.

Klima J, Fitzgerald-Butt SM, Kelleher KJ, et al. (2014) Understanding of informed consent by parents of children enrolled in a genetic biobank. *Genet Med* 16(2):141–148. https://doi.org/10.1038/gim.2013.86.

Kochenderfer JN, Dudley ME, Feldman SA, et al. (2012) B-cell depletion and remissions of malignancy along with cytokine-associated toxicity in a clinical trial of anti-CD19 chimeric-antigen-receptor-transduced T cells. *Blood* 119(12):2709–2720. https://doi.org/10.1182/blood-2011-10-384388.

Kon AA, Shepard EK, Sederstrom, NO, et al. (2016) Defining futile and potentially inappropriate interventions: a policy statement from the Society of Critical Care Medicine Ethics Committee *Crit Care Med* 44(9):1769–1774. https://doi.org/10.1097/CCM.0000000000001965.

Kouros N. (2013) Women inmates in California sterilised without state approval. *Monash Bioeth Rev* 31(2):27–28.

Kuhse H & Singer P. (1990) Individuals, humans, and persons: the issue of moral status. In: JP Lizza (ed) *Defining the Beginning and End of Life: Readings on Personal Identity and Bioethics*. Baltimore, MD: Johns Hopkins University Press.

Larrabee MJ (ed.). (1993) *An Ethic of Care: Feminist and lnterdisciplinary Perspectives.* New York and London: Routledge.

Magelssen M, Pedersen R, & Førde R. (2016) Four roles of ethical theory in clinical ethics consultation *Am J Bioeth* 16(9):26–33. https://doi.org/10.1080/15265161.2016.1196254.

McConkie-Rosell A, Spiridigliozzi GA, Elizabeth Melvin E, et al. (2008) Living with genetic risk: effect on adolescent self-concept, *J Med Genet C* 148C(1):56–69. https://doi.org/10.1002/ajmg.c.30161.

McDougall R, Delany C, & Gillam L. (2018) The value of open deliberation in clinical ethics, and the role of parents reasons in the zone of parental discretion, *Am J Bioeth* 18(8):47–49. https://doi.org/10.1080/15265161.2018.1485773.

National Academy of Medicine, National Academy of Sciences, and the Royal Society. (2020) *Heritable Human Genome Editing*. Washington, DC: The National Academies Press. https://doi.org/10.17226/25665.

National Commission for the Protection of Human Subjects of Biomedical and Behavioral Research (1979) The Belmont Report: Ethical Principles and Guidelines for the Protection of Human Subjects of Research. Washington, DC: US Department of Health and Human Services http://www.hhs.gov/ohrp/humansubjects/guidance/belmont.html Accessed August 26, 2013.

National Society of Genetic Counselors. (2018) National Society of Genetic Counselors Code of Ethics, *J Genet Couns* 27(1):6–8. https://doi.org/10.1007/s10897-017-0166-8.

National Society of Genetic Counselors. (2022) Access to Reproductive Healthcare. https://www.nsgc.org/Policy-Research-and-Publications/Position-Statements/Position-Statements/Post/access-to-reproductive-healthcare Accessed July 1, 2022.

Nurk S, Sergey Koren S, Rhie A, et al. (2022) The complete sequence of a human genome, *Science* 376(6588):44–53. https://doi.org/10.1126/science.abj6987.

Oakley J. (2010) A Virtue Ethics Approach. In: Helga Kuhse and Peter Singer (eds) *A Companion to Bioethics*. Oxford: Wiley-Blackwell, pp. 91–104. https://doi.org/10.1002/9781444307818.ch10.

Ormond KE, Iris M, Banuvar S, et al. (2007) What do patients prefer: informed consent models for genetic carrier testing. *J Genet Couns* 16(4):539–550. https://doi.org/10.1007/s10897-007-9094-3.

Ormond KE, Mortlock DP, Schole DT, et al. (2017) Human germline genome editing. *Am J Hum Genet* 101(2):167–176. https://doi.org/10.1016/j.ajhg.2017.06.012.

Ormond KE. Bombard Y, Bonham VL, et al. (2019) The clinical application of gene editing: ethical and social issues. *Per Med* 16(4):337–350. https://doi.org/10.2217/pme-2018-0155.

Parens E & Asch A (eds). (2000) *Prenatal Testing and Disability Rights*. Washington DC: Georgetown University Press.

Pencarinha DF, Bell NK, Edwards JG, & Best RG. (1992) Ethical issues in genetic counseling: a comparison of M.S. counselor and medical geneticist perspectives. *J Genet Couns* 1(1):19–30.

Quill TE, Lo B, & Brock DW. (1997) Palliative options of last resort: a comparison of voluntarily stopping eating and drinking, terminal sedation, physician-assisted suicide, and voluntary active euthanasia. *JAMA*, 278(23):2099–2104. https://doi.org/10.1001/jama.278.23.2099.

Ross LF, Saal HM, David KL, et al. (2013) Technical report: Ethical and policy issues in genetic testing and screening of children *Genet Med* 15(3):234–245. https://doi.org/10.1038/gim.2012.176.

Ross LF. (1996) Disclosing misattributed paternity. *Bioethics* 10(2):114–130.

Ross LF. (2019) Better than best (interest standard) in pediatric decision making. *J Clin Ethics* 30(3):183–195.

Sawyer KE, Dundas N, Snyder A, & Diekema DS. (2021) Competencies and milestones for bioethics trainees: beyond ASBH's healthcare ethics certification and core competencies. *J Clin Ethics* 32(2):127–148.

Saxton M. (1998) Disability Rights and Selective Abortion. In: Rickie Solinger (ed) *Abortion Wars, A Half Century of Struggle: 1950 to 2000*. Berkeley, CA: University of California Press, pp. 374–395.

Senter L, Bennett RL, Madeo AC, et al. (2018) National Society of Genetic Counselors Code of Ethics: Explication of 2017 Revisions. *J Genet Couns* 27(1):9–15. https://doi.org/10.1007/s10897-017-0165-9.

Shuster E. (1997) Fifty years later: the significance of the Nuremberg Code. *N Engl J Med* 337(20):1436–1440. https://doi.org/10.1056/NEJM199711133372006.

Siegler M. (2019) Clinical medical ethics: its history and contributions to American medicine. *J Clin Ethics* 30(1):17–26.

Silvers WS, Wynia MK, Levine MA, & Himber M. (2021) Teaching health professions students about the Holocaust. *AMA J Ethics* 23(1):E26–30. https://doi.org/10.1001/amajethics.2021.26.

Singer PA, Pellegrino ED, & Siegler M. (2001) Clinical ethics revisited. *BMC Med Ethics* 2:E1. https://doi.org/10.1186/1472-6939-2-1.

Spector-Bagdady K Prince AER, Yu J-H, & Appelbaum PS. (2018) Analysis of state laws on informed consent for clinical genetic testing in the era of genomic sequencing, *Am J Med Genet C* 178(1):81–88. https://doi.org/10.1002/ajmg.c.31608.

Tarzian AJ, Wocial LD, & ASBH Clinical Ethics Consultation Affairs Committee. (2015) A code of ethics for health care ethics consultants: journey to the present and implications for the field. *Am J Bioethics* 15(5):38–51. https://doi.org/10.1080/15265161.2015.1021966.

Thomson JJ. (1971) A Defense of Abortion. *Philos Public Aff* 1(1):47–66.

United States Department of Health and Human Services. (1996) Health Insurance Portability and Accountability Act of 1996. Public Law 104-191. *United States Statutes at Large* 110:1936–2103.

Venter JC, Adams MD, Myers EW, et al. (2001) The sequence of the human genome. *Science* 291(5507):1304–1351. https://doi.org/10.1126/science.1058040.

Wakefield CE, Hanlon LV, Tucke KM, et al. (2016) The psychological impact of genetic information on children: a systematic review. *Genet Med* 18(8):755–762. https://doi.org/10.1038/gim.2015.181.

Wertz DC, Fletcher JC, & Mulvihill JJ. (1990) Medical geneticists confront ethical dilemmas: cross-cultural comparisons among 18 nations. *Am J Hum Genet* 46(6):1200–1213.

Whitney SN, McGuire AL, & McCullough LB. (2004) A typology of shared decision making, informed consent, and simple consent, *Ann Intern Med* 140(1):54–59. https://doi.org/10.7326/0003-4819-140-1-200401060-00012.

Wrigley A, Wilkinson S, & Appleby JB. (2015) Mitochondrial replacement: ethics and identity. *Bioethics*, 29(9):631–638. https://doi.org/10.1111/bioe.12187.

Wynia MK. (2022) Professional civil disobedience - medical-society responsibilities after Dobbs. *N Engl J Med* 387(11):959–961. https://doi.org/10.1056/NEJMp2210192.

Wynia MK & Silvers WS. (2021) A call to commemorate International Holocaust Remembrance Day, January 27, in all health science schools, *AMA J Ethics* 23(1):E75–77. https://doi.org/10.1001/amajethics.2021.75.

Zampas C & Andión-Ibañez X. (2012) Conscientious objection to sexual and reproductive health services: international human rights standards and European law and practice. *Eur J Health Law* 19(3):231–256. https://doi.org/10.1163/157180912x639116.

13

Genetic Counseling Research: Understanding the Basics

Sarah Scollon and Beverly M. Yashar

Research creates an opportunity to expand our understanding of our world, to shine a light on an issue that is either open to deeper evaluation or has not previously been investigated. Designing and successfully implementing an effective research study is filled with numerous opportunities for both success and failure. The process can be demanding, time consuming, and stressful. So why embark on this process? Research allows us to discover something novel, not only in our area of interest but also in ourselves as investigators. Working through a research project creates the opportunity to develop and deepen skills in critical thinking and analysis. More globally, research is an avenue to facilitate change, impact practice and policy, and advance the field of genetic counseling more broadly.

Since research attempts to break new ground, there is no guarantee that it will be successful. While our failures often can tell us as much as our successes, the goal of this chapter is to provide you with guidance that will help you tip the balance towards success. We will be looking at research as a structured process composed of discrete steps (Figure 13-1). Research requires us to be

A Guide to Genetic Counseling, Third Edition. Edited by Vivian Y. Pan, Jane L. Schuette, Karen E. Wain, and Beverly M. Yashar.

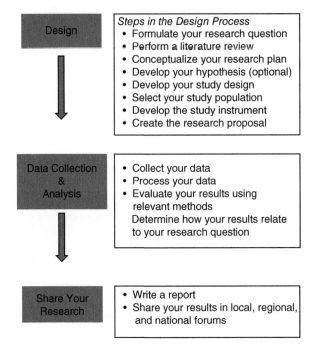

FIGURE 13-1. *The Research Process*

simultaneously creative and practical. In the end (or more accurately from the start) research requires taking a leap of faith into the darkness.

This chapter will touch on all aspects of the process but will focus most heavily on study design and consider potential significant outcomes of your research. We will take a step-by-step approach and provide general guidance to help you successfully approach, navigate, and complete these components. While our perspective will be grounded in the social sciences as opposed to laboratory-focused research, many of the concepts are broadly applicable. A number of excellent textbooks are available that discuss individual topics in more detail. A few of these are listed at the end of this chapter.

If we knew what it was we were doing, it would not be called research, would it?
attributed to Albert Einstein (1879–1955)

WHY DO RESEARCH?

The knowledge that is generated by a research study can provide insights that can be used to effect change and improve our work as genetic counselors. This process is driven by a unique way of thinking that is exemplified in the definition of the word itself. The word "research" is derived from the French word *rechercher* meaning "to seek out, to search closely" (Merriam-Webster Inc., 2019). The prefix "re" means anew or over and over again. Consequently, research is an iterative process in which an investigator is able to answer questions that explore the "who, what, when, where and why" of a phenomenon and develop an understanding of how and why these answers are true. A research project in the field of genetic counseling can help answer questions like:

- What are key ethical, legal, and social implications (ELSI) to consider in the implementation of population based genetic screening programs?
- What approaches to genetic counseling program recruitment and application processes will increase equity and inclusion for all applicants?
- How can genetic counselors incorporate new technologies into practice to respond to an increasing demand for genetic counseling services?
- How can health care providers, researchers, and community organizations partner to increase access to genetic services for all communities?

The iterative component of research refers to the fact that simply asking and answering a question once is insufficient. In the world of research, you have established the "truth" of your answer when multiple experts reach the same conclusion based on independent findings. While researchers are continually striving for objectivity, the process itself and the resulting outcomes are extremely sensitive to error. Consequently, repetition helps to ensure accuracy and allows a researcher to answer a single research question using a variety of approaches. For example, the question "How can health care providers, researchers, and community organizations partner to increase access to genetic services for all communities?" might be explored by asking:

- What barriers are community members (i.e., potential patients) in areas with low utilization of genetics services experiencing in accessing care? What can we learn from community stakeholders to develop novel approaches that increase empowerment of members of a community to access genetic services?
- Are community members more likely to participate in genetic testing and family communication about cascade screening following an educational webinar on genetics services held by their local support group?
- How can genetic counselors build better partnerships with interpreter services?
- What is the impact of chatbots developed with community stakeholder feedback on promoting referral uptake of genetic services?

Completely understanding the larger research question requires exploration from a variety of complementary approaches and generally requires the design and execution of multiple focused research projects in various settings and/or populations. It is not necessary for a single researcher to answer all of these focused questions in order to establish insights into the larger research question. As part of the decision-making process about how to answer the broader research question, individual researchers generally consider their personal interests, their research expertise, the ways in which their approach will reflect the variability in their study population, and available resources.

Genetic counseling research can be focused in multiple directions. These can include the practice of genetic counseling itself, our professional identity, and the varied clinical, social, legal, and ethical issues that both inform patient care and matter to our patients. A quick scan of the tables of content of the *Journal of Genetic Counseling* finds manuscripts that display a range of perspectives. This variety reflects the diverse interests of individuals within the profession and demonstrates that interested researchers have explored a wide variety of questions, employed varied methodologies, and applied novel theoretical lenses to explore and understand the depth and breadth of disciplines in which genetic counselors as researchers bring value. The abstracts presented at the National Society of Genetic Counselors Annual Meeting showcase examples of the diverse research interests of our community, issues that matter to our patients and their care, and a resource for contemporary topics in the field (NSGC, n.d.).

A critical factor unifying these varied approaches is reliance on evidence-based methods. This demands that the researcher forms their clinical research question in response to a recognized need for information, searches for the most appropriate evidence, critically appraises it, seeks to incorporate the results into a strategy for action, and lastly evaluates the outcomes. Evidence-based medicine is formally defined as an approach to health care that promotes the collection, interpretation, and integration of valid, important and applicable patient-reported, clinician-observed, and research-derived evidence (Sackett et al., 1996; Evans and Khoury, 2007; Schaaf et al., 2020; Dungan et al., 2023). High-quality research allows clinical researchers to evaluate the potential impact on genetic counseling practice and can help us to understand and bring about effective change. As stated in our Code of Ethics, genetic counselors are encouraged to participate in actions that have the purpose of promoting the wellbeing of society and access to health care (Senter et al., 2018).

WHAT MAKES SCIENTIFIC KNOWLEDGE DIFFERENT?

Scientific research is a unique activity with its focus on objectivity—holding to this standard can be quite difficult given the nature of being human. Our perspectives on how the world around us works (i.e., the rules that govern our lives) are continually influenced by our personal experiences. These anecdotal experiences are a central part of how we explain and bring order to the world around us and form the basis of a *subjective* perspective in which one's thinking is informed by previous experiences, educational background, discipline of study, philosophy, and sociocultural background. This type of awareness is different from research in which we strive for an *objective* perspective and are working to explore and explain a phenomenon in a way that does not introduce the researcher's (i.e., our own) biases. Objectivity gives research its special character as it can help us to identify and develop consistent and defensible explanations of natural phenomena. However, it may be these same personal experiences, interests, and worldviews that motivate the researcher, inform research questions, and serve as individual strengths of a researcher. Therefore, it is important to leverage these subjective perspectives while ensuring they do not translate into biases in the development or interpretation of your own research.

Attaining objectivity can be considered both a method and a goal when conducting research, yet it may not always be fully achievable. It is easiest to envision achieving research objectivity in a controlled experimental situation that produces the same or similar results; that is, the findings are replicable. In a practical sense, a research result is deemed to be objectively "true" when independent researchers arrive at the same conclusion. This insistence on replication helps protect against researchers' biases. In disciplines like genomics, biostatistics, and clinical research, the process for obtaining objective results (and the reasons why objectivity is so valuable) are relatively easy to understand. The research relies on techniques and tools that have been validated (tested for accuracy) and standardized (shown to produce consistent responses); there are well-defined metrics for interpretation, and it may be relatively straightforward to replicate a study. However, even in these "controlled" research settings, researchers' biases can impact the results as they make choices about which questions are being asked, how they are explored, what data is analyzed, and how it is interpreted. In seeking to pose and answer research questions that are grounded in an individuals' beliefs and motivations (i.e., qualitative research), striving for objectivity is impacted by both the researcher's perspective and the fact that the goal is to understand subjective lived experiences that are inherently variable. In truth, subjectivity and variability are the strengths of qualitative research, and the generalizability of the results (i.e., the ability to apply the findings of a single study to a broader population) arises from the aggregation of these individual inherently variable experiences. Because absolute objectivity can never be achieved, it is critical for the researcher to keep themselves attuned to their biases in all steps of their work. In all research endeavors, the following precepts should be kept in mind:

- Adherence to the scientific method is central to success. This methodology demands you apply a systematic approach to all steps of your investigations, including formulating your research question, generating theories and/or a hypothesis, designing your study, and collecting, analyzing, and interpreting your results.
- The belief that natural phenomena can be understood—even if only in a limited and probabilistic manner.

- Striving for complete honesty in all aspects of your research endeavor. Continually ask yourself what evidence your results provide either for, or against, your hypothesis or research question. Awareness of your assumptions can help guard against bias in all stages of your work.
- Being open to critical inquiry from others and being self-aware at every step in the process. Recognize the potential impact of your personal beliefs and motivations on the process and its outcomes.

This mindset makes it possible to define discrete characteristics of a successful research project and to begin to understand how to approach designing, implementing, and analyzing a research project in which the results are valid and verifiable. Critical factors to remember include:

- All phases of your work, from design through to analysis, should be planned at the outset. This comprehensive research plan serves as the blueprint for the actual work.
- Identify potential alternatives to foreseeable challenges in advance. It is a given that you will need to deviate from your original research plan, it never goes as you expect. While you can't anticipate all roadblocks, the ability to adjust the research plan without sacrificing scientific rigor will lead to success.
- Develop a plan for gathering and analyzing your data that is not only organized and methodical, but also carefully documented.
- As a researcher you should strive for rigor (accuracy and exactness) in all phases of the project. This is especially true in data analysis and interpretation but begins with the design of the project.
- The inherently reductionist nature of research which strives to break down a complex issue into simplified components and outcomes, means that the researcher needs to ask themselves how well their results represent the bigger research question they are seeking to answer. In other words, what do your results tell you about your research question and what do they fail to address?

THE RESEARCH PROCESS

No matter how long or short the time period you have to undertake a research project, it is beneficial to approach your research in a step-wise manner that breaks it down into a process composed of discrete phases: design, data collection and analysis, and sharing your research (Figure 13-1). This approach will help you organize your work and is an important factor in ensuring the success of your research. For illustrative purposes, the design process itself has been broken down into eight discrete sequential steps. The order in which these steps are undertaken can vary from project to project and researcher to researcher and the process is often iterative. The steps as listed provide a general framework, but you may find yourself needing to return to an earlier step or move back and forth between steps as you move through the process. This is okay; and revisions to your plan are an ongoing process. To the novice researcher, it can be difficult to envision where your project will lead. However, dedicating focused time and seeking input from others on your research team to help you anticipate and critically evaluate your end point(s) or desired outcomes, how the steps in your research plan will get you there, and trying to anticipate problems that may arise along the way, mean you will have a higher likelihood of successfully completing a project that provides answers to your questions. The research plan helps you impose a method to a complex process.

Design Step 1: Formulate Your Research Question

The first phase of designing your research plan is to formulate your research question. Where can you find good research ideas? Curiosity is a critical first step in identifying a potential project. What have you been learning about in class, observed in your clinical rotations, heard discussed in conferences, or presented at seminars? What did you find interesting or intriguing and wanted to know more? Your daily professional world is a great place to start (Table 13-1).

Reading current literature can also help you identify topics of interest. Look at the tables of content from journals of interest to genetic counselors, including but not limited to *The Journal of Genetic Counseling, Genetics in Medicine,* and the *American Journal of Medical Genetics.* Importantly, exploring the tables of content and reading articles in journals of interest can help you develop research ideas that refine or extend previous research. Read abstracts from recent genetics professional meetings and those related to your interests. Explore professional forums and social media platforms related to genetics to identify trends in questions or topics that the community is wrestling with. Look at recent projects that have been funded by relevant agencies, like the Jane Engelberg Memorial Fellowship or the Audrey Heimler Special Projects Award at NSGC. What are

TABLE 13-1. Developing Practice-Based Research Questions

Identify areas of your practice that:
you "use" but they don't work effectively
you "use" but you are unsure why they work
you "do" differently from others or the way you were taught
you "see" as an opportunity to improve patient care
you "see" as an opportunity to increase access to genetic counseling services
you "believe" are an opportunity to expand the scope of genetic counseling practice

the research priorities of the professional and patient communities you want to impact? You could start by looking at their website and the requests for proposals (RFPs) from possible funding groups. These documents generally describe new questions that need addressing and identify general approaches that thought leaders in the field see as important. Even if you are not going to be applying to these agencies, evaluating RFPs can be a great way to identify interesting research questions. Let your creative juices flow. Just because the topic you have identified has been previously researched, it does not mean that the specific question you want to explore has been fully asked and answered. Your perspectives will be unique—use them. Lastly, consider your personal interests and motivators. These motivations may be informed by both past and present experiences. What are concepts or topics that matter to you? Finding research that drives you on a personal level will allow you to maintain your motivation over the course of the research project.

Give yourself permission to identify new areas for exploration. This can be a very exciting part of the process. Think big: at first nothing should be out of the realm of possibility. You will have plenty of time to determine what is going to be workable and to evolve the project to ensure success given the constraints of your environment. This is the point in the process where everything is possible. Once you have identified your general area(s) of interest, it is important to consider how interested in this topic you really are. Research projects require a lot of time; make sure that this is something that you really want to do. Is this a topic that you really care about? Ask yourself why you chose this topic and exactly what you want to discover. Make an informed choice. Think through your idea carefully—make sure that you are committed and passionate about it (Box 13-1).

Once you have selected your broad area of interest, you will need to refine the topic into more specific research question(s) that are manageable given the time you have available. You will further refine your research question by creating an objective and specific aim(s) in Step 3. The steps outlined in Table 13-2 provide a practical approach to developing your research idea into research questions that you will enjoy pursuing. Remember that a good topic will address an important issue; however, it is unlikely that your research will be able to provide all the answers you are seeking. Set realistic expectations for yourself and the outcomes of your work.

Design Step 2: Perform a Literature Review

With a good research question in hand, it is important to explore the existing literature so that you can see what is already known about the topic. This search will help you gain a fuller understanding of the history of explorations in your topic. This analysis helps you to figure out what is really known and what is still unknown and where your research results will fit into the current body of knowledge. This review can also help you identify theories or conceptual frameworks that you can use to support your proposed work.

BOX 13-1. CONSIDERING THE SCOPE OF A THESIS OR
CAPSTONE PROJECT

Identifying your thesis topic while in your genetic counseling training program can feel overwhelming, particularly when your proposed research must be completed within the time constraints of your training. While you want your project to be relevant to the field of genetic counseling, it also needs to be manageable. You will want to identify a project that will give you this experience, but is not so large in scope that you will become overwhelmed. A few tips in considering the scope of your research include:

- Be open. You may begin your journey with a specific research topic or study design in mind but find yourself running into hurdles related to feasibility. Be willing to consider other options that may fall within the same area of interest but are more feasible than your original idea.
- Be realistic about the time that each research step will take. If you will need to recruit participants to your study, be sure that the participant population is readily accessible, so your project is not delayed by recruitment. Also, consider the length of time necessary to design a good study instrument and/or to complete your data analysis.
- Consider identifying individuals with ongoing research projects where an option to participate in a sub-study is available. Researchers may have existing datasets that are ripe for analysis and interpretation.
- Be willing to brainstorm with your teachers, your supervisors, and your classmates. The more you can talk about your idea and get varied perspectives on what will work and what won't, the higher the likelihood that you will be successful. These conversations can help you focus your research questions and maintain rigor in your design and analysis.
- Consider the areas of expertise that you will need to successfully complete your project. This will help you assemble your research team (i.e., members with expertise in your proposed research design, a content expert, a statistician, a community stakeholder, etc.).
- Learn from the experiences of others. Talk to senior graduate students or program alumni to learn more about their process.

At first, this search might humble you. You may think that all the good ideas have already been asked and answered. However, this is the time to really use your critical thinking skills. Evaluate what has already been accomplished, identify its strengths and weaknesses, and recognize there are multiple ways of asking and answering a question, each of which, if rigorously developed and applied, will yield complementary insights. What possible gaps or issues are there in the previous research? What future research directions relevant to your topic are raised by

TABLE 13-2. Identifying and Developing a Research Idea

Step	Guidance	Questions to Ask Yourself
1. Identify a broad area of interest and define the purpose of your study.	Work to be as clear and precise as you can. Make sure that you really care about this topic.	Why do I want to work on this research question and what do I hope to achieve?
2. Dissect the broad area into subareas.	This is the time to brainstorm multiple ways of evaluating your research idea.	Have I explored my idea from varied perspectives?
3. Select a subarea.	This should be the idea that you find most interesting.	Do I still really "care" about this idea? Why is it appealing?
4. Raise a specific research question.	Make sure that it relates to your original research idea.	Will this question really allow me to explore my area of interest?
5. Undertake a literature review.	Determine what is already known about your topic. Be sure to consider relevant related areas. This process will help you decided if your question is research worthy.	Has this idea been explored previously? If yes, why is it worthy of replication or follow up investigation? If no, why not?
6. Formulate an objective and specific aim(s) (or subobjectives).	This is derived from your research question and should take the form of action-oriented statements.	Is the specific aim(s) doable and related to my objective?
7. Assess your specific aim(s) in terms of feasibility.	Evaluate if the specific aim(s) and your results will make a difference to you as a researcher and to others. Define the obstacles related to knowledge, available data, time, and cost. Weigh the benefits against the costs.	How much work will this project involve? Is the scale doable? Do I have enough time, money, and access to necessary resources/expertise? Are there ethical considerations regarding the study population and are they accessible?
8. Double-check that you are still interested in your project.	Make sure that the project is relevant, adds to a body of knowledge, and supports your interests.	Am I still interested? Do I agree with my objectives? Do I have the needed resources?

authors in the literature? What is appropriate for future analysis? This review will help you develop objectives (including sub-objectives/specific aims) that are grounded in the literature, doable, and relevant to the field. In some instances, you may find that there is limited literature on your specific topic or population, in this case you can look for a study that resembles your research idea in topic or design and then apply the same critical questions in evaluating the results. You can also consider asking for help from your librarians, they are experts in helping you undertake the most comprehensive literature search.

So how to get started on your review? Ask your advisor, mentor, supervisors, and senior students to help you identify the most credible (usually peer-reviewed) and useful journals and conference proceedings in your area of interest. Also ask for advice on identifying highly influential or "classic" papers that you should definitely read. Ask yourself what other investigators considered relevant in their review of the literature; that is, what information was reviewed in the introduction or discussion of the papers you find in your literature review. Aside from helping you to figure out the current state of thinking about the topic, this will help you identify relevant issues and anticipate common problems; that is, avoid common traps and pitfalls. Many articles will also contain a future directions section which will highlight future research questions as proposed by the authors.

You will need to immerse yourself in the literature so that you can become familiar with the field. In the beginning you will be spending most of your time reading. It's normal to be overwhelmed by the possibilities. It is impossible to read everything that might be relevant; instead, read selectively. Before making the time to read a paper in depth, make sure it's worth it. Scan the title, then the abstract, and then glance at the introduction and conclusions. Before you try to understand all the nitty-gritty details of the paper, skim the whole thing, and try to get a feel for the most important points. If it still seems worthwhile and relevant, go back and read the entire paper. Pay careful attention to the methods and results and evaluate how well they support the conclusions. You may want to take notes while you read. Even if you don't go back and reread them, this process can help you to focus your attention and forces you to summarize as you read. And if you do need to refresh your memory later, rereading your notes is much easier and faster than rereading the whole paper.

One last detail This is the point in planning your research project when you should start to figure out how you are going to keep track of your references, including not just the citations but relevant information gleaned from the articles. There are several excellent online bibliographic management programs, including Citation Manager, EndNote, Mendeley, RefWorks, and Zotero. Some of these may be available for use through your local library. Make an informed decision about which program you want to use and learn how to use it effectively to keep track of your literature search.

Design Step 3. Conceptualize Your Research Plan

While there are many absolutes about the process of designing and implementing a research project, there are also multiple opportunities for you as a researcher to make decisions that are determined by your unique interests. Selection of the experimental approach (choosing a quantitative or qualitative method of investigation) to address your research question is one such example. In a *qualitative* study the investigator is focused on describing variation in a phenomenon, situation, or attitude, and working to understand the deeper meaning of individual experiences. Often the aim is to produce a detailed description that allows us to understand how this meaning influences a person's behavior. In a *quantitative* approach, the research is focused on quantifying variation utilizing precise and generalizable statistical methods and looking for cause and effect, where factors or variables cause outcomes.

In *qualitative studies,* data is generally collected in the form of words as opposed to numbers and results are evaluated in terms of themes or categories using a descriptive rather than an analytical approach (Poth and Creswell, 2018; Miles et al., 2020; Wainstein et al., 2023). The goal is generally discovery, description, understanding, and interpretation. The analysis is interpretive rather than measurable and is highly context dependent. This type of an approach often leads towards the development, rather than testing, of a hypothesis and/or theory. It also may be used in follow-up to quantitative studies to more deeply explore relationships or correlations detected.

A qualitative study can consider details and nuances of subjects' replies and explore multiple interpretations of answers (Table 13-3). The process is highly dependent on communication and observation and subjects generally have freedom in their responses; that is, they can describe their experiences in their own words. Methods of choice can include observation, document analysis, interviews, and focus groups with the latter two more commonly being utilized in genetic counseling research. In both interviews and focus groups, participants are asked to respond to general questions and the interviewer or group moderator probes and explores their responses. During this exploration, you are working to identify and define participants' perceptions, opinions, and feelings about the topic or idea being discussed. Probing in a focus group can have the added goal of trying to determine the degree of agreement that exists within the group. In total, this type of research is exploratory and open-ended. Qualitative research is extremely effective in discovering the meaning events have for the individuals who experience them. It is interpretive in character as the analysis is dependent on interpretation by the researcher. Thus, the quality of the findings from a qualitative research project is directly dependent upon the skills, experience, and sensitivity of the interviewer or group moderator as well as those coding and interpreting the data. While qualitative research could be perceived as more subjective given the fact that it is dependent on individual's perspectives, exploring this subjectivity is one of its goals.

TABLE 13-3. **Features of Quantitative and Qualitative Research**

Qualitative	Quantitative
The aim of this research is detailed descriptions that rely on individual experiences.	The aim of this research is classification, counting, and construction of statistical models that explain your observations.
Can be highly useful in the early phases of research.	Recommended during later phases of research projects.
Researcher may only know roughly what they are looking for in advance of data collection, i.e., it is exploratory in nature.	Researcher decides at the start what they are looking for, e.g. the research may have a hypothesis they want to test.
The analysis plan is iterative and emerges as the study unfolds.	All aspects of the study are designed before data collection starts.
Researcher is a component in the data gathering process.	Researcher relies on tools that collect numerical data, including surveys and data abstraction forms.
Data and results take the form of words, ideas, and themes.	Data are in the form of numbers and statistics.
Qualitative data are richer, results are more time consuming to generate and less generalizable.	Collection of quantitative data can be very efficient. The data can be used to test hypotheses and more generalizable. Of note, these types of studies may miss contextual details.
Researcher can become subjectively immersed in the subject matter.	Researcher can be more objective with regard to the data and results.

Quantitative studies measure characteristics and experiences using numerical and/or categorical groupings that are analyzed statistically. This method may rely on structured questions in the form of a survey with predetermined response options, data collection tools with predetermined data points, or data abstracted from chart reviews or laboratory tests. This approach does not restrict the types of research questions that are being explored; rather it imposes a specific structure on the ways in which the research questions are explored, and the results are gathered and evaluated (Table 13-3). The upside of the quantitative approach is that it is possible to explore the experiences of greater numbers of individuals and could be viewed as more objective. However, in quantitative research, the study instrument can be a source of bias and it is the responsibility of the researcher to assess the study instrument for both validity (i.e., the accuracy of the measurement) and reliability (i.e., consistency or reproducibility of a measurement). If you are gathering data using a survey, it is important to try to use and/or develop questions and response options that have the same meaning to all participants. The best way to achieve this goal is by using measures that have been used in previous research and ideally have been validated. Validated measures have an evidence base to support that they measure what they intend to measure. However, even with pre-existing or validated measures, it is important to understand the settings and the

TABLE 13-4. **Common Survey Measures**

Scale	Measure	Resource
Genetic Counseling Outcomes Scale	Assesses patient-reported outcomes for clinical genetics services.	(McAllister et al., 2011)
Genetic Counseling Efficacy Scale (GCSES)	Assesses genetic counseling self-efficacy which can be used in professional development and training contexts.	(Caldwell et al., 2018; Keller et al., 2020)
State Trait Anxiety Inventory	Assesses trait and state anxiety which can be used in clinical settings to identify clinically significant symptoms of anxiety.	(Spielberger et al., 1983)
Decisional Conflict	Assesses personal perceptions of uncertainly in choosing options, factors contributing to uncertainty, and effective decision-making.	(O'Connor, 1995)
Decision Regret Scale	Assesses regret or remorse after a health care decision.	(Brehaut et al., 2003)
Multidimensional Impact of Cancer Risk Assessment (MICRA)	Assesses the impact of results disclosure after genetic testing. Includes three subscales: distress; uncertainty; and positive experiences.	(Cella et al., 2002)
Family Communication Questionnaire (FCQ)	Assesses four dimensions of family communication for genetic testing: communication of test results; time between disclosure of result and communication with relatives; motivations for communicating or not communicating; and topics discussed with family members.	(Hughes et al., 2002)
The Genetic Psychosocial Risk Instrument (GPRI)	Identifies psychological risk factors that predict distress in patients having genetic testing.	(Esplen et al., 2013)

populations where the validation was performed: an existing measure may not be valid if it is being applied within populations where the research questions are not applicable, relevant, or culturally appropriate. A sample of measures commonly used in genetic counseling practice are included in Table 13-4.

While qualitative research can generate rich, detailed data that provides an in-depth understanding of a topic, quantitative research generates reliable, population-based data and is well suited to establishing relationships between variables, by looking for correlations (statistical associations between the factors or variables you are measuring). The decision whether to choose a quantitative or a qualitative design is both philosophical and practical (MacFarlane et al., 2014). Which method you choose will depend on the nature of the project, the type of information you hope to gather, the context of the study, and the availability of resources (time, money, and human) (Table 13-3). Are you looking to gain new knowledge or develop new theories or methods to apply to the research process itself? Alternatively, is your research going to be focused on applications (also known as clinical or translational research) in which you are trying to understand an area of practice and working towards improvement or change? It is important to keep in mind that these are two different philosophies, not necessarily polar opposites. In fact, elements of both designs can be used together in mixed-methods studies. While combining qualitative and quantitative research is becoming more and more common, it is important to recognize that successfully accomplishing the goals of a mixed-methods study requires design, testing, and analysis of two separate study instruments, which creates an extended time frame for your research.

Combining both types of research can result in:

- Better research development: one approach can be used to inform the other; that is, qualitative research results can be used to develop a quantitative research instrument and the results of a quantitative analysis can be explored in a follow-up qualitative study.
- Increased validity: confirming results from different data sources and different mechanisms.
- New ideas, fresh perspectives, and the identification of contradictions.

Once you have an experimental approach in mind, it is time to transform your research question into a format that will drive the next phase of developing your research plan, your *objective(s)* and *sub-objective(s)* or *specific aim(s)* (Table 13-2). The *objective* defines the overall thrust of your study. It sets the relationships and associations that you want to establish or discover and summarizes what will be achieved by the study in general terms. The objective is derived from your research question. The *specific aim(s)* describes the specific aspects of the topic that you will be investigating. It should break down the general objective(s) into smaller, doable pieces and systematically address the various aspects of your research problem. Each specific aim has a single purpose that is clear and nonredundant and is generally specified in terms that rely on action words like: to determine, to compare, to verify, to calculate, to describe, and to establish. Avoid the use of vague nonaction verbs such as: to appreciate, to understand, or to study. Specific aims are generally focused on key factors that you believe influence or cause the problem (these are identified from your literature search), and they should specify exactly what you will do in your study, and the order in which they will be done. Formulating specific aims will help you focus your study and narrow it down to the essentials. If properly formulated, specific aims will facilitate the development of your research methodology and help orient the collection, analysis, interpretation, and utilization of data. Setting a specific aim(s) should help you organize your study into clearly defined parts or phases and help you avoid collecting data that are not strictly necessary for understanding and solving the problem you have identified (Box 13-2).

BOX 13-2. AN EXAMPLE OF CONCEPTUALIZING YOUR
RESEARCH PLAN

Going back to the research question: How can health care providers, researchers, and community organizations partner to increase access to genetic services
for all communities?
 An objective for a research study could be:
 Identify community-based mechanisms that empower community members
to participate in and promote cancer genetic screening programs.
 A specific aim could be:
 Describe the impact of community-based dialogues about cancer screening
on participants' perception of the value of genetic counseling services and
intention to communicate with family members about these services.

Take care to make sure that the specific aim(s) of your study:

• cover the different aspects of the problem and its contributing factors in a
  coherent manner and in a logical sequence;
• are clearly phrased in operational terms, specifying exactly what you are
  going to do, where, and for what purpose;
• are realistic considering your resource constraints (especially your own time!);
• really allow you to test your hypothesis or provide answers to your research
  question;
• align with your experimental approach.

Lastly, remember that research is an iterative process, and that iteration also
applies to the design process. Consider where your research question fits into the
wheel of science (see Figure 13-2). For instance, as you refine your objective and
specific aims, you may find that an alternate experimental approach is more suitable. If you find your question is more exploratory, you might consider a qualitative
approach. On the other hand, if your research is more confirmatory or tests a
hypothesis, it may be best suited for a quantitative design. Make sure that at each
step in conceptualizing your research plan your decisions are logical, doable, and
support your ultimate goals (Table 13-2). If not, you will need to go back and
revisit the process from an earlier stage.

Design Step 4 (optional): Develop Your Hypothesis

Based on your work to this point in developing your research project (your literature review, critical analysis of previous results and supporting theories, choosing
your experimental approach, and the development of your research objectives and
specific aim(s)), you may have discovered that you can postulate testable explanations for your research question. If so, you can formulate a hypothesis(es) in
addition to the study objective. In some instances, you might choose to establish

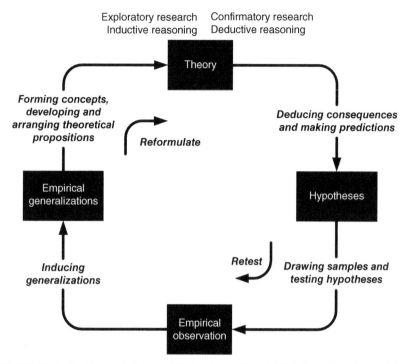

FIGURE 13-2. *The Wheel of Science. Eikebrook and Busch 2016. Based on Wallace, WL (1971). The Logic of Science in Sociology. Routledge*

your hypothesis before you create your objective and/or specific aim(s). Your thesis committee can help you explore these variations and make these decisions.

The *hypothesis* takes the form of a prediction about the results of your research; it defines the relationship(s) between one or more factors (variables) and the problem you are planning on studying in a format that can be tested. It describes in concrete terms what you expect to happen in the study and provides an explanation for the expected results (Table 13-5). In doing so it brings direction, specificity, and focus to your research study and becomes the basis for the subsequent design of your project. The hypothesis generally states what the investigator believes to be the most probable explanation for the phenomenon they are planning on studying. A hypothesis may also inform the type of statistical analysis that will be utilized in analyzing your data.

Consequently, the hypothesis:

* represents the best hunch of the researcher and is simple, specific, and conceptually clear;
* is a tentative proposition, but is related to a body of knowledge;
* has unknown validity, but is capable of being tested and measured;
* specifies a relationship between variables that is one-dimensional; that is, tests one relationship at a time.

TABLE 13-5. Issues to consider in Study Design, Implementation and Analysis

Component	Issues to Consider
Hypothesis	Evaluate the validity of your hypothesis. Ask if it is specific enough to be researchable yet still meaningful. How certain are you of the relationship(s) between variables? *Food for Thought. After you have completed all the subsequent steps in study design is your hypothesis still applicable and relevant? Do you need to partially redesign to make sure it all hangs together?*
Variables	What will you be measuring? What degree of error is acceptable? *Food for Thought. Did previous studies adequately evaluate the variables that you are considering? How can you build greater depth of understanding in your study? If this has never been studied before, look at related studies (you could ask you research committee to help with this) and see if this can guide your assessment of your variables of interest.*
Study Population & Sampling	Which individuals or group will you need to work with to answer your research question? What are the important characteristics of your entire population? How will you choose your sample? How big is big enough? Does your sample need to be representative? If so, of whom or of what, and what degree of accuracy is acceptable? *Food for thought. Take care in designing and implementing your sampling plan. Consider, what types of biases or potential stratification impacted previous studies and what you can do in your study to limit their impact?*
Study Instrument	How will you get the data you need to test your hypothesis? What tools or devices will you use to make or record observations? Are valid and reliable instruments available, or do you need to construct your own? *Food for Thought. Using an instrument that has been validated can help optimize the validity of your results, save time in the design and implementation phases of your research, and make it easier to compare your results to the existing literature.*
Data Collection: Logistics	How will you coordinate the various steps? Will interviewers, observers, or analysts need to be trained? What level of inter-rater reliability will you accept? *Food for thought. What is your timeline? How much leeway do you have?*
Data Processing & Analysis	What combinations of analytical and statistical process will be applied to the data? What will allow you to accept or reject your hypothesis? Do the findings show numerical differences, and are those differences important? What skills do you need to develop or expertise to identify in order to accomplish this? *Food for Thought. A consideration of the methods you plan to use will help ensure that you will be able to answer your research question. In addition, evaluation of your analysis plan during the study design stage will also help you anticipate how you will compare your previously published results.*
Ethical Considerations	Can the data be collected and subjects' rights still preserved? *Food for Thought. Have you incorporated/considered topics of diversity, equity, inclusion, and justice in your study design?*

TABLE 13-5. (*Continued*)

Component	Issues to Consider
The Research Proposal	Make sure to write for your reader and follow all requirements in the final document. *Food for Thought. How can your committee members help you in this process? Think about when you want this input in the process of developing and finalizing your proposal.*
Interpretation & Conclusions	Was your initial hypothesis supported? Did your findings answer your research question? What are the implications of your findings for the theory base, for the background assumptions, or relevant literature? *Food for Thought. What if your findings are negative? What recommendations can you make for public policies or programs in this area? What suggestions can you make for further research on this topic?*

While generating a hypothesis at the start of a research project has the advantage of helping to guide the research project, not all projects are well suited to the strictures imposed by a hypothesis. If an area of research is novel and truly exploratory, generating a hypothesis can oversimplify the investigation and limit the process. Since a hypothesis defines testable relationships, the existing body of literature (either specific to the topic or related) must be sufficient to define testable components of the hypothesis. If your project is going to be the first to explore a topic, then generating a hypothesis will likely not be useful and may need to wait for the generation of appropriate observations.

How do you go about designing your hypothesis? First you need to figure out what concepts you want to understand. These are your variables. They translate your concept into an objective and measurable construct and define the type of data you will be gathering and analyzing. The *hypothesis* states the relationships between variables so that they can be tested experimentally. It may take the form of a cause-effect statement, or an "if X, then Y" statement. Remember that the hypothesis makes *tentative* predictions about how we expect the variables to *covary*. The variable that measures the assumed cause in the relationship is called the *independent* variable (i.e., the variable that is postulated to explain another variable); and the effect or outcome is called the *dependent* variable (i.e., it is affected by the independent variable). While research is inherently reductionist (we are always trying to simplify the issue), it is never so simple as to assume that there are only cause and effect relationships. In generating your hypothesis, it will be important to consider variables that affect, connect, or link the relationship between the independent and dependent variables. *Extraneous* variables can impact the dependent variable but are generally not measured in the study, while *intervening* variables link the independent and dependent variables and are necessary in order for the independent variable to impact the dependent variable. As part of this step in the design process, you also want to think about *confounding* variables, factors that could influence the results but are not going to be part of your final research design. This step in the design process is important in helping you to understand the limitations of your results.

Design Steps 5: Develop Your Study Design

You have decided on your objectives, specific aim(s), and determined if it is appropriate to develop a hypothesis (and, if needed, designed one). What to work on next? You will now need to set up the overall strategy for accomplishing your specific aim(s). In this phase you will have to decide what data you need to collect in order to generate results that meet your research objective(s) and test your hypothesis; that is, decide how to gather and analyze your data. Remember the weeding out and narrowing down that occurred as you moved from identifying your research idea to setting objectives and specific aims? Why did you go through this process? It allowed you to develop an idea for your research project that was valid, verifiable, rigorous, and ultimately doable. Similar critical criteria must be applied to the development of your study design in which you determine how you are going to actually explore, test, and generate answers to your research questions.

Keeping your specific aims and hypothesis in mind, think about your project from start to finish and consider each component individually. This includes your research variables and their relationship to the study instrument, the study population itself (including sampling and recruiting), and the logistics of data collection, storage, processing, and analysis. Table 13-5 identifies questions to consider at this point in the process. During study design, you also want to take a critical look, again, at previous research on your topic. At this point in the design process, you are looking with two new lenses. First, you're evaluating the results from previous research to see where the holes are that you can address in your study. This can often help you focus on variable selection and definition and identification and sampling of your study population. This critical appraisal will help you build on previous research and ensure that your results are novel. Second, you are looking to see what aspects of prior successful research you can repurpose for your work. This often focuses on your study instrument and your analysis plan.

Part of this process includes anticipating potential obstacles and challenges in the design and implementation of your study and identifying alternative approaches. Time considerations are important at multiple steps in design, including planning for the length of time you will need to design and pilot a new study instrument, your timetable for identifying and building a partnership with research participants, or the length of time you will need to complete your analysis. In addition, this is a great point in the design process to revisit the membership of your research team. Think strategically about the types of expertise you will need and when over the course of working on your research project you might need this help; for example, design, implementation, analysis, and/or presentation. As you consider the final composition of your research team, you might also consider how much time they have to actually provide input. While expertise is critical, availability is equally important.

And, finally, figure out what resources you will need. This can include the cost of survey design, participant incentives, statistical consultants, transcription, coding programs, research assistants, communication with participants, and general technology. These practical details can impact the rigor of your results; anticipating them can ensure that you get the answers you are looking for.

Design Step 6: Selecting your Study Population

Often during the process of identifying and designing your research question, you will have defined exactly who you want to include as participants in your study; that is, the members of your study population. For example, if your research will be focused on developing an educational program for genetic counselors that could strengthen their ability to provide gender affirming care, then the broad parameters of your study population have been identified. However, there are times when your research question is developed independent of a specific population. If you are interested in exploring the public's opinion of genomic sequencing in the newborn period, your study population could be quite broad. In either instance, it will be impossible to interact with every potential research participant and you will need to determine how you will identify participants; that is, your sampling strategy. Careful sampling of your population can help ensure that your research provides comprehensive information that is representative of the entire group. However, it is important to be aware that since sampling provides an estimate of your population, it is also subject to error or bias. Depending on the type of research project and the objectives, an investigator may be more or less concerned about this issue.

If you hope that the results from your research project will provide answers that reflect the perspectives of the entire population, it will be important to develop a sample that is representative of the entire population. In the research question exploring "the public's opinion of genomic sequencing in the newborn period" it is going to be impossible to interact with every member of the public, consequently it will be important to apply *random or probability sampling*. This approach selects a subset of individuals in the population that are representative of the entire population. When appropriately applied, *random sampling* provides a solid estimate of the entire study population. This sampling methodology is more commonly associated with quantitative studies and can be used to test a hypothesis and develop population statistics.

When using random sampling in building your study population, it is important to work on minimizing bias. Think very carefully about who comprises the entire population and consider any special structures/strata that may exist in the larger study population that could create bias in your population sample. For instance, in the example above, if you had subsets of the population with high health literacy and others with lower health literacy, you want to ensure you sample from both populations in order to limit bias related to participants' prior knowledge. These substructures may necessitate employing additional sampling precautions, including systematic random, stratified random, and cluster sampling (MacFarlane et al., 2014; Kumar, 2019; Babbie, 2020; Creswell, 2023). Deciding between these options is dependent on a variety of factors that include the stratification of your study population, your research question, available time, and money. As you define your actual sample, it is important to evaluate this issue carefully and comprehensively. This is a great place to seek input from your research team; these discussions may include considerations of time, access to and interest by potential participants, and your analysis plan.

Generally, in exploratory research or in a project that is based on qualitative methodology, the researcher will use a *nonrandom sampling method* that focuses on potential research participants with very specific characteristics in terms of knowledge, experiences, or expertise. For these types of studies, participants are not expected to provide comprehensive perspectives that represent all potential voices or parameters in the study population. Instead, they are able to engage in an in-depth reflective exploration of your topic and generate new insights and hypotheses (Figure 13-2). *Nonrandom sampling* has the benefits of: 1) generating in-depth insights from a focused sample of a population of interest; 2) simplifying research participant identification and enrollment, 4) potentially minimizing expenses; and 5) limiting the impact of population stratification; that is, the presence of subgroups in your population. However, this type of sampling strategy can be sensitive to bias (the quality of a measurement or analysis that results in misrepresentation), both at the level of the population itself (who chooses to volunteer) and with regard to the selection of study participants by the researcher (decisions the researcher makes when they select the population as a whole and select individual participants).

How big a sample do you need?   Sampling provides a means of saving time and minimizing cost. The actual/final size of your sample depends on the type of research design you have selected; the desired level of accuracy in and generalizability of your results; and the characteristics of the population of interest. There are a variety of statistical methods to assess if the sample size is adequate (i.e., power calculations). While this topic is beyond the scope of this chapter, this short introduction to this topic is not meant to minimize the importance of this step in your study design. The references at the end of this chapter provide a starting place to learn about this topic.

How good is your sample?   It is important to realize that there will always be a difference between the sample statistic and the true population mean or average. Error is an inherent byproduct of sampling. The guiding principles of sampling include working to provide the best approximation of the population and avoiding bias in sample selection. While increasing your sample size will increase the accuracy with which it represents a population, bias can still arise either due to nonrandom selection, incomplete or inaccurate representation of the population, (i.e., the sampling frame is wrong), or critical segments of your population that can't be identified or won't participate in your research.

Lastly, take the time to consider your choices about your study population in light of your research objectives. Does your final population still allow you to gain information that is relevant to your research objective? If your research objective is to improve the ways that genetic counselors practice, then your sampling scheme will need to consider the demographics of potential genetic counselor participants, in addition to specifics related to their actual areas of practice. However, if your research is focused on increasing stakeholder engagement in genetic counseling research and your objective is to learn from prospective patients, then your sampling scheme should reflect diverse perspectives in the patient community. You should work towards identifying and including individuals from the diverse communities we serve including those with, or identifying with, varied levels of education and health literacy, socioeconomic backgrounds, ethnic and racial diversity, gender identity, disability, and so on. It is important to note that historically the field of genetic research has demonstrated systematic bias in the sampling of primarily European participants in many research initiatives. It is essential that all researchers, including those within the field of genetic counseling, take responsibility to ensure that all populations are appropriately represented in genetics and genomics research in order to achieve outcomes that benefit all communities. Readers are encouraged to explore focused texts on this topic.

Design Step 7: Developing the Study Instrument

Deciding what study instrument you will use depends on the type of data you want to collect. *Primary data collection* is gathered directly from those who hold the information. This method often includes using surveys, interviews, focus groups, and clinical trials. Alternatively, you can extract your data from *secondary sources*, like clinic forms, chart notes, clinical records. Each method has its own benefits and limitations.

All things being equal (and of course they never are), you should work to ensure that the tool or tools you use to gather your data—your study instrument—provides you with the highest quality data. There are limitations to both primary and secondary data collection in terms of *accuracy* (how well your methods and results measure the true value) and *reliability* (the consistency and stability of your methods and results). Whether you choose to collect your data face-to-face or virtually, first consider the strengths and drawbacks of each approach, how much bias is acceptable, and what type of an error rate you can tolerate. It is also important to think about mechanics, available time, money, skills, and resources. Table 13-6 provides a brief overview of four

TABLE 13-6. A Sampling of Study Instruments and Considerations

	Study Instruments			
Considerations	Survey	Interview	Focus Group	Chart Review
General Use	Participants respond to set prompts with predetermined responses. Additional information can be gathered in open-ended questions.	Participants respond to questions in real time using their own words.	Similar to Interviews. Can be also helpful in community-based participatory research.	A review and analysis of previously recorded data.
Goal	Quantitative data/statistics about a sample in order to make inferences about a larger population.	In-depth qualitative data from purposively selected individuals. These perspectives can seed future research.	Group members interact with each other, reflect on their beliefs in response to others, and build new ideas both individually and collectively.	Answer clinical or administrative questions.
Considerations in Study Design	Ensure that questions/prompts explore relevant variables, have the same meaning to all participants, and consider participant literacy. Can use existing instruments if applicable to your population. If designing new questions, you will need to pilot them.	Develop a series of prompts/questions that will allow you to explore all relevant variables. Questions should be open-ended and avoid bias.	Similar to an interview. Pay attention to the impact(s) of the interactions between participants.	Consider access, accuracy, and specificity of data source(s) (e.g., clinic notes, lab results, pedigrees, etc.). May need to design tools and mechanisms for data collection and consider frameworks that support subsequent analysis.
Study Population Limitations	Can gather data from a large number of individuals. Consider whether sample is representative of larger population and sample size needed (i.e., power calculation) to support analysis plan.	Generally smaller number of participants. Critical to identify those with the correct expertise and consider their willingness to participate in research and the amount of time they could have for the interview.	Similar to Interviews. Be mindful of attributes of focus group participants and how this could impact data collection.	Limited to those who received clinical care.
Data/Results Interpretation	Results are confined to survey content areas/variables. However, data can be compared between participants and between studies and can be generalizable.	Allows for in-depth exploration and identification of new ideas from participants. The goal is often transferability over generalizability.	Similar to interviews.	Depends on the research question, the amount of data that is available in the chart, and the mechanism(s) and consistency by which the data was recorded.

| | Study Instruments | | | |
Considerations	Survey	Interview	Focus Group	Chart Review
Implementation	Data can be gathered quickly. Often, designing the study instrument(s) is the most time-consuming step.	Can be time consuming. May need to develop skills to ensure that there is consistency in data collection, including building fluency with an interview guide and developing interviewing skills so that the process is conversational, responsive to participants' perspectives, and does not reflect researcher's biases or interpretations. May need to perform pilot interviews. Time is also necessary to schedule and conduct the actual interviews.	Similar to interviews, but generally more structured. Consider how you will facilitate and manage group dynamics so that all voices are heard (e.g., establishing and enforcing ground rules and ways to address disagreements). May need additional time for scheduling and running the actual event. Also need to plan for logistics of the event itself, i.e., including schedule, venue, in-person or virtual, mechanism of data capture, and support personnel.	Need to make sure that you have a mechanism to ensure accurate data capture.
Analysis/Needed expertise	May need expertise to help with statistical analysis; this can be costly. If you have developed an analysis plan during study design, this can move relatively quickly.	May need expertise based on proposed qualitative methodology. Will need to determine approach to coding (e.g., inductive coding, deductive coding, or a combination), participants in the coding process and theme generation. Identify coding software and plan for related costs.	Similar to interviews. In addition, will need to decide if you will code the data as a group discussion or based on the responses from each participant.	Often similar to those for a survey.

common approaches to collecting data and highlights important considerations. For all approaches, it is critical to think about the following:

- Defining and testing your variables to make sure that they provide the types of data that will support your specific aim(s).
- The breadth, depth, and reliability of the data you want to generate. Think about the relationships between the questions you are asking participants to respond to with an eye towards your analysis plan; that is, how will you evaluate your results and will this analysis provide the insights you are seeking? Think about how long it will take a participant to complete the study and make decisions about what is essential information to answer your research question. At this step you may also need to go back and evaluate your specific aim, making sure that the current version of your study instrument allows you to attain this goal. Tables 13-5 and 13-6 identify a number of issues that you could consider.
- Whether your instrument is appropriately targeted to your study population in terms of their unique characteristics.

Design Step 8: The Research Proposal

Often a necessary step in the development of your plan is finding support for your project. Convincing someone that your research idea has value (Is the research question you want to answer/explore important/worthwhile?) and is doable (Do you have a plan that will allow you to answer your question?) is a main outcome of writing a research proposal. In addition, a research proposal is usually necessary to apply for and acquire funding that may be essential to successful completion of your research plan.

While the process of writing a proposal may seem onerous and time consuming, it can also be very helpful in ensuring that your research is effectively organized and enables you to answer your proposed question(s) (Locke et al., 2013). If appropriately developed, your research proposal should translate your idea into a work plan that defines what you are going to be doing, how you will be doing it, and when it will happen. It can help you identify where you may run into problems at multiple stages in your research and help you plan for how you will deal with them (Tables 13-5 and 13-6). Writing a proposal can help you to establish a timeline for your project. It can also be useful in generating an application to an Institutional Review Board (IRB). Often the required components and the level of detail are similar to those of an IRB application (see section *The Human Side of the Equation*). Lastly, it can optimize communication with other members of your research committee and working group or, if applying for funding, the granting body. This is a creative process and can help you think about what you wish to achieve with your research and how to effectively communicate your goals and broader vision. An effective proposal should delineate the research problem, provide a convincing argument for why it needs to be explored, demonstrate that your planned approach (i.e., your methodology) is adequate for the task and tailored to your reader and their rationale for requesting proposals.

A well-organized research proposal focuses on both the big picture and the minutiae. This activity can provide you with the opportunity to really think through your project from start to finish. There is no single universally accepted format for creating a proposal, though some funding agencies or institutions may have required or suggested templates. However, there are usually a set number of tasks/components that must be addressed, often in a very condensed format. Generally, a research proposal contains: 1) Introduction or background and significance; 2) Objectives, hypothesis (if appropriate), specific aim(s); 3) Study design and preliminary data (if available); 4) Analysis plan; 5) Timeline; and 6) References.

The *Introduction* section generally serves multiple purposes. In its simplest form it introduces the study and states the research question. In general, this section of a proposal answers the question "What is this study about?" and helps the reader/reviewer understand your research purpose and plan. In addition, the Introduction section answers the question: "Why bother to undertake this study?" by providing a justification for your proposed work. This is usually grounded in previous research. In order to be able to develop this section, you will need to identify and discuss related work (e.g., provide a relevant literature review) that explores how your research question was previously investigated. As part of this review, you will need to address the shortcomings of existing work in the area and demonstrate how your approach will both differ from and either improve upon or add to existing work. This section should remind you of the work that you undertook to develop your research idea. In fact, much of the work that you did while developing research project/idea can be reused to write the Introduction section of your proposal. You may also be asked to include a section that discusses the significance of your research and answers the question "What benefits can be expected from your work?" The focus and content of this section should explore how your research results will add to the existing body of knowledge and/or directly impact practice/clinical care. In some cases, this section will ask you to explore the broader implications of your research.

The content of the sections of your proposal that present your *Objective(s)*, *hypothesis*, and *specific aim(s)* will be derived from the work you did while conceptualizing your research plan. Make sure that the information that is provided in the Introduction section provides adequate justification for these sections of the proposal.

The *Study design (also known as the Methods)* provides information on the mechanics of your research. It defines and justifies the methodology that you will be using to accomplish your research. It generally describes where the work is going to be taking place, how you will gather information (your research instrument), defines your study population (sample size and sampling design), and defines the methods of data analysis. It may also provide details about your budget (including material, people, and equipment support) and define a timeline for accomplishing the proposed work. This section typically contains a discussion of the problems or limitations of the proposed work, identifies possible roadblocks, and provides a plan for how you will deal with these potential issues. The Study design should also include information about relevant resources that you will be utilizing to help you accomplish the proposed work (i.e., additional expertise that will be provided by your committee members, collaborators, or consultants). Finally, it is important to remember to refer to all relevant literature. It is critical that you present your ideas for investigating your research question in as much detail as possible and present a reasonably detailed plan for how you will accomplish this work. Generally, you will be able to reuse parts of the proposal in the preparation of your final write up/thesis/manuscript. This means that a well-written proposal will simplify your work at the end of graduate training.

Lastly, pay close attention to the writing itself. Be sure that your document is logically organized (i.e., do your arguments make sense to someone who is new to your research idea and are they presented so that the reader can evaluate them?). If you present your research plan in a strong, error-free manner, your reader is more likely to take the time and effort to really understand your arguments. If your writing is weak, your reader is more likely to become confused and distracted and it is less likely that they will be won over by your arguments. Work on making your writing as clear and compelling as possible. To that end it is worthwhile to consider the importance of striving for simplicity, clarity, and brevity in your writing. Do not make your writing so complicated that the reader has no idea where you are going. No matter your purpose, work to produce a proposal that is accessible. Often this can be accomplished by enlisting the help of others in reviewing your proposal. This can include individuals who have expertise in your research topic and those who don't. They will read your proposal differently and while it may be challenging to receive this feedback, having input that looks at both the content of your proposal and the clarity of your presentation will help you produce a stronger final document that will support your goals.

DATA COLLECTION AND ANALYSIS

Data collection and analysis is an interesting and exacting discipline in its own right. As you design your research project, it is critical to also think about this part of the process (Tables 13-5 and 13-6). Often, data processing and analysis will require that you develop new knowledge and skills, and depending on the timeframe, scope and focus of your project, and your prior expertise you may want to think about calling on others with this expertise. The content provided below is intended to provide you with a quick introduction to critical concepts.

Quantitative Analysis

In a quantitative analysis, determining the significance of your results depends on applying a variety of mathematical procedures that generate statistics. The first step in this multistep process is to evaluate the completeness and accuracy of your dataset. After downloading your data and transferring it to the relevant analysis program, you will need to identify "holes" in your data and decide how you will address this missing information. Issues to consider include determining how well your participants answered the survey questions; that is, evaluate how long it took each participant to answer individual questions and to complete the entire survey. At this step you will also want to assess how well each question or set of questions in your survey provide a range of responses; that is, the distribution of responses. The answers to these questions will help you decide if any study participants and/ or survey questions should be removed from subsequent analysis.

As part of this process, you should review your research question/hypothesis and decide if the data you have gathered will support answering this question and evaluate/re-evaluate the statistical approaches you want to apply. If you were intending to generate a descriptive dataset evaluating a single variable at one time point, you will be looking at the numbers of respondents/responses, means, standard deviations, and so on. Alternatively, if you were planning on looking at two or more variables at a single timepoint, your analysis will focus on correlations. While if you were planning on looking at many variables at once with a single outcome, your analysis will rely on performing a regression; or if you were hoping to evaluate the relationships between multiple predictors and multiple outcomes, you will need to perform an analysis of variance— ANOVA. As part of this analysis and decision-making process, you will need to decide if you will collapse the responses to individual survey questions. If you set up your questions so that responses could assume any value within a given range (also known as continuous variables) or defined categories of response options (also known as categorical variables that are often measured using a Likert scale), the distribution of responses you evaluated earlier (do the responses follow a normal distribution or is there skewing?) will help you make this determination.

Looking at the size and completeness of your data will allow you to decide if you can follow your initial analysis plan or will need to pivot. As part of this decision-making process, you will also want to make a decision about the level of statistical significance, also known as the P-value, that you will use to evaluate your results. This value allows you to determine how likely it is that your hypothesis (if you have one) is true and measures the probability that any observed differences between two measurements happened by chance. A P-value of 0.5 means that the difference you have measured has a 50:50 (0.5 in 1) of having happened by chance while a P-value of 0.05 means that there is a 0.05 chance (1 in 20) that the result happened by chance. In general, the lower the P-value, the less likely that the difference you measured happened by chance and the higher the significance of the findings. For most studies a P-value of 0.01 (1 in 100 times likely to have occurred by chance) is considered highly significant. One additional point to consider in setting the bar for statistical significance is the optimal size of your sample population. This determination is also known as a power calculation and considers the number of variables you are measuring and the desired level of significance. If the final size of your study population is less than you anticipated in the design process—that is, you are underpowered—you will need to re-evaluate your analysis plan and may not be able to test your planned hypothesis. Since multiple factors can impact your ability to generate results with statistical significance, setting your threshold for statistical significance should be discussed with the members of your committee and rely on input from a statistics expert.

A few words about measurement Since variables provide a way of measuring a concept, they can be operationally defined. Attributes are the specific values or characteristics of a variable. This is accomplished in quantitative research by assigning numbers or categories that are amenable to statistical analysis (age, height, weight, personal beliefs, or preferences). As an example, from the NSGC Professional Status Survey, if the variable were "years employed as genetic counselor," the attributes could be: "<1, 1–4, 5–9, 10–14, 15–19, 20–24" years of experience (Kumar, 2019; Walters et al., 2021). If the variable were degree of job satisfaction, the variables could be: "very satisfied," "satisfied," "dissatisfied," or "very dissatisfied."

There are varied levels of measurement. These variations determine the type of statistical analysis that can be conducted, and, therefore, the type of conclusions that can be drawn from the research. In *nominal* measurements, data can be placed in named categories that have no particular order, like eye color. In *ordinal* measurements, data can be placed in categories that can be ordered from least to strongest but the relationship between individual measurement categories is inexact, like an individual's beliefs about susceptibility to disease. In rank ordered or interval measurements, the interval between response options represent consistent and equivalent differences, like measuring temperature in Fahrenheit or Centigrade. The rules that are used to assign labels to variables (the attributes) are a critical component of measurement. If the rules used to assign the labels are poorly designed, the outcome(s) can be meaningless. In all forms of measurement, the attributes that are used to categorize your variable should form categories that are both *mutually exclusive* and *exhaustive*. *Exhaustive* means that there must be enough categories that all the observations will fall into some category. *Mutually exclusive* means that the categories must be distinct enough that no observations will fall into more than one category.

Qualitative Analysis

Before data collection begins for a qualitative project, there are a few decisions to be made. The first of these is how you will record data, which will be impacted by your study design (Table 13-6). Some qualitative studies may include passive observation or analysis of content of written materials. Here data collection may consist of taking notes or keeping detailed records. However, in many genetic counseling studies, including interview or focus group studies, the researcher may utilize a questionnaire or script to collect participant responses. The researcher needs a reliable way to record participant responses that will later be used for analysis. Options might include having a note-taker, audio-recording, video-recording, or a combination of these. If the study design allows, having a full recording of responses is one of the more robust collection methods. When deciding between audio-only or audio with video, it may be helpful to consider whether having access to nonverbal communication will enrich analysis. For instance, in a focus group where there are multiple participants, it may be helpful to document the nonverbal responses of participants who are not actively speaking. You will also want to consider if data collection will occur in-person, by phone, over videoconference, and so on. This may be influenced by study logistics or study goals. Are your research participants local or are you looking at a national sample? Could there be barriers to study participation if interviews are held in-person? The format the interview is conducted in can also impact elements of the experience such as anonymity. If discussing difficult topics, a phone interview may allow for more anonymity. On the other hand, a face-to-face interview may provide an increased chance to build rapport and trust with the interviewee. It is important to discuss these variables with your research team to determine what is best for your research design or question.

If your data includes audio/video recordings, these will need to be transcribed verbatim into a written document, or transcript. Transcription can be done by the research team or by a professional transcription company. Transcripts need to be checked for errors and "cleaned," or have all personal identifiers removed to anonymize the transcripts for analysis. Individual transcripts can be assigned a code linking them to individual study participants. The key to this code should be kept in a separate document to protect the anonymity of the respondents. Once the transcripts are ready, the coding process or data analysis begins.

Your coding process will be informed by the type of qualitative analysis you have proposed (Saldana, 2015; Miles et al., 2020). This will be determined by your research goals, research paradigm, and proposed methodology (Poth and Cresswell, 2018). It may also be guided by the expertise of your research team. Having early discussions with your research team to define these aspects of your qualitative study design are essential to planning for your data collection and analysis. Once you are ready to move forward with the coding process, you will first need to assemble your coding team. This will include all individuals who will be involved in the direct analysis of the transcripts. Having more than one individual coding the data allows for increased objectivity and accuracy in the interpretation of the data. As a part of the analysis, a coding frame or codebook will be developed. This typically includes a list of codes, typically words used to describe and identify common topics or themes for analysis. Codebooks may also include descriptions of each code and/or examples to encourage consistency amongst coders. The codebook can be developed through an inductive or ground-up approach, where codes are derived from the data itself, or a deductive approach where researchers begin with a pre-set list of codes. The codebook is then utilized for data analysis by applying specific codes to data segments. It is important that each coder agrees on the particular codes assigned to specific blocks of data within the transcripts, or consensus. Therefore, a methodology to achieve consensus must be agreed upon. An example of this might include two coders reviewing the same transcripts and reconvening to compare codes and resolving any areas of disagreement. A quantitative approach to this is calculating inter coder reliability, which is a statistical measure of the agreement between coders, which can also be considered (O'Connor and Joffe, 2020). Coding is often an iterative approach where codes are refined as you work through the data. For this reason, it is important to maintain a detailed account of the steps that were taken during the coding process that can later be included in the reporting of your data (O'Brien et al., 2014). Additional relevant information includes determining when you reached saturation— that is, no new data was needed to explore your research question—in terms of the number of interviews you completed, the development of the codebook, and the linking of codes, such as to themes or theories, dependent upon your methodology, methods, and analysis plan.

THE HUMAN SIDE OF THE EQUATION: ETHICAL RESEARCH

Many research studies that are performed by genetic counselors depend on participation by people, either directly as research participants or indirectly in the analysis of information that is tied to an individual or groups of individuals. For example, in a study "Exploring the impact of community-based dialogues about cancer screening on participants' perception of the value of genetic counseling services and intention to communicate with family members about this knowledge" your research participants could be the community members who engage in focus groups and provide insights into your research question. Before contacting any potential research participants, you will need to attain a review and approval from an Institutional Review Board (IRB) to conduct the study. The IRB will evaluate the study design and outcomes with a focus on protecting the rights and welfare of participants and ensuring they are treated ethically and equitably. The history of regulation around human subjects research is long and checkered (starting in the 1930s both nationally and internationally) (Kim, 2012).

In the United States, multiple branches of the federal government (Office for Human Research Protection, Office for Research Integrity, the FDA—Food and Drug Administration) are focused on protecting the rights of human research participants. The IRB serves as the local face of this regulatory system; its regulations apply to both research participants and researchers. Similar research review boards exist internationally but may have different names and different regulatory structures (PRIM&R et al., 2021; Services, 2022). Highlighted below are some general principles at play in the United States.

What Defines a Human Subject/research Participant?

The federal regulations in the United States define a human subject as any living individual or fetus about whom a research investigator obtains data via interaction or intervention (45CFR46, 2001). This regulation also includes human tissue but excludes deceased individuals and consequently research on them (including their tissue or information) is not protected by IRB regulations. In addition, research that is conducted on individuals participating in public behaviors (observation of anonymous individuals on the street) is not regulated by the IRB.

The federal regulations defining human subjects also apply to identifiable private information and require that researchers carefully consider what constitutes identifiable private information. According to the Health Insurance Portability and Accountability Act of 1996 (HIPAA), private health information is defined as information (including demographic information) about a patient that: 1) is created or received by a health care provider; 2) relates to the past, present, or future physical or mental health of the patient; provision of health care to the patient; or payment for the provision of health care to the patient; and 3) identifies the patient or with respect to which there is a reasonable basis to believe it could be used to identify the patient (Service, 2023). While HIPAA does not directly govern research, it does regulate holders of medical records (e.g., hospitals, physicians, insurers, and health care clearinghouses) that are essential to conducting research.

As a general rule, any research that involves human subjects and relates to private behavior or private information is considered human research and subject to an IRB review. It is critical while you are designing your project that you determine if it will be subject to IRB review and, if so, incorporate the IRB review process into your planning timeline. A careful review of all the information in your institution's IRB website will help you make this determination. This process will educate you about the varied rules and regulations that will govern your research. If necessary, you can contact your local board for a discussion about the specifics of your project and your IRB application.

What is Not Subject to IRB Review?

Since genetic counselors often wear both research and clinical "hats" for their patients, it is important to remember that human research is different from clinical practice in that:

- The purpose is focused on obtaining general/generalizable knowledge rather than on improving an individual patient's health.
- Direct benefit to the participant is possible, but unknown.
- The validity of an intervention is also unknown.
- The short-term goals are focused on new knowledge that may (or may not) ultimately impact patient care in the long term.

It is also important to distinguish research that must be reviewed by an IRB from systematic investigations that fall under the umbrella of *Quality improvement* as these types of projects do not require IRB review. *Quality improvement* projects are also a form of investigation or assessment and rely on the collection and analysis of data but, unlike research that requires IRB review, they are focused on improving the delivery of a health care service in specific settings as opposed to focusing on generalizable scientific knowledge that can support evidence-based care more broadly. In quality improvement, the goal is to solve practical problems that directly and immediately impact patient care and the results are usually specific to a particular medical/organization setting. For example, your clinic may be interested in how to decrease wait times for an appointment in your clinic. Conducting an internal study to improve clinic flow is generating knowledge specific to the institution and would be considered a "quality improvement" project rather than a research project meant to generate generalizable knowledge. Consequently, quality improvement efforts do not seek to generate generalizable knowledge but rather evaluate specific programs or processes. In trying to make this distinction, you might ask yourself the following questions:

- Am I trying to improve practice in my medical center/clinic/institution by creating a practical solution to a problem or evaluating something that is already considered an established practice? If the answer is yes, then this is likely quality improvement research.
- Am I trying to determine if there is a better way of providing care to my patients compared to my current practice and do I believe that my discovery will impact genetic counseling practice? If it will contribute to generalizable knowledge, then it is research that requires IRB review.

It is important to work with your local IRB directly to determine if your project falls under the definition of quality improvement and will therefore be exempt from IRB review.

How to Approach the Process?

At the end of the day, the research review process is focused on protecting research participants from the risks associated with research; consequently, the review process (both from the perspective of the investigator and the participants) is geared towards minimizing potential risks and maximizing benefits (PRIM&R et al., 2021). While the regulations that govern all IRBs within the US are the same, the process of initiating and completing an IRB review can vary from institution to institution. A good first step is to review the IRB website at your institution and take a close look at the actual IRB application. You will see that many sections mirror those in your research proposal. If you have done a good job of developing your research plan and your research proposal, the process of creating the application should be relatively straightforward.

As with all other phases of your research project, work on learning from others about how to successfully navigate this process. This could include talking to the administrators at your IRB or those who are familiar with submitting applications and asking for their help. This is another place where the members of your research committee can be helpful. Lastly, you want to figure out how long the review process typically takes within your institution. This information can help you build appropriate time into your research planning. It is important to recognize that investigations into topics that would be considered sensitive—such as sexual attitudes, preferences, or practices; use of alcohol, drugs, or the like; information that could impact financial standing, employability, or reputation; topics and information that could result in social stigmatization or discrimination; psychological or mental health information; and genetic information or involved participants who could be considered vulnerable—will raise red flags in an IRB review and potentially prolong the review process. Vulnerable populations can include: children, neonates, prisoners, pregnant women, individuals with disabilities, economically, socially, or educationally disadvantaged persons, or institutionalized individuals.

SHARING YOUR RESEARCH WITH OTHERS

Research in genetic counseling often generates new perspectives on our profession. Its value is maximized when it is shared within and outside of the community. Making sure that others are aware of the results of your work is a critical endpoint of the entire research process. Your goal in a research presentation is to share your work with a greater audience so that it can be evaluated against the current standards in the field, incorporated into the broader body of research on the topic, and become a stepping-stone to new ideas and practices. There are multiple opportunities to share your work. These can include: your final write-up, peer-reviewed manuscripts, and book chapters and presentations at local, regional, and national meetings (including both oral platform and poster presentations). In each case there will usually be specific requirements and instructions about the format, content, and length. It is essential that you review these guidelines and follow them as precisely as possible. This will ensure that your proposed presentation receives a comprehensive and fair review.

If you are preparing a thesis, your graduate school will have specific requirements for the content and format of this document. If you are preparing a manuscript for submission to a journal, there are usually instructions on their web page.

Below are some ideas on how to go about developing a research article. A full discussion of this topic is provided by (Resta et al., 2010).

- The *abstract/summary* is designed to tell the reader what your study was about and your conclusions. It should be short (generally a paragraph) and to the point. While it always appears at the start of a paper, it is generally the last thing that you will write since it is based on the content of all the other sections.
- The *introduction* allows you to state clearly what the research is about and includes the relevant background information (i.e., places your research in context, introduces the reader to the topic, provides important definitions).

It should include content that explores your research topic and lays out the central question(s). This section is similar to that contained within the introduction of your proposal but depending on the actual format of your write-up, may be more detailed (a thesis) or more focused (a manuscript).

- The *materials and methods* section describes all aspects of how the study was carried out. It contains information about the study design, participants, procedures for data collection, measures that were used in the data analysis, and the actual process of data analysis. There should be a sufficient level of detail such that others could replicate your work.

- The *results* is a factual presentation of the findings from your analysis. Use tables, graphs, and figures to enhance and clarify your information and results.

- The *discussion/conclusion* section provides a systematic and thoughtful interpretation of your finding and discusses the implications. Start by restating your topic and briefly summarizing your results. Your discussion is the place where you go beyond the summary. Work to provide an answer or answers in light of everything that you have done and discussed. Your conclusions have to be linked to the evidence provided by your results.

- *References.*

- *Figures/tables/appendices/supplementary materials.*

Another important forum for sharing your research can be in professional meetings. These are often competitive and require submission of an abstract that describes your work. Like other forms of research writing, there are often specific guidelines on format and word limits. Look carefully for these instructions, as failure to comply can result in your abstract not even getting a review. When your research is accepted for presentation, there will also be guidance about the format for your presentation (both for talks and posters).

SEEING IT THROUGH TO THE END

It can be very hard to maintain a positive attitude and stay motivated throughout the entire research process. It would not be uncommon at different points in a research project to feel that your project is boring, to worry about how you are going to get it all done or to even feel insecure about the validity of what you are attempting to study. These are all normal feelings and often arise when you have lost focus about the purpose of your project and the endpoint(s) that you are working towards. In order to help you stay focused and motivated, manage your research time so that you are working your project regularly. Procrastination is not your friend. Try to set up daily, weekly, and monthly goals. Make your goals realistic and work hard to attain them. In addition, setting up regular meetings with your advisor can help you stay on track. The more opportunities you create to present and talk about your research, the easier it will be to maintain your momentum: this can include talking to other students, your supervisors and mentors, and planning regular meetings with your committee members. Not only will this help you keep on track, it will also be helpful when you start to analyze your results or if you run into problems with your project. Of course, a natural consequence of all these conversations is that you will receive feedback about your research. This is an innate element of the iterative nature of the research process and central to the success of most projects. The more you can work on bouncing your ideas off of others and getting regular feedback, the higher your likelihood of success.

RESEARCH AS A CAREER: THINKING BEYOND GRADUATE SCHOOL

While there is variability in the degree to which genetic counselors may incorporate research into their own practice following graduate school, research transcends all practice areas and can also support genetic counselors who work in education, laboratory settings, public health, and so on. Research results may directly impact patient care or clinical practice, influence institutional policies, impact genetic counseling training, provide tangible guidance to third party payors, or effect change in more global policies. All practicing genetic counselors are required to be informed consumers of research whether to guide clinical decision-making, pursue professional development, or seek continuing education. However, many genetic counselors may also engage in more focused research initiatives. For some genetic counselors, research may be entwined with their clinical roles (e.g., case reports, chart reviews, patient satisfaction). Scholarly achievements may also be included in the list of elements considered for promotion across disciplines. Genetic counselors may also participate as committee members or mentors for student thesis/capstone projects or may engage in other education-related research initiatives. As seen through these examples, there are several touchpoints at which research can be integrated into genetic counseling practice without specifically choosing research as a primary professional endeavor.

A smaller subset of genetic counselors will choose to focus on research as a significant component of their career. In the 2024 Professional Status Report from the National Society of Genetic Counselors, 19% of respondents reported research as a significant role in their position and 3% had research included in their job title (NSGC, 2024). Genetic counselors take on a variety of research roles including, but not limited to, independent research, research collaborations within their academic institution, roles within national and international research consortia, clinical laboratories, and public health programs. In addition, there are increasing roles for genetic counselors in implementation science, defined as the "scientific study of methods to promote the systematic uptake of research findings and other evidence-based practices into routine practice, and, hence, to improve the quality and effectiveness of health services and care" (Eccles and Mittman, 2006). This discipline is increasingly important in supporting the movement of the latest genomic technologies and precision medicine into health care systems (Chambers et al., 2016). Research roles often involve collaborative science in which the genetic counselors engage with researchers from multidisciplinary backgrounds (i.e., medicine, laboratory sciences, public policy, ethics, biostatistics) to address large-scale research questions. Positions within these teams might include principal investigator, co-investigator, research coordinator, or study genetic counselor. These job positions typically involve protected research time to carry out research initiatives, but may require that researchers attain additional sources of funding in order to support themselves. The NSGC provides grant opportunities such as the Audrey Heimler Special Project Award and Jane Engelberg Memorial Fellowship for members to serve as independent research investigators, particularly for those in the early stages of pursuing their own research initiatives. For the first time in 2020, the NIH announced research grant announcements specific to the study of genetic counseling, opening even more doors for genetic counselors to lead large-scale federally funded initiatives.

Students with professional goals that include a career in research may worry that their graduate school research project will define their career trajectory. While your graduate research work may spark or further your research interest and skillset, you will have an entire career to explore a diversity of research topics, interests, and designs. Additional knowledge and research skills can be gained beyond graduate training through on-the-job training, peer collaboration, continuing education, and additional graduate training. For some, research careers may have a narrow focus that a researcher dedicates the bulk of their attention toward. However, for many others, a career may have multiple foci in response to the ever-evolving questions that genomics can raise. Therefore, a key outcome of completing a research project as part of your graduate training is to experience the research process from start to finish. This will give you the lived experience of a "researcher" and is not meant to define or limit your future research initiatives.

CONCLUSION

Research is a complicated process. The topics that have been presented in this chapter are meant to help you understand the big picture; however, to be successful in this endeavor you will need to delve more deeply into each content area. Why make the effort? Undertaking your own research project will provide you with multiple benefits. Working through a research project will allow you to develop a broader perspective of the current clinical practices in genetic counseling. The skills you will develop include critical thinking, creative problem solving, and oral and written communication. Building these skills will help you successfully complete your research project and will complement your clinical genetic counseling skills. By becoming part of the research community, you will broaden your definition of yourself as a genetic counselor and have the chance to contribute something truly novel to the profession.

REFERENCES

Babbie ER. (2020) *The Practice of Social Research* Fifteenth Edition. Boston, MA: Cenage Learning.

Bedard AC, Huether CA, Shooner K, et al. (2007) Career research interests and training of genetic counseling students. *J Genet Couns* 16(5):645–653. https://doi.org/10.1007/s10897-007-9104-5

Brehaut JC, O'Connor AM, Wood, TJ, et al. (2003) Validation of a decision regret scale. *Med Decis Making* 23(4): 281–292. https://doi.org/10.1177/0272989X03256005

Caldwell S, Wusik K, He H, et al. (2018) Development and validation of the Genetic Counseling Self-Efficacy Scale (GCSES). *J Genet Couns* 27(5):1248–1257. https://doi.org/10.1007/s10897-018-0249-1

Cella D, Hughes C, Peterman A, et al. (2002) A brief assessment of concerns associated with genetic testing for cancer: the Multidimensional Impact of Cancer Risk Assessment (MICRA) questionnaire. *Health Psychol* 21(6):564–572. https://www.ncbi.nlm.nih.gov/pubmed/12433008

Chambers DA, Feero WG, & Khoury MJ. (2016). Convergence of implementation science, precision medicine, and the learning health care system: a new model for biomedical research. *JAMA* 315(18):1941–1942. https://doi.org/10.1001/jama.2016.3867

Creswell J. (2023) *Research Design: Qualitative, Quantitative and Mixed Methods Approaches* Fourth Edition. New York, NY: SAGE Publications.

Dungan JS, Klugman S, Darilek S, et al. (2023) Noninvasive prenatal screening (NIPS) for fetal chromosome abnormalities in a general-risk population: an evidence-based clinical guideline of the American College of Medical Genetics and Genomics (ACMG). *Genet Med* 25(2):100336. https://doi.org/10.1016/j.gim.2022.11.004

Eccles M & Mittman B. (2006) Welcome to Implementation Science. *Implement Sci* 1(1):1–3. www.implementationscience.com/content/1/1/1 Accessed June 5, 2024.

Esplen MJ, Cappelli M, Wong J, et al. (2013) Development and validation of a brief screening instrument for psychosocial risk associated with genetic testing: a pan-Canadian cohort study. *BMJ Open* 3(3). https://doi.org/10.1136/bmjopen-2012-002227

Evans J & Khoury MJ. (2007) Evidence based medicine meets genomic medicine. *Genet Med* 9(12):799–800. https://doi.org/10.1097/gim.0b013e31815bf9b5

Hughes C, Lerman C, Schwartz M, et al. (2002) All in the family: evaluation of the process and content of sisters' communication about BRCA1 and BRCA2 genetic test results. *Am J Med Genet* 107(2):143–150. https://doi.org/10.1002/ajmg.10110

Keller H, Wusik K, He H, et al. (2020) Further validation of the Genetic Counseling Self-Efficacy Scale (GCSES): Its relationship with personality characteristics. *J Genet Couns* 29(5):748–758. https://doi.org/10.1002/jgc4.1202

Kim WO. (2012) Institutional review board (IRB) and ethical issues in clinical research. *Korean J Anesthesiol* 62(1):3–12. https://doi.org/10.4097/kjae.2012.62.1.3

Kumar R. (2019) *Research Methodology: A Step-by-Step Guide for Beginners* Fifth Edition. New York, NY: Sage.

Locke L, Spirduso W, & Silverman S. (2013) *Proposals That Work: A Guide for Planning Dissertations and Grant Proposals* Sixth Edition. New York, NY: Sage.

MacFarlane IM, McCarthy Veach P, & LeRoy BS. (2014) *Genetic Counseling Research: A Practical Guide.* Oxford: Oxford University Press.

McAllister M, Wood AM, Dunn G, et al. (2011). The Genetic Counseling Outcome Scale: a new patient-reported outcome measure for clinical genetics services. *Clin Genet* 79(5): 413–424. https://doi.org/10.1111/j.1399-0004.2011.01636.x

Merriam-Webster Inc. (2019) *The Merriam-Webster Dictionary.* Springfield, MS: Merriam-Webster, Incorporated.

Miles MB, Huberman AM, & Saldaña J. (2020) *Qualitative Data Analysis: A Methods Sourcebook* Fourth Edition. New York, NY: Sage.

National Society of Genetics Counselors (NSGC). (n.d.) https://www.nsgc.org/conference, accessed May 23, 2024.

National Society of Genetic Counselors (NSGC). (2024) 2024 Professional Status Survey. https://www.nsgc.org/Policy-Research-and-Publications/Professional-Status-Survey. Accessed 13 June 2024.

O'Brien BC, Harris IB, Beckman TJ, et al. (2014) Standards for reporting qualitative research: a synthesis of recommendations. *Acad Med* 89(9):1245–1251. https://doi.org/10.1097/ACM.0000000000000388

O'Connor AM. (1995) Validation of a decisional conflict scale. *Med Decis Making* 15(1): 25–30. https://doi.org/10.1177/0272989X9501500105

O'Connor C & Joffe H. (2020) Intercoder reliability in qualitative research: debates and practical guidelines. *Int J Qual Methods* 19:16094069-11989922. https://doi.org/doi. org/10.1177/1609406919899220

Poth CN & Creswell J. (2018) *Qualitative Inquiry and Research Design: Choosing Among Five Approaches* Fourth Edition. New York, NY: Sage.

PRIM&R, Bankert EA, Gordon BG, & Hurley, EA. (2021) *Institutional Review Board: Management and Function: Management and Function* Third Edition. Burlington, MA: Jones & Bartlett Learning.

Resta R, McCarthy Veach P, Charles S, et al. (2010) Publishing a master's thesis: a guide for novice authors. *J Genet Couns* 19(3):217–227. https://doi.org/10.1007/s10897-009-9276-2

Sackett DL, Rosenberg WM, Gray, JA, et al. (1996) Evidence based medicine: what it is and what it isn't. *Brit Med J* 312(7023):71–72. https://doi.org/10.1136/bmj.312.7023.71

Saldana JM (2015). *The Coding Manual for Qualitative Researchers* Third edition. New York, NY: Sage Publications.

Schaaf CP, Betancur C, Yuen RKC, et al. (2020) A framework for an evidence-based gene list relevant to autism spectrum disorder. *Nat Rev Genet* 21(6):367–376. https://doi.org/10.1038/s41576-020-0231-2

Senter L, Bennett RL, Madeo AC, et al. (2018) National Society of Genetic Counselors Code of Ethics: explication of 2017 revisions. *J Genet Couns* 27(1):9–15. https://doi.org/10.1007/s10897-017-0165-9

Spielberger CD, Gorsuch RL, Lushene R, et al. (1983) *Manual for the State-Trait Anxiety Inventory.* https://www.apa.org/pi/about/publications/caregivers/practice-settings/assessment/tools/trait-state. Accessed July 7, 2024.

US Department of Health and Human Services. (2022) Office of Human Research Protections. https://www.hhs.gov/ohrp/regulations-and-policy/belmont-report/index.html. Accessed August 10, 2023.

US Department of Health and Human Services. (2023) Health Information Privacy. www.hhs.gov/hipaa/index.html. Accessed August 10, 2023.

Wainstein T, Elliott AM, & Austin JC. (2023) Considerations for the use of qualitative methodologies in genetic counseling research. *J Genet Couns* 32(2):300–314. https://doi.org/10.1002/jgc4.1644

Wallace W. (1971) *The Logic of Science in Sociology* First edition. London: Routledge. https://doi.org/10.4324/9781315132976

Wallgren A, Veach PM, MacFarlane IM, & LeRoy BS. (2021) Content analysis of Journal of Genetic Counseling research articles: a multi-year perspective. *J Genet Couns* 30(3):774–784. https://doi.org/10.1002/jgc4.1373

Walters S, Campbell M, & Machin D. (2021) *Medical Statistics: A Textbook for the Health Sciences* Fifth Edition. Oxford: Wiley-Blackwell.

U.S. Department of Health and Human Services. (2020). Health Information Privacy. www.hhs.gov/hipaa/index.html Accessed August 10, 2021.

14

Clinical Supervision: Strategies for Receiving and Providing Direction, Guidance, and Support

Monica Marvin

INTRODUCTION

Participation in clinical rotations is often one of the most exciting and rewarding aspects of graduate school. Clinical rotations are where classroom knowledge, case preparation, role play experiences, and critical thinking all come together under the supervision of a practicing genetic counselor. With the excitement of clinical rotations, it is normal for students to also feel anxious, nervous, and uncertain (MacFarlane et al., 2016). As students enter clinical supervision, whether this is their first or last rotation, the general expectation is that genetic counseling students have knowledge to gain, skills to develop, and confidence to build. At the same time, clinical supervision is also a learning opportunity for supervisors, as working with students affords opportunities for self-reflection and consideration of new perspectives. While the timing and sequencing of clinical rotations vary significantly across

A Guide to Genetic Counseling, Third Edition. Edited by Vivian Y. Pan, Jane L. Schuette, Karen E. Wain, and Beverly M. Yashar.
© 2025 John Wiley & Sons Ltd. Published 2025 by John Wiley & Sons Ltd.

graduate programs, the most effective clinical supervision is characterized by student readiness, skilled supervisors, diverse clinical experiences, a positive learning environment, a strong working alliance between supervisor and student, and a curriculum that is built to support learning.

As the profession of genetic counseling has evolved and matured, so has our understanding of the challenges of receiving and providing clinical supervision, as well as the requisite student and supervisor skills and attributes that enable successful clinical supervision relationships and experiences. This chapter provides multiple perspectives on the topic of supervised clinical training (clinical supervision), including guidance for genetic counseling students (students) and for the novice genetic counseling clinical supervisor (supervisor). Ideally, students and supervisors should review and consider the full content of this chapter, including the guidance provided to both members of this supervisory relationship. A mutual appreciation of the perspectives and challenges of both parties can foster a respectful and productive experience.

DEFINING CLINICAL SUPERVISION AND ITS GOALS

Supervised clinical training is an essential and required component of the curricula of graduate programs in genetic counseling (graduate programs). The most cited definition of clinical supervision in the genetic counseling literature is derived from Bernard and Goodyear, who define supervision as an intervention that promotes the transmittal of skills, knowledge, and attitudes of a particular profession to the next generation in that profession (Bernard and Goodyear, 1992). Drawing on mental health professions, they note that clinical supervision ensures that clients receive a certain minimum quality of care from students as they are working to gain clinical skills. Bernard and Goodyear also note that the relationship between the supervisor and supervisee is evaluative and hierarchical, with supervisors also serving a gatekeeping function (Bernard and Goodyear, 1992). Within the context of genetic counseling, the gatekeeping role includes a supervisor's contribution to evaluations of whether a student meets the Accreditation Council of Genetic Counseling (ACGC) Practice Based Competencies, and thus would gain access to the profession (ACGC, 2023a). Weil defines genetic counseling supervision as an activity that helps students develop and gain an increased awareness of ethical issues and their resolution, develop greater awareness of their professional blind spots, and become socialized to the profession (Weil, 2000). The outcome of clinical supervision proposed by Wherley et al. (2015) in the Reciprocal Engagement Model of Supervision is that the "student understands and applies information to 1) independently provide effective services, 2) develop professionally, and 3) engage in self-reflective practice." Taken together, these definitions highlight the varied student outcomes of effective clinical supervision including the development of clinical skills, knowledge, and self-awareness, as well as socialization into the profession.

In contrast to many other health care professions, the most prevalent method used in supervision of genetic counseling students is live supervision, defined as when a supervisor is present for part or all of a student's encounter with a patient (Hendrickson et al., 2002; Lindh et al., 2003). Within the context of live supervision, students may experience different levels of entrustment. As discussed later in this chapter, varying levels of entrustment include how frequently supervisors intervene or "step in" during live supervision, and how often, if at all, supervisors allow students to counsel parts of a session independently when they are not in the room (Lenhart et al., 2023). In addition to what happens within a counseling session, live supervision is typically coupled with supervisor–student discussions of case preparation, the clinical encounter, case presentations, written documentation (letters and clinic notes), and professional growth, all as supervisors work to model the behaviors expected of genetic counselors (McCarthy Veach and LeRoy, 2009).

Familiarity with the ACGC Practice Based Competencies is essential for both students and supervisors as they represent the ultimate goal of graduate training, with clinical supervision representing an "essential vehicle for advancing student development of these Practice Based Competencies" (McCarthy Veach and LeRoy, 2009). By way of review, the ACGC Practice Based Competencies and subcompetencies define and describe the "minimal skill set of a genetic counselor which should be applicable across practice settings" (ACGC, 2023a). As such, the Practice Based Competencies are also commonly used in the development of clinical goals, clinical activities, and clinical assessment tools. Given their centrality to clinical training, students should seek clarification from their supervisors and/ or their graduate programs if there is uncertainty about the definition or assessment of a specific competency. Similarly, supervisors can ask for guidance from their peers, the graduate program, and/or the ACGC if they have questions about the competencies.

SETTING THE STAGE FOR GROWTH AND LEARNING: GUIDANCE FOR STUDENTS

The road to clinical competence will include multiple clinical rotations and experiences. In some ways, students may find starting each rotation similar to starting a new job in that they will be working with new supervisors, new patient populations, new clinical indications, new goals, and new processes. Often, just as students develop confidence within a clinical rotation, it is time to move onto the next. As described throughout this section, there are several general steps students can take to optimize these experiences and transitions, including working to understand expectations, coming prepared to supervision, following through on supervisor assignments and recommendations, being open and responsive to feedback, informing supervisors of specific needs, disclosing important information, asking for assistance as needed, and engaging in honest self-evaluation (McCarthy Veach and LeRoy, 2009).

Getting Started and Establishing a Working Alliance

Open communication with the supervising genetic counselor(s) at the start of a rotation is important for developing a working alliance. At the start of a clinical rotation, students generally meet with the supervising genetic counselor(s) to discuss what they have done in any previous rotations, their goals for the upcoming rotation, expectations—including related to both the student's responsibilities and the supervisor's responsibilities—and any questions or concerns they may have. These discussions of goals and expectations are often guided by Clinical Supervision Agreements, as described later in the chapter. Asking for clarification regarding items in such agreements can be helpful in minimizing misunderstandings and establishing a pattern of two-way communication.

Students will work with many different clinical supervisors throughout graduate school, each with their own supervision style, counseling style, and, in some cases, expectations. Despite this variability, students can generally anticipate relationships with supervisors during a clinical rotation to be hierarchal. Therefore, while establishing a working alliance with a supervisor is dependent on commitment and action from both the supervisor and student, students can typically expect the supervisor to set some of the boundaries and standards that will shape the relationship. Like other hierarchal relationships students may have had with teachers, coaches, employers, and other people, some relationships may be more challenging than others. Given the central role of the relationship between a student and supervisor in effective clinical supervision (Wherley et al., 2015), here we describe a few steps that students can take to foster productive, respectful, and rewarding learning experiences and supervisory relationships. Additional guidance is provided later in this chapter for students that encounter barriers to such relationships (*Seeking Additional Support*), as well as guidance for supervisors.

Students are encouraged to enter each rotation prepared (having reviewed relevant documents), showing curiosity (asking questions), and demonstrating initiative (seeking solutions and new opportunities) and a willingness to listen, to learn and to incorporate feedback. Even if the specialty is not the student's "favorite," it is important to recognize it as a learning opportunity and to value the skills that may be transferrable to other clinical specialties. Furthermore, while students often share with each other about their experiences at rotations at different clinical sites and about individual supervisors, students can strive to enter each supervisory relationship with an open mind, recognizing that each person's experiences are different and colored by their own background, circumstances, and biases.

Students can proactively consider what information they feel safe sharing with supervisors about their personal needs or concerns. Some students may find it helpful to alert a supervisor to a personal or familial experience relevant to the rotation (for example, pregnancy loss, cancer diagnosis, or chronic illness). Are there extenuating circumstances like health concerns for the student or a family member that the student thinks may present unique challenges? Does the student have concerns about reliable transportation? Does the student have caregiving or employment responsibilities that they worry could impact the rotation? Furthermore, students should be attentive to their own boundaries as they work to build relationships and share information with supervisors. While a discussion of the Clinical Supervision Agreement is a great time to approach many of these matters, there may be some topics or situations that students wish to delay discussing with supervisors until there has been time to establish rapport and a basic understanding of the supervisory relationship(s). As students settle into a rotation and get to know the supervisory team, they may find that they feel more comfortable with a specific supervisor than others. Additional guidance is provided below (*Seeking Additional Support*) for students who may continue to feel uncomfortable or unsafe disclosing personal information with supervisors.

It can also be helpful for students to recognize the supervisor's numerous responsibilities. Most supervisors work to support student skill development while they balance multiple roles and responsibilities related to maintenance of quality patient care, clinical schedule constraints, additional learners in the clinic, and other professional responsibilities.

Establishing Goals

There will be multiple types of objectives and goals for any clinical experience, including goals that are developed by the student, goals that are developed by a clinical training site, goals that are developed by the graduate program, and goals that may be specific to a given case. Goals are most effective when they are explicit, specific, measurable, and feasible (i.e., they reflect aims that are within a student's ability range, and there are sufficient opportunities to achieve them). When considering personal goals for a rotation at a clinical site, students should consider how their goals for a first-year, introductory rotation would be different than those from a second-year rotation. The Discrimination Model and Bloom's Taxonomy, described later in this chapter, can be helpful in this respect.

Students generally articulate their own personal goals with their supervisors at the start of the rotation. In many graduate programs, the development of a student's personal clinical goals is guided by discussions with program leadership or other mentors and documented in a form that can be shared by the student with supervisors. In some cases, supervisors or program leadership may ask students to revise their personal goals based on clinic-specific constraints or because the goals are not specific or are too ambitious or too modest in scope. If there is a "disconnect" between any of these goals or uncertainty about any aspects of goals, students and supervisors should not hesitate to seek clarification from the graduate program or colleagues, as appropriate. Once the rotation is underway, students may revisit their personal goals with their supervisors and can consider the need for adjustments in either the scope of the goals or the activities that support reaching those goals.

Adopting a Growth Mindset

A growth mindset is one where students recognize that expertise, knowledge, and abilities (in this case clinical skills) are changeable and that the road to competence is a developmental progression. A growth mindset is distinct from a closed mindset in which students believe their attributes and skills are unchangeable (Dweck, 2006) (Table 14-1). A growth mindset can foster increased willingness to ask questions, make mistakes, and welcome feedback. Because clinical training necessitates that students try new things throughout training, students can begin the journey towards a growth mindset by recognizing existing tendencies to adopt a fixed or growth mindset, recognizing and anticipating what might trigger a more fixed mindset, and setting an intention to

TABLE 14-1. Adapting a growth mindset

Fixed Mindset: Expertise/skills are static	Growth Mindset: Expertise/skills can be adapted
Student avoids challenges: *"This indication is new and complex; I think it is best if I just observe."*	Student embraces challenges: *"This indication is new and complex; I'd like to give it a try with my supervisor there as a backup."*
Student gets defensive or gives up easily when confronted with obstacles: *"I can't seem to meet my supervisor's expectations, I give up."*	Student persists in the face of obstacles and setbacks: *"I haven't figure this out yet, what can I learn or change to improve this?"*
Student sees effort as fruitless: *"I'm not good at this."*	Student sees effort as the path to mastery: *"With more practice, I am seeing a way forward."*
Student ignores criticism/negative feedback: *"I think my supervisor just wants me to be like them."*	Student grows from criticism: *"This feedback is making me think about what I am doing differently. I am willing to try a different approach and see how it goes."*
Student feels threatened by the success of others: *"My classmates are already counseling full cases. I feel so behind."*	Student finds lessons and inspiration in the success of others: *"What can I learn from my classmates?"*

Adapted from Dweck (2006).

challenge oneself. In general, genetic counseling students should strive to ask questions, to challenge their way of thinking, and to be brave as they take on new skills. A growth mindset is valuable not only as a student, but also as a genetic counselor, as lifelong learning is a key component to professional growth and satisfaction.

Receiving and Responding to Feedback

Receiving a combination of positive and corrective feedback from clinical supervisors is to be expected and represents a critical component of clinical supervision. When provided skillfully, feedback can reinforce positive behaviors, explore areas for improvement, establish strategies for growth, and enhance the working alliance between the student and supervisor.

As per the ACGC Standards, students will receive formative feedback throughout the course of the clinical supervision experience, as well as summative feedback at the mid-point and end of the rotation (ACGC, 2023b). Formative feedback focuses on the student's day to day activities, such as case preparation, case presentations, visual aids, journal clubs, live supervision of patient encounters, and written documentation. Formative feedback is intended to help students grow throughout the course of a clinical rotation and identify the need for any adjustment to the expectations, support, or remediation. In contrast, summative feedback is typically provided at the conclusion of a rotation and is intended to summarize an overall assessment of skill development.

For many genetic counseling students, receiving corrective feedback is a new and uncomfortable space. Students are encouraged to consider the following recommendations as related to feedback. Depending on where a student is in training (early or later in training) and the relationship that has been established with their supervisor, students may find it helpful to also discuss approaches to improving the provision and reception of feedback with faculty from their graduate program or other trusted mentors. The following suggestions are provided for students (adapted from McCarthy Veach and LeRoy, 2009).

- Accept positive feedback: Awareness of your strengths is as important as awareness of areas for improvement; do not gloss over positive feedback too quickly. You may want to use this feedback to think of new ways to adapt your strengths to different situations.
- Accept corrective feedback: Remember that corrective feedback is necessary for your development as a genetic counselor. Everyone has areas for improvement, so try to welcome this information rather than avoid it. If you are not receiving corrective feedback, you are often missing out on important guidance.

- Clarify feedback: Let your supervisor know if you understand the feedback; ask for clarification until you do understand. If the feedback does not fit with your perceptions, ask for clarification. If you understand the feedback but disagree with it, consider the pros and cons of "pushing back" versus continuing to reflect on the feedback.

- Reflect on feedback: Take time to absorb, synthesize, and reflect on feedback you have received and think about ways to apply feedback in subsequent genetic counseling sessions. Considering the feedback you have received over time can also be helpful in recognizing where you have grown and what you have learned. If you continue to receive similar feedback, consider what barriers might be making change difficult.

- Share your response: When receiving feedback, you may have both cognitive and affective reactions. If you feel comfortable, let you supervisor know how this feedback makes you feel. If it is difficult to immediately articulate your response to the feedback, consider scheduling a separate time to further debrief. If the supervisory relationship doesn't feel like a safe space to have such a discussion, consider consulting with another trusted supervisor, faculty member, or peer.

- Exercise personal responsibility: As you develop your skills, you will become more aware of your own strengths and weaknesses. Take responsibility by asking for feedback about specific behaviors and issues that are challenging for you. This may be as simple as asking your supervisor to pay attention to how often you use filler words (um, oh, er, so); or about something more advanced, such as your ability to explore new psychosocial tools and approaches.

- Advocate for feedback that works for you: If you feel comfortable in your relationship with your supervisor, consider ways to improve the provision of feedback. Areas where adjustments may be feasible include the amount of feedback (enough to help you grow, but not so much that it is overwhelming), the timing of feedback (immediate enough that you can recall how a session went, but also allowing some time for you to self-reflect) and the content of the feedback (enough positive and constructive feedback to support ongoing growth and confidence). If the volume and/or content of feedback feels overwhelming, consider asking the supervisor to help you prioritize the feedback (Is any of the feedback more critical than others? Does the supervisor consider any of the feedback "fine-tuning" or "stylistic" as opposed to critical to correct?)

- Ask for help from others: If you feel something is not working well and are not sure how to approach the conversation with your supervisor, graduate program leadership, other supervisors, or faculty can often be helpful in considering how to approach these conversations.

Supervisor and Student Roles

As students receive feedback throughout the trajectory of their clinical training experience, they are likely to find that both students and supervisors are moving in and out of different roles depending on the student's needs and the supervisor's style and tendencies. Bernard and Goodyear (1992) define four types of supervisor and student roles: teaching, consultation, counseling, and evaluation.

Teacher/Student Roles   When the supervisor is in the teacher role and the student is in the student role, the primary focus is instruction. The clinical supervisor is a resource who shares information, skills, and strategies. Teaching activities include demonstrating, explaining, and interpreting information and events that happen before, during, and after a session, and identifying appropriate interventions. In this sort of interaction, the supervisor is the "expert" who provides at least some of the answers. This sort of relationship may be what students are most familiar with from previous experiences as an undergraduate student and is often most appropriate for students early in clinical experiences.

Consultee/Consultant Roles   When the supervisor is a consultant and the student is a consultee, they interact collaboratively and the supervisor encourages the student to self-evaluate. Consulting activities may also include brainstorming possible strategies and interventions. The supervisor acts as a facilitator who works with the student to determine effective planning and action.

Counselor/Client Roles   When the supervisor is in a counselor role and the student is in a client role, the primary interaction is one of exploration with the goal of promoting self-awareness and growth. Here the focus is on the student as a person, and thus support is emphasized. The supervisor assists the student to recognize developmental tasks and become aware of personal issues that may affect responses to patients. For example, many genetic counseling students will experience anxiety as they take on new skills (MacFarlane et al., 2016). A supervisor in the counselor role can introduce a discussion of these dynamics and help to normalize them (e.g., "Most students feel some anxiety about their skills. Is that what you are feeling?"). The supervisor plays a role in helping the student identify feelings and defenses and understand how these inner experiences affect their genetic counseling skills and related interactions.

Evaluation Role   When the supervisor is an evaluator and the student is an evaluatee, the primary interaction is the provision of feedback. The supervisor acts as a gatekeeper assessing the student's skills. Evaluation activities include formal and informal assessments, goal setting, and giving and receiving formative and summative feedback.

The following supervisor–student scenario and interactions illustrate how these different sorts of roles might play out within clinical supervision.

Scenario: The student has just completed a genetic counseling session in which the patient started to cry as they heard the results of their genetic testing. The student had responded by repeating extremely complicated information about the test results in a rapid, highly technical fashion, at which point the supervisor elected to take over the session. Later, during a discussion between the supervisor and the student, the case was reviewed, and the issue was discussed.

Teaching Roles

> **Student:** I didn't know what to do. What should I have done?
>
> **Supervisor:** Sometimes when there is so much emotion, it can be helpful to stop providing information and consider changing direction. You can try to take a moment to breathe and try to address the patient's emotion before moving forward. When providing a lot of new information, I try to pay attention to the words I use to make sure it is not too technical and work to define the language in the test report.

Consultation Roles

> **Student:** I missed my chance to address her feelings. I'd like to figure out some ways that I could respond when patients cry.
>
> **Supervisor:** I'm glad you picked up on that and I know this relates to one of your goals for this rotation. Why don't we talk about different strategies? What sorts of approaches were you thinking about?

Counseling Roles

> **Student:** It's not usually like me to ignore a patient's feelings. I don't know what was going on.
>
> **Supervisor:** Let's talk a bit more about this. What were you feeling during that moment? Are there characteristics of the patient that may have played a role?

Evaluation Roles

> **Student:** I think I could have done better when the patient started to cry, how did you feel about this part of the session?
>
> **Supervisor:** I am glad you want to talk about this part of the session. You've demonstrated a lot of growth in your ability to reflect on cases and identify the parts for continued improvement. It seems that you continue to fall into the habit of repeating facts and figures when you get anxious or nervous about a patient's emotions. This is certainly a place for continued growth.

These roles are not necessarily discrete or mutually exclusive of each other and no single role is the absolute "right" role to assume in clinical supervision. Each approach has a place within the supervision relationship, and, ideally, supervisors and students are versatile in their use, shifting among roles as needed.

Seeking Additional Support

In some instances, students can face frustrations, or less commonly, significant conflicts or transgressions in interactions with supervisors or other team members within their clinical experiences. While ACGC mandates that students are provided with the opportunity to anonymously evaluate clinical supervisors (ACGC, 2023b), students should understand what to do if there is a concern that needs to be addressed during a rotation. Often concerns can be resolved through revisiting and clarifying expectations with supervisors. Graduate program leadership, other supervisors, or faculty members can help students navigate approaches to concerns that arise in the supervision experience. However, some concerns may be very difficult for students to discuss directly with individuals in a position of power, especially during a clinical rotation and/or before the student has completed their graduate degree. Mentors external to the graduate program, such as mentors from affinity groups or trusted advisors, may be helpful in these scenarios, recognizing that students should not be expected to suffer through disrespectful or unprofessional treatment. Furthermore, student handbooks/manuals should contain institutional policies and resources related to processing of student grievances and allegations of harassment.

TRANSITIONING FROM STUDENT TO SUPERVISOR

Clinical supervision is a required component of graduate training: maintenance and growth of a qualified genetic counseling workforce is dependent on the efforts of practicing genetic counelors to fulfill supervisory roles for future generations of trainees. For some genetic counselors, supervision of genetic counseling students is a responsibility that is clearly documented in their job description. For others, clinical supervision is not a job requirement, but is an activity they take on voluntarily.

Supervision of genetic counseling students provides an opportunity for ongoing professional development. The process of supervision typically requires deliberate thought about why genetic counselors do what they do in their own practices and consideration of alternate approaches as curious students with unique perspectives and clinical training needs seek guidance and support. In this way, student supervision fosters growth in a supervisor's genetic counseling skills. Furthermore, effective clinical supervision relies on a set of competencies (Eubanks Higgins et al., 2013) that are distinct from the ACGC Practice Based Competencies and provides an opportunity for professional growth. Supervisors who adopt an open, humble, growth mindset can also experience personal growth when they engage in dialogues with their students about different dimensions of diversity and personal experiences, perspectives, and values. In this way, learning and growth can be bidirectional.

Beyond the job satisfaction and personal and professional growth afforded by providing clinical supervision, the NSGC Code of Ethics (NSGC, n.d.) highlights the importance of supervision of genetic counseling students. Among other items, Section III of the Code of Ethics (Genetic Counselors and Their Colleagues) states that genetic counselors work to share their knowledge and provide mentorship and guidance for the professional development of other genetic counselors, employees, trainees, and colleagues (III.1), respect and value the knowledge, perspectives, contributions, and areas of competence of colleagues, trainees and other professionals (III.2), ensure that individuals under their supervision undertake responsibilities that are commensurate with their knowledge, experience, and training (III.4), and maintain appropriate boundaries to avoid exploitation in their relationships with trainees, employees, employers, and colleagues (III.5).

Supervisor Competencies and Requirements

Analogous to ACGC's Practice Based Competencies that define the requisite skills needed to function as an entry-level genetic counselor, competencies for genetic counseling supervision have also been delineated through a Delphi study of clinical supervisors and directors of genetic counseling graduate programs (Eubanks Higgins et al., 2013). These competencies highlight that the process of providing clinical supervision is distinct from the process of providing genetic counseling. Furthermore, the acquisition of competence in supervision should be considered a developmental process, with the supervision competencies providing a roadmap for the novice supervisor.

The six domains of the GC Supervisor Competencies are (Eubanks Higgins et al., 2013):

1. Personal traits and characteristics: *"Genetic counselor supervisors are competent genetic counselors as evidenced by their training, education and certification. They demonstrate a variety of personal qualities and related skills."*

2. Relationship building and maintenance: *"Genetic counselor supervisors demonstrate knowledge and skills that promote a working alliance and a safe and positive learning environment."*

3. Student evaluation: *"Genetic counselor supervisors demonstrate knowledge and skills that reflect awareness of effective management of the evaluative nature of supervision."*

4. Student-centered supervision: *"Genetic counselor supervisors demonstrate knowledge and skills that allow them to work effectively with student individual differences, in particular, student learning styles and developmental levels."*

5. Guidance and monitoring of patient care: *"Genetic counselor supervisors demonstrate knowledge and skills in ensuring students learn to provide a standard of patient care."*

6. Ethical and legal aspects of supervision: *"Genetic counselor supervisors demonstrate knowledge and skills that model ethical and professional treatment of patients and students."*

The reader is referred to Eubanks Higgins et al. for a comprehensive review of these competencies (Eubanks Higgins et al., 2013).

Genetic counselors are often asked to supervise students very early in their careers. Novice genetic counselors working at their first genetic counseling position can advocate for time to gain some self-confidence in their professional role before agreeing to take on substantive supervision responsibilities. Furthermore, ACGC sets standards regarding the qualifications of clinical supervisors, including training in supervision, experience as a clinical genetic counselor, and genetic counselor certification (ACGC, 2023b). When possible, novice supervisors can strive for a gradual progression into supervision. For example, a novice supervisor may supervise students taking on smaller parts of sessions before having primary responsibility for a student taking on full sessions or more advanced skills. It may also be helpful for novice supervisors to observe and then discuss how another supervisor interacts with students during activities like reviewing student goals, clarifying site expectations, or providing feedback.

ESTABLISHING A WORKING ALLIANCE WITH STUDENTS

As defined by Bordin's working alliance of supervision, components of a working alliance include: 1) mutual agreement and understanding of goals between the supervisor and student; 2) an understanding of the task needed to reach those goals; and 3) a bond between the supervisor and student (Bordin, 1983). The strength of the working alliance between a genetic counseling student and supervisor is central to the supervision process and can have an impact on multiple aspects of a student's supervisory experience and progress in a clinical rotation. A strong working alliance (as perceived by the student) is positively associated with trust in the feedback (MacFarlane et al., 2016), an ability to cope with stressors (MacFarlane et al., 2016), self-efficacy to perform specific GC tasks (Caldwell et al., 2018), and less anxiety with patients and the supervisor (MacFarlane et al., 2016).

Getting to Know Each Other

Before considering goals and expectations, it is important to consider how to establish the "bond" between supervisor and student, a process which takes time and deliberate effort, especially in the context of the inherent power differential between a supervisor and student. Students will come to supervision at different time points in training, with unique and distinct personal, professional, and educational experiences, with varying levels of confidence and competence. Even if the supervisor has already been told a bit about the student from the graduate program, spending time getting to know each other is critical to initiate a working alliance.

Supervisors should clarify what the student wants to be called, learn how to pronounce their name, and learn and use their pronouns. Engaging in a two-way conversation about whether the student lives locally or not, where they grew up, and what outside interests they have may help build rapport. Furthermore, given that clinical rotations are just one part of their graduate school experience, asking about classes, research ideas, jobs, or other responsibilities can be informative. Supervisors can also ask what, if anything, might make this rotation especially challenging for the student such as particular academic stressors, other life stressors, or related personal or familial experience with the specialty, such as infertility, pregnancy loss, disability, or cancer. These conversations can help demonstrate to students that supervisors recognize and respect them as a whole person, with valuable skills, experiences, interests, and responsibilities outside of the clinical rotation setting. Such conversations can also help supervisors grow as they gain a greater appreciation for the diversity that exists among their students. As supervisors work to build these connections with students, it is important to recognize that students will have different boundaries that should be respected; some students may feel uncomfortable sharing glimpses into their personal lives in a professional setting. Therefore, flexible approaches to these conversations are important.

Because the student–supervisor relationship is bidirectional, as supervisors work to get to know their students, they can consider sharing a bit about themselves. As appropriate based on each individual's personal and professional boundaries, a supervisor might talk about their professional journey (e.g., where they went to graduate school, how long they've held their current position, previous positions, challenges they experienced as a student), their research interests, or any hobbies. Just as students are asked to share anything that might be a barrier to the rotation, supervisors can also be transparent about factors that may impact the supervision experience that are outside of the student's control, such as short staffing, administrative support, or a tight clinical schedule. These discussions can also create opportunities for students to learn about some of the administrative aspects of clinical practice.

As noted above, the power differential between supervisor and student can make it less likely for students to disclose stressors or worries, especially at the start of a rotation before any trust has been established. This may be especially true for genetic counseling students with minority identities (one or multiple) who may be particularly hesitant to speak up (Carmichael et al., 2020). With this in mind, at the start of a rotation, supervisors can introduce topics of cultural identity, diversity, power, and privilege within the supervisory relationship and recognize these as important issues to be aware of and open to discussing in supervision (ACES, 2011). Acknowledging this tension early in the rotation demonstrates a supervisor's openness to these topics as students grow more comfortable in the supervisory relationship. Furthermore, a Clinical Supervision Agreement (described later) can help elicit information from all students related to topics such as student specific needs, cultural differences, religious observances, and accessibility.

For students with accommodations approved by an institutional disability office, supervisors should work with the program, the student, and the institutional disability office to ensure appropriate, reasonable accommodations are provided. Supervisors should also consider the principle of "Universal Design" so that the clinical supervision experience is designed, to the greatest extent possible, to be accessible to all students. Within the context of a full-time clinical rotation, for example, this might include providing protected time for all students to attend to personal matters and reducing the need for students to self-disclose specific needs (Hayward, 2021).

Finally, given the small size of the genetic counseling profession and the graduate training community, it is not uncommon for students and supervisors to have more than one relationship with each other, with different associated roles and responsibilities. For example, a genetic counselor may be a clinical supervisor, a classroom instructor, a research committee member, and/or a work supervisor for the same student along their journey through graduate school. Supervisors should explicitly discuss the nature of the clinical supervisory relationship and how it may differ, or not, from other relationships.

Establishing Expectations

Clarity around expectations for a clinical rotation is critical to achieving the mutually established goals for a rotation. Each time a genetic counseling student enters a new clinical rotation, they are interacting with new individuals, new indications, new workflows, and likely variable expectations. Many of the areas where clear delineation of expectations is important are defined in the Clinical Supervision Agreement template at the end of the chapter. Relevant topics that should be discussed at the start of a rotation include how case assignments are determined, what is expected for case preparation and when it is due, how counseling roles within a session will be determined, and what is expected in terms of case documentation. Clearly defining expectations for participation in journal clubs, outreach events, special projects, and other activities is also important, as well as determining any potential schedule or other conflicts. Supervisors can also consider and then discuss how expectations might be different for students who are at different stages in training or for students who are completing a full-time summer rotation as compared to one with fewer hours requirements.

Students can also benefit from having clear expectations about how and when they will receive formative and summative assessment feedback. Establishing early on that corrective feedback is to be expected may help normalize the experience of receiving such feedback. An expectation for student self-reflection can also be set early in the alliance. Students can also benefit from understanding what to expect in terms of how a supervisor sees their role as a supervisor and their general tendencies as a supervisor. For example, some supervisors are more prone to jumping in when students seem uncertain, while others have a more "hands off approach." Supervisors who are part of a team can highlight any known similarities or differences between supervisor styles or expectations and acknowledge any associated challenges. Supervisors can also use awareness of their own supervision habits as an opportunity to develop versatility in how they work with different students.

Establishing Goals

While the ACGC Practice Based Competencies define the overall goal of clinical training, the attainment of clinical competence is a developmental process, with growth (and sometimes setbacks or new challenges) occurring in each clinical rotation with contributions from a multitude of supervisors and clinical experiences. For any given clinical rotation, goals provide a framework for supervision as they represent the skills that a student is working to attain (McCarthy Veach and Leroy, 2009). As noted in the earlier section on guidance to students related to establishing goals, there will typically be multiple types of objectives and goals for any clinical experience, including goals that are developed by the graduate program, goals that are developed by the student, goals that are developed by a clinical training site, and goals that may be specific to a given case.

In considering goals that are developed by a student, it can be helpful to ask the student to tell you about the rotations they have completed, the types of roles, if any, the student has taken on in previous rotations, what has gone well and what has not. Considering the responses to these questions in the context of the goals the student is proposing may identify a need for modification of the goals and/or opportunities for additional support.

As a supervisor considering goals for their clinical training site, one can consider the following questions. As a result of this rotation, what should students know? For example, should all students leave the rotation understanding laws and policies related to pregnancy termination? What should they be able to do? For example, should all students leave the rotation with the ability to use specific genomic variant databases? It is important to recognize that some goals and expectations will differ for each student and can by impacted by when the rotation is occurring— early or late in training. The goals established by both the site and the student should be realistic and attainable based on the student's developmental stage. In considering clinical goals in relation to a student's developmental stage, there are a few relevant models and constructs to consider.

The Discrimination Model, developed by Bernard and Goodyear (1997) classifies student goals and skills into four categories based on whether the skills primarily involve overt behaviors or covert feelings or thoughts. Understanding the types of skills a student is working to develop may be helpful in considering the related goals. Examples specific to genetic counseling are categorized as (McCarthy Veach and LeRoy, 2009):

- Process skills: These are "doing skills" that consist of the actual techniques and strategies used in a genetic counseling session:
  - The student obtains appropriate family, medical, and social histories.
  - The student uses open-ended questions to help patients express concerns.
  - The student is able to manage expressions of strong emotions by patients.
- Professional skills: These are "doing skills" that involve adherence to professional standards of behavior, including adherence to ethical standards of the profession:
  - The student comes to genetic counseling sessions adequately prepared.
  - The student seeks consultative help when needed.
- Personalization skills: These are "feeling skills" that pertain to the internal, subjective reactions students have toward their patients, toward genetic counseling, and toward their supervision relationships:
  - The student recognizes how a patient's loss triggers the student's own grief reaction.
  - The student is able to tolerate ambiguity.
  - The student seeks feedback during supervision nondefensively.
- Conceptualization skills: These are "thinking skills" that involve cognitive processes such as case analysis and patient conceptualization:
  - The student formulates appropriate and specific plans and strategies for sessions.
  - The student anticipates patient reactions to genetic information.
  - The student is able to interpret patient response/nonresponse accurately.

For any given rotation, it may be appropriate to have some goals from each of these domains, recognizing that conceptualization skills are often the most advanced and may be more challenging for some students in early rotations.

Bloom's Revised Taxonomy is another helpful model in considering realistic expectations and goal setting for clinical rotations (Anderson and Krathwohl, 2001). Bloom's Revised Taxonomy consists of six levels of cognitive learning: remembering, understanding, applying, analyzing, evaluating, and creating. A novice student is more likely to have memorized basic genetic information and understand some of it, but tends to need to develop skills required for application, analysis, and evaluation to patient encounters. As a student acquires additional clinical

TABLE 14-2. The application of Bloom's Revised Taxonomy to genetic counseling skills

Level	Definition	Goal
Remember	Retrieve, recall, or recognize relevant knowledge from long-term memory	Student knows that exome sequencing is used to look for variants in all of the exons in an individual's genome
Understand	Demonstrate comprehension through one or more forms of explanation	Student articulates that exome sequencing does not identify variants in non-coding regions of the genome, that not all exons are covered at the same depth, and that some structural variants may be missed.
Apply	Use information or a skill in a new situation	Student can apply their knowledge of exome sequencing to describe the testing to a patient
Analyze	Break material into its constituent parts and determine how the parts relate to one another and/or to an overall structure or purpose	Student can discriminate the differences between exome sequencing and other technologies such as chromosomal microarray, disease-specific multigene panels, and whole-genome sequencing and the pros and cons in different clinical situations
Evaluate	Make judgments based on criteria and standards	Student can assess the significance of a positive, negative, or uncertain exome sequencing result in the context of patient's history
Create	Put elements together to form a new coherent or functional whole; reorganize elements into a new pattern or structure	Student designs tools to help patients, providers, or others understand exome sequencing

experience, clinical goals will relate to skills representative of higher levels of the hierarchy. Table 14-2 describes the levels of Bloom's Revised Taxonomy Model and how it can be applied to and assessed in a genetic counseling context, including during case preparation, during a case, during post case discussions, then/or other activities.

PROVIDING ONGOING FEEDBACK AND SUPPORT FOR STUDENTS

Beyond the establishment of a working alliance (establishing a relationship, defining goals, and outlining expectations), supervision involves the provision of instruction, guidance, support, and feedback, all while maintaining quality patient care and navigating other professional responsibilities.

Providing Feedback

Feedback is an essential component of clinical skill development that can reinforce positive behaviors, explore areas for improvement, establish strategies for growth, and enhance the working alliance between the student and supervisor. Providing and receiving constructive feedback can also be challenging for both the supervisor and the student and deliberate thought should be given to this process.

Formative Feedback   Formative feedback focuses on a student's day-to-day activities, such as case preparation, case presentations, visual aids, journal clubs, live supervision of patient encounters, written documentation, etc. Formative feedback is intended to help students grow throughout the course of a clinical rotation and identify the need for any adjustment to the expectations, support, or remediation. Supervisors should inform students that they should expect to receive formative feedback throughout the course of the clinical supervision experience, as well as summative feedback at the mid-point and end of the rotation.

STRATEGIES FOR PROVIDING FORMATIVE FEEDBACK

(Adapted from Ende, 1983; McCarthy Veach and LeRoy, 2009)

- Provide feedback that is timely and expected.
- Discuss feedback in a private, safe setting.
- Prioritize your feedback. Feedback overload can diminish the most important messages. Help students understand what changes are critical to providing quality genetic counseling services and what are stylistic choices that may differ from counselor to counselor.
- Remember the student's developmental level and personal goals. A student who is attempting a new skill for the first or second time cannot be expected to perform the same as a more experienced student.
- Elicit student's impressions first to assess their own insight and promote reflective practice.
- Provide balanced feedback that includes positive feedback and corrective feedback.
- Recognize areas of growth and efforts made by the student (even when additional work is still needed).
- Elicit student's understanding of and response to the feedback. Clarify as needed.
- Develop a plan for moving forward for continued growth, incorporating a growth mindset where the student feels encouraged about their potential.
- Recognize the emotional impact feedback may have on the student.

- Be transparent about aspects of a case that would have been challenging for even experienced practitioners.
- Be objective and focus on the precise behavior that the student either is exhibiting or failing to exhibit.
- Consider a short delay in discussing feedback after a particularly challenging situation. The student and supervisor may both benefit from time to reflect and plan for the discussion.

Summative Feedback/Evaluation In addition to providing ongoing, formative feedback to students, supervisors provide summative feedback regarding a student's progress in formal documentation that is shared with both the student and the graduate program. Such evaluations should be completed at the mid-point and end of a rotation (ACGC, 2023b). Each graduate program maintains specific evaluation forms that are designed for this purpose. While these evaluations include language informed by the practice-based competencies, supervisors should anticipate variation between graduate programs in the items and scale used on these forms, as well as how final "grades" are assigned for a rotation and by whom. Supervisors should ask for clarification from the graduate program about any aspect of the evaluation process that may be unclear.

Summative evaluation typically does not focus on a single case but rather on the student's general skill acquisition and professional development. It is helpful to consider and address the goals (student, programmatic, and clinic specific) that were established at the start of the rotation. Like formative feedback, recognition of where growth has occurred is important and can be empowering for a student as they consider goals for ongoing skill development. In the case of supervisors that are working as part of a team, input should be incorporated from all supervisors that have had substantive interactions with the student. Ideally, if the provision of formative feedback has been ongoing, there should not be any "surprises" in the summative evaluation. Comparing students to their peers or previous students is typically not helpful. Rather, all evaluations and feedback should be centered on the student and their own progress, accomplishments, and areas for ongoing growth.

Summative evaluations should be discussed with the student, leaving space for the student to ask questions and respond. The final evaluation can serve to formally bring the rotation to a close. During this discussion, supervisors can encourage students to provide feedback about their clinical supervision experience, recognizing that some students may remain reluctant to provide critical feedback directly to a supervisor and may instead provide that feedback to the graduate program. Graduate programs must also provide students with the opportunity to provide anonymous feedback about supervisors, with feedback only shared with the supervisor in aggregate once enough feedback has been received to maintain student confidentiality (ACGC, 2023b).

Identifying a Need for Additional Support or Remediation The expectation within a rotation is that all students will require guidance, support, and encouragement. However, occasionally students can have a significant struggle with an aspect of their clinical rotation. Supporting such students requires additional time, consideration, problem-solving, patience, and empathy. It can be difficult for supervisors to determine when additional help is needed beyond the typical mentorship provided within the context of the rotation, as well as the underlying reason for a student's struggle. Keeping an open mind about possible causes of the difficulties is helpful. While it is easy to assume that difficulties in a clinical rotation relate to deficiencies in knowledge, critical thinking, or effort, the literature suggests that the underlying issues are commonly related to confidence, wellbeing, responses to stereotype threats, or external stressors (Sayer et al., 2002). In the context of genetic counseling, students from underrepresented backgrounds may be particularly vulnerable to such stressors (Carmichael et al., 2020).

If concerns about a student's performance arise, it is often helpful to talk to other supervisors within your team to help gauge the scope of the problem, keeping in mind the importance of protecting the student's privacy and maintaining compliance with federal student privacy regulations (https://studentprivacy.ed.gov/). Supervisors should not hesitate to reach out to the student's graduate program to discuss their concerns. Partnering with the graduate program can be very important in helping determine the root cause of the difficulty, the most appropriate course of action, as well as appropriate resources. Depending on the situation, options for additional support may include activities like extra role plays with the student, additional time spent discussing case preparation or post-session feedback, supplemental readings to help with knowledge, exploring whether case outlines and/or visual aids have too much or too little detail, etc. Supervisors should be transparent with graduate programs about their ability to provide additional support to students. In some cases, it may be necessary to scale back or revise the goals for a rotation so that students are still making progress in clinical skills, but with a new "endpoint" in mind. In other cases, a more significant adjustment may be most appropriate, including a "pause" or suspension of clinical activities. These types of decisions are generally made in very close consultation with the graduate program. Therefore, ongoing, honest communication with the graduate program and student is important.

Advocating for Students

As supervisors work to promote an environment where students feel safe sharing information about their multidimensional identities and needs, supervisors are reminded that the genetic counseling profession continues to be homogeneous, with an overwhelmingly white, cis-gendered, female workforce (NSGC, 2022). In this context, students from underrepresented racial, ethnic, educational, and/or socioeconomic backgrounds may face challenges during training (including clinical supervision) that can diminish a sense of belonging, causing them to feel "othered" (Carmichael et al., 2020). Other important dimensions of identity that can lead to inappropriate biases and assumptions that contribute to a diminished sense of belonging within the profession include gender identity, sexual orientation, and religious and spiritual orientation (Exeter Group, 2021), as well as disability status (Darr et al., 2023), chronic illness, and neurodiversity (Hayward, 2021).

Supervisors should speak up when there is inappropriate behavior from members of the health care team, patients, students, staff, and others. The intervention may vary based on whether the student is the recipient, the source, or the witness (bystander), of the inappropriate behavior. In the context of clinical supervision, responding to inappropriate behavior such as microaggressions should be done in a manner intended to create teachable moments, promote allyship, and advance inclusivity in the supervision experience, as well as within the profession (Ackerman-Barger et al., 2021). Supervisors should also remain attentive to student wellbeing as they respond to inappropriate behaviors, recognizing that students are typically the most vulnerable in such circumstances.

Supervisors should commit to be open and responsive to feedback from students about overt macroaggressions, microaggressions, and concerns (regardless of the source), recognizing that the student may not only be seeking listening but also action (Carmichael et al., 2020). While it is easy to feel defensive when a student shares a concern, it is important for supervisors to recognize how difficult it is for a student to speak up and such brave actions should be commended. Furthermore, supervisors can work with colleagues and program leadership to identify contacts for students who would prefer to speak with someone with a shared minority identity (Carmichael et al., 2020).

OTHER RESPONSIBILITIES OF SUPERVISORS

Maintenance of Quality Care

There is often a tension between a supervisor's desire to foster student learning with their duty to ensure quality patient care and their concern for the patient's wellbeing. While some supervisors are hesitant to entrust students with a high degree of autonomy, most genetic counseling students are eager to have more autonomy during patient encounters, hoping it will help with their skill development and confidence (Lenhart et al., 2023). Notably, each supervised genetic counseling session, whether it is a largely observational experience or one where the student is providing most of the genetic counseling, is a learning opportunity for the student. The level of supervision should be "commensurate with each student's documented skills and competencies. A student in the early part of their training must be directly supervised at all times. After the student consistently achieves specific skills, the focus of direct supervision is expected to position the student to develop not-yet achieved or emerging skills"

(ACGC, 2023b). The topic of entrustment is further discussed in the Additional Considerations in Supervision section.

Modeling Ethical and Professional Behavior

The NSGC Code of Ethics serves to "clarify and guide the conduct of a professional so that the goals and values of the profession are best served." Supervisors have a responsibility to model professional conduct, and "walk the walk" defined within the Code of Ethics. There will be instances where a student is witness to or involved in behaviors and interactions that are contrary to the Code of Ethics. Such transgressions may involve the supervisor, other colleagues, patients, staff, and/or the student and may occur within a counseling session, staff room, case conference, etc. As previously described, when supervisors recognize these transgressions and/or a student brings them to their attention, the supervisor should make space to process the occurrence with the student and consider what actions should be taken to further address the situation.

Commitment to Growth as a Clinical Supervisor

Clinical supervision, like genetic counseling, is a process that draws on multiple attributes, skills, and behaviors. Even "seasoned" supervisors can benefit from ongoing attention to supervision skills. There are several steps that supervisors can take to foster continued growth in this important process, including participating in training opportunities like workshops, podcasts, or peer supervision. Supervisors should carefully reflect on the feedback they receive from students and graduate programs. Supervisors can consider the supervisor roles (teacher, consultant, etc.) and consider whether they are "stuck" in a certain role, like that of the "teacher," and identify steps they can take to become more versatile in their approach. Supervisors can engage in ongoing activities that increase awareness of their own biases, knowledge, and skills (Borders, 2014) and engage in activities to learn about injustice related to structural racism, white privilege, ableism, homophobia, sexism, and other forms of prejudice and bias. Additional activities that build skills in the provision of culturally sensitive supervision and clinical care include training in bystander intervention. Each of these approaches can allow for growth in clinical supervision skills, genetic counseling skills, and others.

Maintaining Confidentiality

Just as there are federal laws related to protected health information, there are analogous regulations related to the privacy of student records. The Family Educational Rights and Privacy Act (FERPA) is a federal law that protects the privacy of student educational records. FERPA prohibits educational institutions from disclosing "personally identifiable information in education records" without written consent. In the context of clinical supervision of genetic counseling students, communication between clinical supervisors and with the graduate program is permitted and expected among individuals with a "legitimate educational interest."

Instances may occur where a student is concerned about the confidentiality of information that they share with a supervisor. Students may struggle to decide how open or vulnerable they should be with a supervisor who ultimately will evaluate them. Students may fear that anything they say is "fair game" for the supervisor to share with others. On the other hand, some students believe that everything they say is completely confidential. The supervisor is responsible for clarifying and upholding confidentiality limits, which can be documented in the clinical supervision agreement, as described below. In some cases, information revealed during the supervision relationship needs to be divulged, especially if it places the student, other students, clinicians, patients, or others at risk.

ADDITIONAL CONSIDERATIONS IN SUPERVISION

Student Anxiety

Some level of anxiety, trepidation, or nervousness can be expected as genetic counseling students are challenged to take on new responsibilities in the clinical setting. In fact, experiencing anxiety in the context of live supervision is "fairly universal" among genetic counseling students (MacFarlane et al., 2016). Sources of student anxiety may include being observed and evaluated, being in a new clinical rotation with different clinical indications, and needing to acclimate to new supervisor's expectations. Anxiety can also result from students feeling pressure to prove they can do what they came to graduate school to do (McCarthy Veach and LeRoy, 2009). This insecurity may also be accompanied by imposter syndrome, in which students, despite objective successes, doubt their abilities and fear being exposed as a fraud or imposter (Kolligian Jr. and Sternberg, 1991).

While anxiety within clinical supervision is to be expected, in some cases, anxiety can negatively impact a student's clinical performance and openness to supervision and feedback (Fall and Sutton, 2004). For some students, the anxiety can lead them to feeling overwhelmed or frozen during a genetic counseling session (MacFarlane et al., 2016). Anxiety can also impact a student's overall physical and mental health and performance across multiple domains of the curriculum.

Attention to the strategies described earlier in this chapter can help to mitigate student anxiety. Additional strategies to address student anxiety include working to strengthen the supervisory relationship by encouraging students to talk about their worries (Suguitan et al., 2019). Supervisors can explore whether students are more focused on their supervisor's evaluation of their "performance" than on their patients (MacFarland et al., 2016; Hendrickson et al., 2002) and then help them shift their focus. Supervisors can also work collaboratively with the student to identify practical approaches to lessen their anxiety. Such modifications may include scaling back expectations or goals for individual sessions, decreasing the number of supervisors a student works with, encouraging or incorporating role plays with supervisors or peers as part of case preparation, working to minimize the complexity and/or diversity of clinical indications, and adjusting the seating arrangement of supervisor and student within a counseling session. Supervisors can also normalize anxiety, including consideration of self-disclosing one own's experiences with anxiety during training. Supervisors and graduate programs can also work to model and/or share mindfulness and relaxation techniques.

Supervisors should also consider whether their supervision style or the structure of the rotation may be contributing to the student's anxiety. For example, is there an appropriate balance of positive and corrective feedback? If the student is working with multiple supervisors, are dramatically discrepant supervision styles and expectations contributing to student anxiety? Are other nonstudent related dynamics or stressors, such as being short-staffed, contributing to a more stressful environment?

Entrustment

Supervisors are encouraged to consider ways that they can provide students with increasing entrustment, including in case preparation, during the session, and in follow-up activities. The first time a supervisor allows a genetic counseling student to take on a given role within a session, the supervisor is demonstrating a willingness to take a chance that things may not proceed as planned or desired. There are several opportunities for supervisors to assess their student's preparedness for new roles, including review and discussion of case outlines and visual aids, case presentations, role plays of parts of sessions, personal observation of sessions, discussions with other supervisors from the clinical rotation, and feedback from the patient. These types of ongoing assessments of a student's knowledge and abilities can help supervisors feel more comfortable allowing students more autonomy, while also maintaining quality patient care.

Once a student is entrusted to conduct part of a session, it can be challenging for supervisors to remain passive, especially if the student's approach differs from the supervisor's own. Supervisors are encouraged to weigh the benefits and risks of letting students continue during a challenging part of a session before intervening. Allowing time for the student to try multiple different strategies and skills, waiting for longer time periods prior to intervening, and eventually intervening less during supervised sessions may ultimately increase student's readiness to navigate challenging situations in their own clinical practice (Lenhart et al., 2023). When it is necessary for a supervisor to intervene within a session, supervisors should consider how they can then shift some of the counseling back to the student. These entrustment decisions can be challenging, but allowing students room to navigate challenges under supervision fosters the skills necessary for independent practice.

Remote Supervision

Remote clinical supervision within the genetic counseling profession became more common in 2020, with the COVID-19 pandemic as the driving force behind a dramatic shift in service delivery models (MacFarlane et al., 2021). Similar strategies can be employed for in-person and remote supervision, though particular attention to some aspects of supervision can be critical. When students and supervisors are working from separate locations, relationship building can require more deliberate effort, as there are typically fewer opportunities for spontaneous interactions. Spending extra time to get know students at the start of a rotation may be helpful, as well as making time for more regular check-ins with the student. When students and supervisors are working from separate locations, supervisors should also consider how to keep students engaged and learning about case management tasks, such as completion of test requisitions, making inquiries to laboratories, and consulting with colleagues. Supervisors should also consider whether students working remotely are missing learning opportunities involving case discussions in clinic staffrooms, observing procedures, and interacting with support staff. If this is the case, strategies to compensate for these missed activities can be considered.

When providing remote supervision of clinical encounters, students and supervisors should establish a plan for how a student can signal they need help during a session. Some supervisors use instant messaging for this purpose. Care should be taken to be sure that this is not a distraction to the student (or patient) and that the messaging application is separate from the application being used to communicate with the patient to avoid inadvertently sending messages to the patient. As supervisors strive to give students more autonomy, they can consider muting themselves and/ or turning off their camera to allow the patient to be more focused on the student. In the author's experience, some students rely more heavily on extra notes and outlines opened on their desktop during remote supervision, so it is helpful to talk to students about what tools, cues, or outlines they are using for virtual care and how this may compare to in-person visits. Developing psychosocial skills during remote supervision may also require more explicit attention given fewer nonverbal cues. Supervisors can encourage students to be more direct in asking patients about how they are feeling. Similarly, if students are receiving feedback virtually, supervisors should consider being more direct when asking students about how they feel about encounters.

Supervision of Other Learners

While clinical supervision of genetic counseling students by genetic counselors is the focus of this chapter, it should be noted that genetic counselors participate in other types of clinical supervision. This may include supervision of more novice members of their clinical team, peer supervision where individuals with comparable levels of experience provide support, guidance, and feedback to each other (Zahm et al., 2008), and supervision of other learners such as medical students, residents, fellows, and others. When providing clinical supervision to nongenetic counseling learners, genetic counselors should be deliberate in considering the specific objectives and goals of the supervision, the individual learner's goals, and the objectives defined by the learner's educational curriculum. For example, supervision of nongenetic counseling learners may be geared towards helping them understand the expertise of genetic counselors and how to best partner with them, rather than developing specific genetic counseling skillsets.

CLINICAL SUPERVISION AGREEMENTS

A written clinical supervision agreement is an important tool that can be used to support many of the principles and suggestions described throughout this chapter, including those related to clarity around goals, day-to-day logistics, expectations, the provision of feedback, roles, and responsibilities in supervision. These agreements can be extremely valuable in orienting students to each site, fostering consistency in what students are told, and providing a "contract" for the supervisory relationship that can be referred to as needed (Hendrickson et al., 2002). To fully reap the benefits, a clinical supervision agreement should be seen as a tool that can open a dialogue between the supervisor(s) and student. Without discussion of its content, the utility of an agreement will be limited. Table 14-3 provides a template for a supervision agreement. For sites with multiple supervisors, all supervisors should be aware of the content of the agreement.

WORKING WITH GRADUATE PROGRAMS

Supervisors should look to the relevant graduate programs for support, structure, and guidance. If you are working with students from multiple graduate programs, it is important to recognize that there are program-specific variations in processes such as those related to summative evaluations and approval of cases and/or case logs. There are also program-specific variations in the expectations for student skill development, observation versus active participation in sessions, hour requirements, etc.

Supervisors should consult with appropriate personnel within their institution to understand the rules and regulations related to supervision of clinical trainees. For example, at some institutions, live clinical supervision of students is required at all times. For clinical sites that are external to a student's graduate program, a formal affiliation agreement or memorandum of understanding should be in place that defines the responsibilities of the clinical site's institution, the graduate program's institution, and the student (ACGC, 2023b). These are formal legal documents that should only be executed with appropriate legal guidance and signed by the individuals with the appropriate level of authority. Individual supervisors should be aware of the content of these agreements to assure that all obligations and requirements are fulfilled by the site, graduate program, and student.

TABLE 14-3. **Clinical supervision agreement template**

General Site Information	Site name, address, phone and fax Phone numbers: Include important lab numbers, patient billing, etc.
Your Supervisor(s)	For each supervisor, consider including information about professional experience and credentials. This might include information about the graduate program they attended, current and past jobs, professional activities, and previous supervision experiences. If there are multiple supervisors at a site, it is important to clarify whether there is one genetic counselor that will oversee the rotation and whether there are any specific topics or questions that should be directed to a particular genetic counselor. Supervisors can also share information about their mentorship style, what they find most rewarding about supervising students, how they look at the student/supervisor relationship, etc. Supervisors can also consider whether there are any dimensions of their own identity that may help build rapport with students, acknowledge their privilege, etc.
Other Members of the Clinical Team	Describe the other individuals that contribute to the overall activities of the site, including other health care providers, schedulers, genetic counseling assistants, and support staff. Include a description of their roles and how the student might anticipate interacting with these individuals.
General Schedule	Describe the general hours of operation of the clinic site, clinic schedule (days, patient slots), and hours that students are expected to be present (on-site or virtually), as well as the hours that supervisors are generally available (on-site or virtually). The schedule of other activities including case conferences, staff meetings, journal clubs, etc. should also be provided, as well as clarification of which activities are required or encouraged. It may be helpful to provide a separate student-specific calendar of activities for each student that covers the time they are rotating.
Communication	Describe any preferences related to communication to and from the student. Is email, in-person, phone, teleconferencing, or instant messaging preferred? Clarify expectations regarding sending, receiving, or responding to emails. Should students expect supervisors to see and/or respond to any emails that come in after-hours? Do the supervisors have an "open-door" policy for students (in-person or electronically) when questions arise in between regularly scheduled meetings?
General Goals for the Rotation	As the supervisor(s), are there specific things you think all genetic counseling students at the site should learn or do? These site-specific goals should be documented, including clarifying any differences related to the goals for a student early verse late in training, as appropriate.
Student Specific Goals for the Rotation	Acknowledge that attention will also be paid to the student's individual clinical goals for the rotation and include "space" for students to insert their personal clinical training goals into the document.

TABLE 14-3. (*Continued*)

Student Specific Needs/Requests for the Rotation	Provide space for any statements that are specific to a particular student or rotation. This can be a good place to detail any adjustments that are necessary related to religious observances, medical or other appointments, learning or other disabilities, chronic illness, schedule conflicts, etc. Explicitly asking all students about such needs will help normalize these conversations and remove the burden from the student to initiate such conversations.
Preparation	Describe how the student can best prepare for the rotation. This might include assigning relevant reading or review of specific resources such as lectures, recordings, or case studies.
Student Clinical Expectations and Responsibilities	Be explicit about what is expected of students and how this might differ for students early versus late in training. Examples where clarity is important are as follows: • Case assignments. Define how and when it is decided which patients a student will see. • Case preparation. Define any specific items the supervisor(s) expect to see during case preparation discussions, such as case outlines or visual aids and when and how those will be reviewed with students. • Counseling roles. Define how the roles a student will take on will be decided. • Case presentations. Describe in what settings the student will be expected to give case presentations and general guidelines. • Documentation. Because multiple types of documentation of genetic counseling services are utilized by genetic counselors (Vandenboom et al., 2018), define any specific requirements related to the format of case documentation and when documentation should be completed. For example, to whom should letters be addressed (patient and/or health care provider), are other providers (for example an attending physician) also contributing to part of the documentation, is there a general expectation regarding the length of the documentation? Some supervisors expect students to use their clinics templates and others discourage this. Let the students know the expectations.
Other Student Expectations	Describe any requirements like participation in journal clubs, outreach activities, or special projects, including the timeline and point person for questions.
Expectations of Supervisors	Describe what students can generally expect from the experience, such as timely and constructive feedback, a supportive, respectful, and inclusive learning environment, and opportunities for growth. It may also be helpful to define what they should not expect from their supervisors, such as personal counseling/psychotherapy, which should generally be sought outside of the clinical supervision arena.

(*continued*)

TABLE 14-3. (*Continued*)

Feedback	Describe when and how formative feedback will be provided after clinical encounters and throughout the rotation. Set the expectation for student self-reflection for individual cases and normalize that constructive feedback will be provided.
Evaluation Process	Define the timeline for discussion of the midpoint and final evaluation. If more than one counselor will be supervising the student, how will the final evaluation be completed and reviewed?
Confidentiality	Describe that a students' evaluations or other information will not be shared with other students or outside supervisors. It may be helpful to discuss how clinical supervisors within the rotation collaborate to best support student learning. For example, let students know if it is typical for supervisors to discuss student progress from week to week. Define limits to confidentiality including as related to instances that violate the legal or ethical standards established by the institution or the genetic counseling profession.
Addressing Concerns	Identify individuals that the students can turn to discuss any questions or concerns that they might not feel comfortable speaking with the main supervisor about, acknowledging the power differential between supervisors and students. Such individuals may be other genetic counselors, other members of the clinical team, or grievance departments within your institution. Students can also be encouraged to bring concerns back to their graduate program.
Guidelines for Patient Care	Describe any specific requirements related to the provision of patient care by trainees, (i.e., continuous live supervision).
Statement of Agreement	Like an informed consent document, students and supervisors should discuss the agreement, clarify questions or concerns, and then sign the agreement indicating their understanding and acceptance of the terms described.

Whether the clinical training site is housed within the same institution as the graduate program or not, the graduate program has several responsibilities to support a successful clinical rotation.

Supervisors should expect the following from the graduate program:

1. General information about the student, including what other rotations, if any, they have completed.
2. Graduate program-specific learning objectives for the placement, often based on whether this is a rotation that is early or late in the student's clinical experience.
3. Graduate program's expectations about students' time commitment and number of cases per rotation.
4. Evaluation tools that will be used in the summative assessment, as well as guidance on how and when these should be completed.

5. Information about how students will track their cases and information about what, if any, role supervisors have in approval of cases.
6. Anonymized student feedback about the supervisory experience, typically only "after a sufficient number of students have contributed" (ACGC, 2023b).
7. Access to training opportunities related to clinical supervision.
8. Ongoing support and availability to discuss any concerns related to the rotation or student.

CONCLUDING THOUGHTS

This chapter describes the roles and responsibilities of genetic counseling students and practicing genetic counselors within the context of clinical supervision. Becoming a competent genetic counselor is a developmental process, as is the process of becoming a skilled clinical supervisor. Ideally, as genetic counselors gain confidence and competence in their supervision abilities, the clinical supervision process can lead to professional growth and satisfaction for both the student and supervisor.

ACKNOWLEDGEMENT

The author would like to acknowledge that the foundation and some of the content for this chapter were derived from the writings of Patricia McCarthy Veach and Bonnie LeRoy who authored the chapter in the first two editions of the textbook.

REFERENCES

Accreditation Council for Genetic Counseling (ACGC). (2023a) ACGC Practice Based Competencies. https://www.gceducation.org/forms-resources Accessed October 20, 2023.

Accreditation Council of Genetic Counseling (ACGC). (2023b) Standards of Accreditation for Graduate Programs in Genetic Counseling. https://www.gceducation.org/forms-resources/ Accessed October 20, 2023.

Ackerman-Barger K, Jacobs NN, Orozco R, & London M. (2021) Addressing microaggressions in academic health: a workshop for inclusive excellence. *MedEdPORTAL* 17:11103. https://doi.org/10.15766/mep_2374-8265.11103.

Anderson LW & Krathwohl DR. (2001) *A Taxonomy for Learning, Teaching, and Assessing: A Revision of Bloom's Taxonomy of Educational Objectives*. Boston, MA: Allyn & Bacon.

Association for Counselor Education (ACE) Supervision Task Force. (2011) ACE Best Practices in Clinical Supervision. https://acesonline.net/wp-content/uploads/2018/11/ACES-Best-Practices-in-Clinical-Supervision-2011.pdf. Accessed June 24, 2024.

Bernard JM & Goodyear RK. (1992) *Fundamentals of Clinical Supervision*. Boston, MA: Allyn and Bacon.

Bernard JM & Goodyear RK. (1997) The discrimination model. In: CE Watkins (ed.) *Handbook of Psychotherapy Supervision* pp. 310–327. Hoboken, NJ: Wiley.

Borders LD. (2014) Best practices in clinical supervision: another step in delineating effective supervision practice. *Am J Psychother* 68(2):151–162.

Caldwell S, Wusik K, He H, et al. (2018) The relationship between the supervisory working alliance and student self-efficacy in genetic counseling training. *J Genet Couns* 27(6):1506–1514. https://doi.org/10.1007/s10897-018-0263-3

Carmichael N, Redlinger-Grosse K, & Birnbaum S. (2020) Conscripted curriculum: the experiences of minority genetic counseling students. *J Genet Couns* 29(2):303–314. https://doi.org/10.1002/jgc4.1260

Darr K, McCarthy Veach P, Wurtmann E, & LeRoy B. (2023) Effects of genetic counselor disabilities on their professional experiences: a qualitative investigation of North American counselors' perceptions. *J Genet Couns* 32(1):235–249. https://doi.org/10.1002/jgc4.1637

Dweck CS. (2006) *Mindset: The New Psychology of Success.* New York, NY: Random House.

Ende J. (1983) Feedback in clinical medical education. *JAMA* 250(6):777–781.

Eubanks Higgins S, Veach PM, MacFarlane IM et al. (2013) Genetic counseling supervisor competencies: results of a Delphi study. *J Genet Couns* 22(1):39–57 https://doi.org/10.1007/s10897-012-9512-z.

The Exeter Group. (2021) National Society of Genetic Counselors Diversity, Equity, and Inclusion Assessment: Report of Findings and Recommendations. https://www.nsgc.org/Policy-Research-and-Publications/Justice-Equity-Diversity-and-Inclusion-JEDI/DEI-Resources. Accessed March 20, 2023.

Fall M & Sutton JM. (2004) *Clinical Supervision: A Handbook for Practitioners.* Boston, MA: Allyn and Bacon.

Hayward J. (2021) Where are all the disabled genetic counsellors? *NSGC Perspectives.* https://www.nxtbook.nxtbooks/nsgc/perspectives_2021q4/index.php#/p/10. Accessed August 5, 2024.

Hendrickson SM, McCarthy Veach P & Leroy BS. (2002) A qualitative investigation of student and supervisor perceptions of live supervision in genetic counselling? *J Genet Couns* 11(1)25–49. https://doi.org/10.1023/A:1013868431533

Kolligian Jr. J & Sternberg RJ. (1991) Perceived fraudulence in young adults: is there an "Imposter Syndrome"? *J Pers Assess* 56(2):308–326. https://doi.org/10.1207/s15327752jpa5602_10

Lenhart K, Yashar BM, Sandhu G, & Marvin M. (2023) Entrustment decision making in genetic counseling supervision: exploring supervisor and student perspectives to enhance training practices. *J Genet Couns* 32(6):1288–1300. https://doi.org/10.1002/jgc4.1712

Lindh HL, Veach PM, Cikanek K, & Leroy BS. (2002) A survey of clinical supervision in genetic counseling; a survey of clinical supervision in genetic counseling. *J Genet Couns* 8(1)23–41. https://doi.org/10.1023/A:1021443100901

MacFarlane IM, McCarthy Veach P, Grier JE, et al. (2016) Effects of anxiety on novice genetic counseling students' experience of supervised clinical rotations. *J Genet Couns* 25(4):742–766. https://doi.org/10.1007/s10897-016-9953-x

MacFarlane I, Johnson A, & Zierhut H. (2021) Changes to the genetic counseling workforce as a result of the COVID-19 pandemic. *J Genet Couns* 30(5):1244–1256. https://doi.org/10.1002/jgc4.1488

McCarthy Veach P & LeRoy BS. (2009) Student supervision: strategies for providing direction, guidance and support. In: WR Uhlmann, JL Schuette, & BM Yashar (eds.) *A Guide to Genetic Counseling* Second Edition, pp. 401–434). Hoboken, NJ: Wiley.

National Society of Genetic Counselors (NSGC). (2022) Professional Status Survey. https://www.nsgc.org/Publications/Professional-Status-Survey/Past-Professional-Status-Surveys Accessed August 5, 2024.

National Society of Genetic Counselors (NSGC). (2024n.d.) Code of Ethics. https://www.nsgc.org/Policy-Research-and-Publications/Code-of-Ethics-Conflict-of-Interest/Code-of-Ethics. Accessed March 20, 2023.

Sayer M, Chaput De Saintonge M, Evans D, & Wood D. (2002) Support for students with academic difficulties. *Med Educ* 36(7):643–650.

Suguitan MD, McCarthy Veach P, LeRoy B et al. (2019) Genetic counseling supervisor strategies: an elaboration of the Reciprocal-Engagement Model of Supervision. *J Genet Couns* 28(3): https://doi.org/10.1002/jgc4.1057

Van den Boom E, Trepanier AM, & Carmany EP. (2018) Assessment of current genetic counselor practices in post-visit written communications to patients. *J Genet Couns* 27(3):681–688. https://doi.org/10.1007/s10897-017-0163-y

Weil J. (2000) Introduction. *J Genet Couns* 9(5):375–378.

Wherley C, Veach PMC, Martyr MA, & LeRoy BS. (2015) Form follows function: a model for clinical supervision of genetic counseling students. *J Genet Couns* 24(5):702–716. https://doi.org/10.1007/s10897-015-9837-5

Zahm KW, McCarthy Veach P, & LeRoy BS. (2008) An investigation of genetic counselor experiences in peer group supervision. *J Genet Couns* 17(3):220–233. https://doi.org/10.1007/s10897-007-9115-2

15

Professional Identities, Evolving Roles, Expanding Opportunities

Erica Ramos

INTRODUCTION

The nature of professional identity and development is a lifetime of evolution and change. To write a chapter that encompasses all that a genetic counseling student or genetic counselor needs to know is impossible, as it is impossible to predict where our field or your career will progress to. However, that is not the purpose of this chapter. The purpose of this chapter is to help you to identify key questions and considerations related to your professional development and to establish the fundamentals and a shared lexicon of professional development. Most importantly, it is to firmly establish that you have agency over how you evolve, both personally and professionally, and the impact that you make as a genetic counselor. Be mindful of the professional environment in which you exist today and how that will change over your career. When you encounter strong leaders and environments in which you thrive, consider what you find appealing or supportive. When you

A Guide to Genetic Counseling, Third Edition. Edited by Vivian Y. Pan, Jane L. Schuette, Karen E. Wain, and Beverly M. Yashar.
© 2025 John Wiley & Sons Ltd. Published 2025 by John Wiley & Sons Ltd.

encounter people or situations that are challenging, consider why you are challenged by them. Sometimes you will find that there are experiences that make you want to change for the better. Other times, you will find that you don't need to change yourself but may benefit from changing your environment. This may include simply being aware that something is someone else's issue, not yours. This cycle of assessment and reassessment, both internally and externally, can help you better navigate the present and progress towards a future where you can flourish—as a person and a professional.

The genetic counseling profession has been successful in many ways. Since the last version of this book was published in 2009, our profession has grown from approximately 2500 genetic counselors to more than 6000 and is projected to double in size in the next ten years. Genetic counseling is consistently ranked as a "best job" (US News, n.d.), the average genetic counselor salary continues to increase, and 86% of genetic counselors report that they are satisfied with the genetic counseling profession (National Society of Genetic Counselors, 2023a). Historically, genetic counselors have had very low rates of unemployment or part-time employment except for by choice. However, economic downturns (e.g., the Great Recession of 2007–2009), national emergencies (e.g., the COVID19 pandemic in 2020), and volatility in the biotechnology and laboratory sectors (e.g., 2023–2024) have resulted in furloughs and/or reductions in force/layoffs and challenges in finding employment at various times in our history. In 2008, only 18% of respondents to the National Society of Genetic Counselors (NSGC) Professional Status Survey (PSS) defined their role as nondirect patient care (National Society of Genetic Counselors, 2009). In 2023, that number increased to 27%, with an additional 20% reporting a mixed position. While the percentages varied by position, roles reported across all position types included, but were not limited to, education/teaching, research, customer service/client support, medical writing, variant interpretation, business development, project management, and marketing (National Society of Genetic Counselors, 2023a). Our roles and opportunities have expanded in many interesting ways, most notably in the way that genetic counselors are now embedded in all stages of a patient's genetics journey, including laboratory testing, research, and clinical trials.

THE BENEFITS AND CHALLENGES OF PROFESSIONAL IDENTITY, CONDUCT, AND PROFESSIONALISM

It has been exciting to see the genetic counseling profession grow and develop in such a powerful way, and it is not surprising that many genetic counselors feel a strong connection to the profession and the opportunities it holds. This rapid growth and expansion, pushing the limits of how we apply our skills, is one of many contributors to our professional identity.

Adams et al. define professional identity as "the attitudes, values, knowledge, beliefs and skills shared with others within a professional group" (Adams et al., 2006).

Heled and Davidovitch highlight the critical point that "professional identity has two interconnected components: the interpersonal (group professional identity) which relates to the culture, knowledge, skills, values and beliefs of a profession that the individual has acquired; and the intrapersonal (personal professional identity) which considers the individual's perception of themselves in the context of their profession" (Heled and Davidovitch, 2021). Professional identity can be a valuable part of one's career, particularly personal professional identity as it relates to finding self-meaning connected with one's work (Olesen, 2001). The most important aspects of one's interpersonal professional identity are the ability to self-reflect, master a body of knowledge, practice ethically, display professionalism, and have a lifelong intention to participate in continuing education. However, it is also important to recognize the adverse outcomes that can stem from the establishment of a rigid group professional identity.

The Accreditation Council of Genetic Counseling (ACGC) lays out "the practice-based competencies that an entry-level provider must demonstrate to successfully practice as a genetic counselor" (Accreditation Council for Genetic Counseling, 2019). While genetic counselors have shared training and certification requirements aligned to these competencies and may have similar knowledge and skills, when we graduate our divergent paths in our professional careers create differences and disparities in our knowledge and skillsets over time. As a result, some of these items cease to be part of the professional identity of many individuals over time. For example, a new graduate may strongly identify with the competency of "Integrate knowledge of psychosocial aspects of conditions with a genetic component to promote client wellbeing" because of the intense focus on clinical cases during training. However, a genetic counselor that transitions to a job centered in variant curation for a clinical laboratory may find themselves less tied to that piece of identity over time if it ceases to be part of their daily work.

Additionally, group professional identity is often adapted to highlight the characteristics of the majority. The genetic counseling profession has been historically homogeneous, and although we have seen small improvements in diversity, it remains so today. Per the 2023 PSS, most genetic counselors identify as women (93%), straight/heterosexual (86%), white and non-Hispanic (89%), without a disability (81%), and under age 40 (68%) (National Society of Genetic Counselors, 2023a). Unfortunately, this homogeneity has led to a harmful and exclusionary image of a genetic counselor. In 2020, NSGC engaged with The Exeter Group to conduct an organizational assessment of NSGC and the genetic counseling profession in service of NSGC's diversity, equity, and inclusion (DEI) efforts. A theme that arose was "pressure to fit the mold" with focus group participants highlighting how personality traits ("type A"), physical appearance ("tall, blond, skinny"), and even clothing choices ("a cardigan and pearls") have become both stereotype and culture for genetic counselors (The Exeter Group, 2021). While these personal characteristics are not a problem, they become problematic when they are tightly linked and conflated with professional identity.

Using high-level and limited language to define our group professional identity creates more room for inclusion of different roles, positions, and people. In her 2012 Presidential Address, Brenda Finucane highlighted work from NSGC's Core Skills Task Force to "identify key attributes of genetic counselors," which she summarized as:

- *Deep and broad knowledge of genetics*
- *Ability to tailor, translate and communicate complex information in a simple, relevant way for a broad range of audiences*
- *Strong interpersonal skills, emotional intelligence, and self-awareness*
- *Ability to dissect and analyze a complex problem*
- *Research skills*
- *In-depth knowledge of healthcare delivery.*

Finucane goes on to state, "When I look at these attributes, I can see why so many of us who have gone in different professional directions still maintain our identities as genetic counselors" (Finucane, 2012). This type of group professional identity is deeply tied to what we do and the skills that we have rather than who we are. Who we are is also critical and each individual's identity contributes to a more successful profession, but these qualities and characteristics should neither be standardized nor excluded at the group level.

While one's identity as a genetic counselor may remain important throughout one's career, personal professional identity will change over time, shaped by one's experience with each role, job, manager, and employer. Some genetic counselors may pursue new roles that leverage their genetic counseling training, and their professional identity may evolve to align more closely to characteristics tightly tied to other professions, such as business development or public health. For others, they may feel tightly linked to the genetic counseling profession at all stages in their career. Regardless, we are all genetic counselors.

Professional Conduct

Professional conduct can be considered in two key ways. The first is the standard for how an individual works with colleagues, clients/patients, communities, and others while doing their job. The second includes the official rules and regulations of the professional bodies for a particular profession. Multiple resources guide the professional conduct of genetic counselors. In addition to the specific guidelines of an employer or institution, the NSGC, American Board of Genetic Counselors (ABGC), Canadian Association of Genetic Counsellors, state licensure regulations, and others define the boundaries of professional conduct.

The NSGC Code of Ethics, adopted in 1992 and revised in 2017, helps to define what good professional conduct of genetic counselors looks like. Genetic counselors value competence, integrity, dignity, and self-respect in themselves as well as in each other. Genetic counselors' relationships with other genetic counselors, genetic counseling students, and health professionals from other disciplines are based on mutual respect, caring, cooperation, support, and a shared loyalty to their professional goals. The relationships of genetic counselors to segments of society or to society as a whole include interest and participation in activities with the goal of promoting societal wellbeing. Finally, the counselor–client relationship requires respect for autonomy, informed decision-making, privacy, and respectful provision of services regardless of a client's background or beliefs. This document is not intended to be a comprehensive list of all aspects of professional conduct, nor is it sufficient to cover the scope of all roles that genetic counselors will take in their careers. It is not prescriptive, but rather "a document that attempts to clarify and guide the conduct of a professional so that the goals and values of the profession are best served."

Certification and recertification, and state licensure, create standards for ongoing professional education and conduct and validate that a genetic counselor has achieved a level of education and knowledge deemed necessary for high-quality patient care. Board certification, regardless of the certifying body, and state licensure also contribute to professional conduct standards and regulation. Although not all jobs performed by genetic counselors require board certification, most genetic counselors maintain their certification throughout their career. In the US, the ABGC not only creates the guidelines for that ongoing education, but also maintains The Disciplinary Review Committee, "responsible for review of matters stemming from improper behavior, fraudulent credentials, and/or legal, regulatory and credentialing actions" (American Board of Genetic Counseling, 2019). State licensure sets a professional standard and provides at least a baseline expectation for the quality of services rendered. Licensure serves as one means of protecting public health, safety, and welfare by ensuring a standard of practice, education, and qualification. State licensure also defines the scope of practice for genetic counselors within that state and creates guidelines for the suspension and/or revocation of a license. As such, certification and licensure are two mechanisms by which some significant breeches in professional conduct can be addressed. This is primarily impactful for genetic counselors who are seeing patients; however, even employers of genetic counselors without patient-facing activities tend to look at certification especially as optimal or required.

Professional Conduct and "Professionalism"

Professionalism has multiple definitions encompassing a wide range of activities and attributes and is often used interchangeably with professional conduct. For clarity, professional conduct is specific to a profession, whereas professionalism tends to be a more nebulous concept that includes standards of professional behavior that are universally applied regardless of the job or career. Adhering to professional conduct relevant to your specific role as a genetic counselor and/or any role in a professional environment helps to create a safe and appropriate environment to engage with patients, co-workers, and others. However, there are oppressive expectations encapsulated in interpretations of "professionalism" that must be assessed critically.

Multiple websites reference definitions of professionalism from Merriam-Webster as "the skill, good judgment and polite behavior that is expected from a person who is trained to do a job well" and "the conduct, aims, or qualities that characterize or mark a profession or a professional person" (as of July 2016, per Rowan-Cabarrus Community College, 2024). Interestingly, the first of the two definitions is no longer found on the Merriam-Webster website (Merriam-Webster, n.d.) and this shift is consistent with the fact that there are many viewpoints on the meaning of professionalism. The term has been co-opted to create standards that are centered on values of the historical majority of the business world—namely white, Western, straight, cis-gender men with no disabilities. In a piece on "professionalism standards" that highlights their adverse impact on people from populations that have been marginalized, Aysa Gray states that this "systemic, institutionalized centering of whiteness ... explicitly and implicitly privileges whiteness and discriminates against non-Western and non-white professionalism standards related to dress code, speech, work style, and timeliness" (Gray, 2019). Biases of individuals based on "non-white sounding" names, language, vocabulary, gender, and accents are all given as examples of when falling outside of "the norm" can inhibit a person's work and career opportunities. Physical characteristics, including natural hairstyles, piercings, and tattoos, whether related to an individual's culture or self-expression, are subject to a negative interpretation of "professionalism."

These issues have been validated by individuals from communities that have been marginalized who have shared their experiences in the workplace. Specifically, many report that they are not able to work as their authentic selves if they want to be successful in their chosen careers. One study found that "more than 35 percent of African-Americans and Hispanics and 45 percent of Asians, for instance, say they 'need to compromise their authenticity' to conform to their company's standards of demeanor or style" (Hewlett et al., 2012). The CROWN Research Study (Creating a Respectful and Open Workplace for Natural Hair), which surveyed approximately 1000 Black women and 1000 non-Black women (95% white), found that Black women were 30% more frequently the recipients of grooming policies and 80% more likely to agree with the statement "I have to change my hair from its natural state to fit in at the office" (JOY Collective, 2019). Stemming from these findings, the CROWN Act was signed into California state law in July 2019 and prohibits discrimination by employers and schools, including implementing or enforcing grooming standards that do not allow for natural or protective hairstyles. Similar laws have been enacted in more than a dozen states and, as of March 2022, a federal version of the CROWN Act passed the House of Representatives (CROWN Coalition, n.d.).

The ableist roots in the concept of professionalism have also been critiqued by the disability community. Dr. Shane Neilson, MD, PhD details her experience as a student and with colleagues in the medical community as an individual with a chronic illness and notes that expectations of professionalism can be a bigger issue when working in the medical profession. As a student, she recalls, "Despite the intense bursts of work, I received the predictable feedback applied to a student looking and sounding like me in that era in which the rise of professionalism meant that I was characterized as bad, a problem student" (Neilson, 2020). This has also been studied in the patient–physician relationship regarding how a patient perceives the professionalism of their physician. Jarus et al. (2020) surveyed patients with and without disabilities about how they would imagine the difference in engaging with a disabled versus a nondisabled physician. All patients felt that disabled physicians would be more client-centered and empathetic. Those with disabilities felt that the physician would be a role model for them, and that it would help balance the power dynamics between patient and physician. However, when addressing professionalism, the patients all expressed a concept that the authors deemed "as long as ...". More specifically, the authors summarize, "All participants said they could not foresee the professional behaviour of a healthcare provider being negatively impacted by a disability as long as they are licensed, and there was a good fit between their role, the setting, and the disability." The disabled patients identified another "as long as ...": "that as long as the client does not hold stigma towards disabilities, then the clinician will be perceived as professional" (Jarus et al., 2020). This "as long as ..." mentality likely holds for patients who have providers who are part of the LGBTQIA+ community, come from racial or ethnic minority groups, are immigrants, have language differences, or have other identities that have historically been marginalized.

The issues surrounding professionalism have surfaced in the genetic counseling community as well. Multiple genetic counselors shared their negative experiences related to hair style and piercing "policing" in a series of tweets in response to the ABGC's #ABGCListens Twitter initiative (Bryana Rivers [@GcBry], 2020). Genetic counselors have also written profound posts about how problematic professionalism standards, requirements to conform to binary dress codes, and perceptions of personal relationships result in an erasure of integral parts of the personhood of LGBTQIA+ individuals (Berro, 2019; Zayhowski and Sheridan, 2022). For the first time, the NSGC 2022 PSS assessed questions of inclusivity and belonging for individual groups with minoritized identities, such as those of racial and ethnic minority groups, the LGBTQIA+ community (specifically related to sexual orientation and gender identity), and the disability community. Specifically for the questions "I can be myself without having to compromise or hide any part of who I am" and "people from all backgrounds have equal opportunities to succeed" as they relate to the genetic counseling profession, respondents from each of the groups above ranked these as significantly lower than those in the majority (National Society of Genetic Counselors, 2022).

A 2020 publication reviewed positive and negative professionalism experiences of 268 genetic counselors from the graduating classes of 2015–2019, as they were asked to reflect on their graduate school experience. While the majority expressed satisfaction with their graduate school experience and every participant recalled empathetic and respectful interactions, many negative behaviors were also reported. When asked if they had experienced specific negative behaviors, seen these negative behaviors demonstrated towards another, or both, students reported scenarios where they or others were "made to feel like a burden when participating in a clinic as a student," "publicly embarrassed or humiliated," "subjected to negative or offensive behavior based on your personal beliefs or personal characteristics other than gender, race/ethnicity, or sexual orientation," "subjected to racially or ethnically offensive remarks/names," and "subjected to offensive sexist remarks/names." Equally concerning is that "Of the 158 individuals who experienced or saw an inappropriate behavior, 64.6% did not report inappropriate behaviors to any authority, agency, or program leadership" (Aamodt et al., 2021).

Given the biases inherent in standards of "professionalism," awareness and intolerance of abusive or discriminatory behaviors is critical. As a community, we must be aware that students and colleagues are experiencing these abusive behaviors and create reliable and safe ways for them to be confronted. As we strive to create a diverse, inclusive environment, from the application period through a genetic counselor's career, we must apply standards of professional conduct with careful awareness to their origins and impact. As we believe that the profession of genetic counseling benefits from members who express their whole, authentic selves, we must support their diversity in gender, sexuality, culture, disability, and other attributes that are part of that whole.

As you reflect on this section:

- Consider what you see as the group professional identity of genetic counselors. Are there components that might be exclusionary? If so, how can you take steps to change those things?
- Reflect on any personal professional identities that you may have had in the past or have today. What aspects of your personhood do you want to have reflected in your work? How has that changed based on your personal development or the evolution of the jobs that you've held?
- Think about whether you've experienced situations where standards of professionalism kept you or someone around you from authentically expressing yourself/themselves in your work environment. How did that feel? Are there standards of professionalism that should change? How would you define professionalism?

PROFESSIONAL DEVELOPMENT, FULFILMENT, AND ADVANCEMENT

Professional development is important within the individual genetic counselor's place of employment, both for personal fulfillment and to achieve professional goals. The skills genetic counselors possess can be applied in many ways across the genetic counseling ecosystem and these opportunities are key to genetic counselor satisfaction. Genetic counselors rank, intellectual stimulation, learning opportunities, diversity of roles, and personal and professional growth fall amongst the items with the highest satisfaction regardless of role (Figure 15-1).

While these data help us to quantify the profession's satisfaction across different metrics, no single item is necessary or sufficient to generate satisfaction, fulfillment, or advancement for any individual. As the roles that genetic counselors fill have evolved and broadened, the opportunities for growth are vaster than ever. That is great news for those pursuing a career in genetic counseling or advancing their careers, but it can be overwhelming as well. While we summarize some of

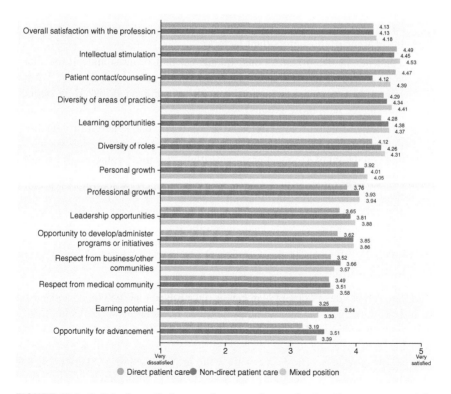

FIGURE 15-1. *Satisfaction with the genetic counseling profession. Figure courtesy of the National Society of Genetic Counselors, 2022 Professional Status Survey (Professional Diversity, Inclusion and Satisfaction)*

the many paths that can lead to professional fulfillment and advancement, it is an individual journey that will likely take many twists and turns over a career and requires careful consideration of the advantages and disadvantages of each path and one's own values and goals.

As you read this next section:

- Consider the items in Figure 15-1. What areas are important to you? What areas feel less critical for your fulfillment? What have you seen or heard from other genetic counselors who may be further along in their careers?

- How have you planned for your career? Consider making a two- or five-year plan, or even a list of skills, experiences, interests, and job requirements that you would prioritize for your next job.

- Think about the importance of development and fulfillment in your professional environment. What is most important to you in a job? In your career? How can you make sure that a potential job will meet those standards? Can other things, like volunteerism and networking connections, fulfill some of those important factors?

- Think about the organizations, initiatives, and professional efforts that you've read about in this book. What efforts are you drawn to? What efforts do you envision supporting with your unique skills? How might you engage with those groups?

- Create your networking circles. Who have you encountered in your life that might help you get questions answered or get an introduction to someone you would like to meet professionally? Who could you support in their networking?

- Reflect on managers, mentors, and/or leaders that you've had in the past. If you had a positive experience, what made it good for you? If you had a negative experience, what made it bad for you?

Career Planning

Creating a career development plan can be a useful exercise as you consider your path through the genetic counseling profession. There are many ways to create a plan. Some people find the exercise of creating a two-, five-, or ten-year plan to be valuable, even when there will likely be shifts as time goes on. Long-term planning allows you to see how you want your priorities, skills, experiences, and opportunities to evolve over time given your current position and how your career may change with your personal life. Layering in aspects of your personal life can help you create a plan that is balanced and feasible, such as including where you might live, how you might want to raise your children, or what financial priorities you have. Revisiting and revising these plans require that you reassess your goals and consider how you and your priorities may have changed over time. For others, their career plan may be more nebulous. You may not have a specific timeframe in which you want to accomplish steps in your career but have a checklist of experiences or skills that you want to acquire over time. While a timeline can be useful in putting those things in a logical order, the order may be less important to you. Regardless of your approach, this is an opportunity for self-exploration that increases in value if you do it regularly and mindfully. There are many templates for career development and career action plans available online, including those that merge short-, mid-, and long-term goals and your personal and professional goals. Also consider getting feedback from mentors, colleagues, and people who are doing the jobs that you are interested in to make sure that you are considering as many aspects of your career as possible.

Career planning can be particularly valuable when you are considering or actively seeking a change in your career, whether you're evaluating a promotion, an opportunity with a new employer, or if you are just ready for something new due to burnout, a lack of challenges, feeling undervalued, or your personal priorities. You may find that you are not fulfilled in your current role, even though you once were. Throughout your career, you will become a different person with different priorities and interests. Aligning these priorities with changes to your existing role or a bigger change can help prevent burnout, frustration, and a lack of fulfillment.

Promotion

Regardless of the institution or role, the first opportunity for advancement for many is promotion within their current place of employment. Generally, there are two key components to assessing someone for a promotion: can the person do the job; and is there a need to have someone at that level or role? The first addresses whether the individual is a strong candidate to advance into a role with more responsibility and greater complexity. The second is sometimes ignored, but despite someone's readiness for promotion, there may not be an identified reason to promote into a higher role. This disparity can lead to disappointment when people know that they want and can do the job that is next on the ladder, but the opportunity has not been solidified.

In some cases, an employee may see the need for a higher-level role before the employer. This provides an opportunity to create this position by collecting data about why the position is needed, including the benefits that the position would bring to the organization and the risks if that position weren't created. If the position is not mapped to an existing career ladder, the skills, knowledge, achievements, and experience that the role requires should also be documented. Finally, you can advocate for yourself to fill this role, either now or in the future. One career coaching company lays out a four-step approach to prepare yourself for a promotion: clarify expectations; ask for feedback; track and report on your success; and discuss goals, strengths, and motivators (Marlow Group Inc., n.d.).

This can be an intimidating process and following these steps can help you break it down into smaller, more manageable pieces.

Career ladders typically define the specific set of skills, activities, and requirements needed to satisfy a particular level in a work setting. Career ladders can be specific and documented or may be subject to institutional knowledge where "you know it when you see it." Documented career ladders are beneficial when they create quantitative measures of skills and responsibilities that someone would have to meet to be eligible for that level or role but must be carefully structured either within a department or across an institution. Kofman et al. highlight their experience in developing a career ladder for genetic counselors across the institution, regardless of role. Their ladder had four steps (i.e., GCI, GCII, GCIII, GCIV) and up to three stages at each level (e.g., Basic, Intermediate, Advanced). Steps included "aspects of patient care, student training, professional development, or mentorship. Each of these individual steps requires different degrees of professional expertise and skills in a specific area." Compensation bands were assigned to each step and level and a committee was formed to support the annual review process, where the committee would review a self-assessment by the genetic counselor and an optional recommendation for promotion from a supervisor or physician, and vote for what step and level the counselor will stay at or move to (Kofman et al., 2016).

A more modern approach to the career ladder is the career lattice. The purpose of defining clear skills, goals, and activities remains the same but a career lattice allows for lateral and diagonal career advancement. For some genetic counselors and companies, this is an optimal way of considering career growth as roles for genetic counselors have expanded in business, marketing, market development, product management, project management, and others, and these roles may not be the first that genetic counselors have in an organization. Additionally, this approach can help people visualize movement from one specialty area to another in patient-facing roles. For instance, the leveling of a position might not change when someone moves from a cancer to cardio genetic counseling role (i.e., lateral movement). However, in this example, the knowledge base is not the same and additional work may need to occur for a genetic counselor to make that transition.

For some individuals, neither of these models will be quite the right fit. The first person to explore a new position leveraging their genetic counseling skills will be leading the way for others but has to clear that path themselves. Additionally, this will look different from employer to employer. The critical pieces for genetic counselors are to be aware of the different paths to advancement, know what they are for their employer or prospective employer, and consider how to use them for their career growth.

Faculty Appointments

One specific type of advancement in academic settings is the opportunity for faculty appointments. According to the 2023 NSGC PSS, 25% of respondents hold a faculty appointment. Among those with faculty appointments, 60% are at their institution of employment and the rest are at an institution other than where they are employed (National Society of Genetic Counselors, 2023a).

Faculty appointments can be tenure-track or nontenure-track, primary or adjunct. At your institution, faculty appointments may not be offered, but if you regularly teach students at another institution, you may qualify there for an adjunct appointment. Generally, academic institutions can appoint faculty on instructional, clinical, or research track (these may be identified by other names at your institution). Faculty appointments may be granted at the time of hire or later in your career. Faculty appointments are based on your professional track record and can take into consideration clinical work, teaching, scholarship, service (organizational and institutional committees, administrative and leadership positions), and publications. Associate- and Professor-level faculty appointments generally require a regional or national reputation and depend on evaluations from impartial external sources. There will be set expectations for faculty appointments, reappointments, and promotion that will vary depending on the faculty track and the institution.

The requirements and rewards of a faculty path are person- and institution-dependent. Faculty status can be desirable because it brings opportunities for participation in campus governance, educational programs, continuous appointment in a nontenure stream, sabbaticals, and higher salaries. Counselors who are interested in scholarship and service, want to improve the teaching quality of their institution, or advocate for their clinical service and the genetic counseling profession within their institution may find that faculty status helps them reach these goals. However, the ability to be granted faculty status is highly variable. Some institutions have existing paths for genetic counselors, either in clinical or nonclinical paths. At other institutions, genetic counselors may have to advocate for faculty appointments and the requirements, timing, and availability of faculty appointments are highly dependent on the division or department that you work in. For those interested in faculty paths, leveraging your institution's faculty career center and talking with your departmental chair and dean can help you to be aware of the pathways for promotion, as well as the benefits and limitations of these roles.

On-The-Job or Academic Training

The multidisciplinary nature of genetic counseling provides many avenues for professional development. Some genetic counselors find that their graduate training sufficiently equips them to learn new material through self-study or other means, while others may take courses, obtain a second Master's, or a more advanced degree. Genetic counselors have pursued advanced education in bioethics, business, public health, policy, psychology, sociology, and many other disciplines. For example, a genetic counselor might obtain a Master's degree in marriage and family counseling as a means of expanding their practice to include long-term psychotherapy for individuals and families dealing with genetic disorders. Another might obtain a Master of Business Administration (MBA) to learn the skills to start their own genetic counseling services company. Overall, PhDs in various related fields and Masters of Public Health (MPH) and MBA degrees are the most frequently pursued by genetic counselors (National Society of Genetic Counselors, 2023a).

While there has been concern that advanced degrees will cause competition with Master's prepared genetic counselors, a study by Wallace et al. suggested that there is an employment niche for individuals who have a PhD in genetic counseling that is complementary to those with a Master's degree (Wallace et al., 2008). PhD opportunities for genetic counselors have grown over time and about 3% of genetic counselors have PhDs (National Society of Genetic Counselors, 2023a). In response to a desire from some students to start on the PhD track from the beginning, several institutions now offer a PhD in Human Genetics with a focus in genetic counseling as single or dual degree programs. Some genetic counselors return to school for their PhD after getting their genetic counseling degree, often while working. In a 2007 study of genetic counselors with PhDs, genetic counselors were asked about motivations for pursuing a PhD after their Master's. The top reasons noted were a desire to do research and to ensure new and more flexible job opportunities. Genetic counselors with PhDs, regardless of the order in which they received their degrees, reported the key differences in work activities between a genetic counselor with a PhD and a Master's-level genetic counselor were an increase in research (87% versus 31%) and teaching (77% versus 61%). When asked about the advantages of a doctoral degree, 58% (18/31) reported greater knowledge and skills, 55% (17/31) reported performing research, 48% (15/31) reported additional opportunities in leadership and academia, 35% (11/31) reported greater respect and recognition, and 16% (5/31) reported tenure eligibility or greater autonomy (Atzinger et al., 2007). For genetic counselors interested in this path, X and other social media platforms are excellent places to connect with others working on or with PhDs and get practical feedback on the opportunities and challenges of this endeavor.

The development of a genetic counseling PhD and/or clinical doctorate (ClinD) has been assessed extensively as a supplement to PhDs in other fields. The critical issues in this debate have been related to employability and the practicality of having an advanced degree for genetic counselors, including the potential negative impact of changing from a profession in which the Master's is the entry-level degree (i.e., genetic counselors would be required to have a ClinD as the standard). NSGC convened a task force to study the impact of having the ClinD as the entry-level degree for genetic counseling versus as an optional advanced degree. Of the 1956 practicing counselors and 225 students surveyed by the task force, 81.1% (1753/2161) of respondents advocated "maintaining the Master's degree as the current entry level and terminal degree at this time." The survey also highlighted concerns about potential barriers for individuals practicing with Master's degrees if the ClinD became the standard, including the time and expense of "catching up" by going back to school to get a ClinD, attrition of practicing counselors who chose not to get a ClinD, and limitations in training options (Nagy et al., 2015).

These concerns were echoed by the program directors who reported that 18 of the 27 programs reviewed would close or be at risk to close (Reiser et al., 2015) and the general consensus has been not to replace the Master's with a ClinD as the entry-level or terminal degree.

Certificate programs can supplement on-the-job training without requiring an expensive, time-consuming commitment to ongoing education. Many provide very targeted training in a short period of time and can be accessed through large e-Learning platforms, such as Coursera, Udemy, and edX. Many are free, and those that aren't are often a few hundred dollars or less per course. Certificates in business classes, technology skills (e.g., coding), and process engineering (e.g., Lean Six Sigma) are popular with genetic counselors who are working in the corporate space, but can also have benefits for counselors managing clinics, developing and growing programs, and other project/program leaders. Additionally, there are certificate programs to enhance comfort and knowledge for specific roles, like variant curation/variant science, which are aligned with genetic counseling skillsets but for which people may have had variable degrees of formal training.

Obtaining an additional academic degree is not the only way to advance or gain new skillsets. Many genetic counselors working in product management/development, marketing, market development, business development, and sales did not learn the tricks of their trades in a classroom. Rather, they have sought opportunities in these areas and acquired the needed knowledge, often with the opportunity to learn on the job. By leveraging their genetic counseling skills, the roles they step into often intersect with the counselor, patient, and family journey in genetics, but may require additional training for success. This training will vary by role and by company type. The technology, culture, pace, and even lexicon of the corporate world, particularly in start-ups, can be much different from that of academic, clinical, and even large company employers (Rabideau et al., 2016).

The evolution of the typical genetic counseling position is ongoing. A 2011 study reviewing roles of laboratory genetic counselors reported that the two most common roles were serving as customer liaison (95%) and test results delivery (88%). While 44.2% reported signing lab reports, the roles of "variant interpretation" or "variant classification" do not appear in the paper (Christian et al., 2012). Just five years later, a follow-up study found that at least 90.9% of respondents reported the roles of "interpretation and result reporting" and at least 88.9% reported a role of "test development/performance" with varying degrees of frequency across all lab types (molecular, cytogenetics, biochemical, maternal serum, newborn screening, and hospital send-out) (Waltman et al., 2016). Some of this shift in roles is likely due to the rapid growth of next-generation sequencing (Swanson et al., 2014). In response, many training programs dedicate time to skill development in relevant areas such as variant interpretation.

It's also important to note that genetic counselors learn more than new skills on the job. Runyon et al. highlight that genetic counselors report that they gained self-efficacy (the belief in one's ability to succeed in a specific situation or with a specific task); a stronger understanding of the intersection of professional and personal life experiences and how they influence each other; releasing control and managing values, biases, and opinions; assessing and managing job satisfaction; and finding comfort in uncertainty. The paper also provides a summary of advice for students just starting in their careers, although it has valuable guidance for people at all stages (Table 15-1) (Runyon et al., 2010).

TABLE 15-1. **What advice would you give to genetic counseling students just starting their career?**

Theme	Representative Quote
Remain Flexible	"Be open to new experiences and not to be rigid. If you learned something one way it does not necessarily mean it's the only way to do things."
Be Psychosocially Focused	"When in school one might feel that they have to learn all the 'facts' of genetic counseling—all the medical details. When you've been practicing awhile you realize that one might have it backwards, that is ... medical details you can always look up. It's the counseling/ psychological/sensitivity issues you most need to work on in school and after."
Learn from Patients	"Be humble and open to learning just as much from the individuals and families you see as you do from your professional colleagues and the so-called 'experts.'"
Cultivate Empathy	"Never take a situation for granted and always place the patient first ... each encounter you have with a patient can make a lasting impression on them (i.e., will they view themselves as a 'mutant' or a 'carrier'). As a student, there are times to leave your 'agenda' alone and really concentrate on the patient as a person ... as a sister with cancer ... or a mother with a baby with a birth defect. Empathy and listening go a long way in the long-term wellbeing for the patient."
Find a Mentor	"Find a mentor and, in turn, mentor others as you gain more experience. Share what you know with peers. Give freely of yourself so others may grow."
Network	"Find colleagues, former classmates, GCs elsewhere with whom you can share your experiences and learn from them ..."
Learn from Other Staff Members	"Utilize case conferences and discussions with other genetic counselors to the fullest extent possible, it builds your confidence in how you're handling your own cases, and allows a great deal of additional exposure and lessons from other people's cases."
Find Satisfying Work	"Don't sell yourself short on your salary, job benefits, and respect that you should have/earn from those who work with you. Genetic counselors may not have the most recognized, coveted jobs, but they are very important. Always accept the praise and recognition you are given by patients and colleagues."
Try Something New	"Learn how to network, negotiate, do administrative tasks, write grants, etc. Things that are not immediately relevant to clinical counseling, but are incredibly relevant to career-building. Assume that no job is safe and keep in mind that the delivery of genetic medicine is rapidly changing."

TABLE 15-1. (*Continued*)

Anticipate Obstacles to Job Satisfaction	"In school you often learn about 'ideal' genetic counseling, or what you should do or expect in a session and job with appropriate time, staff support, value in your skills, and political climate. Unfortunately, the working world is not always ideal and we must work hard to do what we can for our patients, even if it is not what we would consider ideal or complete genetic counseling. Take small steps, and many of these things may come with time. Be patient!"
Get Help When You Need It	"This is pretty trite, but I think it is very important. Don't be afraid to ask questions and don't be afraid to say 'I don't know, but I'll look it up and get back to you.' The longer I work, the more it seems like people who don't ask questions are the ones who need to ask them the most!"
Find Your Way	"You are only 'half baked' when you get out of graduate school. You have a skillset, but that skillset undergoes considerably more refinement in your first years of practice."
Be Personally Accountable	"Good counselors continue to evaluate themselves and their handling of cases throughout their careers. Not all cases will go well."

Volunteerism

Our profession has a long strong history of volunteerism to advance the goals of genetic counselors and genetic counseling. Volunteering with genetic counseling professional organizations, at local, state, or national level, also creates an excellent opportunity for fulfillment and career advancement.

There are many opportunities to volunteer for roles in the major professional genetics organizations. A "Call for Volunteers" is generally sent out by each organization on an annual basis via email and social media, or when specific roles need to be filled. The roles for volunteers can vary from a very focused and shorter-term effort (e.g., writing a blog post or speaking in a webinar) to a multi-year leadership role with a broad scope (e.g., a committee chair or a Board of Directors position). One benefit to responding for some annual "Call for Volunteers" is that the application will give you the chance to highlight your skills and interests without requiring that you specifically request a particular volunteer opportunity. The organization will take your answers and match them to specific efforts that need support. However, if there is a committee, special interest group, webinar, or other effort that you have a specific interest in, you can consider reaching out to a member or leader in that group to express your interest.

There have been many articles written about the benefits of volunteering broadly but volunteering in your profession may have additional advantages. It enables you to widen your professional network and meet fellow genetics specialists who may share a specific set of interests or passions. It can be an opportunity to create relationships with individuals who may work where you want to work or do the job that you want to do, but without the specific weight of creating a relationship just for that purpose.

Volunteerism does not have to be limited to our professional organizations. Patient support and advocacy groups and other genetics interest groups can gain huge benefit from the genetics and clinical expertise that genetic counselors possess. If there is a condition that you are particularly interested in or an advocacy group that moves you, reach out through their website or social media to introduce yourself and ask how you might be able to support their work.

Many genetic counselors also volunteer their time in support of genetic counseling training programs. Working with programs may begin as a volunteer opportunity and then expand to paid work. Roles with training programs may include supervising students, lecturing, participating on admissions panels and other committees, or providing general support to the students of a program. Another important volunteer opportunity is to support people who are interested in becoming genetic counselors. Engaging with them on social media, having a 30-minute call for them to talk to you about your job, mentoring a student (discussed in more detail below), or, if you are able, letting them shadow you with patients or at your job are all ways to volunteer your time to improve the future of the genetic counseling profession.

While volunteerism has been a strong contributor to the success of the genetic counseling profession, it is also important to view volunteerism through the lens of equity and systemic bias. Disparities in the ability to volunteer time and energy must be addressed and, while the onus to create an inclusive and equitable volunteer structure is on the organization, we can all help focus attention on barriers to an inclusive volunteer environment, including limitations on time, fear of tokenism, biases in awareness of volunteer opportunities, and financial barriers (Johnson, 2021).

Volunteer efforts take varying amounts of time, and everyone must determine for themselves how to balance those efforts with other commitments in their lives, including paid opportunities to support the genetic counseling profession. In the 2023 PSS, 69% of respondents reported that their employers supported work on professional activities during work hours. This was less common in roles that were purely patient facing than those that are nonpatient facing or mixed (National Society of Genetic Counselors, 2023a). If your employer would benefit from the outcomes of your volunteerism (e.g., advocacy for Medicare reimbursement so that they can bill for services, name recognition from working on projects) or they are supportive of broadening your professional boundaries, they may be open to you contributing to some or all of your volunteer activities during work hours or as a part of your job.

Networking and Social Media

The importance of connection in your professional career is paramount. Networking has long been the broad term for making many of these connections, either as the person who is looking to benefit from a connection or to give support to a connection. As our genetic counseling and affiliated communities grow, networking will be increasingly valuable in finding professional opportunities. Unfortunately, networking can be challenging for different people for different reasons. For introverts and others who find large social engagements challenging, networking can conjure images of uncomfortable conference or "speed networking" events that don't provide the best environment to shine. For the tech-phobic, the idea of updating and sharing information on a professional networking page may be overwhelming. Not every avenue for networking is ideal for all, and while you may not always be able to overcome the discomfort of some situations, there are many ways to engage with your colleagues and build professional relationships in a productive—and not totally painful—way. However, a balance of modalities can be useful and developing strategies for any situation is key.

For those who struggle in large groups, unstructured social scenarios, places where they don't know anyone, or other events, there are many great tips and tricks to help you break the ice and find some comfort. An online search for "introvert expert" Susan Cain, will yield many great interviews and posts about this topic. In one blog post, she shared seven tips to love networking, including "collect kindred spirits" (forget about the networking and find people who you enjoy talking with), "choose your people" (research the specific people you want to talk to, reach out in advance, and plan one-on-one time to meet), and "pace yourself, and be strategic" (find the topics that interest you most and the times of day where you are at your best) (Cain, 2015).

It is also important to recognize that people are challenged by social networking situations for reasons other than introversion. People with visible and invisible disabilities face discrimination and barriers in large social events in many ways. It may be an inaccessible space for those using mobility aids, loud rooms for those with hearing difficulties, or dark rooms for those with visual impairments. It may be photosensitivity, noise sensitivity, prolonged eye contact, or the concern of not meeting social cues for those who are neurodivergent (Page, n.d.). It may be an environment that centers around alcohol when someone is sober or doesn't drink for religious or cultural reasons (Moss, 2021). These are just a handful of the many challenges that different people may face with networking or professional events. Therefore, in the spirit of community and communication, consider how you might be able to provide support when setting up or attending such events.

Online networking is one way to get around some of these challenges—or at least make them less challenging. Online networking is more than just connecting with people to schedule an in-person meeting. It is a way to share information, find new people who share common goals, interests, or jobs/careers, use existing connections to create new ones, and to build and maintain relationships over time. Networking circles are well suited for online networking and connections. The idea of a networking circle is to cluster people based on relationship, shared interest, or other factors. It can also be time-based (e.g., connections from high school, college, grad school). Many social networking sites allow you to create lists, friend groups, or filters based on how you know different people, which can allow you to selectively share information that may be of most interest to those groups and choose how to spend your time engaging with their posts. While some sites are promoted as professional sites, most social media platforms can be used for professional networking when set up and used properly. Social media use in the genetic counseling community for patient care and other uses has been an ongoing topic of discussion and while specific platforms fade in and out of popularity and use, the fundamentals remain solid.

In discussions of social media use in health care, the possibility and unique requirements of patient and provider connection must be assessed. Moore et al. (2018) surveyed practicing genetic counselors and patients regarding mutual engagement via social media. Patients were more likely to agree that social media had the potential for improving patient–provider interactions and that communication with patients within social media can be safely accomplished. Patients were also more likely to note case-specific interactions (e.g., giving/receiving/discussing test results) as helpful social media interactions and had lower levels of concern about these interactions compared to the genetic counselors despite more than half of the genetic counselor respondents being age 30 or younger (Vogels, 2019).

For genetic counselors who are looking for additional guidance on creating accounts and engaging for professional purposes, NSGC has a social media toolkit and other social media resources available for members (Jaracz, n.d.; National Society of Genetic Counselors, n.d.a) and regularly provides a toolkit for specific events (e.g., Genetic Counselor Awareness Day) or action requests (e.g., federal advocacy support). Genetic counselors should be fully aware of their employer's social media policy, both broadly and as it is related to interactions with patients or potential patients. Additional resources to guide these interactions include the American Medical Association's Professionalism in the Use of Social Media (American Medical Association, n.d.).

Networking via social media has become one of the primary tools for many genetic counselors and has spawned research collaborations, presentation ideas, thesis projects, new jobs, and new friendships across the genetic counseling community. Everyone can choose to engage at various levels, from viewer (for purposes of remaining up to date about current and key issues within the community) to an active participant and content generator. Creating a professional social media presence does not mean leaving your personality and personal life behind. Most guidance around a professional social media presence highlights that, while you likely will not share all of the things that you would in your personal circle, authentically presenting yourself and including personal interests and passions will help people get to know you and help you collect those kindred spirits that Susan Cain mentioned.

Mentorship, Management, and Leadership

Mentoring, management, and leadership are three key components to professional development and advancement. All three require overlapping but distinct skills and are often incorporated into the professional development opportunities detailed above, including promotion within career ladders/lattices and faculty appointments. Each of these three categories is a course of study on its own and warrants further investigation for opportunities within your career, workplace, affinity groups, and other communities.

Mentorship Mentorship is the act of engaging with one or more individuals to provide or be provided with guidance, counsel, and/or coaching at any stage in career or personal development. The traditional relationship is that of a single mentor and single mentee, where the mentor is a more senior and experienced advisor to the mentee. However, peer mentorship, where two or more individuals are at similar levels of experience, can also be highly beneficial. Mentoring can be structured in several ways. There are formal mentorship programs, often hosted by an organization or employer, where mentoring may occur in a specific timeframe and within another structure (e.g., frequency of meetings, setting specific goals). Mentoring can also be informal, particularly when a trusted relationship develops that can be leveraged over time for specific circumstances. Participating in a mentoring relationship has benefits for all involved and can be a highly beneficial resource for personal and professional development and advancement. For the mentee, this can include insight into what is called the "hidden curriculum," defined as knowledge and awareness about a profession or employer that is not taught broadly, but rather consists of the unwritten rules, standards, values, and customs that are passed on informally. The "hidden curriculum" has been assessed in detail in medical education and contributes to bias and discrimination within the profession, with a disproportionate negative impact on trainees from communities that have been marginalized (McClinton and Laurencin, 2020).

There are currently two broad mentorship programs for genetic counselors. The first is NSGConnect, which is available for all members of the National Society of Genetic Counselors, including genetic counseling students. The second is for members of the Minority Genetics Professionals Network (MGPN), which was created in support of current and future genetic counselors who are from racial or ethnic minority groups (Mann, 2020). This mentoring program was set up to support longer-term structured mentoring engagements or a one-time "flash mentoring" for a specific topic. All MGPN members can participate in the mentoring program, including those who are considering genetic counseling as a career, actively applying to programs, and genetic counseling students (Minority Genetic Professionals Network, n.d.).

An extension of mentorship is sponsorship, which can provide even more benefits for the mentee/person being sponsored. Sponsorship may include aspects of mentorship but requires that the sponsor make specific efforts to promote the professional or career advancement of the person being sponsored. As sponsorship generally requires that the sponsor is in a position of influence and uses their power and network to drive advancement; it may not be possible in all mentoring relationships. Feedback from genetic counselors highlights the desire and need for both (Baldwin et al., 2022).

Management   Management implies a role of responsibility and oversight for people, programs, or products. Management is often a requirement for promotion, regardless of whether one is employed by for-profit, nonprofit, or academic organizations. Top-level managers, also referred to as "upper management" or "executive management," are a limited number of individuals who are accountable for the success of the organization and who lead strategic planning and decision-making for an organization. This includes "the C-suite" (Chief Executive Officer or CEO, Chief Operating Officer or COO, Chief Academic Officer or CAO, Chief Medical Officer or CMO, and others), and may include a President, Senior Vice Presidents (SVPs), and/or Vice Presidents (VPs), depending on the organization. Middle management is the next level, and these individuals typically have responsibility for specific divisions or functions within an organization. Titles might include Directors, Department Manager/Head, or Division/Regional Manager. These individuals are typically experts in their specific functions and ensure strong communication between the executive levels and the rest of the company. They are also typically "managers of managers," so optimally they not only are strong managers themselves, but can mentor and develop the other managers who work for them. First-line managers typically have a single team within a defined area of the company. Titles might include Supervisor, Office Manager, Manager, or Assistant Manager. These management roles are common for genetic counselors, with 9% of 2023 PSS respondents identifying as first-line managers, 7% as middle management, and 1–2% as upper management or executive management (National Society of Genetic Counselors, 2023a). Academic institutions will generally have similar levels of management but may have different titles. For instance, managerial titles may include Provost, Chancellor, or Vice-Chancellor at the level of institutional administration, Dean at the level of a college or school within the institution, and Chair at the level of a department.

In addition to the management of individual direct reports, people managers also typically have responsibilities related to the team's management (e.g., recruitment, hiring, performance reviews) and the team's performance (e.g., adherence to budget, setting and meeting/exceeding team goals in support of employer initiatives and targets, ensuring cross-functional collaboration when needed). Management opportunities may also extend to specific products or projects, with management roles sometimes referred to as "team leaders." These individuals are typically assigned to manage specific efforts and are responsible for developing timelines, ensuring people meet deadlines, team communication, training, and being the key link between middle or upper management and the team.

Student supervision may be one of the first opportunities for new genetic counselors to learn and practice the skills of people management. Assessments of the characteristics of a strong supervisor (e.g., accessible, transparent, collaborative, empathetic, and self-reflective) and the competencies needed for the successful supervision of students (e.g., an awareness of how to work with individuals of different backgrounds and personal characteristics, the ability to resolve conflicts and addressing interpersonal dynamics, addressing performance with clear and specific feedback, and creating open communication with the student) are highly overlapping with the characteristics of a strong people manager (Eubanks Higgins et al., 2013; Suguitan et al., 2019).

Leadership Unlike management, where a position or title dictates the role, leadership can come from anyone. Leadership is broadly defined as the ability to guide and influence others, but the ways in which people lead or what they seek to accomplish is highly variable. Leaders create a vision for the future, communicate that vision to others to get their buy-in and support, generate the environment for the vision to succeed, and develop and empower the team that can execute. There are hundreds of lists of the essential characteristics or qualities of a good leader, but those that come up most frequently include authenticity, self-awareness, strong communication skills, high emotional intelligence, empathetic, resilient, supportive, empowering, accountability, and vision. Many of these characteristics overlap with the qualities of a successful genetic counselor! There are also many styles of leadership, meaning that there is a lot of space for individuals with different strengths to be leaders.

Since leadership is defined by the ability to influence others, leaders are not limited by their age, background, title, or training. Leaders themselves may be extroverted, enthusiastic, and boisterous, or they may be introverted, quiet, and pensive, or anywhere in between at any given time. There is an oft-cited phrase that "Leadership is taken, not given," which simply means that no one can make you a leader and you shouldn't wait around to be granted the designation of "leader." But the converse of that is also true: "Leadership is given, not taken," because people must choose to follow you. Both are important reminders for genetic counselors as they proceed through their careers.

Although there are many traits of leadership that may seem innate, there are many courses on cultivating the skills and approaches that support strong leadership. In addition to the resources listed below, there are many free courses on leadership on large e-Learning platforms. Employers may also offer courses or leadership coaching, and ABGC has launched the Leadership Education Advancement Development (LEAD) Academy to offer training to certified genetic counselors ("ABGC LEAD Academy," n.d.).

Selected Resources for Leaders

1. Dare to Lead by Brené Brown – book, podcast, and course on leadership (Brown, n.d.)
2. PurpleSpace – "the world's only networking and professional development hub for disabled employees, network and resource group leaders and allies from all sectors and trades" (PurpleSpace, n.d.)
3. TED Topics in Leadership (TED, n.d.)

4. Books on becoming a leader and leadership:
   - *Crucial Conversations* by Kerry Patterson, Joseph Grenny, Ron McMillan, and Al Switzler
   - *Diversity in the Work Place: How to be an Inclusive Leader, Manage Diversity in the Work Place, Tackle Unconscious Bias, and Foster Inclusive Conversations* by Erika Nielsen Brown
   - *Five Dysfunctions of a Team* by Patrick Lencioni
   - *Harvard Business Review*'s Must Reads Boxed Set
   - *Lead from the Outside: How to Build Your Future and Make Real Change* by Stacey Abrams
   - *Leading Change* by John P. Kotter
   - *Master Mentors – 30 Transformative Insights from Our Greatest Minds* by Scott Jeffrey Miller
   - *Professional Troublemaker* by Luvvie Ajayi Jones
   - *Quiet: The Power of Introverts in a World That Can't Stop Talking* by Susan Cain
   - *The Leader's Guide to Unconscious Bias: How To Reframe Bias, Cultivate Connection, and Create High-Performing Teams* by Pamela Fuller and Mark Murphy with Anne Chow
   - *The Memo* by Minda Harts
   - *True North* by Bill George
   - *Wolfpack* by Abby Wambach

MANAGING PROFESSIONAL CHALLENGES

Despite the overall high levels of professional satisfaction for genetic counselors, everyone will encounter professional challenges during their career—beginning in graduate school through to retirement. There is no perfect and challenge-free path. But there are tools that can help you to avoid some challenges and mitigate others, so that these challenges don't weigh as heavily when they appear, and we can move through them more quickly.

As you read this next section:

- Think about the concept of "work–life balance." What things in your personal life are important to keeping you centered and resilient? What things would you never give up for work?

- Consider your core values and what types of work environments would/ would not match up well to how you want to work. You can find many "core value activities" online that can help you define and refine your core values, including:
  - Taproot's Live Your Core Values: http://webmedia.jcu.edu/advising/ files/2016/02/Core-Values-Exercise.pdf
  - The Good Project Value Sort Activity: https://www.thegoodproject. org/value-sort
  - Think2Perform Values Cards Exercise: https://www.think2perform. com/our-approach/values/new
- Have you experienced times of moral distress in your career? What triggered that response? What coping strategies might you use if this comes up in the future?
- Reflect on bystander intervention. Have you been in a situation when someone intervened on your behalf or when you intervened for someone else? How did that make you feel? How might you intervene for a colleague in the future?

Burnout

Did you know that "burnout" has its own ICD code? Burnout was initially added to ICD-10 and in 2019, in ICD-11, the World Health Organization revised the definition to the following:

> *Burn-out is a syndrome conceptualized as resulting from chronic workplace stress that has not been successfully managed. It is characterized by three dimensions:*
>
> - *feelings of energy depletion or exhaustion;*
> - *increased mental distance from one's job, or feelings of negativism or cynicism related to one's job; and*
> - *reduced professional efficacy.*

(WHO, 2019)

While reduced efficacy, negativism, and cynicism can occur in many parts of one's life, burnout is specific to one's job. As such, there may be provocative factors and stressors that one does not typically have to address in their personal life and the impacts and outcomes may also be distinctive from other situations. Stress, exhaustion, depression, and overwhelm all overlap with burnout, so by recognizing that burnout is specific to work, it can be addressed more directly and hopefully, more successfully.

Burnout is an active area of study in the genetic counseling community and will be critically important as our profession grows and evolves, particularly given the high frequency of self-reported signs of burnout. Those who experience burnout at any level should know that they're not alone in their struggles: 24% of 2023 PSS respondents stated "I am definitely burning out and have one or more symptoms of burnout, such as physical and emotional exhaustion" and an additional 10% reported more significant levels of burnout (National Society of Genetic Counselors, 2023a). An early study of burnout demonstrated that genetic counselors demonstrated significantly higher levels of burnout than genetic nurses, with emotional exhaustion most frequently reported (Bernhardt et al., 2009). Subsequent studies have also assessed the relationship between burnout and stress (Johnstone et al., 2016), burnout and clinical supervision roles (Allsbrook et al., 2016), and factors contributing to burnout and the consequences of burnout in genetic counselors (Caleshu et al., 2022). They report multiple positive and negative associations with burnout, summarized in Table 15-2, highlighting that these may be targets for prevention and intervention. Mindfulness has been a particular area of interest, as it is a simple and efficient activity. One study (Silver et al., 2018) found a negative association with mindfulness and compassion fatigue and burnout, and a positive association with empathy. A randomized clinical trial of mindfulness in genetic counselors (Me-GC) may help to identify if mindfulness is another coping mechanism for burnout (Campion, 2021).

Workplace Ethics and Moral Distress

NSGC's Code of Ethics addresses the professional ethics that guide genetic counselors. However, workplaces have their own set of documented and undocumented workplace ethics and integrating personal morals and ethics into those

TABLE 15-2. **Factors that can impact burnout**

What can exacerbate burnout?	What can prevent or alleviate burnout?
Stress	Feeling valued
Anxiety	Administrative support/Operating at the top of one's scope of practice
Depression	Autonomy
Emotional exhaustion	Mindfulness
Depersonalization	Self-care behaviors (e.g., cognitive awareness, professional support, life balance)
Lack of professional accomplishment	Reflection and discussion with a trusted mentor and/or peer group
Distress (e.g. personal values conflicts, collegial distrust, burden of professional responsibility, negative patient regard, patient dread)	Connection with patients
Inauthenticity	Resilience
Work volume and overload	

(Bernhardt et al., 2009; Johnstone et al., 2016; Silver et al., 2018; Campion, 2021; Caleshu et al., 2022)

environments can sometimes be challenging. That can be internal to the workplace itself (i.e., how people within the workplace interact with each other) or due to the relationship that the workplace or your role have with external touchpoints (i.e., how people within the workplace interact while doing business with other organizations or individuals).

It is important to recognize that behaviors in the workplace that many would deem unethical can be accepted or even encouraged in some environments. Behaviors like taking credit for the work of others, verbal harassment, gossip, and nepotism can be a part of a company's (typically unspoken) culture that can create a very negative work environment. Even illegal actions like sexual harassment or discrimination of those who fall into protected classes, including race, religion, sex (including sexual orientation or gender identity), age, and disability status, may not be managed in the correct ways.

When considering a new position, there are approaches that you can use to assess for a work culture that may not suit you, including those that are negative or "toxic." Some approaches to recognize a toxic work culture include (Walters, 2020):

1. Ask about feedback. Understanding how feedback is provided and received can give you insight into how you might be treated as you adapt to a new role and if you will be supported, even if things aren't going perfectly.
2. Examine their core values. Comparing posted core values (e.g., a mission statement on the company website) with what interviewers state as their core values, or what you may read about the company, can tell you if the company's actions are aligned with what they say they care about.
3. Get the lay of the land—or the office. If you will work in person, a tour of the work facilities can give you a sense for how people work together on a daily basis. If you will work remotely, ask about tools that the company uses to connect remote workers and how remote workers fit into the company culture, particularly if there is a mix of onsite and remote employees.
4. Ask an employee their opinion. Ask to speak to people in the department that you'll be working in, particularly if there are people doing the job that you'll be doing.
5. Gauge the pace of the process. Very fast or very slow interview processes can be indicators of difficulties in the workplace.

Additionally, workplace review websites provide reviews by people who have interviewed and/or worked at a particular company, providing another level of insight into the company culture. However, keep in mind that companies may have a presence on these sites and can incentivize their employees to post reviews, and anonymity may be a challenge for employees of a smaller organization, so this should be just one way to assess a company.

Moral distress is a response to the conflict between an individual's ethics and judgment and how they must act. One oft-referenced definition is that moral distress is "the experience of knowing the right thing to do while being in a situation in which it is nearly impossible to do it" (Jameton, 2017). Multiple barriers to doing "the right thing" exist in health care, including institutional regulation, local, state or federal laws, financial and insurance limitations, and other systemic issues. Sources of moral distress in genetic counselors can include the competence or bad practice of other providers, conflict of interest related to family members, privacy/rights, treatment/testing decisions and duty to warn, professional responsibility related to legal concerns, institutional policy, regular practice and scope of practice boundaries, personal beliefs related to pregnancy termination and testing, and patient access issues related to insurance coverage and opportunity for pregnancy termination (Wadman et al., 2022). Coping strategies of those surveyed ranged from seeking social support (20%) to leaving their position (6%). When asked to recommend "ways to alleviate moral distress in the future," strategies including forming a peer support group, joining an ethics committee, speaking to a therapist, practicing self-reflection/mindfulness, changing jobs, and exercising were all mentioned (Wadman et al., 2022).

A related topic is that of conscious clauses. A conscious clause is a law that provides protection for "health care providers who refuse to perform, accommodate, or assist with certain health care services on religious or moral grounds" (Office for Civil Rights (OCR), 2010). For genetic counselors, this is most typically associated with the provision of services related to abortion. Oklahoma, Nebraska, and Virginia have conscious clauses related to abortion for genetic counselors, with no requirement to disclose their objections to the patient or refer to another provider in Oklahoma (Genetic Counseling Licensure Act, 2006). Bonine et al. were the first to publish on genetic counselor awareness of conscious clauses and they highlight that although the Accreditation Council for Genetic Counseling requires genetic counseling training programs to incorporate the NSGC Code of Ethics, which is not a legally binding document, (Accreditation Council for Genetic Counseling, 2019), it is unclear how many programs also train about conscious clauses. This study found that just more than half of the genetic counselors surveyed were aware of conscious clauses (53%) but did not know that such clauses existed for genetic counselors (90%). The paper goes on to examine how genetic counselors feel about conscious clauses, finding a spectrum of opinions about whether conscious clauses could align with the ethics of the profession (Bonine et al., 2021). Given the contribution of ethical conflicts to burnout and moral distress in genetic counselors, and the significant shift in abortion laws after the Dobbs ruling— which eliminated the federal right to abortion before fetal viability (Alito, 2022)—conscious clauses may become increasingly common, and balancing the benefits to the genetic counselor with the needs of the patient will be paramount.

Interpersonal Issues

Interpersonal conflict in the workplace can cover a broad range of person-to-person engagements, some of which are addressed in the professional conduct section. There are many resources online that address common causes of conflict and share strategies on how to address conflict successfully, including the Managing Workplace Conflict toolkit from the Society for Human Resource Management (Society for Human Resource Management, 2022). Crucial Conversations, mentioned in the "Resources for Leaders" section, can also be a very useful tool for workplace conflict.

There are times where interpersonal conflict should be brought to the attention of management/leadership and/or human resources, most critically when the conflict is illegal based on local, state, or federal laws regarding harassment and discrimination. The US Equal Employment Opportunity Commission (EEOC), which "is responsible for enforcing federal laws that make it illegal to discriminate against a job applicant or an employee because of the person's race, color, religion, sex (including pregnancy, transgender status, and sexual orientation), national origin, age (40 or older), disability or genetic information," has a list of federally-prohibited employment policies and practices (Equal Employment Opportunity Commission, n.d.). Additional resources are available at the state and local level and are generally referred to as Fair Employment Practices Agencies. Complaints of discrimination or harassment by employers, unions, or labor organizations can be filed with one or both when not addressed by the employer.

Bullying and microaggressions are amongst the more insidious areas of interpersonal conflict in the workplace. While bullying can be overt when done publicly or when there is a repeating pattern of aggression that can be documented, both bullying and microaggressions can be subtle while still having a significant negative impact on the recipient. Dr. Derald Wing Sue, PhD defines microaggressions as "everyday verbal, nonverbal, and environmental slights, snubs, or insults, whether intentional or unintentional, which communicate hostile, derogatory, or negative messages to target persons based solely upon their marginalized group membership" (Sue, n.d.). Microaggressions may be a component of bullying but are also different and distinct acts. Unfortunately, while microaggressions may fall under laws prohibiting targeted harassment, they may be difficult to document in this way. For instance, Dr. Sue provides the example of "An Asian American, born and raised in the United States, who is complimented for speaking 'good English.' Although this can be a damaging and an 'othering' thing for people to hear – 'You are not a true American. You are a perpetual foreigner in your own country' – both the speaker and others in a workplace environment may assume it is complimentary" (Sue, n.d.).

One thing that everyone can do to support a harassment-, bullying-, and microaggression-free environment is to engage in bystander intervention. Right To Be (formerly Hollaback!), which offers bystander intervention training, developed "The 5Ds" (Distract, Delegate, Document, Delay, and Direct), which are direct and indirect methods of supporting someone who is being subjected to harassing language or actions, including microaggressions (Right To Be, n.d.). While not everyone may feel comfortable with each of the interventions—either due to their personality, their relationship with the individuals involved, or the dynamics of their workplace—at least one is likely to be useable in most situations. Anti-harassment and bystander intervention trainings with a focus on the workplace are valuable in increasing confidence using these techniques.

Imposter Syndrome

Have you ever felt that you were fooling everyone who thinks you are competent, intelligent, and good at your work? That they are overestimating your abilities and that it is just a matter of time before they realize it? These are common thoughts with imposter syndrome, or imposter phenomenon. This concept was first explored by psychologists Pauline Rose Clance and Suzanne Imes in 1978, when they studied 150 high-achieving women from a Midwestern college who were primarily ages 20–45, white, and middle- to upper-class. Clance and Imes noted four types of behaviors that perpetuate the imposter phenomenon: diligence and hard work to prevent them from being "discovered," intellectual inauthenticity by failing to provide their true ideas and opinions, using "friendliness, charm, looks, humor" to win approval, and holding onto the idea of being less intelligent in response to the risk of social rejection. When assessing the four behaviors through a societal lens, one might see that these behaviors are not purely internal but rather a response to misogynistic societal influences. They quote cultural anthropologist Margaret Mead who noted that the successful, independent woman "is viewed as a hostile and destructive force within society" (Clance and Imes, 1978). Latina theologian and writer Prisca Dorcas Mojica Rodríguez has also commented, "Women are socialized to be docile, appeasing, welcoming, humble, not opinionated, and deferential to men. Men are socialized to be aggressive, competitive, bold, and proud; they are groomed for power, dominance, and success. When women began to be recognized for their professional successes, impostor syndrome led them to believe what they had been socialized to believe—that any accomplishments resulted from luck, teamwork, and outside help" (Dorcas Mojica Rodríguez, 2021). Although imposter syndrome has become a widely accepted concept and one that is claimed by many famous and successful individuals, the idea that the person must "fix themselves" and work to overcome this lack of confidence has come into question. Calls to focus on repairing the male-centered and biased workplace cultures rather than focusing on centering the blame on imposter syndrome, further positions imposter syndrome as a systemic issue rather than solely a personal one (Tulshyan and Burey, 2021).

When society and/or those around you are discounting your competence and success, is it really imposter syndrome to experience self-doubt or feel like a fraud? The concepts of testimonial injustice and credibility deficit are important issues in assessing the true nature and cause of imposter syndrome. Dr. Rageshri Dhairyawan describes these related concept thus: "Testimonial injustice occurs when the listener discounts the credibility of the speaker's word due to prejudice about their social identity, and is often associated with gender, ethnicity, class, sexuality or religion. The speaker experiences a credibility deficit" (Dhairyawan, 2020). While not all feelings related to imposter syndrome are due to testimonial injustice or credibility deficit, when they arise, these issues should be explored.

Similarly, there are unique ways where what looks like imposter syndrome manifests in people from identities that have been marginalized. In telling her story of reframing her presumed imposter syndrome, Ms. Mojica Rodríguez reflects,

> We rarely have control of the ways impostor syndrome traps people of color. To assimilate requires erasing your ethnicity; you have to perform in a way that puts white people at ease, to the point where you earn honorary whiteness: 'You're not like the others.' Students like myself who choose not to erase their ethnicity, or who cannot downplay their differences, are othered and quietly outcast. Succeeding through Americanized, white definitions of success means performing to reinforce, or to spite, the greatness of whiteness. We either reinforce or upset the low expectations built by white supremacy. And many of us develop anxiety and other mental illnesses when we are daily asked to compromise ourselves, all while trying to juggle schoolwork, or do our jobs, or live our lives. We dared to believe that degrees and promotions meant success, but no one ever said that success came at the cost of our well-being.
>
> (Dorcas Mojica Rodríguez, 2021)

Working to thrive, or even exist, in a world that is not centered in your success can feel like imposter syndrome, but is truly a reflection of the environment rather than the person.

This is not to say that imposter syndrome can't exist as an independent issue regardless of background and it remains important to address it when it appears. Imposter syndrome isn't limited by gender, race, or other identities and can interfere with your mental wellbeing and success. In the case of imposter syndrome, looking for the four behaviors discussed by Clance and Imes, assessing whether they are perpetuating your imposter syndrome; seeking additional support and guidance may be valuable. Additionally, getting feedback from peers or mentors may help you differentiate between doubt sowed by testimonial injustice and imposter syndrome.

Overall, there are many ways in which genetic counselors can experience challenges in the workplace. Awareness of when and where these issues may appear, along with a toolkit of mitigating actions and activities, will help genetic counselors at all career stages address and overcome these barriers to fulfillment.

LOOKING TO THE FUTURE

If you asked most genetic counseling students entering the profession 40   or even 20—years ago to describe how they thought the profession would be today, it's likely that the response would be a dramatic underestimate of what we are actually doing now. That's because while many of our internal and external drivers are predictable, much in the genetics ecosystem is not. The constant is change, and a significant amount of this professional evolution has been influenced by external forces. Whereas a 2009 genome, at a cost of $50,000–100,000, was only available to an exclusive few, technological developments have enabled exome and genome sequencing to reach the mainstream; so much so that as of July 2023, the Medicaid programs of eight states in the United States pay for rapid genome sequencing for critically ill infants ("GeneDx Commends the States of Arizona and Florida for Adding Rapid Whole Genome Sequencing (rWGS) as a Covered Benefit for Medicaid Pediatric Patients | GeneDx," n.d.), with bills proposed in several other states. Decreased costs of sequencing paired with expanding consumer interest in ancestry and personal genomics have spawned multiple billion-dollar corporations to provide genetic testing for more than 35 million people outside of the health care system. A recognition that genomic data paired with clinical records could drive drug development and other discoveries has generated multiple population-scale sequencing programs at the health system, state, and national level. Genetic counselors have stepped up and stepped in to fill the numerous roles that require our specialized training, ability to translate complex genetic concepts, and deep understanding of the clinical applications of genomics, and today genetic counselors hold diverse positions in clinical care and across industry.

In addition to these extraordinary external influences, our colleagues within the genetic counseling profession are pushing change from within. We have strengthened and broadened our efforts in advocating for state and federal policy to improve recognition of genetic counselors as unique and critical health care professionals, increase reimbursement for genetic services, and improve access to care. In 2008, only four states had licensure (National Society of Genetic Counselors, n.d.b); compared to the 32 states issuing licenses, and three additional states with bills passed and/or are in rulemaking, in 2023 (National Society of Genetic Counselors, 2023b). We are promoting the hiring of genetic counselors, administrative support, and genetic counseling assistants by generating business cases and publishing on the downstream revenue generated by our services. We are leading the development of genetic and genomic testing products and services, ensuring that the voice of the clinician, patient, and their family are represented at all stages of the development cycle. Most importantly, an increasing number of genetic counselors are demanding change in how we must center diversity, equity, inclusion, belonging, and accessibility in all things for our patients, communities, and ourselves. This is an opportune time to be a genetic counselor with unprecedented opportunities for professional growth and development. But we will need to continue to adapt to the changing needs of our colleagues, patient populations, and employers. Many of the topics addressed in this book are difficult and challenge a status quo that has been accepted (and successful) for 40+ years, but it is for the love of a great profession that we must strive for change.

Fundamentally, this chapter has focused on the importance of advancing the profession by advancing the people in it. The best future for our profession includes one where each individual leaves their mark and changes the dynamic of what it means to be a genetic counselor. The way in which you leave that mark is up to you, driven by your passions and priorities, and the manner in which you engage with and support your colleagues, patients, and community.

ACKNOWLEDGEMENTS

I am grateful to fellow genetic counselors Dr. Jehannine Austin, PhD, MSc, CGC and Kim Zayhowski, MS, CGC for sharing their insights and expertise where mine was lacking and for always advocating for our profession to be better through their words and actions.

REFERENCES

Aamodt P, Wetherill L, Delk P, et al. (2021) Positive and negative professionalism experiences of genetic counseling students in the United States and Canada. *J Genet Couns* 30:478–492. https://doi.org/10.1002/jgc4.1334

ABGC LEAD Academy (n.d.) https://www.abgc.net/for-diplomates/abgc-lead-academy/ Accessed August 28.2022.

Accreditation Council for Genetic Counseling. (2019) *Practice-Based Competencies for Genetic Counselors*. McLean, VA: Accreditation Council for Genetic Counseling https://www.gceducation.org/wp-content/uploads/2024/01/ACGC-Practice-Based-Competencies-Rev.-June-2019.pdf Accessed June 6, 2024.

Adams K, Hean S, Sturgis P, & Clark JM. (2006) Investigating the factors influencing professional identity of first-year health and social care students. *Learn Health Soc Care* 5:55–68. https://doi.org/10.1111/j.1473-6861.2006.00119.x

Alito SA, Jr. (2022) Dobbs v. Jackson Women's Health Organization. https://www.supremecourt.gov/opinions/21pdf/19-1392_6j37.pdf Accessed June 6, 2024.

Allsbrook K, Atzinger C, He H, et al. (2016) The relationship between the supervision role and compassion fatigue and burnout in genetic counseling. *J Genet Couns* 25:1286–1297. https://doi.org/10.1007/s10897-016-9970 9

American Board of Genetic Counseling. (2019) The American Board of Genetic Counseling, Inc. By Laws. https://www.abgc.net/Portals/0/ABGC_Bylaws.pdf?ver=fD K0uo9C44jw9WTQLZ5QNA%3D%3D Accessed July 3, 2024.

American Medical Association (n.d.) Professionalism in the Use of Social Media. https://www.ama-assn.org/delivering-care/ethics/professionalism-use-social-media Accessed August 6, 2022.

Atzinger CL, Blough-Pfau R, Kretschmer, et al. (2007) Characterization of the practice and attitudes of genetic counselors with doctoral degrees. *J Genet Couns* 16:223–239. https://doi.org/10.1007/s10897-006-9062-3

Baldwin A, Berninger T, Harrison B, et al. (2022) Assessing barriers to the career ladder and professional development for ethnic minority genetic counselors in the United States. *J Genet Couns* 31(5):1032–1042 https://doi.org/10.1002/jgc4.1574

Bernhardt BA, Rushton CH, Carrese J, et al. (2009) Distress and burnout among genetic service providers. *Genet Med.* 11:527–535. https://doi.org/10.1097/GIM.0b013e3181a6a1c2

Berro T. (2019, April 7) Guest Post: We Can Do Better – The Experience of a Minority Genetic Counselor. The DNA Exchange. https://thednaexchange.com/2019/04/07/guest-post-we-can-do-better-the-experience-of-a-minority-genetic-counselor-by-tala-berro/ Accessed August 28, 2022.

Bonine S, Bell M, Fishler K, et al. (2021) Conscience clauses in genetic counseling: awareness and attitudes. *J Genet Couns* 30:1468–1479. https://doi.org/10.1002/jgc4.1414

Brown B. (n.d.) Dare to Lead Hub. URL https://brenebrown.com/hubs/dare-to-lead/ Accessed August 6, 2022.

Bryana Rivers [@GcBry]. (2020) @ABGCertifiedGCs Also, when it comes to appearance as it relates to professionalism, many people knowingly or not, associate straight hair and hairstyles commonly worn by White people as the standard for professionalism. Stop that. #ABGCListens #GCChat. Twitter.

Cain S. (2015) 7 Tips on How to Learn to Love Networking. https://www.psychologytoday.com/gb/blog/quiet-the-power-of-introverts/201506/how-to-learn-to-love-networking Accessed August 6, 2022.

Caleshu C, Kim H, Silver J, et al. (2022) Contributors to and consequences of burnout among clinical genetic counselors in the United States. *J Genet Couns* 31:269–278. https://doi.org/10.1002/jgc4.1485

Campion MW. (2021) Me-GC: A randomized controlled trial of meditation to reduce genetic counselor burnout and genetic counseling student stress (Clinical trial registration No. NCT03723018). https://clinicaltrials.gov./study/NCT03723018?term=ME%20GC&rank=1 Accessed June 6, 2024.

Christian S, Lilley M, Hume S, et al. (2012) Defining the role of laboratory genetic counselor. *J Genet Couns* 21:605–611. https://doi.org/10.1007/s10897-011-9419-0

Clance PR & Imes SA. (1978) The imposter phenomenon in high achieving women: Dynamics and therapeutic intervention. *Psychother Theory Res Pract* 15:241–247. https://doi.org/10.1037/h0086006

CROWN Coalition (n.d.) The CROWN Act. https://www.thecrownact.com/about Accessed July 3, 2024.

Dhairyawan R. (2020) Reframing imposter phenomenon. *BMJ Leader*. https://blogs.bmj.com/bmjleader/2020/10/08/reframing-imposter-phenomenon-by-rageshri-dhairyawan/ Accessed August 28, 2022.

Dorcas Mojica Rodríguez P. (2021) Assimilation and erasure: how imposter syndrome traps people of color. *Literary Hub* https://lithub.com/assimilation-and-erasure-how-imposter-syndrome-traps-people-of-color/ Accessed August 22, 2022.

Equal Employment Opportunity Commission. (n.d.) Prohibited Employment Policies/Practices. https://www.eeoc.gov/prohibited-employment-policiespractices Accessed August 8, 2022.

Eubanks Higgins S, Veach PM, MacFarlane IM, et al. (2013) Genetic counseling supervisor competencies: results of a Delphi study. *J Genet Couns* 22:39–57. https://doi.org/10.1007/s10897-012-9512-z

Finucane B. (2012) 2012 National Society of Genetic Counselors Presidential Address: maintaining our professional identity in an ever-expanding genetics universe. *J Genet Couns* 21:3–6. https://doi.org/10.1007/s10897-011-9466-6

GeneDx. (2023) Press Release. GeneDx Commends the States of Arizona and Florida for Adding Rapid Whole Genome Sequencing (rWGS) as a Covered Benefit for Medicaid Pediatric Patients. https://ir.genedx.com/news-releases/news-release-details/genedx-commends-states-arizona-and-florida-adding-rapid-whole/ Accessed July 30, 2023.

Gray A. (2019) The bias of 'professionalism' standards. *Stanf Soc Innov*. https://ssir.org/articles/entry/the_bias_of_professionalism_standards Accessed June 6, 2024.

Heled E & Davidovitch N. (2021) Personal and group professional identity in the 21st century case study: the school counseling profession. *J Educ Learn* 10:64. https://doi.org/10.5539/jel.v10n3p64

Hewlett SA, Jackson M, Cose E, & Emerson C. (2012) *Vaulting the Color Bar: How Sponsorship Levers Multicultural Professionals into Leadership*. Los Angeles, CA: Rare Bird Books

Jameton A. (2017) What moral distress in nursing history could suggest about the future of health care. *AMA J Ethics* 19:617–628. https://doi.org/10.1001/journalofethics.2017.19.6.mhst1-1706

Jaracz H. (n.d.) NSGC Social Media Toolkit 63. https://www.nsgc.org/Portals/0/x211001%20Member%20Social%20Media%20Toolkit.pdf Accessed July 3, 2024.

Jarus T, Bezati R, Trivett S, et al. (2020) Professionalism and disabled clinicians: the client's perspective. *Disabil Soc* 35:1085–1102. https://doi.org/10.1080/09687599.2019.1669436

Johnson T. (2021) Addressing Issues of Equity in Volunteerism: Where to Look & What to Do. Tobi Johnson & Associates. https://tobijohnson.com/equity-in-volunteerism/ Accessed June 11, 2023.

Johnstone B, Kaiser A, Injeyan MC, et al. (2016) The relationship between burnout and occupational stress in genetic counselors. *J Genet Couns* 25:731–741. https://doi.org/10.1007/s10897-016-9968-3

JOY Collective. (2019) The CROWN Research Study. Unilever plc/Unilever B.V. https://static1.squarespace.com/static/5edc69fd622c36173f56651f/t/5edeaa2fe5ddef345e087361/1591650865168/Dove_research_brochure2020_FINAL3.pdf Accessed May 31, 2022.

Kofman L, Seprish MB, & Summar M. (2016) Climbing the ladder: experience with developing a large group genetic counselor career ladder at Children's National Health System. *J Genet Couns* 25:644–648. https://doi.org/10.1007/s10897-016-9967-4

Genetic Counseling Licensure Act. (2006) Licensure, accreditation, certification not contingent upon acceptance of abortion as treatment option. https://www.ok.gov/health2/documents/Title%2063%2011-1-19.pdf. Accessed June 6, 2024.

Mann S. (2020) Creation of the Minority Genetic Professionals Network to increase diversity in the genetics work force. *J Genet Couns* 29:202–205. https://doi.org/10.1002/jgc4.1248

Marlow Group Inc. (2020) Want a promotion? Advocate for yourself. https://getmarlow.com/article/want-a-promotion-advocate-for-yourself--1587575057845x238346497723727870 Accessed June 5, 2022.

McClinton A & Laurencin CT. (2020) Just in TIME: Trauma-Informed Medical Education. *J Racial Ethn Health Disparities* 7, 1046–1052. https://doi.org/10.1007/s40615-020-00881-w

Merriam-Webster (n.d.) "Professionalism" definition & meaning. https://www.merriam-webster.com/dictionary/professionalism Accessed May 31, 2022.

Minority Genetic Professionals Network (n.d.) Mentoring Program Overview. https://mgpn.chronus.com/ Accessed August 27, 2022.

Moss H. (2021) How I navigate networking events as a person who doesn't drink. Fast Co. https://www.fastcompany.com/90653140/how-i-navigate-networking-events-as-a-person-who-doesnt-drink Accessed August 6, 2022.

Nagy R, Peay H, Hicks M, et al. (2015) Genetic counselors' and genetic counseling students' attitudes around the clinical doctorate and other advanced educational options for genetic counselors: a report from the Genetic Counseling Advanced Degree Task Force. *J Genet Couns* 24:626–634. https://doi.org/10.1007/s10897-014-9785-5

National Society of Genetic Counselors. (n.d.a) Social Media Start-up Guide. https://www.nsgc.org/Portals/0/x211001%20Member%20Social%20Media%20Toolkit.pdf Accessed June 7, 2024.

National Society of Genetic Counselors. (n.d.b) NSGC Timeline. https://www.nsgc.org/About/About-NSGC/Timeline Accessed August 4, 2022.

National Society of Genetic Counselors. (2009) 2008 Professional Status Survey.

National Society of Genetic Counselors. (2022) 2022 Professional Status Survey: Professional Diversity, Inclusion and Satisfaction. https://www.nsgc.org/Portals/0/Executive%20Summary%20Final%2005-03-22.pdf Accessed June 7, 2024.

National Society of Genetic Counselors. (2023a) 2023 Professional Status Survey. https://www.nsgc.org/Portals/0/2023%20PSS%20Executive%20Summary.pdf Accessed June 7, 2024.

National Society of Genetic Counselors. (2023b) State Licensure Map https://datawrapper.dwcdn.net/xNc1w/2/ Accessed July 30, 2023.

Neilson S. (2020) Ableism in the medical profession. *Can Med Assoc J* 192:E411–E412. https://doi.org/10.1503/cmaj.191597

Office for Civil Rights (OCR). (2010) Conscience Protections for Health Care Providers. U.S. Department of Health & Human Services. https://www.hhs.gov/conscience/conscience-protections/index.html Accessed August 8, 2022.

Olesen H. (2001) Professional identity as learning processes in life histories. *Journal of Workplace Learning* 13(7/8):290–298.

Page R. (n.d.) Networking and neurodiversity | LinkedIn https://www.linkedin.com/pulse/networking-neurodiversity-robert-page/ Accessed June 8, 2022.

PurpleSpace. (n.d.) About Us. https://www.purplespace.org/about Accessed August 6, 2022.

Rabideau MM, Wong K, Gordon ES, & Ryan L. (2016) Genetic counselors in startup companies: redefining the genetic counselor role. *J Genet Couns* 25:649–657. https://doi.org/10.1007/s10897-015-9923-8

Reiser C, LeRoy B, Grubs R, & Walton C. (2015) Report on an investigation into an entry level clinical doctorate for the genetic counseling profession and a survey of the Association of Genetic Counseling Program Directors. *J Genet Couns* 24:689–701. https://doi.org/10.1007/s10897-015-9838-4

Right To Be (n.d.) The 5Ds of Bystander Intervention. https://righttobe.org/guides/bystander-intervention-training/ Accessed August 28, 2022.

Rowan-Cabarrus Community College. (2024) Nursing Education Programs Professional Behavior Policy: Health & Education. https://www.rccc.edu/healtheducation/nursing-education-programs-professional-behavior-policy/ Accessed May 31, 2022.

Runyon M, Zahm KW, Veach PM, et al. (2010) What do genetic counselors learn on the job? a qualitative assessment of professional development outcomes. *J Genet Couns* 19:371–386. https://doi.org/10.1007/s10897-010-9289-x

Silver J, Caleshu C, Casson-Parkin S, & Ormond K. (2018) Mindfulness among genetic counselors is associated with increased empathy and work engagement and decreased burnout and compassion fatigue. *J Genet Couns* 27:1175–1186. https://doi.org/10.1007/s10897-018-0236-6

Society for Human Resource Management. (2022) Managing Workplace Conflict https://www.shrm.org/resourcesandtools/tools-and-samples/toolkits/pages/managingworkplaceconflict.aspx Accessed August 8 2022.

Sue DW. (n.d.) Microaggression: More Than Just Race. https://www.psychologytoday.com/gb/blog/microaggressions-in-everyday-life/201011/microaggressions-more-just-race Accessed July 3, 2024.

Suguitan MD, McCarthy Veach P, LeRoy B, et al. (2019) Genetic counseling supervisor strategies: an elaboration of the Reciprocal-Engagement Model of Supervision. *J Genet Couns* 28:602–615. https://doi.org/10.1002/jgc4.1057

Swanson A, Ramos E, & Snyder H. (2014) Next generation sequencing is the impetus for the next generation of laboratory-based genetic counselors. *J Genet Couns* 23:647–654. https://doi.org/10.1007/s10897-013-9684-1

TED (n.d.) Ideas about Leadership, https://www.ted.com/topics/leadership Accessed June 8, 2022.

The Exeter Group. (2021) National Society of Genetic Counselors Diversity, Equity, and Inclusion Assessment: Report of Findings and Recommendations. https://www.nsgc.org/Portals/0/Docs/Policy/JEDI/NSGC%20DEI%20Assessment%20Report%20of%20Findings%20and%20Recommendations%20-%20Executive%20Summary.pdf?ver=7yIXuQLddI61mqulWw2VVA%3D%3D Accessed June 24, 2024.

Tulshyan R & Burey J-A. (2021) Stop telling women they have Imposter Syndrome. *Harv Bus Rev* https://hbr.org/2021/02/stop-telling-women-they-have-imposter-syndrome?utm_medium=paidsearch&utm_source=google&utm_campaign=intlcontent_bussoc&utm_term=Non-Brand&tpcc=intlcontent_bussoc&gad_source=1&gclid=CjwKCAjw34qzBhBmEiwAOUQcF6fAW70tfHhRSihtrSI_EevP5OCpyxVu63xunGNZnsde7aNHZ9rt7hoCCnEQAvD_BwE Accessed June 7, 2024.

US News. (n.d.) Genetic Counselor Ranks Among Best Jobs of 2023. https://money.usnews.com/careers/best-jobs/genetic-counselor Accessed June 11, 2023.

Vogels EA. (2019) Millennials stand out for their technology use, but older generations also embrace digital life. Pew Research Center. https://www.pewresearch.org/fact-tank/2019/09/09/us-generations-technology-use/ Accessed August 6, 2022.

Wadman E, Conway L, Garbarini J, & Baker M. (2022) Moral distress in genetic counseling: a study of North American genetic counselors. *J Genet Couns* 31:836–846. https://doi.org/10.1002/jgc4.1551

Wallace JP, Myers MF, Huether CA, et al. (2008) Employability of genetic counselors with a PhD in genetic counseling. *J Genet Couns* 17:209–219. https://doi.org/10.1007/s10897-007-9123-2

Walters L. (2020) 5 Ways to Recognize a Toxic Work Culture During an Interview, 2020. Blue Signal Search. https://bluesignal.com/2020/07/07/5-ways-to-recognize-a-toxic-work-culture-during-an-interview/ Accessed June 14, 2022.

Waltman L, Runke C, Balcom J, et al. (2016) Further defining the role of the laboratory genetic counselor. *J Genet Couns* 25:786–798. https://doi.org/10.1007/s10897-015-9927-4

WHO. (2019) Burn-out an "occupational phenomenon": International Classification of Diseases https://www.who.int/news/item/28-05-2019-burn-out-an-occupational-phenomenon-international-classification-of-diseases Accessed 9 June, 2024.

Zayhowski K & Sheridan N. (2022, June 27) Queer erasure in standards of professionalism. NSGC Perspectives. https://perspectives.nsgc.org/Article/queer-erasure-in-standards-of-professionalism Accessed August 28, 2022.

16

Examining our Work through Case Presentations

**Richard Dineen, Logan B. Karns, Matthew J. Thomas,
and Barry S. Tong**

INTRODUCTION
(Jane L. Schuette and Beverly M. Yashar)

We are concluding this textbook with case presentations where genetic counselors recount and examine an actual "case," as this is the best way to capture the nature of the genetic counseling process. Such presentations are meant to facilitate discussion and exploration, thereby enhancing learning and appreciation for the complex nature of the genetic counseling interaction. The process of case presentation is essential to student skill acquisition and development. It is also an opportunity for all of us to look at our work in new ways. As the reader reviews the unfolding of the interaction, it is then that they begin to understand the intricacy of balancing information, communication, the exploring of options, decision-making, and support for choice.

The following cases were prepared by genetic counselors with expertise in their specialties: pediatric genetics, reproductive genetics, cardiovascular genetics, and cancer genetics. Their perspectives provide insights into the breadth of clinical practice settings that involve genetic counseling and highlight both fundamental and novel aspects of providing care. Additionally, these cases allow us to

A Guide to Genetic Counseling, Third Edition. Edited by Vivian Y. Pan, Jane L. Schuette,
Karen E. Wain, and Beverly M. Yashar.
© 2025 John Wiley & Sons Ltd. Published 2025 by John Wiley & Sons Ltd.

experience the unique and distinctive approaches experienced clinicians use to support their patients through the genetic counseling process. The importance of self-reflection for ongoing professional growth is also demonstrated. Individually and in totality, the cases exemplify the complexities, challenges and benefits of genetic counseling and we thank the contributors for sharing them.

THE THINGS WE DON'T SEE: PRENATAL GENETIC COUNSELING (LOGAN B. KARNS)

Introduction

Presenting a case of your own can be an intimidating exercise—even for an experienced genetic counselor. While years of practice hone your counseling skills, each new case presents different challenges; sometimes cases go well, and sometimes they don't. So, when asked to contribute a prenatal case for the 3rd edition of this book, I pondered my options. I was tempted to look for a case that had gone exactly according to plan. No surprises—no "what ifs." My perfect case. I quickly realized that I would be searching in vain for that case. In 34 years, there haven't been any cases like that.

If you are open to it, the cases that are not "perfect" are some of the best learning experiences you can have as a professional. This was one such case for me. The technical aspects of this case are interesting—and that information has changed my practice—yet the most powerful message of this case for me was in awareness. Awareness of patients and all that they bring to a brief encounter, and awareness of myself and what I bring to my work. But awareness also means the ability to look at your work, and yourself, with compassion; the ultimate goal being to have a "living" practice: one that grows with experience, and changes over time.

To frame this case, I am going to use a first-person narrative. And, while I realize that some people do not use this terminology, I will refer to my patient as a "patient," rather than a "client," because my work in a prenatal diagnosis clinic more closely reflects a traditional medical model. In presenting her story to you, I have disguised and changed certain things about her, and her family, to protect their privacy.

This case, while not an easy one, provided me with the opportunity to grow in my practice. Everyone who reads this will see it differently, therefore I have chosen not to dissect this story, or suggest all of the possible different "beginnings" or "endings," but rather leave that as the journey for the reader.

Unique elements of prenatal genetic counseling

Perhaps the best way to introduce this case is to begin by considering what makes prenatal genetic counseling different from other areas of our practice. While genetic counseling as a profession embraces a set of paradigms that transcend job descriptions, each specific area of genetic counseling practice presents unique challenges. One of the most complicated facets of prenatal genetic counseling is the inevitable importance of timing. A full-term pregnancy lasts from the first day of a patient's last menstrual period to 40 weeks of gestation; and it is divided into three trimesters. Most genetic testing is offered during the first, or second, trimester. During that timeframe there is both the need to offer, and execute, the appropriate testing; and, if the results are abnormal, to help facilitate a patient's decision-making regarding pregnancy management—including pregnancy termination. Further complicating the decision-making process is the fact that the information that any patient will have on which to base these decisions is sometimes incomplete, or uncertain. At the end of the day, many individuals and couples find themselves struggling to make important choices in a narrow window of time, sometimes with a paucity of information, and under considerable stress. Virtually no one is fully prepared for these moments.

In addition to these challenges—and certainly not unique to prenatal genetic counseling—other factors can increase the complexity of a session. Some cases involve language barriers that can make it complicated for providers to convey information, and for families to assimilate it. Some patients face economic and social challenges that can have an impact on their decision-making. These, and other barriers to health care, when combined with time constraints and complicated decision-making paradigms, can result in highly stressful situations for both patients and providers.

Lastly, reproductive rights—including the choice about whether or not to have children—is central to the ethos of prenatal genetic counseling. Working with individuals facing complicated choices about continuing or ending a pregnancy is an integral part of what we do, and those issues are never easy. When the Supreme Court overturned *Roe v. Wade* in June of 2022, it ignited a nationwide controversy regarding abortion in the United States. Since that time multiple states have enacted laws that restrict the reproductive rights of individuals, and other states are poised to follow suit. The resulting patchwork of laws will inevitably create unequal access to care, and limit the options we, as providers, have to offer patients. Limiting access to medical care unfairly disadvantages many groups of people, including individuals and families of color, and those who have limited financial resources. This issue will substantively define the practice of prenatal genetic counseling in the years to come.

So why this case?

This particular case was the intersection of all of the elements that make a prenatal genetic counseling case different, and especially challenging. It also called me to examine myself, and my work— an exercise in self-reflection that can be uncomfortable for any of us. So, perhaps for all of these reasons, the case that I have chosen to present is *my* "perfect" case.

Setting the stage: Initiation of care and goal setting

Most of the patients I see for genetic counseling are referred by our obstetric clinic, and they are already pregnant. Each patient will typically have had an initial telephone visit with a nurse at which time a pertinent medical history is reviewed and a routine set of laboratory testing is ordered. The nurse also reviews extensive educational material and informs them about the availability of genetic counseling services and the possibility of genetic screening and testing. Any patient who expresses interest in meeting with a genetic counselor is then scheduled for a separate appointment with me, or a colleague of mine.

Most genetic counseling sessions begin with contracting to elicit the patient's goals for the session. This creates a framework to structure the session and clarify what questions or concerns need to be addressed. The remainder of the session then includes a combination of the patient's goals and the genetic counselor's goals. A common indication for a prenatal genetic counseling session is routine prenatal screening and diagnostic testing. In these types of sessions several elements are typically addressed. A three-generation family history is elicited, as well as a previous pregnancy and medical history. This conversation is then followed by a discussion of screening and diagnostic testing for aneuploidy and genetic carrier testing, including the risks, benefits, and limitations of these testing modalities. Testing can be conducted in that session, or postponed until a later time, depending on the patient's gestational age and the specific testing desired. Results are then given to the patient in a manner that has been contractually arranged between the genetic counselor and the patient. The vast majority of screening test results are negative. Negative—or normal—results are typically called to the patient or sent via the electronic medical record. Whenever possible, abnormal results would always be called to the patient. It is not a routine practice in most prenatal genetic counseling settings to schedule a follow-up appointment to disclose all results (normal and abnormal) in a face-to-face meeting.

Professional society recommendations for prenatal genetic counseling and testing

An important goal of many prenatal genetic counseling sessions is providing the patient with enough information to facilitate an informed decision about which screening and testing options, if any, will give them the information that they are seeking. The American College of Obstetricians and Gynecologists (ACOG) Practice Bulletin 162 states that "The objective of prenatal genetic testing is to detect health problems that could affect the woman, fetus, or newborn and provide the patient and her obstetrician–gynecologist or other obstetric care provider with enough information to allow a fully informed decision about pregnancy management" (Norton and Jackson, 2016). While gathering information for planning purposes can certainly be a goal of prenatal screening and testing, some individuals do not approach this type of testing with the intention of changing the management of their pregnancy in the event of an abnormal result; rather, they can be seeking information to prepare themselves to take care of a child that may have special needs. Everyone feels very differently about why this information either would, or would not, be helpful to them. One objective of pre-test counseling, therefore, is to elicit the patient's goals so that they can be balanced together with the genetic counselor's goals and a framework developed to structure the session so that all of the important elements are addressed.

ACOG recommends that all patients be informed that "prenatal genetic testing cannot identify all abnormalities or problems in a fetus, and any testing should be focused on the individual patient's risks, reproductive goals, and preferences." They further state that "It is important that patients understand the benefits and limitations of all prenatal screening and diagnostic testing, including the conditions for which tests are available and the conditions that will not be detected by testing" (Norton and Jackson, 2016).

Multiple screening and testing modalities are available to patients, and each has a different sensitivity and specificity. For many patients, the volume and complexity of this information is overwhelming, and contributes to the challenges they face in making decisions. Education and informed consent are therefore *prima facie* goals of pretest genetic counseling in any genetic counseling specialty. ACOG, along with other genetics organizations including the National Society of Genetic Counselors (NSGC) and the American College of Medical Genetics and Genomics (ACMG), makes recommendations which guide the profession regarding what screening and testing is standard of care to offer all patients (Wilson et al., 2013; Gregg et al., 2016; Rose et al., 2020).

ACOG Practice Bulletin 226 regarding screening for fetal chromosomal abnormalities states: "Prenatal genetic screening (serum screening with or without nuchal translucency [NT] ultrasound or cell-free DNA screening) and diagnostic testing (chorionic villus sampling [CVS] or amniocentesis) options should be discussed and offered to all pregnant patients regardless of maternal age or risk of chromosomal abnormality. After review and discussion, every patient has the right to pursue or decline prenatal genetic screening and diagnostic testing" (Rose et al., 2020).

NSGC recommends, among other things, the following for all patients:

1. Providers should offer the options of maternal serum screening (MSS) and diagnostic testing for chromosome aneuploidy to every patient.
2. Providers should engage in a discussion with their patients about the benefits, limitations, and risks of MSS and diagnostic testing so that patients may make informed and autonomous decisions.
3. Providers should be aware of factors that may impact the options available to their patients, such as the patient's gestational age, insurance coverage, and access to services and providers. (Wilson et al., 2013)

Background

Ms. S is a 35- year-old patient who presented for her initial genetic counseling appointment at 13 weeks and 4 days gestation by last menstrual period. The following history was obtained from her electronic medical record prior to the appointment.

Ms. S and her husband have had a total of five pregnancies and have three living children. Ms. S is originally from Bhutan and has lived in the United States for five years. Prior to moving to the United States, she lived in a refugee camp in Nepal for 19 years. Her native language is Dzongkha, but she also speaks Nepali fluently, and is conversant in English.

Ms. S's first pregnancy ended in a neonatal demise following a premature labor and delivery in Nepal. She reported that the pregnancy had been progressing well, until approximately 23 weeks when her "water broke" and she went into labor. She reported that the baby was born and survived for only a few minutes before passing away. At the time, she and her husband were not given an explanation for the pregnancy loss, and no records from that pregnancy were available. Her second pregnancy was uncomplicated and ended in the birth of their oldest son in Nepal. He is now 7 years old and healthy. Ms. S. and her husband then moved to the United States as refugees. They had a third uncomplicated pregnancy and have a healthy daughter who is now 5 years old. Their fourth pregnancy resulted in the birth of their second son, T, who is now 3 years old.

Ms. S and her family were relocated to our community two years ago by the International Rescue Committee (IRC). She and her husband, and their three children, live in a house they rent just outside of town. She does not work outside of the home. They have one car that her husband takes to his job at a construction company. They have Medicaid insurance, a federally-funded program, provided to them by the state based on their refugee status. Ms. S speaks English fairly well and prefers to converse in English whenever possible. Her husband's primary language is Nepali. He does not speak English.

My goals for the session

Before meeting with any patient, I try to spend a few moments considering what goals I have for the session. Specifically, is there any medical or social information that I need to ascertain? What medical/genetic information do we need to discuss? Are there any decisions that may need to be made? What barriers to health care might impact this process? In this particular case I had identified several issues that I wanted to address after reviewing information available to me in the medical record:

1. Ms. S is at increased risk to have a pregnancy with chromosome abnormalities, based on her age.
2. Ms. S has the option of having prenatal genetic screening or diagnostic testing for chromosome abnormalities, and there are several options to

discuss with her. Some of these options have time constraints and, based on her current gestational age, there may be limits on what we will be able to offer her.

3. Ms. S's Medicaid insurance may not cover all of the testing options that we will discuss, and additional resources, such as the hospital financial screening program, may not be available to cover the cost of this testing.

4. In order for Ms. S to make an informed decision about testing, we will need to discuss complex medical and genetic information. As English is not her first language, an interpreter may be able to help facilitate this process.

Initial Genetic Counseling Session

Ms. S presented to the genetic counseling session by herself. Ms. S speaks Dzongkha—the official language of Bhutan—but she also speaks fluent Nepali. A certified Nepali interpreter was provided by the IRC and met her in the waiting room at the clinic. Ms. S accepted the presence of the interpreter but stated that she preferred to speak in English whenever possible. We had a conversation at the beginning of the session to determine what specific role the interpreter would have in the session. Typically, the interpreter would restate word for word any dialog either of us would say to the other. This, of course, lengthens the session. Interpreters may remain present, but only translate when clarification of information is needed, if this is the preference of the patient. Ms. S felt that she was fluent enough in English that it would be reasonable for us to conduct the session in English, and for the interpreter to be available only when needed.

Contracting—and why it is important

At the beginning of the session, I asked Ms. S what she had been told about genetic screening and testing, and what she hoped to get out of our meeting. She replied that she had not been given much information regarding the appointment, and came to the session because "my doctor told me to do that." She reported that this pregnancy had not been planned and that she was under considerable stress at home caring for her family. She stated that she was not happy about being pregnant but reported that she was trying to "get used to it."

She further stated that she believed the reason her doctor referred her must be related to her son, T's, diagnosis of "autism." This was new information that had not been included in the initial indication for her referral. When I asked her for more details about her son, she reported that he had previously been evaluated by a medical geneticist and diagnosed with autism. She reported that "a lot of testing had been done" but that "no reason for his problem" had been found. After requesting her permission to access his medical record, I briefly reviewed his medical records to see if any specific genetic diagnosis had been made. At the time of his medical genetic evaluation, T had been diagnosed with autism and global developmental delay. The records indicated that a microarray and fragile X testing had been ordered, and both were negative. Based on these results, additional testing was recommended, but, as of the date that I saw her, had not been done. I reviewed these negative results with her and tried to explore her feelings regarding the medical genetic evaluation and what they knew about his condition at this time. Ms. S seemed to welcome the opportunity to talk about it. She stated that she found the lack of an "answer" despite "all these tests" to be very confusing and difficult to accept. She found it very hard to understand why "no one knew" what was causing his behavioral issues and developmental delay. She wanted very much to understand what had caused her son's difficulties and what they could do about it. She further wanted to know if this baby could be similarly affected.

At this point in the session, I began to be concerned that our discussion would take longer than I had anticipated, and that we would eclipse the time scheduled for her ultrasound appointment, which was to follow. The conversation regarding her concerns needed to be given the space it deserved; however, the ultrasound was also important because if she wanted to have a screening test, certain fetal measurements may be necessary. It was also becoming increasingly clear to me that her goals for the session were not necessarily what I had expected, or prepared for. She wanted to talk about her son and explore her fears and concerns for him; and it is understandable that these issues might resonate with the advent of another pregnancy. My goals for the session, however, did not seem to be synchronous with hers. In addition to supporting her, I was also concerned about her later gestational age and providing her with information in a timely fashion so that she could decide whether to have screening or diagnostic testing for aneuploidy—something she was also at an increased risk for due to her age.

While I felt that we needed to discuss her risk of having a child with a chromosome abnormality, it was quickly becoming obvious that routine screening was not her primary concern. Furthermore, continuing to discuss chromosomal aneuploidy and genetic screening appeared to be distracting and confusing to the conversation she wanted to have. Ms. S kept circling back to her anxiety about her son, and to her need for a diagnosis for him. She stated that she found it difficult to imagine that the screening testing that we were discussing related to this pregnancy would not somehow offer them the opportunity to discover what had caused her son's autism. As she continued to talk, she expressed her great fear that this baby would also have the same issues that her son has.

Moment of reflection

This was obviously not a "typical session." The introduction of new information regarding her son's diagnosis of autism was changing the direction of the session, and I was beginning to find it challenging to balance my goals for the session with her agenda. In hindsight, I was allowing my concerns about timing to dictate the focus of the session. I was concerned that everything I thought we needed to discuss would not be addressed and we would run out of time. She would then miss an opportunity to choose to have prenatal screening. Ms. S also had an ultrasound appointment following our session. This would be the first ultrasound that she had had in this pregnancy, and I wanted to be certain that she got that procedure as having accurate dating for the pregnancy was essential.

As the conversation became more complicated and nuanced, Ms. S seemed increasingly reluctant to accept the translational help of the IRC interpreter. I had anticipated that using an interpreter—which we had discussed at the beginning of the session—would help the process, but Ms. S appeared not to want to engage the interpreter, continuing to raise her questions or clarify a point in English. I was beginning to feel frustrated and confused about how to proceed.

There are moments during a complicated session when an awareness of my own internal feelings has great meaning for me; but managing your own emotional process during a session is a learned skill, and one that is easier to channel with years of experience and practice. Even then it is not always an easy thing to do. The feelings that we as providers experience in the course of our interactions with patients have the potential to impede our work with them, but an awareness of our own feelings, reactions, and behaviors allows us the opportunity to use that information in productive ways.

Countertransference

Countertransference was first introduced by Freud in 1910, as a process whereby the patient's behavior influenced the analyst's unconscious emotional feeling, "We have begun to consider the 'counter-transference', which arises in the physician [analyst] as a result of the patient's influence on his unconscious feelings …" Freud believed that countertransference impeded the work between a therapist and a client and should be consciously avoided "… and we have nearly come to the point of requiring the physician [analyst] to recognize and overcome this counter-transference in himself" (Freud, 1910). In the years since, much has been written about counter-transference, including in the genetic counseling literature (Kessler, 1992; Reeder et al., 2017; Weil, 2000). Reeder et al. quote Kessler as saying that

> "the unconscious projections of the counselor, consisting of the attitudes, beliefs, anxieties, and fears stimulated by the counselees and the issues with which the counselees are dealing, constitute the countertransference. As long as the countertransference remains unconscious, the counselor is likely to misunderstand and distort the counselees' needs. Once they are brought into … consciousness, the counselor can begin to use his/her own feelings as a vehicle for understanding the counselees."
>
> (Reeder et al., 2017)

Kessler's view of countertransference suggests that, if an awareness can be brought to the process, it can be used in productive ways when working with patients.

Countertransference occurs often in therapeutic relationships and can be conscious, or unconscious (Redlinger-Grosse, 2021). Kessler refers to two types of countertransference: associative and projective (Kessler, 1992). Associative countertransference occurs when the behavior of the patient triggers feelings, thoughts or behaviors in the counselor—some of which can be uncomfortable. Experiencing these feelings in a session is often a distraction that can cause the counselor to focus his or her attention away from the patient's experience, and toward their own internal feelings and emotions (Reeder et al., 2017). Projective countertransference occurs when the counselor "over-identifies" with the patient due to a shared, often painful or complicated, experience (Reeder et al., 2017; Redlinger-Grosse, 2021). This may then lead the counselor to assume that they have an understanding and appreciation of the patient's emotional experience that is unrealistic or inappropriate. While countertransference can lead to greater empathy in working with patients, it can also lead the genetic counselor to redirect the session away from the important unique needs, experiences and agenda of the patient.

Recognizing countertransference—as it is happening—is a learned skill that requires the ability to listen without judgment to your own emotional experience. Awareness of your own responses to emotional triggers created by the patient's behavior can help you to understand your own behavior and how it can potentially impact your work.

I realized that I was feeling frustrated. It seemed that the session was losing focus, and I was becoming concerned that we would not have the time to discuss her options related to genetic screening and testing. But, in reality, was the session really losing focus—or was her focus just different from mine? Why was I finding this so challenging?

Commentary

Flexibility is an important part of genetic counseling, but it is often difficult in a clinic setting to adjust the time you have with any one patient. This is particularly true in a prenatal setting when your session is often followed by a procedure, or an office visit with another provider. Some sessions will take more time than others, and other providers with whom you work may not be able to adjust their schedule to accommodate the additional time a particular patient may need. This cannot always be predicted. One thing that can be anticipated, however, is that sessions that involve language barriers are usually longer. Unfortunately, the health care system is often not nimble enough to pivot in these moments to adjust to patients and families with different needs.

Session continued

Ms. S seemed to have deep feelings of sadness and confusion related to her son's diagnosis of autism that were re-awakened by this new pregnancy. The lack of a genetic explanation for his diagnosis was fueling her frustration and creating anxiety about the health of the new baby. We had not determined for her why her son had autism, and we had no testing to offer them in this pregnancy that would determine if this baby was also affected. As the session continued, our individual agendas began to drift apart.

Health care in this country is often not flexible and fails to accommodate the individual needs of everyone seeking care. This is especially true for individuals and families with various health care barriers. It is easy to wonder now if her past interactions with the health care system had somehow failed her. When her son was seen for an evaluation, was the appointment time convenient for her, and long enough to meet her needs? Was the medical information difficult to understand, and were interpreting services available if she needed them? Were her fears and anxieties explored at that time, and did she feel listened to and respected? Had she felt "heard"?

Regardless of the reasons for her feelings, my concern with the time constraints of her later gestation age and the clinic schedule was causing me to become more internally focused, rather than focused on her. What eluded me in that moment was the realization that what she was experiencing might be a "do-over." I wasn't listening to her either.

As the session continued it became more and more unfocused as we each tried to take the agenda in a different direction. As time slipped away, I was beginning to feel ineffectual, and the session started to feel like a tightly wound rubber band that was ready to break.

Commentary

There are several interventions one might consider in this situation, and no one choice is typically more helpful than another. But, regardless of the approach you take, the use of any intervention initially requires an awareness of the situation.

I was focused on the time constraints of our clinic schedule and my desire to offer her screening and testing that is standard of care, and that she might want to have. This was causing me to adopt a more pressured pace, which failed to prioritize the real needs that she was presenting. This discordance was a driving force in our struggle together.

Body language is an important indicator of the emotional tenor of any interpersonal interaction. It can be used both to assess the situation, and to adjust it. I noticed that our body postures and voices had become more rigid. I consciously chose to adopt a more relaxed and thoughtful body language and voice, relaxing my physical posture in the seat and lowering my voice. Most importantly, I also chose to pause and reflect to her what I was "seeing." I attempted to validate her feelings of frustration and worry regarding her son's obvious health care needs, and the concerns she had for the health of this baby.

Session continued

It seemed that our appointment had provided Ms. S with an opportunity to re-address needs that were unmet from her son's earlier evaluation. I attempted to validate those unmet needs and suggested that it might be appropriate for her to pursue the follow-up appointment that had been recommended for her son in the medical genetics department. I explained why I felt that it would be important to order additional testing, and what that could mean for this pregnancy. Specifically, if we had a molecular diagnosis for her son, then genetic testing in this pregnancy might be possible. I offered to facilitate that appointment if she would like to pursue it.

At this point, I attempted to realign the goals for the session to include a discussion about various genetic testing that was available to her and would address the risk of chromosome anomalies. As this was one of my initial goals for the session, I believed that it was important to ask her if she would like to discuss it. Ms. S was interested in exploring various screening and testing options and so we began to discuss options including: cell-free DNA screening, or non-invasive prenatal screening (NIPS), First Trimester Screening/Integrated Screening, and QUAD screening.

We also discussed the benefits and risks of diagnostic testing. Diagnostic testing enables a patient to get a definitive answer by examining fetal cells directly—either by molecular genetic testing or a standard karyotype. The two most common diagnostic tests are chorionic villus sampling (CVS) and amniocentesis. CVS is typically offered between 11 and 13 weeks, and amniocentesis is typically offered after 15 weeks of gestation. Both of these tests have procedure-related risks of miscarriage that are considered low but are not zero.

Ms. S was concerned about the cost of screening and testing, and she was reassured that her Medicaid insurance would cover all of the options presented to her.

Ms. S's family and past pregnancy history were also reviewed, and, with the exception of her first pregnancy loss and her son's diagnosis of autism, were unremarkable. Ms. S reported that she and her husband were non-consanguineous. We discussed carrier testing for genetic conditions, both as single gene testing and as expanded carrier screening, and she declined testing.

Following our discussion, Ms. S chose to have NIPS testing and she had her blood drawn that day. I told her that the turn-around-time (TAT) was typically 5–7 days and I further explained that I would call her with results when available using a telephone Nepali interpreter in case we needed to clarify any information. She was still contemplating a follow-up appointment for her son and wanted to discuss this with her husband, but she told me that she would let me know if I could refer them.

Results

Ms. S's NIPS results were available in 7 days and were unusual and complicated. The report was negative—or normal—for both trisomy 18 and 21, indicating a "low risk." The results for chromosome 13, however, were reported as "indeterminate." The report indicated that there was extra chromosome 13 material present in the sample, and that it was "likely of maternal origin." The amount of the extra material was not enough to represent an entire extra chromosome; therefore, the prediction was that this represented a copy number gain of genetic material from chromosome 13.

Additional information regarding cell-free fetal DNA testing

Cell-free fetal DNA testing, or NIPS, involves isolating and quantifying DNA from specific chromosomes that are circulating in maternal blood. The fetal fraction of the total sample is determined by comparing the length of DNA fragments—maternal fragments tending to be slightly larger—and a certain threshold amount of fetal DNA is necessary to obtain a result. The source of fetal DNA is primarily apoptosis of syncytiotrophoblast cells from the placenta. (Sekizawa et al., 2000) The majority of laboratories use a ratio study in which maternal and fetal DNA are measured together and then compared to a normal control sample. The results are either read as "positive," "negative," "nonreportable," or, as in this case, "indeterminate." Nonreportable results may occur due to poor sample quality, low fetal fraction, or atypical results that make analysis of the total sample impossible. Indeterminate results suggest that partial results are possible, but that certain portions of the testing may not be complete. At the time of this case, NIPS testing was relatively new and the sensitivity/specificity of results in low-risk populations was still being established. As NIPS testing became more widely accepted, unusual incidental findings, while rare, began to be reported. Multiple reports are now available in the literature of unexpected maternal findings identified by NIPS testing, including copy number gains and losses, and maternal malignancy (Snyder et al., 2015; Zhou et al., 2017; Carlson et al., 2018).

Moment of reflection

This result was unexpected, and very complicated. I anticipated that it would be challenging to discuss these results over the telephone, but, as we had agreed that I would call her, I felt that to do otherwise would create more anxiety for her. In hindsight, contracting for a different protocol in the beginning would have been more thoughtful of the language barrier and her situation at home.

Disclosure of results

I called Ms. S to discuss the test results, and, as we had agreed, a telephone Nepali interpreter was present in case we needed it. When she answered the telephone, I could hear children's voices in the background and the audio connection we had was not consistently clear. I explained that I had the results of her testing and inquired if this would be a good time to talk. She reported that she was alone with the children, and that her husband was at work, but that this would be a good time to talk. I told her that the test results were now complete and that the majority of the results were normal; however, a portion of the test had identified an abnormality. I began to explain the results, but the poor telephone connection made it very difficult for us to hear each other. At this point, I suggested that we meet in person to discuss the result, and this was arranged for late the next afternoon. I encouraged her to bring her husband to the appointment, if at all possible, and I told her that I would have a Nepali interpreter available to translate for him.

Session 2

Ms. S got a ride from a Medicaid cab and came to the appointment by herself the next day. I inquired about her husband, and she reported that her husband had to work that day and was unable to attend the appointment with her. She explained that it was important that he not miss a day of work as his income was their sole source of support. She felt that she would be able to discuss the appointment with him that evening. She had arranged to have someone take care of her children, but doing so was challenging for her as they did not have a robust support system in the community. She reported that she only had a short amount of time for the appointment, and then she had to get home to relieve the babysitter.

I had requested an IRC Nepali interpreter be present for the appointment, but no one was available. A telephone interpreter was engaged but Ms. S preferred to speak in English.

Language Barrier

The language barrier in this case raised significant challenges at many different points during our work together and created a conflict for me between respecting Ms. S's autonomy, and my fiduciary duty as her provider to act in her best interests.

According to hospital policy, Ms. S is able to refuse a native language interpreter as long as it does not "impede her care." The definition of impede is to delay or prevent, therefore, the purpose of an interpreter, in part, is to facilitate understanding in order to ensure timely and appropriate medical care and autonomous decision-making. Over the course of several appointments, Ms. S was offered testing that would provide her with information that could lead to complicated decisions about additional testing and pregnancy management. She had a right to that information. The information could present choices. She had a right to those, too. I wanted to ensure that she understood the information well enough that she could make choices that were in concert with her personal, family, and moral values.

Session continued

The results of her NIPS test were discussed with her. I reassured her that the risk that the baby had either trisomy 18 or 21 was now low. However, the laboratory had detected extra genetic material (a gain) on chromosome 13 that exceeded the fetal fraction. This would suggest that, at least in part, this extra material was maternally derived. The exact size of the gain on chromosome 13 was unclear at this point. We discussed drawing her blood for a microarray, which would determine if she had this copy number gain on chromosome 13. If she did, it would give us insight into the unusual NIPS results; however, the only way to determine if the baby had this extra material would be to have a diagnostic test.

Ms. S was also concerned that this finding was related to her son's diagnosis of autism. I again reviewed his microarray results with her and explained that he had already been tested to determine if he had any extra or missing genetic material, and that none had been found. I explained that this atypical NIPS result appeared to be a completely independent result that had no connection to her son's diagnosis of autism. I also explained that we would need more information—determined through additional testing—to help us understand what these results might mean, if anything, for this pregnancy.

Ms. S expressed continued confusion and frustration that we had uncovered another "abnormality" that we could not explain. As the conversation continued, I realized that my focus up to that point had been primarily on the medical aspects of T's diagnosis, and less on the impact of the situation on their family structure. I asked Ms. S to tell me a little more about her son, and how he interacts with the family.

Ms. S reported that her son is now three and a half years old and has significant behavioral issues including hyperactivity and self-stimulation behaviors that the family feels are socially inappropriate. He also requires constant supervision to prevent him from running away. Recently, Ms. S has found it impossible to take him out in public as she is constantly worried that he will hurt himself. Because of the increasing care needs that he has, Ms. S is concerned about her ability to care for another child with a disability. She expressed her worry and feelings of sadness for her son, and her concern for his future. She reported that she spends a lot of time worried about what would happen to him after she and her husband are gone. The rest of their family is still living in Nepal, with no plans to immigrate to the United States. They have no family support here and are struggling to manage all of the needs of their immediate family. As a result, she was feeling overwhelmed and anxious. Ms. S talked for a long time about her feelings but eventually began to feel anxious about getting home to relieve the babysitter and wanted to leave. She declined a prenatal diagnostic test at that time but elected to have a blood sample drawn for a microarray to further characterize the indeterminate NIPS results. We made a follow-up appointment to discuss her results in person when her husband could be present. I explained that she would be able to have a diagnostic test (amniocentesis) at her next appointment if she wished to.

Session 3: maternal microarray results

The microarray results were available in 10 days and confirmed that Ms. S has a duplication of genetic material from the long arm of chromosome 13. It is a large (5 megabase) copy gain that includes several known disease genes. At the time of the report, none of the listed genes had been associated with a clinical phenotype when duplicated; however, no information to suggest that this duplication was a normal variant had thus far been reported. The clinical significance of this duplication was, therefore, determined to be unknown.

Ms. S and her husband came to the clinic to discuss her microarray results, and an IRC Nepali interpreter was present to provide assistance with interpretation. As this was her husband's first appointment in our clinic, I reviewed the information that Ms. S and I had discussed during her previous appointments and outlined the process that she had already completed for testing in this pregnancy, including the NIPS results. The IRC Nepali interpreter translated all of the conversation for her husband which allowed for both of them to hear the information together.

I then began to discuss the results of Ms. S's microarray testing. I explained that the testing showed that Ms. S has a duplicated portion of genetic material on one of her chromosomes—chromosome 13; and, while this extra material was present in all the cells that we tested, we could not rule out a mosaicism. Furthermore, while it did not appear that Ms. S was having any physical or developmental problems related to this extra material, not a lot of information had been reported about other people who had the same extra material on chromosome 13. I explained to them that there would be a 50% chance with any pregnancy that the baby could inherit the gain of chromosome 13 material. And lastly, while we could be somewhat reassuring, based on her clinical phenotype, that a child would be unaffected, we would never be able to completely rule out that a child might be in some way affected by this extra genetic material.

The IRC Nepali interpreter translated all of the conversation, and her husband asked many thoughtful questions. For her husband's benefit I again discussed their son's previous genetic evaluation and we reviewed that his microarray testing had been normal. Therefore, because he had not inherited this copy number gain from her, we did not think that his diagnosis of autism was related to it. I reviewed that it is possible their son has a genetic condition that was not identified by the testing he has already had. I also discussed with them that it is possible that they could have another child with similar issues, and that it was difficult to tell them exactly what the chance of that might be because we do not have a specific identified genetic etiology.

Autism spectrum disorder (ASD) has been estimated to affect 1% of the population and is more common in males than in females. In the case of isolated ASD of unknown etiology, recurrence risk is based on empirical data. The recurrence risk for autism in first-degree relatives is estimated to be between 5–10% for one affected child, and 33–50% if there are two or more affected children (Griesi-Oliveira and Sertie, 2017). In this situation, because a specific genetic cause for their son's autism had not been found, we could not test for it in this, or any other pregnancy. Lastly, if his difficulties were caused by an, as yet undiagnosed, autosomal recessive genetic condition, then the risk could be as high as 25%.

They had many questions about what the NIPS result could mean for the current pregnancy. The NIPS test is a complicated screening test that includes a measurement of both her DNA and the fetus' DNA. As it is a screening test, the results are not diagnostic. Furthermore, the NIPS results cannot definitively determine whether the baby also has this copy number gain. The only way to do that would be through diagnostic testing, which, at this gestational age, would mean an amniocentesis. The risk of procedure-related miscarriage was quoted to be less than 1 in 200, or 0.5%. I explained to them that while we could definitely tell them if the baby had inherited this duplication, we could not guarantee what effect, if any, the duplication would have on the baby. Testing of their two oldest children might be helpful. If one or both of their children also had this copy number gain and are asymptomatic, like Ms. S appears to be, then we would feel more reassured. In order to test their two other children, we would need to refer the family back to the medical geneticist.

It is important that all patients be offered all of the options that are available to them and, at the time of this session, her options included pregnancy termination. I tried to explore their feelings about continuing the pregnancy with uncertain information, and we discussed termination. Ms. S and her husband reported that termination was not a choice that they would make, and that they did not want to discuss it further.

Ms. S was approximately 17 weeks pregnant at this time. She and her husband elected to decline an amniocentesis. They stated that they did not want to take the risk of losing this pregnancy if we could not give them clear, definitive information. They expressed extreme frustration with our inability to give them clarity about whether this current child would be "healthy" or not.

They left with our contact information, and I explained to them that they could call at any time if they had questions or wished to schedule a procedure. They had a 20-week anatomic ultrasound scheduled in three weeks, at which time we agreed to talk again.

Follow-up

Ms. S and her husband returned to the clinic three weeks later for a routine 20-week anatomic survey and a Nepali telephone interpreter was present for this appointment. The ultrasound was unremarkable. We counseled them that while a normal ultrasound is reassuring, ultrasound is essentially another screening tool and we could not guarantee that the baby would be perfectly healthy by these results alone. Furthermore, autism is not something that could be detected by ultrasound. Ms. S and her husband reported that they were reassured by the ultrasound findings and again chose not to have an amniocentesis.

Several weeks went by without any communication with Ms. S, or her husband. Following Ms. S's next routine obstetrical appointment at 24 weeks, her provider contacted me and told me that she had had a long conversation with Ms. S and that she and her husband had decided that they wanted to end the pregnancy at this time. They were requesting a referral for a termination.

Regulations on abortion

At the time, the law in our state regulated abortion after the 2nd trimester and only made exceptions for the life of the mother. Ms. S's gestational age, therefore, made it impossible to offer her this option in our state. Furthermore, had we been able to offer this to her at our institution, Medicaid—a federally funded program in the United States—would not cover the cost of this procedure. At the time of this case, other options for patients were available out of state, but the procedure was extremely expensive and there would be the additional costs of travel and lodging. Some resources were available through private funding, but are typically not enough to cover the cost of the procedure.

Session 4

This was an unexpected development, and uncomfortable for me. I reviewed the conversations that we had had over the course of the last several weeks and wondered if I had missed something.

I contacted Ms. S and had a telephone Nepali interpreter present. While she had continued to express her preference to speak in English, I wanted to have the option of interpretation if needed. I explained to her that I had spoken to her provider and that she had relayed Ms. S's conversation with her earlier that day, and her wish now to end the pregnancy. I asked Ms. S to tell me more about how she was feeling at this point.

She confirmed that she and her husband had talked at length about their concerns regarding the results and decided that they wished to end the pregnancy at this time. She stated that their son, T's, behavioral issues were becoming increasingly more challenging for the family. They had taken him shopping recently and he got angry and broke a glass jar in the grocery store, cutting his arm and requiring five stitches and hours in the emergency room. Ms. S reported that T was beginning to have more frequent anger episodes and that she worried about his safety and the safety of the new baby. She was also very concerned that the new baby could have autism and "anger" issues, and she did not feel that she, or the family, could manage that.

Ms. S stated that if we could not be absolutely sure that this baby would be healthy, they did not want to take the risk of having another child with physical or developmental disabilities. They felt that they had everything they could handle in taking care of T and were concerned about the welfare of their two other children and worried that they would not be able to provide the time and resources that this baby might need. As Ms. S began to relate how she was feeling, she began to cry. While it was difficult to understand everything that she was saying, it was easy to hear her emotional distress. As the conversation got more complicated, Ms. S moved back and forth between speaking in English and Nepali. At times the interpreter had difficulty keeping up with the flow of the conversation and we had to repeat much of what she was saying for clarity.

I reviewed the restrictions and limitations on abortion in our state. I explained that I could refer her to a provider in another state but that the cost would not be covered by her insurance and would have to be paid at the time of the procedure. We discussed the typical cost for this procedure out-of-state, and Ms. S reported that they would never be able to finance the cost of the procedure and travel-related expenses. In addition to the financial concerns, Ms. S related that they could not travel outside of the community for any health care as they would not have anyone to watch their other children. We had a lengthy discussion, and I attempted to answer her questions. I offered her another in-person session to discuss this, and explained that we could do that immediately, or I could be present at her next obstetrical appointment if that would be easier. I explained that I thought it would be important to have this conversation with her husband present and I would do whatever I could to try to make that possible for her. She told me that she would talk to him that night and asked if I could call her the next day.

I called her the following morning and she reported that she and her husband had discussed it, and in light of the cost of the procedure and travel-related expenses, they had decided that they could not afford it. I offered to refer her to an outside provider for a discussion regarding termination and available additional financial resources, and she declined. She also did not want to make a follow-up appointment to discuss this issue with her husband present, and she declined a meeting with a social worker for assistance and support.

Moment of reflection

Sometimes it is easy, when a patient changes course, to think that you were not fully present for the process. That you missed something important along the way. And sometimes this might be true. It is also possible that something has changed for them, or that your conversations have provided them with an opportunity to explore their feelings and beliefs—and pivot towards a different outcome. You may never know. What is challenging in a prenatal setting is the timeline. They may not have the time to pivot.

Follow-up

Ms. S continued the rest of her obstetrical care in our department. The remainder of her pregnancy was uneventful, and she was admitted to Labor and Delivery at 37 weeks following a nonreassuring nonstress test. Based on her past pregnancy history, and her age, a recommendation for induction of labor was discussed with her and she agreed. She had a normal vaginal delivery of a 2820 g male infant with Apgars of 7 and 9. He was discharged home with her on day 2 of life.

At the baby's 8-month pediatric visit, he was developing normally and was being followed by the same pediatrician who sees their other children. At the time he had not had any genetic testing and the family had not returned to the medical genetics department for a follow-up appointment for their older son.

Summary

Pregnancy is a timeline from conception to delivery, and it travels from beginning to end like a moving sidewalk: you get on, and you get off, but you can't stop it along the way while you make decisions. Because of the dynamic nature of this process, an urgency often exists around decision-making. Ms. S presented for prenatal care late in the first trimester of her pregnancy, and this created a narrow window of time for her to make choices about genetic testing. Her later entry to care may have been related to the many barriers she faced in accessing the health care she needed. Families who lack adequate social support systems, and have economic challenges and language barriers, at times have complicated experiences accessing a health care system that is often not flexible enough to meet their needs. These experiences become a part of their story and can inform future encounters with other providers. Ms. S's past experiences with the medical community, and the emotional turmoil it created for her, were a significant component of our work together, but were largely invisible at the beginning of the relationship. It was only through contracting and exploration that this important concern was illuminated.

Ms. S and her husband were struggling to meet the needs of their family with little outside support. This new pregnancy seemed to intensify her anxiety regarding a cause for her son's autism, and resulted in the understandable fear that this new baby would be similarly affected. Their son consumed a disproportionate share of the family's financial and emotional resources, and they had become increasingly worried about his behavior. It was hard for her to imagine how they could take care of another child who would have the same developmental concerns. Furthermore, the lack of an identifiable genetic cause for his issues, despite multiple tests, had stretched their trust in the medical system that they hoped would help them.

Ms. S's complex genetic test results would have been challenging for anyone to understand, and the language barrier that we faced made our conversations more complicated. She had a right to make decisions based on complete information, and I had a fiduciary duty to provide her with that information in a way that would allow her to make informed and autonomous choices.

Lastly, throughout our work together it was very difficult for Ms. S and her husband to believe that these two different medical concerns—their son's diagnosis and her results—were not related. This confusion put an additional strain on their trust in the health care system, and the resulting distrust permeated the current genetic counseling relationship.

Final Reflections

Have you ever asked yourself the question, "What of myself do I bring to my work?" It seems like a simple question, yet maybe the journey to answer that question will take you the entirety of your professional life—just as it has me. And maybe, like me, you will decide that, while it is a simple question, it still begs a thoughtful and meaningful answer.

We are all a product of the journey of our lives—the bumps and curves, and mountains and valleys that bring us to this moment. And our patients also have their own journeys that bring them to that hour or so of time that we spend with them. We know some things about them, and they know less about us. We intersect at a moment in time that is sometimes one of the most fragile of their lives. I consider it a blessing to be witness to it. But all of our life stories— what "makes us"—sometimes influence our work with them. It is a challenge then, and perhaps a calling, to examine ourselves and what we bring to our work.

Ms. S and I collided on an afternoon that I was expecting to be routine. It wasn't. I naively thought that I had the agenda for the session mapped out, and that what I expected her to "need" was what I was prepared to give. It wasn't. Her story, which was not completely known to me at the beginning of the appointment, greatly influenced her hopes and desires for that time with me. As our work together got more complicated, the barriers she was facing to equitable health care became more painful for her, and contributed to the challenges we faced together in meeting her needs. Finally, the health care system that created the framework that shaped our interactions, was not, and is not, nimble enough to meet the needs of everyone whose wellbeing is often defined by barriers to health care. Barriers that I have not experienced in my own life.

I have heard it said that prenatal genetic counseling is the adrenaline sport of the practice, and there are some weeks that I believe that. Trying to help someone make a permanent and life-altering decision, in a narrow window of time with uncertain information, is breathtaking. It creates anxiety about doing the best job we can—being our "best self." And you can get lost in your efforts. In those moments, the support of colleagues and mentors is crucial.

Revisiting this case and committing it to paper has been an enlightening experience, and a gift to me. In the process of having colleagues and editors read it, and comment, I have been challenged to examine my process, beliefs, and also my language. Ultimately, it has deepened my awareness of what I bring to my work. And this will help me—even in the last few years of my practice.

Genetic counseling is often challenging, and sometimes difficult work—and it can affect us. As the years go by, we appreciate the relevance of this as we live the experience of doing the work. But practicing any profession with intention creates a pathway that you can navigate, based on that lived experience. Those bumps and valleys affect us, but they also provide opportunities for growth and change. The journey to create a "living" practice requires one to believe in the importance of continued growth and self-reflection—*and to act intentionally to foster it*. Each of us may have our own way to do that, but for me it will always be to ask the question, "What of myself do I bring to my work?" I am still asking.

CASE EXAMPLE (GANAB PKD): ADDRESSING MULTIPLE EVOLVING GENETIC COUNSELING ISSUES IN A PEDIATRIC POLYCYSTIC KIDNEY DISEASE CASE (RICH DINEEN)

This case will illustrate the multifaceted role of the pediatric genetic counselor. Traditionally, genetic counselors have been paired with a medical geneticist to provide care in a pediatric setting. However, pediatric genetic counseling has become increasingly specialized with many genetic counselors having a more independent role. While the patient in a pediatric genetic clinic is the child, this case will demonstrate that there may be multiple family members benefiting from genetic counseling. This case will also reveal the limitations of genetic testing and the ambiguities of information often provided to families. Presenting uncertain results, explaining puzzling concepts, and leaving families with unanswered questions are all difficult, as families desire definitive test results and concrete answers. Anything less presents a challenge.

Case Management

Referrals to a pediatric genetic clinic typically come from the primary care provider. Depending on the geographical location of the clinic, it is not uncommon for an appointment with a medical geneticist to be scheduled months in the future. Some children may have already been seen by multiple specialists and have had multiple evaluations and laboratory studies while others are referred with essentially no work up having been initiated. Pediatric genetic counselors often spend significant time obtaining and reviewing medical records in preparation for a clinic visit.

The Case

Brian was a 7- year- old male who had a history of slow growth but was otherwise believed to be in good health. While always smaller than his peers, his mother noted her son had not outgrown clothing that had been purchased the previous year. In pediatrics, a child with poor growth may be described as having "failure to thrive." After the mother raised this concern to his pediatrician, his growth was tracked more carefully for several months, but due to minimal improvement, the pediatrician recommended some general laboratory studies consisting of a comprehensive metabolic profile (CMP) and complete blood count (CBC).

These studies revealed abnormalities in kidney function indicated by elevations in the blood urea nitrogen (BUN) and creatinine levels. Given these results, the child's pediatrician contacted a pediatric nephrologist for referral and interim recommendations. The pediatric nephrologist recommended additional laboratory studies as well as an abdominal ultrasound prior to the scheduled clinic visit. The abdominal ultrasound revealed bilateral renal cysts and a genetics evaluation was also recommended. Although wait times to see a medical geneticist can involve months as previously noted, there had been a last-minute cancellation, allowing the family to be seen in genetics prior to the initial visit in pediatric nephrology. This visit was scheduled with a medical geneticist and a genetic counselor.

Case Management

In some centers, it is possible that such a patient may only be seen by a genetic counselor as a targeted genetic counseling visit to coordinate genetic testing for cystic kidneys. Another aspect of care that may vary from center to center is when the initial intake and family history are obtained. At some centers, all information is obtained on the day of the clinic visit, while other pediatric centers attempt to obtain an initial intake by telephone prior to the actual visit. At times, pre-clinic intakes may be obtained by genetic counseling students or genetic counseling assistants. The benefit of this approach is more ample time to obtain information with the ability to fill in gaps of unknown details later. If the intake is performed by a genetic counselor, contact prior to the clinic visit allows the counselor to begin to develop rapport with the family. Particularly in the case of a child, the genetic counselor can inquire what the child may know about the upcoming appointment and determine if there are any sensitive topics and how best to deal with those on the day of the clinic visit.

Case/First session

Brian was brought to the initial clinic visit by his mother and father. During the session, it was learned that his father was a sales manager and his mother worked in a hospital as a speech pathologist. Although both parents were surprised by the finding of cystic kidneys, their level of concern was relatively low given Brian's history of good health. A three-generation family history was obtained. Brian had one younger sister who was reportedly healthy and had normal growth. The remainder of the family history was significant for a paternal grandmother with a single renal cyst, detected incidentally. The family history was negative for any other family member known to have kidney disease or renal failure. No other areas of concerns were identified in the family history. A physical examination was performed by the medical geneticist and revealed no additional findings aside from the child's small size for age. Given the findings on examination, the geneticist recommended a multigene panel for cystic kidney disease. The parents consented for Brian's genetic testing, and a buccal sample was obtained and sent to a commercial genetic testing laboratory for a polycystic kidney disease panel.

Commentary

It is important to involve a child in a pediatric genetic counseling session in an age-appropriate manner. Some sessions may have particularly sensitive topics, such as a child losing developmental skills or the possible consideration of a life-shortening medical condition. In this case, Brian was relatively quiet during the session and asked few questions; however, a few different topics could have been explored. As there had been concerns about Brian's size, inquiring about being smaller than his peers might have been a possible topic for discussion. Any attempts to involve the child can also elicit whether there are concerns that the child may not have expressed to the parent, such as "Am I sick?" or "Am I going to be OK?"

A common question asked by parents in a genetics clinic is how a sample for genetic testing will be collected. With the development of buccal and salvia collection for genetic testing, the need for venipuncture has been nearly eliminated at many centers. This can be very relieving to parents and the child, as many children who have seen multiple specialists may have encountered multiple blood draws. In fact, if such information can be shared prior to the appointment, this will often reduce anxiety for the child who may be anticipating a blood test, allowing the parents to focus attention on other aspects of the session.

Case Management

There are several responsibilities for the genetic counselor in this case. Gathering and assessing the family history is one such important task. While there was one paternal relative with a single renal cyst, this finding is relatively common in the general population. (In this case, Brian's parents were told that the grandmother's single cyst was not likely related to their son's cystic kidneys.) The genetic counselor is also responsible for being familiar with common syndromes in which cystic kidneys are a feature, such as Alport syndrome. Such knowledge would allow the genetic counselor to develop a list of targeted family history questions to screen for other affected family members with different clinical but potentially relevant features such as hearing loss. This family health history is of value for establishing a differential diagnosis and assists the medical geneticist as they evaluate the child for features that may be suspicious for a syndromic etiology for the bilateral cystic kidneys. Typically, such physical examinations would be looking for minor physical anomalies and/or dysmorphic features that may not have been observed or documented by the primary care provider and would help to guide genetic testing or other medical evaluations. For example, if the geneticist observed several hypopigmented lesions on physical examination, this finding may warrant further evaluation for tuberous sclerosis, a condition that may have cystic kidneys as a feature.

The genetic counselor may be responsible for identifying laboratories that offer appropriate genetic testing options for this child. As the results of the child's examination would not be known until the clinic visit, the genetic counselor would need to be prepared for multiple testing scenarios. For example, if the child were found to have other findings on physical examination, providing support for a syndromic disorder, genetic testing might begin with chromosome microarray or exome (ES) or genome sequencing (GS). If there were no additional findings on exam and the child was developmentally normal, considering a multigene panel associated with cystic kidney disease would be appropriate. Gene panels for cystic kidney disease vary by laboratory with some including genes associated with both syndromic and nonsyndromic cystic kidney disease. Working with a laboratory offering reflex testing to ES or GS if panel testing is negative would also be an important consideration.

Genetic counselors may also be responsible for discussing the billing aspects of genetic testing. Families will commonly inquire about the cost of genetic testing and whether insurance will cover these costs. While there are a variety of billing methods for genetic testing depending on the individual center, the genetic counselor is often responsible for being familiar with this information and presenting it to the family.

A genetic counselor may be involved in the actual processing and shipment of the specimen collected from patients and family members. However, at many centers, the responsibility of sending specimens is handled by laboratory staff. Completion of laboratory requisition forms and sending requested clinical information and/or a copy of the pedigree is often part of this process. Many laboratories have moved to online testing portals for test ordering and collection of medical records. A process for tracking laboratory samples should also be in place to ensure proper receipt of specimens.

Finally, the genetic counselor should develop a plan for communication of genetic test results, when available. An important consideration is whether both parents want to be present when receiving results. For this case, as both parents were employed, determining a time of day when they were available to receive a telephone call was an important consideration.

Case/Results disclosure

Genetic testing in Brian revealed a novel intronic variant in the *GANAB* gene that was classified by the laboratory as pathogenic using ACMG criteria, consistent with autosomal dominant polycystic kidney disease type 3 (ADPKD3) (Harris and Torres, 2022). The reported variant was predicted to result in a null allele and loss of function is a known disease mechanism for *GANAB*-related ADPKD (Porath et al., 2016). Additionally, the laboratory noted that the variant was absent in controls and was a phenotypic fit with the genotype given testing of other PKD genes revealed no additional variants. Based on information available at the time, the clinical course for individuals with ADPKD3 was reported to be typically milder than the more common ADPKD1 & 2 (Harris and Torres, 2022). The laboratory recommended targeted parental studies to determine if the variant had occurred *de novo* or was inherited from one of the parents. There was no cost to the parents for these studies.

I contacted the mother by telephone and informed her of these results. At the time of the call, I learned that the mother was driving home from work and offered to call later. I also offered to perform a three-way call so that the father could be involved in the result disclosure, but the mother declined this offer. The mother shared that since Brian's appointment in the genetics clinic, he had now been seen by pediatric nephrology and there was additional information available regarding his clinical status. Brian's kidney disease was assessed to be severe with the recommendation for a kidney transplant within the next several months. Both parents were being considered as potential kidney donors, but neither had yet had any type of renal evaluation. Parental testing now had the additional significance of determining if one of the parents should be excluded as a donor based on the presence of the causative variant. The call ended with plans to send genetic test kits to the parents so that testing could be completed.

Commentary

The information regarding Brian's need for a kidney transplant was unexpected. Neither his past clinical course nor his evaluation in the genetics clinic indicated something so serious. This updated information brought new intensity to this case. The mother had just recently learned of her son's need for kidney transplant and was still clearly upset by this news. Her demeanor changed during this telephone call and subsequent calls. While cheerful and rather talkative during the initial clinic visit, she now had a very serious tone to her voice, and her responses were brief. She was very task-oriented and focused on the potential turnaround time for results and making sure that nothing would slow the process of identifying a potential kidney donor. Possibly this reflected her need to establish some control over a situation for which she felt very little control.

I anticipated the call would be a discussion of the test results and known clinical information surrounding the identified gene and associated disorder. However, the call quickly evolved into crisis counseling. Significant time was spent acknowledging the difficulty of learning unexpected information. Providing reassurance that the next step of the testing process should proceed relatively quickly seemed to reduce the mother's anxiety.

One topic I did not address during this call was preparing for the possibility that one of the parents might carry the same gene variant as their child. While this topic may seem an obvious one to cover during such a telephone call, other issues predominated, and I was focused on attempting to reduce the mother's level of anxiety. This failure is pointed out here to remind genetic counselors that not all patient encounters are handled in an ideal manner, and even experienced counselors may have difficulty addressing all issues due to a variety of factors.

Case Management

As a genetic counselor is often responsible for the coordination of the parental genetic studies, they should be aware of the associated costs and inform the parents of this information. Some laboratories offer targeted variant studies at no cost, while others may charge depending on case specific factors. Testing kits were sent to the home to complete this testing.

Following the results disclosure, I shared the new information about Brian's clinical status with the medical geneticist. While the parental studies were being coordinated, there was time to perform additional research on the genetic results and the disorder. Of particular interest in this case is the question of the natural history of ADPKD3, variable expressivity of the disorder, and whether there is anything known with respect to genotype/phenotype correlation. A review of the medical literature to determine if there were individuals reported with severe disease requiring early kidney transplant revealed a few individuals with earlier ages of onset; however, the medical literature related to the *GANAB* gene was very limited and information regarding genotype/phenotype correlation was not available. The possibility of digenic inheritance was suggested in one case (Waldrop et al., 2019). In addition to searches of medical literature, a genetic counselor can consider resources such as professional discussion groups to inquire whether others have encountered a similar case not published in the medical literature or reported in available variant databases. Some laboratories may have internal data, such as clinical information on other patients with a similar variant, that can be shared to help in the assessment of a gene variant.

Case/Second results disclosure

Parental genetic studies revealed that Brian's father possessed the same pathogenic variant. The mother's studies were negative. For the second telephone call, attempts were made to have both parents available to review results. However, again the results were reported exclusively to the mother. One might wonder why, in both instances, test results were provided only to the mother. Initially, I thought the mother was taking additional responsibility for the medical aspects of Brian's case given her health care background. Over time, I suspected she was attempting to take control of a situation for which she felt a loss of control. Prior to reviewing the genetic testing results, she informed me that she and her husband had had renal ultrasounds performed. Her husband was found to have a single renal cyst; her ultrasound was normal. No additional studies regarding parental kidney function had yet been performed.

When the mother received the results of the genetic studies, the level and intensity of her voice changed, and she immediately began asking several questions. Why was her son's kidney disease so much more severe than her husband's? Would her husband also require a kidney transplant? If so, when? Should Brian's younger sister be tested? If the daughter had positive genetic testing results, would she have kidney disease like Brian or have a course like her father's?

A significant amount of time was spent presenting information that was known and unknown regarding *GANAB*-related kidney disease. We reviewed the possibility of autosomal dominant inheritance with variable expression. At the time of this case, there were very limited reports of early presentation of the disorder. Although there were no reports of autosomal recessive *GANAB*-related disease at the time, we also reviewed that Brian could possess a second variant in *GANAB* in trans that was not detected by current testing methods. We also discussed the potential interaction of the pathogenic *GANAB* variant with another gene. While this theory was proposed in one pediatric case, the underlying mechanism was not known or proven (Waldrop et al., 2019). Based on the available information at that time, we discussed that dominant inheritance with variable expression was the most likely explanation.

During this call, the mother's anxiety increased. Simultaneously confronting her son's upcoming kidney transplant, her husband's new genetic status, her own new status of being the likely kidney donor, and her daughter's at-risk status appeared to be overwhelming her. Recognizing this, I attempted to assist the mother in prioritizing each of these concerns to reduce the level of her anxiety. The most pressing issue of which parent would be an acceptable kidney donor had been answered by genetic testing and renal ultrasounds. We discussed how the subsequent steps of completing the remainder of her evaluations would determine whether she could be the donor; this would then impact when Brian's kidney transplant could proceed.

We further discussed that while Brian's father was found to possess the pathogenic *GANAB* variant, he was several decades older than his son and appeared to be in good health. No additional concerns beyond a single cyst were identified on his renal ultrasound. We discussed the need for him to have further follow-up. I reviewed the recommendation that Brian's younger sister be tested. Given the early onset of kidney disease in this family, early identification of an affected family member could impact medical care by determining surveillance and potential treatment of the disorder. We also reviewed the importance of discussing this information with other paternal at-risk family members.

We talked about issues pertaining to guilt and blame when one parent is found to have contributed a disease-causative variant to their child. Although the father was not present for this telephone call, we discussed that a "carrier" parent may feel responsible for their child's illness. In this instance, I emphasized that since there was no family history of kidney disease nor did the father have a history of medical issues, there was nothing alerting this family to this possibility. We also discussed that the "noncarrier" parent might experience feelings of blame toward the other parent. The mother denied having such feelings, but I suggested the possibility that feelings regarding such issues may change over time.

At the completion of the call, I explained that the results of the parental studies would be sent to Brian's transplant team as soon as possible. I would also review with the medical geneticist whether this would be an appropriate time to coordinate the younger sister's genetic studies.

Commentary

The second telephone call illustrates the complementary roles of the genetic counselor as an information provider and as a counselor. I needed to balance clinical information regarding the genetic test results and their implications for the husband and daughter, as well as devise a strategy for addressing what

I anticipated to be the mother's potential emotional reaction (alarm, disbelief, and overwhelming concern for her husband and daughter). In this case, addressing the psychosocial issues at the onset of the discussion was essential to addressing the other more clinical and technical questions later asked by the mother. It is unlikely that a discussion of technical information prior to focusing on the mother's immediate concerns would have been of much value to her. Furthermore, it's essential to continue to provide psychosocial support throughout the delivery of information; this is often as simple as conveying genuine caring and support throughout the session. Psychosocial counseling and the provision of information should weave together with blurred transitions back and forth between what is informational and what is supportive. This is typically a skill obtained with practice.

When self-reflecting about this case, I believe the delivery of the parental test results was suboptimal. Ideally, the father should have been part of the telephone call as many pertinent issues pertained directly to him. I should have recommended following up with the family either later the same or following day to assess the father's reactions to his results. An in person appointment for results disclosure may have solved some of these issues. However, multiple recent appointments for Brian and the distance required for attending them made an additional visit undesirable.

An additional point for consideration is that preparing patients and families in advance for the possible outcomes of genetic testing may help to facilitate their coping mechanisms when receiving unwelcome news. Had I discussed the possibility of one of the parents possessing the pathogenic variant during the initial results disclosure, it is possible there may have been less anxiety when receiving the unexpected positive paternal results. Discussing the possibility of receiving information that is uncertain or difficult to interpret may also assist with preparing families for receiving unwanted news. Uncertain results can be uncomfortable and challenging. Although the mother asked very reasonable questions regarding the implications of the father's test result, many were not answerable. This can be unsettling for both the patient as well as the provider, who is expected to be the "genetics expert," and I felt that many of my responses were inadequate. Having a discussion about a possible ambiguous outcome is often of value.

Case Management

Following the second telephone call, I reviewed testing of Brian's younger sister with the medical geneticist. Given Brian's presentation of kidney disease at a young age, the geneticist recommended that testing be initiated as soon as possible while acknowledging this was not the ideal time to perform testing because of the current stress the family was experiencing, particularly if results were positive. I placed testing orders for Brian's younger sister and a testing kit was sent to the family's home.

Case/Last result disclosure

Brian's sister tested negative for the familial *GANAB* pathogenic variant. The mother was contacted by telephone with the results. The mother expressed relief at her daughter's negative results. Compared to the two previous telephone conversations, this telephone call was relatively brief. The mother confirmed that the transplant team had received the results of the parental studies. Plans for a kidney transplant using the mother as a donor were proceeding although a specific date for transplant had not been determined.

The mother was much calmer during this final telephone call. Learning her daughter's negative results was likely a contributing factor. Compared to the number of questions and issues during the second telephone call, there were relatively few issues raised during this call. I attempted to learn if Brian's father had any questions or reactions to learning his genetic testing results. The mother reported that he had been initially surprised to learn that he possessed the same pathogenic variant but neither of them had discussed the matter further. The mother continued to inquire about the long-term prognosis for Brian's father and she was informed that this information was not known with certainty. Ongoing follow up for Brian's father was recommended.

We also discussed genetic testing for other extended family members in the paternal family. Although there was still limited ability to predict the clinical course in someone who was found to have the familial pathogenic variant, such information could be used for early identification and to guide future medical management.

Commentary

I anticipated a lengthy third telephone call. The mother seemed to now be focusing on Brian's upcoming kidney transplant with the additional issues discussed during the previous telephone call being of lesser importance. Learning her daughter's negative results seemed to have given her a renewed strength to focus almost exclusively on the transplant. Unfortunately, in this case the father was never contacted directly regarding his impression of his own test results. Ideally, I should have made the effort to contact the father later to obtain his thoughts.

The "ending" to this case illustrates how many pediatric genetic cases seem to end abruptly. As our center does not perform kidney transplants in children, the family transferred care to a different hospital and Brian had no further follow-up with the genetics clinic. There were no inquiries for testing of additional family members. While the family was supplied with copies of all test results, a specific family letter to be used for targeted variant testing was not provided. Many centers supply such a family letter and upon review of this case, this would have been an important addition. Some pediatric centers will automatically schedule or recommend follow-up in such cases in order to serve as an ongoing resource for the family, to address unresolved issues, and to provide updates on variant interpretation and information about the natural history of the disorder and expanding phenotypes, if available. Given the lack of information pertaining to *GANAB*-related kidney disease at the time of diagnosis, such follow up could be helpful.

Conclusions

This case was presented because it illustrates several points particularly common to pediatric genetic counseling.

Although Brian was the original patient in the case, the entire family became "the patient." This is often the case in pediatrics from both the clinical and counseling perspectives, and the genetic counselor should be prepared for this possibility. Although a pediatric patient with obvious symptoms and signs of a disorder may be the first family member to receive a formal diagnosis, other family members may be diagnosed subsequently. Brian's mother became the primary focus later in this case given her level of anxiety and concern over multiple different issues. Additionally, the father would have benefited from his own genetic counseling session after learning of his positive test results. Additional follow-up calls to the parents may have provided more clarity to the situation and helped to determine whether additional support during this time period would have been beneficial.

Finding a balance between the provision of information and psychosocial counseling is an ongoing challenge for the genetic counselor. In this case, it would not have been possible for the mother to adequately process the implications of the test results until some of her other concerns were addressed. Identifying signs in an individual who is experiencing emotional tension and making appropriate accommodations for the delivery of information is a necessary skill of the genetic counselor.

This case also illustrates some of the limitations of genetic testing and available information in the medical literature. Despite autosomal dominant polycystic kidney disease being a well-described medical condition and the identification of a disease causative, pathogenic variant in this family, there were several unanswered questions due to the limitations of our knowledge about the natural history, phenotype/genotype correlation, and factors contributing to variable expressivity and incomplete penetrance of the disorder. Uncertainty is a challenge in genetic counseling and requires a level of comfort on the part of the genetic counselor which comes with experience. In this case, uncertainty about the provided diagnosis given the limited information available about the condition and variable presentation within the family was a particular challenge for the mother. Preparing families for the possibility of uncertain results as well as possible uncertainty even in the face of definitive results (as in this case) may help to ease some of the disappointment and/or discomfort that often accompanies uncertainty. Scheduling return visits, or formulating a plan for staying in touch so that families can be apprised of updated information, may create a sense of hopefulness that uncertainty may be resolvable in time.

CARDIOVASCULAR GENETIC COUNSELING: SUPPORTING A FAMILY FOLLOWING A SUDDEN UNEXPLAINED DEATH (MATTHEW J. THOMAS)

The death

In March of 2019, April Smith received a call from a police officer no parent would ever want or expect. She learned that her eldest teenage daughter, Bonnie, was found deceased in the stairwell of an apartment building hours after visiting her friend there. Since there were no known witnesses to this event, lifesaving measures including cardiopulmonary resuscitation (CPR) were not an option. Even though foul play was not suspected, the police opened an investigation as there were no obvious causes of Bonnie's death at the scene. After Bonnie was found, her body was transported to the regional medical examiner's office for an autopsy as medical examiners and/or coroners are required by law to perform an autopsy in most states and jurisdictions following the unexpected and sudden death of a young person. This is when the investigation into the cause of Bonnie's death began. The goal was to find an answer to a conceptually inexplicable event: why an otherwise healthy young woman would die suddenly and unexpectedly. Genetic counseling and genetic testing played a critical role in the pursuit for answers.

The request for help and initial conversation

I met April in August 2019 when I returned a message left at our cardiovascular genetics office asking for help. The Smith family lived in a rural and medically underserved area of our state, and she found our number while researching options closest to their home. Since April was an 8-hour round trip drive from our medical center, or any other genetics clinic, I offered to work with her and her family via telehealth. I relied on phone calls for our encounters as this was prior to the adoption of video telehealth applications at our institution.

When April answered the phone, I confirmed that she was available to talk for an extended period and was in a comfortable physical and mental space to do so. I expressed my condolences for her loss before asking her how I could help. April thanked me for calling her back quickly and acknowledging her loss. She immediately transitioned to discussing the details of her daughter's death and her desire for postmortem genetic testing.

April reviewed the accumulation of evidence leading her to believe Bonnie died from an inherited heart disease: 1) Bonnie's prior signs and symptoms; 2) medical records she collected and reviewed; and 3) the preliminary outcome of her daughter's autopsy. Based on April's independent research, she learned postmortem genetic testing may find the cause of her daughter's death if it is unable to be determined by autopsy. She found my contact information online as the cardiovascular genetics specialist closest to her.

In the first 15 minutes of our conversation, April relayed to me that she thought her daughter died from an inherited arrhythmia known as "catecholaminergic polymorphic ventricular tachycardia" or CPVT. Prior to this conversation and in the years since, I cannot recall hearing a patient use the full or abbreviated name for CPVT unless they were affected by or had a known family history of this rare inherited heart condition. This level of detail suggested April may have a medical background and/or she or someone in her life did extensive research into what may have caused her daughter's death.

After April walked through the work she had done, her thought process, the condition she most suspected, and what brought her to call my office, I relayed how impressed I was with all the effort she had taken. I expressed my admiration by telling her that she approached her investigation into Bonnie's death in the same manner that I and my colleagues in cardiovascular genetics would have. While complimenting her on the quantity and quality of her efforts thus far, I concisely summarized the details she provided to ensure I understood her correctly. She confirmed my interpretation, and disclosed her nursing background, which included years of caring for patients with cardiovascular diseases. This confirmed a source of her high level of health literacy demonstrated by the terms she used and the quality of her proposed differential diagnosis.

In what continued to be a theme throughout my time working with April, her instincts and judgment almost always found the appropriate next steps for finding Bonnie's cause of death. For me to support her efforts to accomplish this goal, I needed to obtain more data about Bonnie's medical history, family history, circumstances of her death, and the findings of the medical examiner. We transitioned our conversation through each of these topics.

Bonnie's medical history: A single warning sign/red flag

We began reviewing Bonnie's medical history prior to her death rather than starting our conversation with the details of her death to allow me an opportunity to establish more of a relationship with April prior to discussing the inherently distressing topic. Bonnie's medical history was remarkably normal with one major exception: a fainting spell that happened when she was out to dinner with her parents five months before her death.

In November 2018, the Smith family went out for what would typically be an uneventful Sunday dinner. On this particular evening, Bonnie arrived at a restaurant to see that her recent ex-boyfriend was at another table on a date. Immediately after seeing them together, Bonnie collapsed and appeared to have a seizure. After a short yet unspecified amount of time, she spontaneously regained consciousness without any medical intervention. When paramedics arrived, they took her to the emergency department for an evaluation. Before releasing her home with a clean bill of health, the emergency physicians recommended she see a cardiologist and a neurologist. Her outpatient appointments were coordinated in the weeks following the emergency department visit, and her evaluations were considered normal.

Prior to her fainting spell at dinner, Bonnie was a competitive high school athlete with no known symptoms while playing sports or training for them. After graduating high school, she no longer played competitively, but stayed physically active and exercised regularly. April expressed confusion about why Bonnie had many years of high intensity athletics without any events like fainting or other concerning symptoms of a heart problem. Sudden cardiac arrest and death may be the first manifestation of an inherited heart disease in some patients, but there are often warning signs that occur in weeks, months or even years prior to diagnosis or sudden death. Unfortunately, the red flags for an inherited heart disease are often nonspecific (Table 16-1) and the conditions may be challenging to diagnose even when suspected. I acknowledged how many of us in cardiovascular genetics struggle to understand why the initial symptoms can be so sudden and severe in some individuals. Reduced penetrance and variable expressivity are common features of most inherited heart diseases, but when the most extreme phenotype is the sudden death of a young person, those genetic concepts are a woefully unsatisfying explanations for families and providers alike.

April proved to be a reliable and accurate medical historian, but having all of Bonnie's cardiology records was critical in determining the conditions I would add to her differential diagnosis. After a death, obtaining records often requires extra effort by the next-of-kin (i.e., a person's closest living relative through biological or legal relationships), as they need to have documentation of being legally able to access medical information on the decedent. As before, April gathered this information prior to our conversation. I reviewed records from Bonnie's primary

TABLE 16-1. **Red flags for inherited heart disease in patients and/or their family members**

Deaths	sudden
	unexplained
	premature (<50 years old)
	sudden unexpected infant death (SUID)
	late fetal demise
	drowning of those who can swim
	unexplained motor vehicle and other accidents
Symptoms or diseases	cardiac arrest
	fainting *aka* syncope
	seizures or epilepsy
	worsening shortness of breath
	exercise interolance
	chest pain with exertion
	obvious inherited heart diseases (e.g., hypertrophic cardiomyopathy)
Medical procedures	implantable cardioverter-defibrillator (ICD) placement
	pacemaker placement
	open heart surgery
	heart transplant

care doctor, emergency department visit, and her subsequent cardiology and neurology evaluations. Her primary care records detailed a healthy young woman with no comorbidities or signs of an inherited heart disease. Cardiology office notes summarized the results of a normal baseline echocardiogram, electrocardiogram (ECG or EKG), and ambulatory heart monitor (i.e., a 24-hour Holter monitor). Although she had a thorough evaluation, some cardiology tests were not performed as a part of her evaluation: an exercise stress test (often helpful to diagnose CPVT and long QT syndrome) and cardiac MRI (often helpful to diagnose arrhythmogenic cardiomyopathy or ACM). Her neurology evaluation was normal with no concern for a seizure disorder.

The circumstances of Bonnie's death

I gently introduced the conversation surrounding the details of Bonnie's death. I explicitly acknowledged how difficult it can be for parents to review the details of their child's death and deliberately took a moment to pause and confirm she was comfortable having this conversation now rather than returning to this later. She was comfortable moving forward with this topic, so we did so.

The last person to see Bonnie alive was her friend whom she was visiting a few hours before her body was found. According to her friend, there was nothing out of the ordinary about Bonnie that evening as they were just hanging out at her apartment watching TV after having dinner. Bonnie did not complain about feeling sick to her friend that evening nor to her mother when they talked a few days before her death.

A critical detail of sudden death investigations is to know what the decedent was doing when they died, which often means there needs to be a witness or camera to document the event. For example, when the sudden death of a young person happens during exertion some conditions are higher on the differential diagnosis (e.g., CPVT or long QT syndrome types 1 and 2) than if it happened during sleep (e.g., Brugada syndrome or long QT syndrome type 3). Bonnie's death was not witnessed as she was found at the bottom of a stairwell hours after leaving her friend's home. Therefore, we do not know if there was a potential trigger at the time of her death including emotion, physical exertion, loud noise, and so on. The presumption was that she suffered a cardiac arrest while walking down the stairs headed to her car. Even though Bonnie died almost six months prior, the police were still investigating the cause of Bonnie's death to ensure there was no foul play as they waited for the medical examiner's report to be finalized.

A nondiagnostic autopsy

I asked what April learned from the medical examiner's office. Ideally, medical examiners (MEs) or coroners communicate by phone with the next of kin, especially if they suspect an inherited condition that may impact the health of the family. MEs often take many months to "close" a case and determine (or not determine) the cause of death in a formal and signed autopsy report. Bonnie's autopsy report had not yet been finalized in written form six months after her death, but April was verbally told by the medical examiner that they did not find a definitive or likely cause of death. In other words, her toxicology testing (e.g., checking for illicit drugs and other substances that could be lethal), heart, brain, and other organs were considered normal with no abnormalities explaining why she died. Bonnie's case is similar to the roughly one third of sudden deaths of children and young adults, which remain unexplained after comprehensive autopsy (Stiles et al., 2021).

Similar to obtaining medical records, I prefer to speak directly with the ME and review the final autopsy report. When I spoke to the ME, I learned the same information April did: she expected to conclude Bonnie died from a presumed cardiac arrhythmia of unknown etiology but was waiting for toxicology labs to return before signing the report. The ME did not request a dedicated cardiac pathology consult for Bonnie's case to help identify more difficult to detect inherited heart conditions like arrhythmogenic cardiomyopathy—ACM. I asked whether an independent cardiac pathology study could be requested now or in the future. This was denied due to the lack of available heart tissue. At the end of my conversation with the ME, I thanked her and requested the finalized ME's report when it becomes available. A few weeks later I received the autopsy and toxicology reports and there were no significant differences from our conversation.

Family history and the limitations of self-report

After discussing Bonnie's medical history with April, I transitioned to Bonnie's family history. I explained that the purpose of reviewing the family history in detail is to not only look for signs of an inherited heart disease, but determine who may be at risk for an inherited heart disease in the family. I started and ended the three-generation pedigree by reviewing a list of red flags for an inherited heart disease (Table 16-1). April, Bonnie's father, and Bonnie's older full sister are all generally healthy and live together. No one in the Smith family had obvious signs or symptoms of an inherited heart disease nor sudden death. Although Bonnie's "normal" family history supports a *de novo* form of heart disease, the family's knowledge of the heart health of their relatives may be inaccurate.

A patient/family member-reported family history is a required component of cardiogenetic counseling, but it's critical to recognize the limitations of self-reported family history. First, patients often refer to any cardiovascular event in the family as a "heart attack," when it may truly be a cardiac arrest, stroke, arterial dissection, or something else entirely. In a multigenerational study based on the participants from the Framingham Heart Study where the family history was confirmed with medical records, researchers found that reportedly abnormal family histories of heart disease are usually accurate, but normal or negative family histories are often inaccurate (Murabito et al., 2004).

Another limitation of a "normal" family history is the aforementioned reduced penetrance and variable expressivity of most inherited heart diseases. Therefore, one or more of Bonnie's surviving family members may unknowingly be at risk to develop or be affected by an undiagnosed inherited heart disease only detectable by cardiology evaluation and/or genetic testing. To compensate for the limitations of patient-reported family history and undiagnosed disease in sudden death cases, I attempt to obtain documentation of the cardiology evaluations of immediate family and any documentation of reported or suspected cardiac events in more distantly related affected family.

Cardiology evaluations of the Smith family

An essential aspect of a cardiovascular genetic counseling practice, especially after a sudden death, is the integration of cardiology surveillance and management into the assessment of the family. Ideally, clinical cardiology screening of the close relatives (usually first-degree relatives) and any symptomatic surviving family should be performed *in addition to and not instead of* any postmortem genetic testing of the decedent. The reason for doing prompt cardiology testing in the family is due to the potential of one or more relatives being affected by previously asymptomatic, subclinical disease. Given that most inherited heart conditions associated with sudden death are autosomal dominant, the risk to family members is significant. An expert consensus statement from the Heart Rhythm Society summarizes the ideal cardiology evaluations for at risk family members if a cause of death is unknown/uncertain or due to a suspected inherited heart disease based on autopsy or medical history (Stiles et al., 2021). If cardiology screening identifies one or more affected surviving family members, medical management may be initiated immediately, which can include medication (e.g., beta blocker therapy for long QT syndrome and CPVT), procedures (e.g., ICD placement in someone at high risk for SCA), and education/counseling about risk factors to avoid (e.g., QT-prolonging medication, competitive athletics).

In addition to detecting and promptly treating previously undiagnosed family, cardiology evaluations also account for the scenario when genetic testing of the proband is nondiagnostic or unable to be performed. For example, if Bonnie had CPVT that was elusive to genetic testing, a stress test performed in her parents and sister may be the only way to identify signs of disease that would warrant treatment to reduce their risk of a life-threatening arrhythmias.

By the time April spoke to me, the Smith family, including their surviving daughter Dina, Bonnie's father Charles, and April had already undergone cardiology evaluations. Unfortunately, April felt dismissed by the cardiologist when she and Charles were seen. April said the cardiologist explicitly told them "I don't understand why you came to see me." I assured April that she did exactly the right thing to bring her family in for a prompt cardiology evaluation. April admitted feeling some reassurance about her family's normal testing (including Dina's stress test), but the feeling of safety was limited since Bonnie's evaluation after she fainted was also considered normal.

Differential diagnosis

After reviewing Bonnie's medical history and postmortem evaluation, the details of her death, family history, the cardiology evaluations of her family, and her postmortem evaluation, I discussed the differential diagnosis. As April anticipated and based on the description of Bonnie's fainting spell at dinner, I shared her concern that Bonnie may have had an inherited arrhythmia like CPVT or long QT syndrome. In addition to those diagnoses, I described one other possible inherited condition—arrhythmogenic cardiomyopathy (ACM)—which includes arrhythmogenic right ventricular cardiomyopathy (ARVC). Although cardiomyopathies are expected to be diagnosed on an autopsy, ACM can be missed especially when dedicated cardiac pathology is not performed, like in Bonnie's case. Even with the most advanced cardiac pathology, some patients with genetically-confirmed ACM found on postmortem genetic analysis will have no clear evidence of cardiomyopathy on expert cardiac pathology. The breadth of the differential diagnosis influences the scope of the family's cardiovascular screening and the postmortem genetic testing that should be performed.

Postmortem genetic testing

We transitioned to discussing the postmortem genetic testing process and I began by asking April an open-ended question about what she understood about the process. She knew that in order to do genetic testing, the medical examiner needed to submit a sample to a lab where DNA testing for inherited heart diseases would be completed. Our discussion of postmortem genetic testing was a balancing act between presenting: 1) the promise of genetic testing to find answers and determine who else may be at risk in her family; and 2) the limitations of even having a quality source of DNA to test, let alone finding a pathogenic variant if sequencing and analysis were successful.

The promise of postmortem genetic testing   For April, there was intrinsic value in finding a genetic diagnosis to help her understand why this tragedy happened. Her desire for answers is consistent with qualitative and quantitative studies of surviving families following the unexpected sudden death of a loved one, who express a need to understand why something inexplicable happened (van der Werf et al., 2014; McDonald et al., 2020). Genetic testing also has the potential to correct a misdiagnosis (e.g., ACM may masquerade as isolated myocarditis) or limit feelings of guilt if a parent felt something they did or didn't do led to their child's death.

The primary benefit of a molecular diagnosis is to determine the risk of disease to Bonnie's surviving family. If we found a pathogenic or likely pathogenic variant associated with Bonnie's sudden death, then cascade genetic testing of her parents and other close relatives would determine if anyone else in the family is affected or at risk. A second or even third sudden death in a family who has an inherited heart disease magnifies the first tragic loss exponentially. Since cardiology testing is not 100% sensitive for most inherited heart diseases, cascade genetic testing of a pathogenic variant is currently the only way to definitively clear a relative from the risk of an inherited disease in their family.

The limitations and drawbacks of postmortem genetic testing Like any other genetic test for a suspected inherited condition, the sensitivity of postmortem genetic testing is limited. Families and providers alike may be disappointed when all signs point to an inherited heart condition, but a clear diagnosis remains elusive to even the most advanced autopsy practices, including postmortem genetic testing. A diagnostic rate of up to 25% is best-case scenario when the cause of death is undetermined on autopsy (Wilde et al., 2022). Therefore, it was critical for me to emphasize the most likely outcome of Bonnie's postmortem genetic testing: her death remains unexplained. April dedicated dozens to hundreds of hours and likely immeasurable mental energy attempting to find the cause of her daughter's death, and I needed her to process the high probability of us being unable to find that answer. When I discussed this, she expressed a cognitive understanding that we might not know what happened. But this didn't necessarily reassure me that if the outcome of testing was nondiagnostic, April would be able to emotionally live with that outcome, at least in the short term. I still had the sense that she expected genetic testing to be successfully performed and that it would give her an answer.

Another challenge of any genetic testing panel or exome/genome sequencing is the detection of one or more variants of uncertain significance (VUSes). VUSes are to be expected given the large number of genes in cardiovascular genetic testing panels or in exome/genome sequencing. Even though a VUS may be reclassified as pathogenic in the future, historical data suggests that the great majority of VUSes that are reclassified are downgraded to "likely benign." Therefore, I discussed the importance of not overreacting to a VUS. This is to avoid other members of her family being inappropriately tested for a VUS and labeled as being affected and receiving unnecessary treatment like medication or even the placement of an implantable intracardiac defibrillator (ICD). Patients have inappropriately received implantable ICDs after a variant was errantly classified as pathogenic (Gaba et al., 2016) . I knew April had high hopes and expectations of receiving genetic diagnosis, so I needed to lay the foundation that if we only find one or more VUSes, we would unlikely find a genetic answer to Bonnie's death.

Even if we were to find a diagnosis via postmortem genetic testing, there may be unintended psychological consequences for the family. For example, if we identified a pathogenic variant in Bonnie proven to be inherited by April, this had the potential to exacerbate existing feelings of guilt. I asked April whether she had considered how she would feel if this occurred. She told me she was aware of this possibility but did not feel as though it would be a result she would anticipate struggling with. Her priority was an explanation for what happened and plan for her surviving daughter.

Alternatively, if a pathogenic variant is found to be *de novo,* it would be very reassuring for the surviving family members who are negative. However, survivor guilt remains a possible emotional reaction. This was not an psychological outcome I explored with April, but one I was prepared to discuss if this was the result of the testing.

The unique challenges of postmortem genetic testing In addition to setting expectations for no diagnosis or inconclusive results, I reviewed additional aspects of postmortem genetic testing that may serve as barriers to a diagnosis.

First, genetic testing is not possible without a DNA sample of adequate quality and quantity from the decedent, which cannot be taken for granted. In contrast to genetic testing in clinic—where sources of DNA are readily available via a blood sample, buccal swab, or saliva sample—in the postmortem setting finding a single source that has enough high quality and quantity DNA may not be possible. Professional recommendations for postmortem sample retention for genetic testing by MEs and coroners are available and detail possible samples where DNA may be extracted for testing (Middleton et al., 2013; Stiles et al., 2021). Despite this guidance, sample collection and storage practices vary dramatically state-by-state and even county-by-county. In my experience, the single greatest barrier for postmortem genetic testing once I've connected with a family is the availability of a sample that is suitable for DNA extraction and testing. Therefore, in addition to reviewing possible test results (i.e., abnormal, inconclusive, normal), I review the possibility of not receiving any results due to a lack of a quality sample.

Fortunately, the ME was exceptional and retained multiple samples from Bonnie's autopsy: 1) a tube of blood in EDTA in a refrigerator; 2) another EDTA tube in a freezer; and 3) frozen liver tissue. Therefore, we had up to three reliable sources for DNA extraction and testing for Bonnie.

Second, testing any postmortem sample requires appropriate legal consent by the next of kin, which is usually a parent/guardian (if the decedent is a minor or not married), spouse/partner, siblings, or other person designated by the decedent's stated wishes or applicable law. After establishing the person(s) who can approve the request to transfer and test a sample, there are state, county/city, and even ME office-specific requirements for the documentation needed to send a sample out for genetic testing. April was prepared to sign all required paperwork and had all documentation needed that established her as the next of kin.

A patient's health insurance coverage ends at their death, so the cost of postmortem genetic testing most often falls to the family. Like other forms of genetic testing, the cost of postmortem genetic testing has dropped significantly due to advances in sequencing technology and laboratory competition. Although the cost has declined from thousands of dollars to hundreds of dollars for a standard postmortem genetic testing gene panel, either the expense or the perception of expense remains a barrier for some families who may benefit from it. For some families who have difficulty affording testing, another third party may bear the cost (e.g., medical examiner's office, research grant, support organization). Bonnie was prepared and able to pay for her late daughter's testing.

Finally, because of the aforementioned intricacies of postmortem testing, the turnaround time for results after a genetic counseling appointment is often longer. In clinic, a sample may be drawn and shipped the same day with minimal effort; whereas, postmortem testing requires the coordination of multiple parties to get a sample to the lab for testing. If a first sample fails quality control, then a second one needs to be sent. Therefore, it typically takes at least a few weeks longer than testing does in clinic, and I prepared April for this timeframe.

Selecting the genetic test and the lab

After determining Bonnie's differential diagnosis and confirming the existence of samples, I determined the ideal testing to order and the lab to send the sample to. The first decision was what test should be ordered: cardiovascular gene panel(s) of various sizes versus exome or genome sequencing. Outside of the research setting, exome or genome sequencing is seen as not having benefit or not recommended for the investigation of unexplained sudden death according to guidelines written primarily by and for cardiologists (Stiles et al., 2021; Wilde et al., 2022). This recommendation is based on the increased out-of-pocket cost, the lack of guaranteed full coverage for the most critical genes associated with SCD-causing conditions, and the greater potential to misinterpret variants of uncertain significance. Eventually, I believe exome/genome sequencing will become the standard test in postmortem genetic testing like in most other clinical situations, but in this setting, I started with a comprehensive panel of genes associated with inherited arrhythmia and cardiomyopathy conditions.

Given the limited number of samples available from Bonnie's autopsy and the preciousness of these samples, I prioritized choosing a lab with a track record of performing genetic testing on postmortem samples. Labs communicate the sample types they accept, what they do when samples are not stored in ideal conditions or for extended periods of time, what they do if a sample failure occurs through the process (i.e., specifically whether a family is billed if testing fails, which may be an insult-to-injury situation if a family is not prepared for this), and if they expect to have leftover DNA that could be used for DNA banking. DNA banking of leftover DNA or from DNA extracted from other postmortem samples, is recommended following a sudden and unexplained death of a young person especially if the cause of death is not determined by initial genetic testing efforts. Banked DNA samples offer the hope that we may later find diagnosis through future testing techniques (e.g., exome or genome sequencing) performed clinically or on a research basis.

April had no additional questions or concerns about the testing process, so we wrapped up a plan to initiate the transfer of the retained sample from the ME's office to the diagnostic lab for testing. We agreed on the best way for results disclosure, which April preferred for me to do in the same manner we previously worked together—by telephone.

Genetic test results—trust but verify the reported variants

Two months after my initial conversation with April and following the process of transferring the sample from the ME's office to the lab, I received Bonnie's genetic test results. The lab reported a variant of uncertain significance (VUS) in the *RYR2* gene, which is the gene associated with CPVT. A second VUS in the *MYH6* gene was also detected.

Not all VUSes are created equal, and on first glance the *RYR2* variant initially felt like it must be truly pathogenic. Early in my cardiovascular genetics career, I often fell victim to the bias that "this VUS must be the answer because it's in a gene associated with a condition that matches the phenotype." However, after receiving a few dozen VUS results in large gene panels, I quickly adapted the "innocent until proven guilty" approach to VUSes. The *RYR2* gene is huge (over 100 exons) with a high background rate of rare variants that are mostly not causative of CPVT or any other disease. The VUS rate for *RYR2* is even higher for those who are underrepresented in population databases, so this is one area where knowing a patient's ancestry may help with variant interpretation.

There were other reasons to be cautious of the pathogenicity of the *RYR2* variant. Even though CPVT was high in the differential diagnosis and the *RYR2* gene is the most prominent gene linked with CPVT, Bonnie was not clinically diagnosed with CPVT. Her true phenotype was unexplained sudden death which is a nonspecific phenotype with a differential diagnosis where "idiopathic" or unknown SCD accounts for the largest percentage of deaths even with the highest quality autopsy. We did not have any cardiology data on Bonnie or her family specifically suggestive of CPVT. Admittedly, this absence of clinical evidence may be because Bonnie did not have an exercise stress test as a part of her cardiology workup.

Although I have a high level of trust in the labs where I send genetic testing and their expertise, I always perform some level of independent variant research like many other clinical genetic counselors (Reuter et al., 2018; Wain et al., 2020). As a nonlaboratory genetic counselor, I did not have professional training in variant interpretation. Therefore, I deliberately attended conference sessions such as NSGC's Annual Conference on this topic and found other professional development opportunities to learn and develop this skill (e.g., ClinGen Variant Pathogenicity Curation).

In the process of researching Bonnie's specific *RYR2* variant, I found that it was reported in a recent publication that was not cited in the lab report. In this publication, three unrelated individuals with a clinical diagnosis of CPVT and/or SCD had the same *RYR2* variant with two of the *RYR2* variants being *de novo* after parental testing. I reviewed the publication in as much detail as possible and wrote up a short summary that I sent to the lab for their opinion.

When the lab received my message, they replied immediately thanking me for the additional information and submitted it to their variant scientist team to review. In a few days, the lab contacted me to let me know they changed the classification of the variant from a VUS to likely pathogenic given the additional evidence.

Therefore, Bonnie now had an *RYR2* variant interpreted as likely pathogenic, which supports the conclusion she had CPVT that likely led to her fainting spell at the dinner with her family and her premature sudden death. A key term here is "likely" pathogenic as the interpretation is still not 100% certain as variant interpretation often happens on a continuum rather than a binary decision of abnormal versus normal. Fortunately, familial testing could offer additional support for the *RYR2* variant's pathogenicity if the variant was proven to be *de novo* after testing April and Charles. Pathogenic *RYR2* variants are estimated to be *de novo* in 30-40% of patients with CPVT (Napolitano et al., 2004). Alternatively, if the *RYR2* variant was inherited, close phenotyping of those found to have the variant may support variant-phenotype segregation if stress testing was abnormal.

The *MYH6* gene was included in the large cardiomyopathy and arrhythmia panel as it had a weak association with inherited heart disease. In other words, the gene itself is more like "gene of uncertain significance" and was later designated as having a limited association with hypertrophic and dilated cardiomyopathy by ClinGen after a comprehensive and systematic review of the literature (Ingles et al., 2019; Jordan et al., 2021). This was not available to me at the time of our consultation but given the phenotype weakly associated with the *MYH6* gene was not found on Bonnie's autopsy (i.e., hypertrophic or dilated cardiomyopathy), this VUS seemed highly unlikely to be an explanation for her sudden death in my assessment. A few years later, I received variant reclassification notification for Bonnie. The *MYH6* variant was downgraded from VUS to likely benign due to new population frequency data.

Results disclosure and initiation of family genetic testing

For results disclosure, I called April and spoke with her and her husband, Charles. They placed me on speakerphone so that I could review results with both of them. I started my results disclosure conversation asking whether they were ready to receive the results and if they had any questions or concerns before I got started. There were none, and they were ready to receive results.

I started the conversation by saying that the lab found a variant in the *RYR2* gene that is likely to be the answer we have been looking for. I told them that I believe the results mean that Bonnie had the condition April suspected all along: CPVT. After this brief disclosure, I paused to await their feedback. Sometimes when I pause, I am anticipating an emotional response, like tears or elation but this time I heard the question "are you still there?" This moment highlighted a challenge of telephone counseling versus in-person or video visits. The lack of nonverbal cues made it difficult for them to recognize that I was still very much present with them. Instead, I verbally acknowledged I was still on the phone and explained the reason I stopped talking was to give them time to process and reveal their initial impressions with me. Another potential way to assess their initial impressions in this call would be to ask an open-ended question about their thoughts and feelings after hearing these diagnostic test results.

April had no major positive nor negative emotional reaction, which I anticipated due to her previous emotional engagement (or lack thereof) we had by phone. One possible reason for her somewhat matter-of-fact response was that this was the diagnosis April was suspecting all along. She believed Bonnie had CPVT before our first phone call, so these test results confirmed her long-held expectations. Charles remained silent throughout the call and deferred most of the conversation to April.

April expressed relief knowing there was likely a cause of death she could share with loved ones. When a young person dies, some in the community may make assumptions about the cause of death (e.g., overdose, suicide) in an attempt to explain something so rare, tragic, and unfamiliar. A death is not only traumatic for the immediate family and friends, but it can be for the community whose members may make presumptions that are difficult for parents to hear.

Since the interpretation was more complicated than simply "we found the answer, case closed," I went into more detail on how genetic test results are interpreted on a continuum from pathogenic to benign. I expressed the lab's and my current belief that while this variant was previously considered uncertain on the original report, it was reclassified to likely pathogenic based on new information we discovered. I re-reviewed the role and value of parental variant testing: 1) it may determine if either April or Charles are affected by or at risk to develop CPVT; and 2) it could also help reinforce the likely pathogenic classification of the variant if it was *de novo*. I prepared them that even if they were both negative, I would strongly encourage their daughter to be tested due to the possibility of germline mosaicism.

I walked April and Charles through the impact of their two possible results. A positive result would suggest one of them is affected by or at risk to develop CPVT and would need to establish care with an electrophysiologist (EP) who is a cardiologist who specializes in heart rhythm disorders. The EP would ideally have a strong background in inherited heart diseases. I reviewed general diagnostic and management recommendations for CPVT, which would be determined by their EP and likely include an exercise stress test, beta blocker therapy, and certain changes to exercise and activities. This couple is not particularly active in exercise or sports, so activity restriction would not be expected to change their lives dramatically. However, the psychological burden of knowing that one of them could have passed this risk/condition to a child was a larger concern for me. For this reason, I attempted to engage in a conversation by asking each of them individually how they might feel if they tested positive similar to our pre-test counseling conversation. Although I asked a question attempting to assess emotion, they responded with the behaviors they would take (i.e., see a cardiologist for testing and treatment, ensure other family was tested). I did not have success engaging in a conversation about how they'd feel if one of them knew they might have passed down the condition associated with their daughter's death.

I obtained their informed consent and mailed at-home test kits for sending their saliva samples to the lab where Bonnie was tested.

A month later, April and Charles's results came back negative, confirming the *RYR2* variant was *de novo*. Paternity testing was not included in the analysis by the testing lab, but Bonnie's father tested positive for the VUS in the *MYH6* gene. With this new parental data, the interpretation of the *RYR2* variant was upgraded from likely pathogenic to pathogenic.

I emphasized that their results further reinforced the likelihood that Bonnie's death was from CPVT given the accumulation of all the data we have. I acknowledged that genetic testing, like other medical testing, is imperfect and the interpretation of a result may change in the future with new knowledge. This is a reason why integrating cardiology testing with genetic test results is critically important to ensure that family members are as phenotypically normal as their genetic test results suggest. This means April and Charles would ideally benefit from an exercise stress test to confirm they have no signs of an arrhythmia during exertion. Fortunately, they were willing to follow up with their cardiologist for exercise stress testing and their normal test results were routed to me by their cardiologist.

After disclosing their results, Bonnie's older sister, Dina, joined the phone to discuss her own testing. Like Charles, she remained very quiet and my efforts to engage with her were minimally successful. In retrospect, I would have ideally reached out to Dina to offer her the ability to meet one-on-one for her pre-test counseling. I anticipated that she would choose to have her mother attend the appointment based my experience with the family, but I did not give her the opportunity to decide that.

However, it was clear her mother served as her "genetic counselor" and had explained the role of familial variant testing as she understood the implications of a negative or unexpectedly positive result with minimal education on my part. When I asked what Dina thought her risk of testing positive would be, she replied "low," which I agreed with given her parents' normal test results, her normal cardiology evaluation (including a stress test), and the lack of a concerning medical history. Therefore, since "stakes" did not feel as high with the likelihood of her testing positive being much less her parents, I made the decision to concisely discuss the impact of a positive test result on her medical care and life overall rather than a longer pre-test session like the one I had with her parents.

As hoped and expected, Dina tested negative for the likely pathogenic *RYR2* variant a few weeks later. I disclosed these results with April and Dina by speakerphone and there was an audible sigh of relief. Both thanked me for sharing the good news.

Closing the loop on postmortem genetic testing beyond the family

Since Bonnie's postmortem genetic testing was diagnostic and found the likely cause of her death, I shared the results with the medical examiner verbally and in writing. This genetic diagnosis allowed the medical examiner to reclassify the cause of Bonnie's death from unexplained to a cardiac arrhythmia secondary to

CPVT. In addition to explaining Bonnie's death, this experience demonstrated the benefit of postmortem genetic counseling and testing to the medical examiner for future cases. Since medical examiners are often at the front line of a sudden unexplained death of a young person, they have the potential to facilitate postmortem genetic testing and counseling. Without being notified by a medical examiner or coroner, parents and other surviving loved ones may never be aware of this testing even being an option.

Although I'm unfamiliar with any objective data on the frequency of postmortem genetic testing offered to those who had died suddenly at young ages, my experience tells me it's incredibly underutilized. In other words, I anticipate only a small minority of families who have experienced a sudden death are connected with genetic counselors who can offer postmortem genetic testing and other family evaluations. Although individual encounters between medical examiners and genetic counselors will likely improve this, larger-scale interventions are needed. The growth of multidisciplinary inherited heart disease clinics and centers may help, but these tend to be exclusively located in larger academic medical centers and in larger cities. The Postmortem Working group of the NSGC Cardiovascular Genetics SIG initiated a project to connect genetic counselors in cardiology with their local medical examiner's office in order to help break down this knowledge barrier and recognize our role in improving public health by preventing a second sudden death.

Finally, a few weeks after speaking with the ME, the police officer responsible for investigating Bonnie's death called me with questions after receiving Bonnie's updated autopsy and death certificate. Although he generally understood the cause of death had been determined, he wanted more detail so he could confidently decide to close his death investigation, which he was ultimately able to do.

Psychological assessment and support

Throughout the months I worked with April and her family, I attempted to assess her psychological state and find ways to support her. After the sudden unexpected death of a young person, almost half of family members report psychological morbidity, including prolonged grief and posttraumatic stress disorder (PTSD) symptoms with the highest risk found in mothers and those who witnessed the death (Ingles et al., 2016). As demonstrated by all the work April did to investigate her daughter's death prior to meeting me, she clearly intellectualized the loss by pursuing answers and funneling at least some of her grief and anguish into action. Her goal was to find an answer using her medical background and to gather and analyze all the data she could find. These efforts were objectively successful and ultimately led to the diagnosis she suspected Bonnie to have.

However, there were a few areas where I found April to be potentially struggling. First, I believe she felt some level of guilt as she asked questions about what could or should have been done differently to diagnose Bonnie after she fainted. April knew that if Bonnie had been diagnosed with CPVT while she was alive, there would likely have been a treatment to prevent her premature death. I know I can't take away a patients' feelings of guilt even when I objectively tell them, as I did April, that the tragedy of deaths like Bonnie's is that there are often no signs or only signs that are understandably missed. In Bonnie's case there was a major red flag (i.e., syncope with emotion), but this was addressed as best a parent could by ensuring she was promptly seen by a cardiologist and a neurologist who both offered reassurance.

Beyond identifying some of her feelings of guilt that she may have missed a red flag, I sensed that April was angry. She was mad that she, her husband, and her surviving daughter seemed to be dismissed by the cardiologist who saw them after Bonnie died. It made her question herself and if she was overreacting. I explicitly said she did what she should have done and exactly what I recommend for families to do following a sudden death—getting her family a thorough evaluation by a cardiologist.

April was also distressed and angry that the cardiologist who saw Bonnie may have missed a potentially treatable inherited heart disease. Questioning what Bonnie's cardiologist did not diagnose was a recurring theme throughout the months I worked with the family. When we first began working together, I had no cardiology or other medical records from Bonnie, so I truly didn't know if anything might have been missed. Furthermore, not being a cardiologist, I can't interpret or overread studies, so I would need a cardiologist experienced in inherited heart diseases to review any available imaging to conclude if a study may have been abnormal or if symptoms warranted an additional test like an exercise stress test. Even if I did find out something was "missed," this is a sensitive topic with emotional and medicolegal implications. Ultimately, I answered her questions with transparency by explaining that a stress test might have provided a diagnosis and my uncertainty about whether most cardiologists would have known to order this test in their evaluation of April.

Fortunately, the cardiovascular genetics community has made progress in the recognition and treatment of families experiencing distress including PTSD and prolonged grief. This is demonstrated in the recent consensus statement guidelines for the investigation of decedents following a sudden unexplained death where a multidisciplinary group of authors (e.g., cardiologists, psychologists, and genetic counselors) dedicate an entire section on how to best assess and support those impacted by a sudden death (Stiles et al., 2021).

April did not express overt signs of PTSD, prolonged grief, or a major depressive disorder that I was able to recognize in our time working together. She was not having problems sleeping and returned to work after a typical bereavement leave. Although she was still appropriately grieving the loss of her daughter, she told me that she felt she was in a place where she would expect any mother to be after the death of a child. In the time since working with April, I have learned about objective instruments that measure PTSD and prolonged grief that may warrant inclusion in a cardiovascular genetics service in the intake and evaluation of those who are being evaluated after the sudden death of a loved one (Prigerson et al., 2021; APA, 2023).

I attempted to assess her support. She said her husband and daughter have been there for her and she's been there for them. Other extended family and their church community also pitched in when they've needed more practical help like meals. She was offered grief counseling shortly after Bonnie's death and declined. In the years after I worked with the Smith family, we have added a PhD psychologist to our team with expertise and experience working with patients with inherited heart disease and families who have lost relatives to sudden unexpected death. They have been an invaluable addition to our multidisciplinary team for those in need who accept the referral. For those working with patients expected to have a high rate of significant mental health disorders, having a trusted colleague who can offer short or long-term therapy and other psychological treatment is critical.

Since Bonnie declined meeting with a therapist, I offered support in the form of the preeminent organization that serves families affected by sudden death—whether the cause of death is determined to be genetic or not—the Sudden Arrhythmia Death Foundation (SADS) Foundation. Given the rarity of premature sudden death and the rural and medically underserved area where the family lived, I did not expect to nor did I find a local support groups in their area. Therefore, I most often rely on national organizations that serve families via social media platforms and through private forums. By the time I spoke with Bonnie, she had already connected with the SADS Foundation, which is where she obtained my contact information and the recommendation to connect with me to discuss genetic testing. This was a reminder of how valuable it is for genetic counselors to connect with the organizations who serve our patient populations, as those organizations can help patients and their families find us. This referral and others I have received from the SADS Foundation over the years have been for patients and families who were often at the greatest risk. Additionally, it's reassuring to know there is an organization I can confidently direct patients to who can offer support beyond what I'm able to due to their shared experience of tragic loss and/or living with an inherited heart condition. Finally, partnering with organizations like the SADS Foundation has offered genetic counselors the opportunity to collaborate on research projects for recruitment or intervention, create educational materials, provide education to larger medical and patient audiences, and learn about state-of-the-art information from other medical specialists who have expertise in this area.

How postmortem genetic testing and counseling helped a family find meaning in a tragedy

In one of our last phone calls working together, April told me she was thinking about a way she could reduce tragic sudden deaths like Bonnie's from happening to another family. I expressed my admiration of her for trying to make a change to help others in the future and asked what she had in mind. One thing she considered was partnering with the SADS Foundation or creating her own group to raise money for cardiovascular screening programs or genetic testing to find young people who are unknowingly affected by inherited heart conditions. She also wondered if there was a way to educate cardiologists to recognize inherited heart diseases like CPVT. Ultimately, we finished our call with a lot of ideas, and I was confident that she had the capacity to make meaningful change in whatever area she chose. Little did I know, April would lead a state-wide initiative.

Families with the ability, support, and resources to do so often find ways to direct their grief towards efforts such as creating their own foundations to honor their lost loved one, by establishing scholarships in their memory, or fundraising for cardiology screening, medical research, or defibrillators for local schools and gyms. Almost three years after I first met with April, I learned what April ultimately decided to do to honor Bonnie and to help other families facing the same devastating circumstance. Along with the police officer dedicated to her daughter's case, April channeled her skill and passion to create a bill requiring postmortem genetic testing in all young people who die unexpectedly in their state. The officer who investigated Bonnie's death notified me about this bill and connected me with the sponsoring state senator. I was able to provide some background information to the sponsoring senator and the chief medical examiner about the process, benefit, and costs of a postmortem genetic testing program. Eventually, I was asked to briefly testify in support of the bill. Eventually, her bill passed both the Senate and the House and was signed into law. April's efforts will ensure that other families facing these terrible circumstances are offered the same services she was to find answers and prevent others in the family from unknowingly being affected and untreated.

Summary

Providing genetic counseling to families who have experienced the sudden and unexpected death of a loved one is simultaneously the most challenging and rewarding aspect of the cardiovascular genetics specialty. Working through a single postmortem case with a family often takes many hours of time outside of the genetic counseling session itself. The process requires navigating multiple initially unfamiliar systems like an ME's office, tracking down medical records and samples to be used for testing, obtaining the required legal documentation to support communication and request testing, and ongoing correspondence with the family and all parties involved. All of this coordination of care happens within the context of serving a family who has experienced the worst moment of their lives and the psychological and emotional impact of a death.

Fortunately, our training as genetic counselors provides a unique combination of skills to help a family navigate through a tragedy with a goal of seeking answers that may prevent more suffering. We know how to communicate with people in a variety of roles, both medical and nonmedical, and how to navigate sensitive family dynamics during an incredibly stressful time. We can discern the most appropriate genetic test(s) to offer and ensure the results are assessed critically to avoid misdiagnosis and more harm. We can listen empathically and can work productively through crisis situations. We can identify those family members who are experiencing distress and connect them with therapists and support organizations to address their grief and bereavement. And even when genetic testing doesn't provide an explanation, we can help a family adapt to uncertainty while ensuring they are appropriately evaluated by cardiologists to ensure their health and safety.

SUPPORTING PATIENTS' DECISIONS IN A CANCER SETTING: FAMILY MATTERS (BARRY S. TONG)

Germline genetic testing has become an integral component of the care for many patients with cancer due in part to the availability of targeted therapies for individuals with certain germline pathogenic variants in cancer predisposition genes (Stadler et al., 2021). To address this, many clinics have implemented methods for offering germline testing to all patients with certain malignancies, including ovarian cancer, with high rates of acceptance (Bednar et al., 2017; Konstantinopoulos et al., 2020). However, patient acceptance of testing and its implications may vary among patients, particularly those that prefer alternative approaches to their cancer care or have different opinions about the role of cancer screening and prevention on their health. In these scenarios, genetic counseling may be especially important to help the patient understand the utility of germline testing, adapt to results. and facilitate family communication.

In my current clinical practice, most patients with a new diagnosis of ovarian cancer are offered germline testing by their Gynecologic Oncology team via different service delivery models that may involve a genetic counselor but not necessarily include pre-test counseling. However, the following case begins with a referral specifically for pre-test counseling and highlights the potential complex decision-making and implications of working with a family through learning about and testing for a hereditary cancer predisposition. The opportunity to understand and respect a patient's autonomy in their decision to pursue testing can occasionally be at odds with a genetic counselor's desire to recommend the best medical course of action. When that is the case, the tools and methods I rely on, which heavily emphasize knowledge and education as the basis for informed decision-making, can become unconstructive or, at worse, coercive. The subsequent genetic counseling sessions I had with the family members of my proband, Beth, also exemplify the complex family dynamics of cascade testing and the different ways people in the same family can come to a decision about genetic testing.

Beth's Pre-test Counseling Session

Beth was a 68-year-old woman, assigned female at birth, with a newly diagnosed, metastatic, high-grade, serous ovarian cancer, referred by her gynecologic oncologist and alternative medicine provider to discuss germline testing for inherited cancer risk given her diagnosis and Ashkenazi Jewish ancestry. She arrived at the in-person counseling visit with her husband, Jim, and stated they were present only because their providers, including the medical oncologist, gynecologic oncologist, and alternative medicine oncologist, had all recommended germline genetic testing.

Beth and Jim clearly stated at the start of the visit that they were adamantly against using chemotherapy and were not pursuing the gynecologic oncologist's treatment recommendations.

Beth and Jim had also recently traveled across the state to work with an oncologist with a natural and Eastern medicine focus. They were exploring opportunities to cure the cancer through diet, herbal medicines, and acupuncture. However, they acknowledged that even the natural medicine oncologist had recommended genetic counseling, given Beth's diagnosis and ancestry. I suspected it was because of their trust in this provider, or perhaps that genetic counseling and testing had been recommended by multiple specialists, that they chose to keep their appointment with me.

At the beginning of each session, I initiate contracting by confirming the referring provider. This helps me identify where a patient's care is being managed and where they are in the treatment process based on recent appointments. This also demonstrates to the patient that I'm up to date on their care and that I am a part of their health care team.

From the start of this session, I recognized several of Beth's perspectives on cancer treatment would be challenging for me: her disagreement with the evidence-based standard of care, her disbelief in the benefit of chemotherapy, and her belief that alternative medicine approaches could cure her cancer. It reflected similar opinions I had heard from my immigrant Chinese family when I was younger that led me to pursue a career "in" Western medicine, and I suspected, for this patient, this disbelief or mistrust potentially impacted her perception of the utility of genetic counseling and genetic testing as well. Recognizing this countertransference, I actively chose to use a motivational interviewing approach of "rolling with resistance," or reflecting and restating the patient's views even when they go against recommended medical advice, rather than countering or immediately correcting with facts (Resnicow et al., 2022). *The purpose was to better understand Beth's values and how she came to approach this perspective without conveying judgment or promoting fear that her views were invalid. As I listened to Beth's reasons, I began cataloging what was being voiced as important to her, to use later in support of her decision-making around genetic testing.*

After establishing our genetic counseling agenda, I reviewed Beth's cancer history, asking how she first learned about her cancer, and then summarized and confirmed what I had identified from her medical records. Briefly, her first symptom was mild abdominal pain and bloating that was intermittent for a few months. After several appointments with her primary doctor and a gastroenterologist, that included imaging and an elevated serum CA-125, a blood test that can be used to screen for ovarian cancer, Beth was referred to medical oncology. More imaging and a sampling of abdominal fluid confirmed her diagnosis, and she was referred to a gynecologic oncologist to discuss treatment options.

Symptoms of ovarian cancer are often nonspecific initially, presenting as bloat-ing, changes in weight, urinary urgency, or pain, even in the setting of an advanced or metastatic disease. I suspected this was the reason why Beth felt the severity of her stated disease was discordant with her symptoms. For many ovarian cancers that are too advanced to proceed to surgery directly, neoadjuvant chemotherapy (chemother-apy given prior to surgery) is recommended (Armstrong et al., 2022), as it helps shrink the size of the tumor so surgery can be more successful. While this is the exper-tise of my oncology and surgery colleagues, as a genetic counselor working with patients undergoing complex treatments, knowledge of general approaches to cancer care and etiology can aid in understanding the patient's perspective of their treat-ment and decisions about the timing of genetic testing, which in turn can influence treatment decisions.

Beth and her husband reiterated that they did not want chemotherapy in any scenario and expressed a desire for surgery upfront. However, her gynecologic oncologist had explained that there was no clinical benefit (does not extend life) to upfront surgery with the type of cancer in Beth's case.

By exploring Beth's and Jim's perspectives, I learned that they viewed chemo-therapy as unnatural and toxic, believing more natural remedies likely existed. Additionally, Beth claimed she felt "fine" and had no major symptoms of ovarian cancer, contributing to her disbelief of the extent of her disease. I reflected back that the contrast between how she felt, and the very aggressive and, literally, toxic nature of the recommended treatments likely felt discordant to her. To this state-ment, I did not notice any discernible change in her affect, but her pause led me to suspect she was a little surprised to hear me validate her perspective.

Her gynecologic oncologist's clinical notes also stated that Beth had declined standard-of-care approaches to treatment and was exploring alternative therapies by seeking other providers, including natural medicines and herbal medicines. When describing these alternative therapies, Beth and her husband also expressed interest in clinical trials, particularly around immunotherapies.

At this point I had identified a few educational gaps in the couple's under-standing of Beth's options, in particular clinical trials and immunotherapy. Her lack of desire for chemotherapy, yet interest in trials and immunotherapies (which, at the time, were often given in conjunction with or after traditional chemother-apy), demonstrated to me that she didn't quite understand all of her treatment options, yet was still searching for different options for her care. Importantly, she was not resigned to letting her cancer spread or foregoing treatment, which meant she likely had hope for a cure. I planned to use this to guide the conversation around genetic testing.

Beth's Pre-test Counseling Session: Family History

To continue Beth's risk assessment, I collected her family history by constructing a three-plus generation pedigree (not shown) in the order provided in Table 16-2. For the pedigree, I started with obtaining the number, gender, and ages of her

TABLE 16-2. **Beth's family history**

Family member (name), status, age	Medical History	Notes
Daughter (Alex), living, age 36	Alive and well (a/w)	Father is Jim, Beth's current partner, who is not of AJ ancestry
Daughter (Emily), living, age 44	a/w	Father is Beth's ex-husband, who is of AJ ancestry
Daughter (Talia), living, age 48	a/w	Father is Beth's ex-husband, who is of AJ ancestry
Brother 1, living, age 69	a/w	
Brother 2, deceased, age 58	motor vehicle accident, cause of death	
Nephew, deceased, age 34	brain cancer diagnosed 29y, cause of death	Son of brother 2. No prior genetic testing
Maternal		
Mother, deceased, age 64	breast cancer initially diagnosed age 61, triple negative pathology, metastasis to brain, cause of death	Mother was an only child. No prior genetic testing
Maternal grandfather, deceased, age 70s	Lung disease, cause of death	AJ ancestry
Maternal grandmother, deceased, age 70s	Lung disease, cause of death	AJ ancestry
Paternal		
Father, deceased, age 56	Brain aneurysm, cause of death	
Paternal aunt, deceased, age 75	Cancer, primary site unknown, metastatic, diagnosed age 70	
Paternal grandfather, deceased, age 85	No history of cancer, died of old age	AJ ancestry
Paternal grandmother, deceased, age 67	Stroke, cause of death	AJ ancestry

children, individually asking about any cancer history or other relevant medical history she felt was pertinent to cancer risk. I repeated the process with any grandchildren and siblings, parents and so forth. For family members with a cancer diagnosis, I asked about the primary site, age at diagnosis, key pathologic features (e.g., cell type, receptor status, genomic indicators), clinical course (e.g., early stage, in remission, metastatic), and if prior genetic testing had been done, knowing that many of these details are often not known by family members. For deceased family members, I also obtained age and cause of death, if due to cancer progression or not.

Depending on the indication, noncancer or pre-cancerous findings associated with hereditary cancer predispositions may be relevant to assess (e.g., colon polyps, breast density, head circumference, dermatologic findings, benign growths, and tumors).

As communication and knowledge about a family member's health can vary tremendously from person to person, I practice multiple strategies in using lay language to obtain the information above, including:

1. *clarifying where a cancer started, if known, versus where it spread to;*
2. *obtaining rough estimates of family member's ages if not known, particularly emphasizing milestones relevant to risk assessment guidelines; for example, if they were younger (before age 50) or older (after age 50);*
3. *asking to understand how certain the consultand is of the cancer history, which may invite an understanding of their relationship with that family member, their involvement (or lack thereof) in their care, and other family narratives;*
4. *assessing cancer screening or health behaviors in family members to understand disease presentation or progression/course;*
5. *refocusing the consultand on what they know about treatment history if the primary site, pathology, clinical course, or progression is not known (e.g., where and how much surgery, chemotherapy versus daily medication)*
6. *normalizing that communication of health information is variable across many families and reassuring that it's okay to not know certain details, particularly when hearing from families or cultures where certain health conditions like cancer can be stigmatized;*
7. *acknowledging the emotional impact of recalling and reliving the cancer histories of a family, or the emotional impact of not knowing due to family migration, estrangement, political or social unrest, or other multidimensional reasons.*

Beth's Pre-test Counseling Session: Risk Assessment, including Cancer Epidemiology

Reviewing the family history in total, I assessed from Beth's personal and family history several indicators or red flags of hereditary cancer predisposition, and mentally catalogued their relevance to risk assessment, including prevalence of inherited etiologies and guideline recommendations for genetic testing:

1. Beth was diagnosed with a high-grade, serous ovarian cancer. An inherited cancer predisposition is identified on genetic testing in approximately 20–25% of individuals with an epithelial ovarian cancer, regardless of ancestry or family history (Walsh et al., 2011; Norquist et al., 2016). Germline genetic testing is clinically indicated based on national medical guidelines for anyone with a diagnosis of epithelial ovarian cancer (Armstrong et al., 2022).

2. Beth's mother was diagnosed with triple negative (negative for estrogen receptors, progesterone receptors, and HER2, or human epidermal growth factor receptor 2, proteins) cancer. Inherited cancer predisposition syndromes are identified in approximately 20% of individuals with triple negative breast cancers. Personal or family history of triple negative breast cancer is also a clinical indication for germline testing (Daly et al., 2020).

3. Both sides of Beth's family are of Ashkenazi Jewish ancestry (AJ). Hereditary Breast and Ovarian Cancer Syndrome (due to germline pathogenic variants in *BRCA1* and *BRCA2*) are found at a higher prevalence in individuals of Ashkenazi Jewish ancestry due to a founder effect. The combination of a personal or family history of breast or ovarian cancer at any age and Ashkenazi Jewish ancestry is also an indication for germline testing (Daly et al., 2020).

4. Beth's nephew was diagnosed with a fairly early-onset brain tumor, although the pathology or additional details about the tumor type were unknown. The combination of a central nervous system tumor, early age of onset, and family history of breast cancer is vaguely suggestive of Li-Fraumeni syndrome, but does not meet any formal or historic testing criteria. Therefore, this did not add to the risk assessment or clinical suspicion, but further reinforced the option of considering testing in the context of a multigene panel that included Li-Fraumeni syndrome, which is recommended per national guidelines regardless.

To communicate my risk assessment to Beth, I first recontextualized Beth's diagnosis by providing education about the epidemiology of breast and ovarian cancers (approximate incidence, typical age and stage at presentation, and common risk factors). I used this baseline to frame why the presentation of the red flags in her family stood out from other cancers in her family that had a lower association with hereditary predisposition. From there, I shared that genetic testing was clinically indicated per national guidelines and gave her a subjective approximation of the likelihood she would be identified with a hereditary cancer predisposition on genetic testing. In this case, I recall quoting her "at least 20%, if not higher" based on the combination of multiple red flags in her personal and family history.

I believed this approach to the risk assessment served multiple purposes. The verbal description:

1. *normalized that cancers are common, and the majority are due to nongenetic, multifactorial, or unknown etiologies;*

2. *identified cancers in her family that could have a genetic etiology due to identified hereditary cancer predisposition syndromes, and which did not;*

3. *provided a platform for sharing the current medical guidelines for genetic evaluation and testing in the context of her family history, and where my recommendation was derived from;*

4. *primed her for the potential outcomes of germline testing.*

At this point, I paused in my education-heavy risk assessment to gauge if clarification was needed. Beth and Jim replied they were "mostly familiar" with the information. I then asked if they had heard of Hereditary Breast and Ovarian Cancer Syndrome (HBOC), or more commonly the *BRCA1* and *BRCA2* genes. Beth stated it sounded "vaguely familiar," but very peripherally, and she didn't know much about the condition.

At their prompting, I briefly reviewed that HBOC was an inherited condition that significantly increased the risk of developing both breast and ovarian cancers, as well as other cancers including pancreatic, prostate, and melanoma. However, this was one of many hereditary cancer predisposition syndromes that included ovarian cancer, so the approach to genetic testing was typically through a multigene panel that includes many relevant genes and conditions.

Beth's Pre-test Counseling Session: Possible Results of Testing and Implications

To further describe HBOC in the context of her care and to emphasize the relevance and potential impact of doing genetic testing, I described the possible results of genetic testing. I delineated the impact of the results of genetic testing by answering three questions: 1) Does the genetic test result explain the etiology of the cancer diagnosis and inform the treatment plan?; 2) What is the future risk of developing cancer?; and 3) What is the cancer risk and recommended management for family members?

For Beth, a positive or "abnormal" genetic test impacted the following.

1. Treatment for her ovarian cancer. In this case, results could identify her eligibility for targeted therapies at a later point in treatment (i.e., PARP-inhibitors) or clinical trials including immunotherapies, which Beth and Jim had previously expressed an interest in pursuing.

2. Management of future or second primary cancer risk. This included discussing the recommended surveillance and risk-reduction options available for other cancers. Since my index of suspicion was elevated for HBOC, I described breast cancer screening and risk-reduction methods as examples. While this would not be appropriate for an individual with terminal disease, in Beth's case, I felt that describing future opportunities for cancer prevention aligned with her perception that her ovarian cancer was not as advanced as described (Zhong et al., 2015).

3. Cancer risk information for family members. Genetic test results could allow for cascade testing and subsequent cancer screening and risk-reduction for the family. I emphasized that each daughter could have a 50% chance of inheriting a pathogenic variant if one was identified in Beth.

While I did not specifically know or discuss the inheritance pattern of Beth's presumed hereditary risk, I typically assume simple autosomal dominance in the pre-test setting, as most identifiable cancer predispositions are. However, in this family, we would soon learn this assumption was not entirely correct.

I then reiterated the higher likelihood of a negative result, given that most individuals with ovarian cancer test negative (Walsh et al., 2011). We reviewed the implications of a negative result which could include:

1. no change in the treatment recommended by her gynecologic oncologist;
2. likely no significantly elevated risk for a second or future cancer, depending on family history;
3. a lower likelihood of an increased risk for her daughters for developing ovarian cancer, although not a zero risk.

I also briefly explained that occasionally genetic testing would reveal uncertainties, such as a variant of uncertain clinical significance, given the diversity of humans and our incomplete understanding of the genome. I explained that "variations" in our genetics were normal and part of what makes us different, but the laboratory's ability to identify and determine the pathogenicity of each variant was imperfect. Without overemphasizing, I reassured Beth that the lab could identify known pathogenic, or disease-causing, variants readily, and that we could address any uncertainties if they arose.

After describing the implications of testing and possible results, I asked Beth if she was interested in pursuing testing. She stated she desired genetic testing to protect her three daughters. She recalled the experience of her own mother, dying from metastatic cancer, attributing it to the failure of Western medicine, chemotherapy, and diagnostics. Beth reiterated that she had not yet decided on her own course of treatment, and that these results likely wouldn't change her ultimate treatment choice, even in the context of targeted medications. However, the information about risk to her daughters was important enough to pursue testing.

I noted, but did not state, yet another potential mismatch in Beth's perception of the extent and severity of her disease vis-a-vis her proactivity and concern for her daughters. Beth was clearly aware of the adverse effects of chemotherapy and had witnessed the lack of response of her mother's cancer to treatment. I suspected this mismatch was because she was still grappling with the advanced nature of her own disease: suppressing or denying the likely outcome of her cancer. Although I chose not to point this out in my session with Beth, I have found that opportunities to empathetically support other patients that are further along in their decision-making to not to treat their advanced cancers. For example, I may provide reflections that reiterate their prioritization of their current and near-term quality of life, which can be just as or more important than decisions focused on the potential prolonging of life via treatment.

Beth's Pre-test Counseling Session: Decisions About Testing

Jim, at this point, chimed in stating that they (inclusive of Beth) did not believe in cancer screenings, and a more naturalistic approach to health was what was preferred in their family. Beth was silent in response, and I sensed that she did not fully agree with Jim's perspective. Due to the time constraint of the hour-long appointment, we did not explore his comment further and instead initiated the testing process by collecting a saliva sample for a multigene cancer panel. We agreed to an in-person results disclosure, given that they felt they had a higher *a priori* likelihood of finding a germline pathogenic variant.

Beth's Results Disclosure: Personal and Family Implications

Three weeks later, the lab issued Beth's genetic test report. The test identified two pathogenic Ashkenazi Jewish founder variants: one in BRCA1 and a second in BRCA2.

The results disclosure was scheduled exactly one month after our initial counseling visit, and both Beth and her husband attended. We very briefly discussed what changes had occurred in the past month. They were still exploring natural therapies but had not decided on any definitive treatment. They had not returned to the medical oncology or gynecologic oncology teams for follow-up and were now exploring potential alternative medicine providers outside of the state. Beth stated she was eager, but not anxious, to learn the results, which I suspected was due to her perception that the results had more future-focused implications for her daughters, rather than immediate implications for her.

We jumped right to a discussion of the test results. I stated that we had identified two Ashkenazi Jewish founder pathogenic variants in *BRCA1* and *BRCA2*. Following a sequence similar to the pre-test counseling results discussion, I first emphasized that the results entirely explained *why* she had developed ovarian cancer. In regard to the impact on her treatment, I encouraged her to discuss the prognostic implications of the results as well as opportunities and timing for PARP-inhibitor therapies or other clinical trials with her gynecologic oncology team, despite knowing she had thus far chosen not to pursue treatment with the team.

Beth's decision to decline standard-of-care therapy triggered a tension between the desire to respect her autonomy and my knowledge of the clinical benefits of treatment. Ovarian cancer treatment trials have demonstrated an improved survival in individuals with a germline BRCA1 *or* BRCA2 *pathogenic variant when treated with platinum chemotherapy, which is standard-of-care (Armstrong et al., 2022). Additionally, the prospect of targeted therapies like PARP-inhibitors in improving survival in people with germline variants is the cornerstone of personalized medicine in cancer treatment. Beth's continued "resistance" to treatment, in light of the potential benefit to prolonging life, was very difficult to accept as a health care provider. In this case, I chose education and information in an effort to persuade Beth to consider/think about treatment, recalling her interest in clinical trials. However, with Jim in the room, who had voiced a very strong opinion against treatment, this was not a topic I wanted to address very deeply at this point in time. I anticipated that Beth would need Jim's support as we moved on to discuss the impact of the positive results on their daughters.*

We then briefly reviewed possible future cancer risks, describing her breast and other cancer risks associated with the pathogenic variants in *BRCA1* and *BRCA2* (Kuchenbaecker et al., 2017). However, knowing the advanced nature of her ovarian cancer, I did not overemphasize the cancer screenings or risk-reduction opportunities for secondary cancers. Additional cancer screenings are typically determined by the treatment team in the near-term, balancing the primary cancer treatment and imaging needs.

I then transitioned to discussing the implications for Beth's family, knowing that the main reason she chose to pursue testing was to understand her daughters' risks. Given the two variants identified, her daughters each had a 25% chance for having inherited neither variant, a 25% chance for having inherited the *BRCA1* variant only, a 25% chance for the *BRCA2* variant only, and a 25% chance for having inherited both the *BRCA1* and *BRCA2* variants. This meant an overall 75% likelihood for each daughter to possess at least one of the variants.

Recalling Beth's desire to "protect" her daughters, I described in extensive detail the medical management implications should her daughters test positive. While overwhelming, my purpose in providing this level of detail was to emphasize the immediacy of potential action for her daughters. I reviewed the options for breast imaging, breast cancer risk reduction including surgery, the limitations of ovarian cancer screening, and the strong recommendation for surgical removal of the ovaries and fallopian tubes for ovarian cancer risk-reduction. I noted that, if positive, her daughters were at an age to initiate breast imaging, and importantly her older daughters should consider surgical risk-reduction for ovarian cancer.

Beth's Results Disclosure: Processing

At this point in the session, Beth did not have much to say. She nodded and stated she wanted to make sure her daughters received the information about the genetic test result and would want them to pursue testing. We discussed a family letter that Beth could provide to her daughters, although they lived locally and she saw them often. Jim, however, became agitated during the conversation about medical management for the daughters, stating that he would not want this information for *his* daughter, specifically singling her out. He did not want all this "doom and gloom" for her and stated that he "knew her." He explicitly stated that he didn't want his daughter to learn about this, stating, "She wouldn't want to pursue all the recommended surveillance and medical management." Having not yet met this daughter, I speculated this perspective was a projection of Jim's denial of the inherited nature of Beth's diagnosis, as well as a reflection of his views on Western medicine.

Beth, my patient, whose care was my primary responsibility, recognized the gravity of the two BRCA1/2 *variants and what they meant for her daughters. She believed the next step was to help them learn about their risks. By this second meeting, I sensed she knew the likely disease course for herself, and her quietness signaled this resignation. I perceived this depression to be a possible step in her grief process. Jim, on the other hand, was still grappling with identifying solutions to his wife's diagnosis and was clearly angry with the information received. I suspected his vocalized desires for his daughter was a way to reassert control in a situation that was otherwise entirely outside of his control. I also suspected Jim was driving the conversations about treatment. However, in the effort to center the discussion around Beth's needs and desires for her daughters, I focused the remainder of our session on the logistics of family communication, ensuring that Beth could pass these results on to her daughters.*

This was the last time I met with Beth and Jim, as is the case with many of my patients whom I've completed germline testing with. Unbeknownst to me at the time, I would soon learn much more about this family in my subsequent visits with each of Beth's three daughters.

Talia's Pre-test Counseling Session

Within weeks of Beth's results disclosure, Beth's oldest daughter, Talia, scheduled an in-person appointment for predictive testing. Talia, an obstetrics nurse, stated outright her trust in the Western medical establishment. She blamed her stepfather for most of her mother's beliefs in natural medicine and alternative therapies. She shared that she had outwardly disagreed with her mother's choice to not pursue standard-of-care therapies, knowing that the herbal medicines and alternative therapies would do little to cure her ovarian cancer. Her sadness, driven by understanding this would lead to continued metastatic progression of her mother's disease, was very present. However, she felt unable to alter her mother's actions and had needed to step back from involvement in her mother's care.

Much of our pre-test genetic counseling session was spent validating Talia's perceptions of the lack of proof in the alternative therapies her mother was pursuing and acknowledging the reality of her mother's prognosis. She came well prepared with a reasonable understanding of Hereditary Breast and Ovarian Cancer Syndrome, and had decided to do testing, with a stated goal of preventing the cancers that were in her family.

I noted how different this conversation with Talia was from that with her mother and Jim, which likely reflected the very different circumstance that she was in. Talia was otherwise healthy and was very motivated by both her mother's insistence that she learn about her risk status and by her personal beliefs about the benefit of this information. She was eager to pursue genetic testing, which was initiated at that visit. Talia felt powerless to help her mother and had exhausted her ability to influence her mother's care. Yet, she recognized her own ability to make decisions regarding her own health and was exercising that ability.

As Talia's genetic counselor, I felt I was able to support her decision to learn about and pursue testing, and provide an empathetic ear to her difficulty with her mother's diagnosis and treatment decisions.

Talia's Results Disclosure

Talia's test report was negative for both pathogenic variants, which she was relieved to hear. However, at the time of the results visit, Talia shared that she was now estranged from her mother and Jim, choosing to remove herself from her mother's ongoing care. She stated that Jim's influence over her mother's choice of treatment course was causing her to physically decline and would ultimately lead to her death.

I acknowledged to myself that Talia may be projecting her feelings about the quick progression of her mother's disease toward her stepfather, blaming him for her rapid decline. Alternatively, I hypothesized that Talia, being the only "medical" person in the family, felt her knowledge and desire to help her mother was not being received in the way that she thought it should. In the moment, I chose not to reflect or highlight these perceptions in the counseling visit beyond offering an empathetic ear and listening. I found myself reflecting on Beth's original goal of wanting to "protect" her daughters, and instead, I wanted to channel Talia's passion towards something that would have a potentially more impactful effect on the family as a whole: encouraging her sisters to test.

I emphasized the role Talia could play as the older sister by recommending and guiding her sisters to consider testing. I also provided the anticipatory guidance that her negative status for both variants could potentially elicit feelings—positive and negative—in her sisters when they learned of their own results. Talia reassured me that she would be aggressively encouraging her younger sister, Emily, to pursue genetic counseling and testing, but that her half-sister, Alex, likely would follow Jim's recommendations. She said she'd try her best.

Emily's Pre-test Counseling Session

Emily was the next daughter to schedule an appointment for predictive testing. Emily, who worked in restaurant hospitality, had quit her job and was now solely responsible for making all her mother's meals—enacting the dietary recommendations provided by her mother's natural health providers. At our pre-test visit, her investment in her mother's care was readily apparent. Emily expressed the desire to learn the results of germline testing for her own health, but did not state any specific actions she would take should the results identify a *BRCA1* or *BRCA2* pathogenic variant. I emphasized the opportunities for action given her age if she were to test positive for one or both pathogenic variants, including breast cancer screening (she had never had a mammogram), as well as surgical risk-reduction for ovarian cancer. She acknowledged the opportunities for action but did not indicate whether she would pursue them.

Emily shared that she knew her older sister had tested negative but didn't express her feelings about this status. I sensed she was consumed by helping her mother, both physically and psychologically.

Emily's approach to testing can be considered through the Health Belief Model, which theorizes that individual beliefs about an illness (such as perceived susceptibility, severity, benefits, barriers, and self-efficacy) contribute to health actions (Becker, 1974). In this case, Emily was clearly in the position to recognize the severity of her mother's ovarian cancer and to grasp her susceptibility risk (the 75% likelihood she had at least one pathogenic variant). However, it seemed in our discussion that the perceived benefits and risks of pursuing testing or taking action based on the results were less important to Emily. Because of this, I was able to justify focusing on information provision and counseling in her pre-test session.

Emily's Results Disclosure

Emily's genetic test identified only the *BRCA1* variant, which meant she had a high risk of developing ovarian cancer, like her mother. However, at the results disclosure session, Emily was in a hurry to return to her tasks for her mother and she received her positive results with little response. We explored how she was feeling about the result. She stated she was not alarmed or scared and had understood the likelihood that she would have at least one of the variants. I attempted to focus our conversation on action steps that Emily could now consider, and she stated she would eventually get to them. But her clear focus was continuing to care for her mother. She declined my referral for a further conversation about her risk and management to our high-risk clinic and said she'd follow up later with her own doctor.

I recognized that Emily's response to put aside this result, compartmentalize her personal risk, and to focus on the daily needs of her mother was potentially a coping mechanism. Additionally, I perceived her withdrawal and inaction might have represented a denial or blunting in her grief process. Despite my efforts to emphasize proactive actions through cancer screening and risk-reduction, this was clearly not her immediate goal. Unfortunately, I did not hear from Emily again, and she did not return to our clinic for follow-up.

Alex's Pre-test Counseling Session

Half a year later, Alex scheduled a genetic counseling visit with me. She attended the in-person appointment with her fiancé, who was visibly supportive throughout the conversation, although mostly silent. I learned through Alex, as she cried and became emotionally distraught, that her mother had died just two months prior. Alex shared that it was her mother's dying wish that she pursue genetic testing. To better understand her involvement, I asked Alex what role she played in her mother's care, to which she said she was her sole caregiver towards the end of her life.

Based on Alex's reasoning for the visit, its timing, and her body language, I sensed that her attendance at our genetic counseling visit was not fully voluntary. I asked Alex what she hoped to get out of genetic testing. She shared she had already been thoroughly informed of the implications by her mother and her sisters. She reiterated that she was only here because her mother requested it— that if it were entirely up to her, she wouldn't be seeking genetic testing. Like her sister, Emily, there was no clear, stated goal beyond information.

Similar to the approach I used with her sisters, I leaned heavily on providing education on the implications of testing and the importance of immediate action should she test positive, despite knowing that she was likely already familiar. This would be a typical approach with any of my patients presenting for predictive testing: to review the medical implications of testing positive to both assess for understanding and provide anticipatory guidance based on possible results. We reviewed the likelihood of a pathogenic finding, the associated cancer risks, and the medical management implications of having a *BRCA1* or *BRCA2* pathogenic variant. At my usual check-in for understanding after providing education, Alex stated she did not know what, if anything, she would do if results revealed a pathogenic variant.

I interpreted through her statements that doing nothing would be a likely outcome for Alex. I offered the possibility that she may want to decline testing, highlighting reasons why people choose to not know. In doing so, I hoped to give her space and a final opportunity to not do the test. However, she kept reiterating that it was her mother's last request, and she had already decided she wanted to have the genetic testing. We proceeded with a saliva sample collection in the office. Offering a few options for results disclosure, Alex requested a phone visit to discuss the results, which we scheduled.

Alex's Results Disclosure

Alex's genetic test revealed she had inherited both of her mother's *BRCA1* and *BRCA2* pathogenic variants. Our phone encounter was extremely short and to the point. I recall that she sounded like she was holding back tears as she listened to me reviewing the immediate medical management recommendations I had for her and the chance for passing the variants to future children. I asked her what she might do with the results and, like before, she stated she didn't know, didn't want to do anything with them, and that she was only doing the testing at her mother's request. I asked her permission to place a referral to our high-risk clinic for long-term management and surveillance, which she agreed to, and she asked to end the call.

At the time of writing this case-study (more than five years), Alex still had not scheduled a visit with our clinic for risk management.

Reflection on Genetic Counseling for Alex

From the beginning, I could see that Alex dreaded the counseling process, the difficulty of having to recall her mother's disease and death, and the possibility of learning that she had inherited her mother's pathogenic variants. Unlike her oldest sister, whose motivation for testing was concordant with her proactive medical beliefs, this was not the case for Alex and despite my intentions, I did not succeed in emphasizing this reason for Alex through education in creating a call to action.

With Alex, because of her uncertainty and likely refusal of medical intervention, I lost what felt like my primary tool to alleviate the immediate sting of her test results. Additionally, the weight of her mother's recent passing, compounded with the reproductive implications on her future family (although I did not ask specifically about her desires for having children), told me this was all too much for Alex at that time.

I am still processing my counseling decisions and trying to understand what I could have done to allow Alex to feel supported and confident in a decision to not pursue testing or how to make a difference for Alex in spite of her final decision to pursue testing.

After a few years of reflection, I think my surprise when Alex came to genetic counseling, whom I had never expected to see given her father's statements, created a misplaced or projected optimism that she would be willing to medically address her hereditary cancer risks through knowledge-seeking and preventive action. I took Alex's willingness to pursue genetic testing at her mother's request as an opportunity to change her mind about medicine, cancer prevention, her perspective of what defined health, and frankly, anything else I could grasp to do what I felt was the right thing for Alex. In reality, these were failed attempts on my end to obtain the outcome I desired for this family, and not necessarily reflective of Alex's immediate values or needs.

I look back and wonder if my approach to counseling Alex was also an attempt to overcorrect for Jim's reactions in the protected environment of my individual counseling session. Concurrently, I also recognize that the final request from Beth to Alex was a form of coercion, making it very difficult for Alex to make her own decision about testing. As her mother's genetic counselor as well, I found myself providing the counseling that I believed Beth wanted for Alex and Emily, supporting Beth's decision and not necessarily what the daughter in front of me wanted or needed. I held on to Beth as my consultand, embodying her desire to "protect" her daughters in my role as her daughter's counselor.

Despite offering the option of not-testing and giving space for Alex to accept that, I could have more intentionally explored Alex's reasons for proceeding with testing solely based on her mother's request, knowing that it was against her personal belief, calling this out in our conversation. As her counselor, should I have overemphasized reasons she might not want to pursue testing, the opposite of overloading opportunities for action? Or should I have created additional space for Alex to resolve her conflict around testing by telling her that I did not think it was a good time for her to make a decision?

Summary Reflection

Through the writing of this case, I have been able to reflect on the perceived utility and consequences of the education I provide to patients. I've often felt that discussing cancer epidemiology, etiology, and the underlying rationales for cancer prevention are a hallmark of my counseling style. It has become an important tool in my genetic counseling skillset that I adjust in complexity according to my assessment of a patient's desire for information, health literacy, and numeracy. I've also recognized, informed by my brief professional experience in medical sales, that providing education can also be used to disproportionately emphasize the importance of a particular outcome and to coerce a specific behavior from a client. However, the provision of education to a patient is not inherently neutral. Most often, this is not something I need to assess in my genetic counseling sessions as most patients' goals around cancer prevention by the time they've surpassed the barriers to access a genetic counseling visit are in alignment with my goal of reducing the burden of cancer. In cases where a patient may not have an aligned desire to prevent cancer or to learn information about their risk, education could be discouraging, coercive, or even smothering.

In this case, I also provided education about medical interventions as an opportunity to "fix" the bad news I was delivering and to provide hope. Presenting opportunities to theoretically regain control through medical action may not be sufficient nor appropriate to counter the significant negative implications of knowing or managing a hereditary cancer predisposition, unless informed by the patient directly. In doing so, I now see that my actions were to make myself feel better or feel that I had done everything to align the patient to a cancer prevention focus. Instead, I missed numerous opportunities to provide reassurance, understanding, and support that my patients were making the right decision for themselves without indirectly questioning their rationale through providing more education. With Emily and Alex, I could have more directly supported their decision to test AND not take preventive action. In doing so, perhaps I would have found an opportunity to better align with their goals for genetic counseling and testing.

REFERENCES

American Psychological Association (APA). (2023) PTSD Assessment Instruments. https://www.apa.org/ptsd-guideline/assessment Accessed June 1, 2023.

Armstrong DK, Alvarez RD, Backes FJ et al. (2022) NCCN Guidelines(R) Insights: Ovarian Cancer, Version 3.2022. *J Natl Compr Canc Netw* 20(9):972–980. https://doi.org/10.6004/jnccn.2022.0047

Becker M. (1974) The Health Belief Model and personal health behavior. *Health Educ Mono* 2:324–508.

Bednar EM, Oakley HD, Sun CC, et al. (2017). A universal genetic testing initiative for patients with high-grade, non-mucinous epithelial ovarian cancer and the implications for cancer treatment. *Gynecol Oncol* 146(2):399–404. https://doi.org/10.1016/j.ygyno.2017.05.037

Carlson LM, Hardisty E, Coombs CC, & Vora NL. (2018) Maternal malignancy evaluation after discordant cell-free DNA results. *Obstet Gynecol* 131(3):464–468.

Daly MB, Pilarski R., Yurgelun MB. (2020) NCCN Guidelines Insights: Genetic/Familial High-Risk Assessment: Breast, Ovarian, and Pancreatic, Version 1.2020. *J Natl Compr Canc Netw*, 18(4):380–391. https://doi.org/10.6004/jnccn.2020.0017

Freud S. (1910) *International Association of Psychoanalysis Congress*. Nuremberg, March, 1910. p.144–145.

Gaba P, Bos JM, Cannon BC, et al. (2016) Implantable cardioverter-defibrillator explanation for overdiagnosed or overtreated congenital long QT syndrome. *Heart Rhythm* 13:879–885. https://doi.org/10.1016/j.hrthm.2015.12.008.

Gregg AR, Skotko BG, Benkendorf JL, et al. (2016) Noninvasive prenatal screening for fetal aneuploidy, 2016 update: a position statement of the American College of Medical Genetics and Genomics. *Genet Med* 18(10):1056–1065.

Griesi-Oliveira K & Sertié AL. (2017) Autism spectrum disorders: an updated guide for genetic counseling. *Einstein* (Sao Paulo) 5(2):233–238.

Harris PC & Torres VE (2022) Polycystic kidney disease, autosomal dominant. In: MP Adam, GM Mirzaa, RA Pagon, et al. (eds.) *GeneReviews*® [Internet]. Seattle (WA): University of Washington, Seattle; 1993–2023.

Ingles J, Spinks C, Yeates L, et al. (2016) Posttraumatic stress and prolonged grief after the sudden cardiac death of a young relative. *JAMA Internal Medicine* 176:402–405. https://doi.org/10.1001/jamainternmed.2015.7808.

Ingles J, Goldstein J, Thaxton C, et al. (2019) Evaluating the clinical validity of hypertrophic cardiomyopathy genes. *Circulation: Genomic and Precision Medicine* 12:e002460. https://doi.org/10.1161/CIRCGEN.119.002460.

Jordan E, Peterson L, Ai T, et al. (2021). Evidence-based assessment of genes in dilated cardiomyopathy. *Circulation* 144:7–19. https://doi.org/10.1161/CIRCULATIONAHA.120.053033.

Kessler S. (1992) Psychological aspects of genetic counseling. VIII. Suffering and countertransference. *J Genet Couns* 1(4):303–308.

Konstantinopoulos PA, Norquist B, Lacchetti C, et al. (2020) Germline and somatic tumor testing in epithelial ovarian cancer: ASCO Guideline. *J Clin Oncol* 38(11):1222–1245. https://doi.org/10.1200/JCO.19.02960

Kuchenbaecker KB, Hopper JL, Barnes DR, et al. (2017) Risks of breast, ovarian, and contralateral breast cancer for brca1 and brca2 mutation carriers. *JAMA* 317(23):2402–2416. https://doi.org/10.1001/jama.2017.7112

McDonald K, Sharpe L, Yeates L, et al. (2020) Needs analysis of parents following sudden cardiac death in the young. *Open Heart* 7:e001120. http://dx.doi.org/10.1136/openhrt-2019-001120.

Middleton O, Baxter S, MacLeod H, et al. (2013) National Association of Medical Examiners position paper: retaining postmortem samples for genetic testing. *Acad Forens Path* https://doi.org/10.23907/2013.024.

Murabito JM, Nam B, D'Agostino RB et al. (2004) Accuracy of offspring reports of parental cardiovascular disease history: the Framingham Offspring Study. *Annal Inter Med* 140:434–440. https://doi.org/10.7326/0003-4819-140-6-200403160-00010.

Napolitano, C., Mazzanti, A., Bloise, R., *et al.* (2004). Catecholaminergic Polymorphic Ventricular Tachycardia. *GeneReviews [Internet]*, https://www.ncbi.nlm.nih.gov/books/NBK1289/ Accessed June 1, 2023.

Norton ME & Jackson M. (2016) Practice Bulletin No. 162: Prenatal Diagnostic Testing for Genetic Disorders. *Obstet Gynecol* 127:e108–e122.

Norquist BM, Harrell MI, Brady MF, et al. (2016) Inherited mutations in women with ovarian carcinoma. *JAMA Oncol* 2(4):482–490. https://doi.org/10.1001/jamaoncol.2015.5495

Porath B, Gainullin VG, Cornec-Le Gall E, et al. (2016) Mutations in GANAB, Encoding the Glucosidase IIα Subunit, Cause Autosomal-Dominant Polycystic Kidney and Liver Disease. *Am J Hum Genet* 98(6):1193–1207. doi: 10.1016/j.ajhg.2016.05.004.

Prigerson HG, Boelen PA, Xu, J, et al. (2021) Validation of the new DSM-5-TR criteria for prolonged grief disorder and the PG-13-Revised (PG-13-R) scale. *World Psych* 20:96–106. https://doi.org/10.1002/wps.20823.

Redlinger-Grosse K (2021) Countertransference: making the unconscious conscious. In: BS LeRoy, P McCarthy Veach, & NP Calanan (eds). *Genetic Counseling Practice: Advanced Concepts and Skills.* Second Edition. Oxford: Wiley Blackwell, pp. 153–175.

Reeder R, McCarthy Veach P, MacFarlane IM, & LeRoy BS. (2017) Characterizing clinical genetic counselors' countertransference experiences: an exploratory study. *J Genet Couns* 26(5):934–947.

Resnicow K, Delacroix E, Chen G, et al. (2022) Motivational interviewing for genetic counseling: A unified framework for persuasive and equipoise conversations. *J Genet Couns* 31(5):1020–1031. https://doi.org/10.1002/jgc4.1609

Reuter C, Grove ME, Orland K, et al. (2018) Clinical cardiovascular genetic counselors take a leading role in team-based variant classification. *J Genet Couns* 27:751–760. https://doi.org/10.1007/s10897-017-0175-7.

Rose NC, Kaimal AJ, Dugoff L, & Norton M. (2020) Screening for fetal chromosomal abnormalities: ACOG Practice Bulletin, Number 226. *Obstet Gynecol* 136(4): 48–69

Sekizawa A, Samura O, Zhen DK, et al. (2000) Apoptosis in fetal nucleated erythrocytes circulating in maternal blood. *Prenat Diagn* 20(11):886–889.

Snyder MW, Simmons LE, Kitzman JO, et al. (2015) Copy-number variation and false positive prenatal aneuploidy screening results. *N Engl J Med* 372:1639–1645.

Stadler ZK, Maio A, Chakravarty D, et al. (2021) Therapeutic implications of germline testing in patients with advanced cancers. *J Clin Oncol* 39(24):2698–2709. https://doi.org/10.1200/JCO.20.03661

Stiles MK, Wilde AA, Abrams DJ et al. (2021) 2020 APHRS/HRS expert consensus statement on the investigation of decedents with sudden unexplained death and patients with sudden cardiac arrest, and of their families. *Heart Rhythm* 18:e1-e50. https://doi.org/10.1016/j.hrthm.2020.10.010.

van der Werf C, Onderwater AT, van Langen IM, et al. (2014) Experiences, considerations and emotions relating to cardiogenetic evaluation in relatives of young sudden cardiac death victims. *Euro J Human Genet* 22:192–196. https://doi.org/10.1038/ejhg.2013.126.

Wain KE, Azzariti DR, Goldstein JL, et al. (2020) Variant interpretation is a component of clinical practice among genetic counselors in multiple specialties. *Genetics in Medicine* 22:785–792. https://doi.org/10.1038/s41436-019-0705-9.

Waldrop E, Al-Obaide M, & Vasylyeva, T. (2019) *GANAB* and *PKD1* Variations in a 12 years old female patient with early onset of autosomal dominant polycystic kidney disease. *Front Genet* 10:44. doi: 10.3389/fgene.2019.00044.

Walsh T, Casadei S, Lee MK, et al. (2011) Mutations in 12 genes for inherited ovarian, fallopian tube, and peritoneal carcinoma identified by massively parallel sequencing. *Proc Natl Acad Sci USA* 108(44):18032–18037. https://doi.org/10.1073/pnas.1115052108

Weil J. (2000) *Psychosocial Genetic Counseling.* New York, NY: Oxford University Press.

Wilson KL, Czerwinski JL, Hoskovec JM, et al. (2013) NSGC practice guideline: prenatal screening and diagnostic testing options for chromosome aneuploidy. *J Genet Couns* 22(11):4–15.

Wilde AA, Semsarian C, Marquez MF et al. (2022) European Heart Rhythm Association (EHRA)/Heart Rhythm Society (HRS)/Asia Pacific Heart Rhythm Society (APHRS)/ Latin American Heart Rhythm Society (LAHRS) Expert Consensus Statement on the State of Genetic Testing for Cardiac Diseases. *Heart Rhythm* 19:e1-e60. https://doi. org/10.1016/j.hrthm.2022.03.1225.

Zhong Q, Peng HL, Zhao X, et al. (2015) Effects of BRCA1- and BRCA2-related mutations on ovarian and breast cancer survival: a meta-analysis. *Clin Cancer Res* 21(1):211–220. https://doi.org/10.1158/1078-0432.CCR-14-1816

Zhou X, Sui L, Xu Y, et al. (2017) Contribution of maternal copy number variations to false-positive fetal trisomies detected by noninvasive prenatal testing. *Prenat Diagn* 37(4):318.

Index

A Guide to Genetic Counseling, Third Edition. Edited by Vivian Y. Pan, Jane L. Schuette,
Karen E. Wain, and Beverly M. Yashar.
© 2025 John Wiley & Sons Ltd. Published 2025 by John Wiley & Sons Ltd.

Printed and bound by CPI Group (UK) Ltd, Croydon, CR0 4YY

16/10/2024

14574596-0001